**HEART DISEASE KILLS SOMEONE IN THE U.S.
EVERY 33 SECONDS.**

HDL, LDL, triglycerides, homocysteine, and C-reactive protein—what do they all mean for your health? Annette B. Natow, Ph.D., and Jo-Ann Heslin, M.A., R.D., C.D.N.—professional nutrition educators—help you lower your cholesterol and reduce your risk for heart disease, providing the most up-to-date information and advice you can trust.

You have the power to change the way you eat and live your life:

- Understand your blood cholesterol numbers and work to bring them into normal range
- Rate your risks and make your lifestyle work for you, not against you
- Use the handy tables, worksheets, and comprehensive food lists inside to track your cholesterol intake
- Understand the importance of exercise, fiber, and medications to help control cholesterol

Living a healthy lifestyle is the key to reducing your risk for heart disease—begin today!

THE CHOLESTEROL COUNTER, 7th EDITION

. . . an essential reference for healthy living

D0021139

Books by Annette B. Natow and Jo-Ann Heslin

The Calorie Counter
(*Fourth Edition*)

The Cholesterol Counter
(*Seventh Edition*)

The Complete Food Counter
(*Second Edition*)

The Diabetes Carbohydrate and Calorie Counter
(*Third Edition*)

Eating Out Food Counter

The Fat Counter
(*Sixth Edition*)

The Healthy Heart Food Counter

The Healthy Wholefoods Counter

The Most Complete Food Counter
(*Second Edition*)

The Protein Counter
(*Second Edition*)

The Ultimate Carbohydrate Counter

The Vitamin and Mineral Food Counter

Published by POCKET BOOKS

THE
CHOLESTEROL COUNTER

Seventh Edition
20th Anniversary Edition

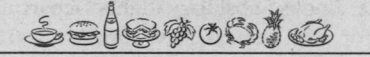

Annette B. Natow, Ph.D.
Jo-Ann Heslin, M.A., R.D.
With the Assistance of Karen J. Nolan, Ph.D.

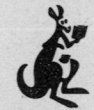

POCKET BOOKS

New York   London   Toronto   Sydney

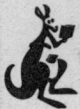

Pocket Books
A Division of Simon & Schuster, Inc.
1230 Avenue of the Americas
New York, NY 10020

Copyright © 1988, 1989, 1993, 1996, 1998, 2004, 2008
by Annette B. Natow and Jo-Ann Heslin

All rights reserved, including the right to reproduce this book or portions thereof in any form whatsoever. For information address Pocket Books Subsidiary Rights Department, 1230 Avenue of the Americas, New York, NY 10020

This Pocket Books paperback edition January 2008

POCKET and colophon are registered trademarks of Simon & Schuster, Inc.

For information about special discounts for bulk purchases, please contact Simon & Schuster Special Sales at 1-800-456-6798 or business@simonandschuster.com.

Cover design by Heather Kern
Cover photo by Karl Newede/Getty Images

Manufactured in the United States of America

10   9   8   7   6   5   4   3   2

ISBN-13: 978-1-4165-0985-1
ISBN-10:   1-4165-0985-2

To our families, who support us
through every project:

Harry, Allen, Irene, Sarah, Meryl, Marty, Laura,
George, Emily, Steven, Rebecca, Joseph, Kristen,
Brian, Karen, and John

ACKNOWLEDGMENTS

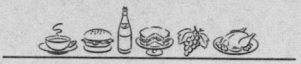

For graciously sharing her knowledge, Karen J. Nolan, Ph.D.

For all her continuous support and help, our agent, Nancy Trichter.

For her suggestions and editing skills, Sara Clemence.

Without the tireless cooperation of Stephen Llano and the production department at Pocket Books, *The Cholesterol Counter, 7th Edition* would never have been completed.

A special thank you to our editor, Micki Nuding.

And, we'd like to thank all our readers for their suggestions and questions. Your input helps us to provide you with the most useful information.

"If only half a dozen foods were available the matter would be quickly settled."

Mary Swartz Rose, Ph.D.
Feeding the Family
The MacMillan Company, 1919

CONTENTS

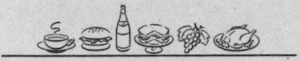

THE
CHOLESTEROL COUNTER

INTRODUCTION

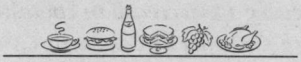

If you are looking at this book, chances are:

- You just found out your cholesterol is high.
- Someone you care about has high cholesterol and you want to help them.
- Someone in your family has heart disease and you want to lower your risk.

Heart disease—or more correctly, cardiovascular disease (CVD)—is very common in the U.S. The number one cause of death for both men and women, it kills one person every 33 seconds! And heart attacks and strokes disable even more people than they kill—more than the number of people who die from all forms of cancer put together.

Heart disease has been called a lifestyle disease of developed countries—it's prevalent because we can afford cars instead of walking and we eat lots of unhealthy foods. Although we still have much to learn, what is clear is that if you are willing to change the way you eat and live, you can lower your risk for heart disease. And the more willing you are to change your lifestyle, the more you can reduce your risk for a heart attack or stroke.

High cholesterol levels are directly connected to your

1

risk for heart disease. The higher your cholesterol, the greater your risk. Lowering your cholesterol lowers your risk.

For every 1% decrease in cholesterol,
your risk for heart disease drops 3% to 4%.

UNDERSTANDING YOUR NUMBERS

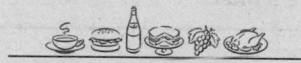

Everyone over the age of 20 should get their cholesterol levels measured at least once every 5 years.

The numbers on your blood test are important to predict your future heart health. If they fall within the normal range, your doctor will recommend another screening in a year or more. If your numbers are up, your doctor will recommend lifestyle changes or even medication. What do those numbers really mean?

Total Cholesterol

Desirable: less than 200 mg/dl
Borderline high: 200 to 239 mg/dl
High: 240 mg/dl or higher

Total cholesterol is just that—the amount of cholesterol in a given volume of blood. It is measured as the number of milligrams (mg) of cholesterol in 1 deciliter (dl) of blood, which is slightly less than a half cup. For example, 222 mg/dl = 222 milligrams of cholesterol per deciliter of blood. To make things simpler, your doctor may give you just the number, 222, rather than the more complete measurement. To reduce your risk for heart disease, you want your level to be below 200.

YOU SHOULD KNOW—

Cholesterol levels change with the season and are highest in the winter.

High cholesterol does not cause any symptoms, so the only way you know if your cholesterol levels are too high is through a blood test. High cholesterol quietly does damage to your body, building up on the wall of your arteries. Over time, this buildup can cause the arteries to harden, a process called *atherosclerosis*. Your blood carries oxygen to the heart; if arteries get narrowed, blood flow to the heart muscle is slowed down and may even be blocked. If not enough blood and oxygen can reach your heart, you may have chest pains. A blocked artery to the heart can cause a heart attack. A blocked artery to the brain can cause a stroke.

Blood is mainly made up of water. To travel through blood, cholesterol, a fatlike substance, is coated with a protein. The combination of fat and protein is called a *lipoprotein*. If your total cholesterol values are high, your doctor will want to know the amount of LDL (low-density lipoprotein) cholesterol and HDL (high-density lipoprotein) cholesterol, as well.

You doctor will order a lipid profile, which will measure the amounts of total cholesterol, LDL cholesterol, HDL cholesterol, and triglycerides. It's important to get a full lipid profile because a simple total cholesterol number can be misleading.

> **YOU SHOULD KNOW—**
>
> *It's wise to fast for at least 8 hours before getting your blood drawn for a lipid profile. Eating a high-fat meal within 4 hours of a blood test can affect the results by raising blood fats.*

LDL Cholesterol

The lower the number, the better.

>Normal: less than 100 mg/dl
>Near or slightly above optimal: 100 to 129 mg/dl
>Borderline high: 130 to 159 mg/dl
>High: 160 to 189 mg/dl
>Very high: 190 mg/dl and above

LDL is the major carrier of cholesterol in your bloodstream. Low-density lipoprotein (LDL) compounds contain very little protein but a lot of cholesterol. If too much LDL cholesterol circulates in the blood, it can stick to the walls of the arteries leading to the heart and brain. This eventually forms plaque—thick, hard deposits that clog arteries. That's why LDL cholesterol is often referred to as "bad" cholesterol. The lower your levels of LDL, the lower your risk of heart disease.

HDL Cholesterol

The higher the number, the better.

>High: 60 mg/dl or higher
>Average for women: 50 to 60 mg/dl
>Average for men: 40 to 50 mg/dl
>Low: less than 40 mg/dl.

About one-third of the blood's cholesterol is carried by HDLs. High-density lipoprotein (HDL) compounds have a lot of protein and very little cholesterol. Experts believe HDL cholesterol carries cholesterol away from the arteries back to the liver, where it is broken down and removed from the body. This process is called *reverse cholesterol transport* and it helps prevent the growth of plaque. For this reason, HDL is referred to as "good" cholesterol.

It may be more important to know if your good HDL cholesterol is too low (less than 40 for men and less than 50 for women) than if your LDL cholesterol is too high. Encouraging lifestyle changes and developing drugs that raise HDL cholesterol is the newest focus in the battle against heart disease. For every 1 point increase in HDLs, there is a 2% decrease in heart attacks and stroke for men, and a 3% decrease for women.

YOU SHOULD KNOW—

Regardless of race, ethnicity, or sex, high HDL cholesterol protects you against the risk of having a stroke, especially if you are over age 65.

Cholesterol Ratio

TC/HDL: total cholesterol to HDL cholesterol
Good: 5:1
Optimum: 3.5:1

Your "ratio" is found by dividing HDL cholesterol into total cholesterol. For example: If your total cholesterol is 200 and your HDL cholesterol is 50, your ratio is 4:1. Experts believe that your total cholesterol-to-HDL ratio

(TC/HDL) may be more important than cholesterol alone for monitoring your risk for heart disease.

Triglycerides

Normal: less than 150 mg/dl
Borderline high: 150 to 199 mg/dl
High: 200 to 499 mg/dl
Very high: 500 mg/dl or higher

Triglycerides are the main type of fat found in food and the major storage form of fat in your body. They are transported through the bloodstream to cells where they are either burned for energy or stored for future use. High levels, over 150 mg/dl, can be a risk factor for heart disease. Your risk for high triglycerides goes up if you are overweight, do little exercise, drink too much alcohol, eat a high-carbohydrate diet, especially refined carbs, smoke, or have diabetes.

YOU SHOULD KNOW—

Dyslipidemia—dys (problematic), lipid (fat), emia (in blood)—*refers to high levels of total cholesterol, high levels of triglycerides, high levels of LDL cholesterol, or low levels of HDL cholesterol. People with dyslipidemias often develop high blood pressure. Abnormal blood fats can be used to identify those at risk for heart disease before they have symptoms.*

If your family history, your blood cholesterol levels, or triglyceride values put you at moderate to high risk for heart disease, your doctor may evaluate two other blood values: homocysteine and C-reactive protein.

Homocysteine

Normal: values between 6 and 12
Moderate risk: values between 12 and 30
High risk: values over 30

Elevated levels of the amino acid homocysteine increase your risk for heart attack and stroke because they encourage plaque to form on artery walls. Generally, levels below 7 are associated with the lowest risk—but not always. Some studies have showed a reduction in heart disease when homocysteine levels went down. But in other studies, when homocysteine levels were reduced the incidence of heart disease stayed the same. Obviously we still have more to learn. But in the meantime, lowering your homocysteine levels by taking a multivitamin rich in B vitamins and eating more fruits and vegetables may help and won't hurt you.

C-Reactive Protein (CRP)

Low risk: levels below 1
Average risk: levels between 1 and 3
High risk: levels over 3

Elevated levels of C-reactive protein (CRP) can triple your risk for heart disease and have been linked to the development of high blood pressure. It's been estimated that 26% of the population have elevated levels and risks increase as weight goes up. For postmenopausal women, CRP levels may be more accurate than cholesterol in predicting heart disease.

CRP is an indication of inflammation in the body. Research has suggested that as heart disease damages arteries, the damage causes inflammation, and this inflammation increases the production of CRP by the body. Almost all healthy lifestyle changes are helpful in lowering inflammation and CRP levels—weight loss, exercise, smoking cessation, blood pressure control, and reduced alcohol intake. Taking a daily antioxidant multivitamin may also be helpful.

YOU SHOULD KNOW—

What are your numbers?

Total cholesterol:	_____	*Aim for 200 or less.*
LDL cholesterol:	_____	*Aim for 100 or less.*
HDL cholesterol:	_____	*Aim for 60 or higher.*
Triglycerides:	_____	*Aim for 150 or less.*

Knowing your numbers and working to get them to healthy levels is an important step in protecting your health and lowering your risk for heart disease. Discuss your numbers and your potential risk with your doctor to be sure you are doing all you can to manage your health.

RATING YOUR RISKS

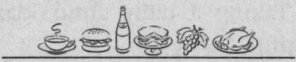

Heart disease often gives you no warning signs.
That's why prevention is so important.

Do you smoke?	Yes	No
Is your total cholesterol high?	Yes	No
Is your LDL cholesterol high?	Yes	No
Is your HDL cholesterol low?	Yes	No
Are your triglycerides high?	Yes	No
Do you have high blood pressure?	Yes	No
Do you have diabetes?	Yes	No
Do you do less than 30 minutes of exercise each day?	Yes	No
Are you overweight?	Yes	No
Men—is your waist measurement greater than 42 inches?	Yes	No
Women—is your waist measurement greater than 35 inches?	Yes	No
Do you drink 3 or more alcoholic drinks a day?	Yes	No
Are you frequently stressed?	Yes	No
Are you 55 or older?	Yes	No
Do you have a close relative with heart disease?	Yes	No

The more times you answered yes, the higher your risk for heart disease. Every no answer lowers your risk. Let's see what you can do to turn some of the yes answers to no answers.

Understanding Risks

The concept of risk factors related to disease is relatively new in medicine. We didn't even consider lifestyle as part of your risk for heart disease until the 1960s. But now we know that many things you do can increase your risk for heart disease. The factors that you said yes to on the quiz are your risks that increase your chance of getting heart disease. And risks tend to cluster and build on one another, creating an even more powerful negative effect on your health. If you have 2 or more risk factors, your risk for heart disease is quadrupled. Three or more makes your risk of heart disease 8 to 20 times higher than if you had no risk factors at all.

While you can't do much about your relatives or your age, you can control other risk factors. Changing the way you live and eat can reduce your chances of developing heart disease, and simple changes can have surprisingly big effects. The sooner you know what puts you at greater risk, the sooner you can do something about it.

Smoking

This is a risk factor you can reduce to zero. If you smoke, try to quit. If you don't smoke, don't start. Heart disease is the cause of 35% to 40% of all smoking-related deaths. And heart disease causes 8% of all deaths caused by secondhand smoking exposure.

YOU SHOULD KNOW—

Understanding % Risk

A 10% risk means for every 100 people, 10 people will be affected by the risk.

If 35% to 40% of all smoking-related deaths are from heart disease, that means for every 100 smokers who die, the cause of death for 35 to 40 of them will be heart disease.

Simply convert the % risk to that number out of 100 people.

(50% risk = 50 out of every 100 people)

Dyslipidemias (problematic blood fats)

High total cholesterol, high LDL cholesterol, low HDL cholesterol, and high triglycerides all increase risk for heart disease. Exercising, losing weight, eating well, drinking moderate amounts of alcohol, and not smoking all help to bring blood fats into the normal range.

High Blood Pressure

One out of 3 adults in the U.S. has high blood pressure, and the higher your blood pressure the more prone you are to heart disease. Blood pressure is measured by the systolic (top) number over the diastolic (bottom) number. For every 20-point rise in the top number or for every 10 point rise in the bottom number over 115/75, your risk for heart disease doubles. People with high blood pressure also frequently have high cholesterol. All the lifestyle changes that lower blood fats will also lower high blood pressure.

> **YOU SHOULD KNOW—**
>
> *Living a healthy lifestyle is a key to reducing your risk for heart disease.*

Diabetes

Over 18 million Americans have diabetes and 75% of all deaths related to diabetes are caused by heart disease. The best way to lower this risk is to avoid getting diabetes, of course. Second best is to keep the condition under control by managing blood sugar, blood pressure, and blood fats. It can be done with lifestyle changes and medication.

Exercise

Few Americans are as active as they should be—only 22% of adults do light exercise daily. Not exercising can increase your risk of heart disease substantially, as much as smoking a pack of cigarettes every day. Fortunately, it's easy to start moving; all you need to do is walk. Start with simple things like not using the drive-thru, parking at the end of the lot, or walking around the mall once before you start shopping. Exercise also makes you feel good, can help you lose weight, lowers blood pressure, and may even improve your sex life.

Weight Loss

This one is the biggie—no pun intended. Over 70% of adults weigh too much and being overweight increases your chances of having high cholesterol, high triglycerides, high blood pressure, diabetes, and heart disease. An overweight 45-year-old man will, on average, die 6 years before his lean counterpart and suffer from heart disease 3 years longer. An overweight 45-year-old woman will die almost 8.5 years before her lean counterpart and suffer from heart disease for an additional year and a half.

You're at an even higher risk if you have the type of body that stores extra weight around the belly. Abdominal or belly fat has been linked to a higher risk for heart disease, diabetes, and hypertension. Belly fat is active and works like a mini-factory producing triglycerides and C-reactive protein.

The good news: When you lose weight, cholesterol goes down, triglycerides go down, high blood pressure goes down, and HDL cholesterol goes up. Your belly gets smaller and CRP levels drop. Losing as little as 5% to 10% of your current weight reduces your risk for heart disease. Lose more and your risk profile gets even better.

Your Age and Your Relatives

You can't become younger or disown Uncle Sol or Aunt Bessie, no matter how hard you try. But it is important to know what diseases your close relatives currently have or what they died from: the information can help your doctor make judgments about your care. Brothers, sisters, and parents count more heavily than second-generation relatives like aunts and cousins.

YOU SHOULD KNOW—

Though men may show symptoms 10 years earlier, heart disease is still the number one cause of death for both women and men.

Alcohol

The question isn't whether you drink, but how much. Studies have shown that 1 to 2 drinks a day can reduce the risk for heart disease by raising HDLs. But more than that—3 or more drinks a day—increases the risk for high blood pressure and heart disease. Moderation is the key.

YOU SHOULD KNOW—

One drink equals a 5-ounce glass of wine, a 12-ounce bottle of beer, or a shot (1.5 ounces) of hard alcohol such as gin, whiskey, scotch, or vodka.

Stress

We once thought that driven people, type A personalities, were more prone to heart disease. But the evidence is inconclusive. Many ambitious, hard-working, busy people are perfectly healthy. It does appear that people who experience a good deal of anger may be at higher risk of developing heart disease. And some of the things experts suggest to lower stress—exercising and drinking less, for example—are good for your heart, too.

MAKE YOUR LIFESTYLE
WORK FOR YOU

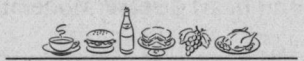

You can lower your cholesterol by:

- Losing weight
- Exercising
- Eating less cholesterol
- Eating more fiber
- Eating more cholesterol lowering foods
- Taking cholesterol lowering medication when indicated

Counting calories, being active 30 or more minutes each day, eating foods lower in cholesterol, eating fiber-rich foods, and carefully following your doctor's advice are all important lifestyle changes. Like risks, healthy behaviors tend to cluster and build on one another, exerting a powerful, positive effect on your health. Many of these lifestyle changes will not only protect you from heart disease—they will also lower your risk for cancer, diabetes, and osteoarthritis.

Losing Weight

Losing weight is hard. If it weren't, we'd all be thin. But you don't have to slim down to your high school weight; losing just 5% to 10% of your current weight will lower your cholesterol. That means if you weigh 175 pounds, losing between 9 and 18 pounds will lower your cholesterol. Cutting calories and being more active is the best way to start.

YOU SHOULD KNOW—

Simple Swaps to Save 100 Calories

- *Use mustard, salsa, or fat-free mayonnaise in place of 1 tablespoon of regular mayonnaise.*
- *Eat 1 slice of toast for breakfast instead of 2.*
- *Order a cup of soup instead of a bowl.*
- *Try a plain baked potato with pepper instead of sour cream.*
- *Eat cereal with skim milk instead of whole milk.*
- *Swap breaded and fried chicken fingers for broiled.*
- *Use tuna packed in water rather than oil.*
- *Swap a regular soda for a diet soda.*
- *Enjoy a glass of wine instead of a martini.*
- *Have a chocolate kiss instead of a chocolate bar.*

How Many Calories Do You Need?

When you cut calories, taking in less energy than your body needs to run each day, it uses stored fat to make up for the shortfall. Over time, as that extra fat gets used up, you lose weight.

To find out how many calories you need each day, you

need to do two things. First figure out how much you want to weigh. Not your current weight, but your target weight—the weight you would like to be. Then select an activity factor that fits your current activity level.

1. Your target weight is: _____

2. Your activity factor is: _____

   20 = Very active men
   15 = Moderately active men or very active
        women
   13 = Inactive men, moderately active women
        and people over 55
   10 = Inactive women, repeat dieters, seriously
        overweight people

3. Target Weight x Activity Factor = Calories needed
   each day.

For example, if your target weight is 130 and you are a moderately active woman (factor 13), you need about 1600 to 1700 calories a day.

130 pounds X 13 = 1690 calories

Eating this amount of calories each day guarantees weight loss, because you are getting only enough calories to support your target weight, not your current heavier weight. Couple this calorie intake with some added exercise and the weight will come off even faster.

Exercise

You don't need to run a marathon. You don't even need to join a gym—though you might enjoy it. Just think of ways to include activity in your life. Everything counts, from mowing the lawn to vacuuming the house to taking a walk on a beautiful afternoon. We like to refer to these activities as "everyday fitness."

Let's look at what you can gain from 10 minutes of activity a day. If you weigh 150 pounds, 10 minutes of lying on the couch watching TV burns about 15 calories. If you sit up, you'll burn 20 calories. Walking in place for 10 minutes burns 40 calories; jogging bumps you to 90. Just adding a leisurely 10-minute walk to your daily routine can burn 14,600 calories a year—the equivalent of 4 pounds. All day, every day, there are opportunities for you to be more active—just move!

Everyday Fitness

- Pace while you're talking on the phone.
- Deliver memos and messages in person rather than by e-mail or phone.
- Go window shopping.
- Clean your house—washing floors, vacuuming carpets, washing windows, and scrubbing bathrooms equals vigorous exercise.
- Garden—weeding, hoeing, cutting the lawn, raking, and trimming bushes burns as many calories as a game of tennis.
- Turn your lunch break into an exercise excursion.
- Carry a basket when shopping for a few items—it's like a free weight that keeps getting heavier and heavier; switch arms for a maximum workout.
- Sign up for a charity walk, bike, or run.
- Turn off the TV one night a week and plan something active.

- Make exercise a hobby—take golf, tennis, or skating lessons.
- Park your car at the far end of the parking lot.
- Take the stairs—you burn 10 calories for every flight you climb; over a lifetime that uses up thousands of calories.
- Dance—salsa, polka, tango—square dancers can cover 5 miles in an evening.
- Grocery shop—one hour in the supermarket, pushing, lifting, bending, uses as many calories as a half hour on a treadmill.
- Spend rainy weekend afternoons walking around a museum; when the sun shines, go to the zoo.
- Wash the car.
- Go bowling instead of to the movies.
- Walk the dog.
- Push the baby in a carriage; take the kids to the playground.
- Be an active spectator; walk the circumference of the soccer field while the kids are playing.
- Play games as a family—badminton, volleyball, stickball, croquet.

YOU SHOULD KNOW—

Every trip counts!

Researchers found that women who climbed stairs for as little as two minutes a day had lower cholesterol levels and improved resting pulse rates.

Eating Less Cholesterol

You get some cholesterol every time you eat animal foods—meat, poultry, fish, eggs, milk, yogurt, cheese, and butter. Egg yolks are a major source of cholesterol, with 211 milligrams. Egg whites don't have any. Your liver also makes cholesterol. In fact, most people make three times more cholesterol than they eat in food.

There is no cholesterol in plant foods—vegetables, fruits, nuts, seeds, cereals, grains, and oils.

KEEP IT SIMPLE—

If a food grows in the ground, it has no cholesterol.
If a food has a face, it has cholesterol.

Using the "Keep It Simple" rule, which of the following foods have cholesterol?

FOOD	YES	NO
Cheddar cheese		
Chicken leg		
Egg		
Hamburger		
Lobster		
Milk		
Salmon		
Almonds		
Apple		
Avocado		

(continued)

FOOD	YES	NO
Bran flakes		
Olive oil		
Peanut butter		
Rice		
Tomato		
Watermelon		

The first 7 foods all contain cholesterol. Hamburger comes from cattle. Salmon and lobster are seafood. Chicken legs and eggs come from chickens. Cheddar cheese and milk come from cows. All of them have faces!

The rest are from plants that grow in the ground. They have no cholesterol. Almonds, avocado, olive oil, and peanut butter all have fat, but it's vegetable fat that does not contain cholesterol.

The Cholesterol Counter lists the amount of cholesterol in over 20,000 foods. Even if a food is not listed, you can still determine if it is a source of cholesterol by simply asking, "Does it have a face?"

If you are like most people, you didn't give a lot of thought to what you ate until your doctor told you to "watch your cholesterol." But what does this really mean?

If your numbers are good—total cholesterol is close to 200, LDL cholesterol is close to 100, and your HDL cholesterol is between 40 and 60—you can eat a moderate-cholesterol diet, which contains no more than 300 milligrams of cholesterol a day.

If any of your numbers are less than desirable, or if your doctor has prescribed a cholesterol-lowering medication, you should eat a low-cholesterol diet, with less than 200 milligrams a day.

That doesn't mean turning your life upside down, but it does mean making smarter choices. For example, many of the foods listed below are made with whole milk, cheese, or butter, all of which contain cholesterol. But there are tasty alternatives that can help you keep your cholesterol down.

INSTEAD OF THIS:	TRY THIS:	MILLIGRAMS CHOLESTEROL SAVED
Omelet, plain	Sunny-side-up egg	553
Egg salad sandwich	Tuna salad sandwich	320
7-layer salad	Tossed salad w/ avocado	119
Creamed spinach	Leaf spinach	100
Chow mein, shrimp	Chow mein, vegetable	92
Cheesecake	Angelfood cake	86
Potato salad	Mashed potatoes	83
Hamburger patty	Veggie burger patty	77
Zabaglione	Flan	73
Coconut cream pie	Pumpkin pie	55
Burrito with beef, beans, and cheese	Burrito with beans	51
Chicken breast, battered and fried	Chicken breast, roasted	36
Pound cake	Pound cake, fat free	32
White toast with butter	Whole wheat toast with margarine	30

(continued)

INSTEAD OF THIS:	TRY THIS:	MILLIGRAMS CHOLESTEROL SAVED
Pork skins	Popcorn	27
Vanilla ice cream cup	Orange sherbet	20
Latte with whole milk	Latte with skim milk	16
Sour cream	Sour cream, fat free	15

Easy Steps to Lower Cholesterol

- Use liquid vegetable oils—olive, canola, corn, soybean, sunflower, and safflower.
- Limit servings of meat, poultry, fish and shellfish to 3- to 4-ounce portions.
- Use lean cuts of meat and trim off all visible fat.
- Eat poultry without the skin.
- Whenever possible, cook without adding fat.
- Bake, broil, or roast.
- Use more beans and vegetables to make up for smaller servings of meat, fish, and poultry.
- Substitute two egg whites for one egg with yolk.
- Use lowfat or nonfat milk, cheese, yogurt, and ice cream and fat free sour cream.
- Use soft margarine instead of butter.
- Use lowfat or fat free salad dressings and gravies.
- Eat fiber-rich foods—beans, whole grains, bran, brown rice, dried fruits, fruits, and vegetables.

- Eat more cholesterol-lowering foods—nuts, soy foods, and antioxidant-rich fruits and vegetables.
- Use more foods fortified with plant sterols.
- If your doctor prescribed a cholesterol-lowering medication, take it daily, even when your cholesterol values return to normal.

Eating More Fiber

Getting enough fiber is especially important for people who need to lower their risk for heart disease. Switching to a fiber-rich diet can lower cholesterol levels by 20% or more. In a study of 6,000 men and women, those who ate the most fiber had significantly lower blood pressure, triglycerides, and homocysteine.

Fiber is the part of plants your body cannot break down and use. So how does it lower cholesterol? Your body uses cholesterol to make bile, which helps you digest fat. Most bile is recycled by the body, but fiber binds with bile and stops it from being recycled. As a result, your body uses up more cholesterol to make more bile. As you continue to eat fiber-rich foods that interfere with bile recycling, your cholesterol goes down.

Whole grains, oat bran, beans, and psyllium are great sources of fiber, but there is fiber in all plant foods. Most of us eat too little fiber. We eat more sugar (soda and candy) and refined carbohydrates (white flour and white bread), and too few fruits, vegetables, and whole grains. That is changing, though, with more fiber-rich foods, like whole grain pasta, appearing on grocery shelves. There is even a whole grain white flour for diehard white bread lovers.

We should eat about 25 grams of fiber a day, but most of us get 15 or less. To reach 25 grams of fiber, aim for 3 to 5 servings of whole grain breads and cereals, 3 servings of fruit, and 3 servings of vegetables a day. *The Cholesterol Counter* gives you the amount of fiber in most of the foods listed so it will be easy for you to see if you are getting enough.

YOU SHOULD KNOW—

Got Oatmeal?

75% of households have oatmeal in the cupboard. Eating oatmeal or another oat-based cereal, like Cheerios, *every day can help lower total cholesterol and LDL (bad) cholesterol.*

It's Easy to Add Fiber

- Eat fruits and vegetables instead of drinking juice.
- Eat the fiber-rich skins of cucumbers, apples, pears, potatoes, and zucchini.
- Eat more berries—blueberries, blackberries, raspberries, strawberries.
- Choose whole grains—brown rice, oatmeal, cracked wheat, barley, and whole wheat pasta, cereal, and bread.
- Eat beans and lentils a few times a week.
- Try soybeans in every form—soy nuts, tofu, tempeh, edamame.
- Snack on lowfat popcorn or unsalted whole wheat pretzels.
- Have vegetarian meals a few times a week.
- Eat dried fruits and raisins.
- Eat bran and wheat germ.
- Try some of the new fiber-fortified foods.

- In addition to eating fiber-rich foods, you may want to try a fiber supplement.

YOU SHOULD KNOW—

Fiber can be added to food to boost its fiber value. Inulin, fructan (also called fructooligosaccharides or FOS), and methylcellulose are found in some brands of yogurt, pudding, and cottage cheese.

Eating More Cholesterol-Lowering Superfoods

It's not just high-fiber foods that will help lower your cholesterol. Studies have shown that soy foods raise HDL (good) cholesterol. Using edamame, tofu, soy milk, soy nuts, or meat substitutes made of soy will not only cut down on some high-cholesterol foods you normally eat, but also provide the extra heart-healthy benefits found in soybeans.

A number of studies have shown that vegetarian diets can reduce cholesterol as effectively as cholesterol-lowering drugs. Many of us are not willing to make such a big dietary change, but adapting some vegetarian habits will help bring your cholesterol down. Try a few meatless meals a week. Eat more beans—on salads, as a side dish, or mixed with pasta or rice. Eat more fruits and vegetables. Aim for at least 5 servings a day. Most are naturally low in calories and rich in antioxidants, and none have cholesterol.

Eat nuts or seeds—a handful, not a canful—daily. They are rich in natural phytosterols, which lower cholesterol.

Nuts and seeds are also rich in fat, but since they grow in the ground, it is the cholesterol-free type.

> **YOU SHOULD KNOW—**
>
> *Sunflower seeds, pistachios, pumpkin seeds, pine nuts, flaxseed, almonds, macadamia nuts, walnuts, pecans, cashews, peanuts, peanut butter, hazelnuts, and Brazil nuts are all rich in natural plant sterols.*

Plant sterols are another natural substance that reduce the absorption of cholesterol in your body. They are being added to more and more foods—margarine, orange juice, milk, cereal bars, chocolate, and yogurt. When eaten regularly, these foods help to lower total cholesterol and LDL (bad) cholesterol. Studies show that getting 2 to 3 grams of plant sterols daily can reduce total cholesterol by 5% to 13% and LDL cholesterol by 6% to 24%. Couple this with other healthy habits and the total effect could be impressive.

Cholesterol-Lowering Medication

Of the 65 million Americans who need to lower their cholesterol levels, about half should be able to do it solely by making lifestyle changes. The rest need medication, too. If you take a cholesterol-lowering medication, it's still important to eat healthy foods, exercise, and avoid smoking to make your medication more effective. Unfortunately, many people don't take their medication daily and some stop taking it altogether when their numbers return to normal. It is important to follow your doctor's instructions and take your medication every day.

COMMON CHOLESTEROL-LOWERING MEDICATIONS

Statins
Altocor
Crestor
Lescol
Lipitor
Mevacor
Pravachol
Zocor

Bile Acid Sequestrants
Colestid
Prevalite
Questran
Welchol

Fibrates
Anatara
Lofibra
Lopid
Tricor

Absorption Inhibitors
Vytorin

Niacin
Niacolar
Niacor
Niaspin
Slo-Niacin

Combination Drugs
Caduet
Zetia

There are several types of cholesterol-lowering drugs on the market today, and more are being developed. Statins slow down your body's absorption of cholesterol, lower total and LDL (bad) cholesterol, and slightly raise HDL (good) cholesterol. Bile acid sequestrants, also known as resins, lower LDL cholesterol and total cholesterol. Fibrates help lower total cholesterol by reducing the amount of triglycerides in the body and increasing HDL cholesterol. Cholesterol absorption inhibitor drugs lower your cholesterol by reducing the amount that is absorbed in your intestines. When given in very large doses, niacin, a B vitamin, can lower triglycerides and LDL cholesterol and increase HDL cholesterol. Even though you can take niacin without a prescription, you shouldn't take it in large amounts to lower your cholesterol unless a prescription form of the vitamin is recommended by your doctor. The National Institutes of Health is funding a large study to determine if a statin-niacin combination would be more effective than a statin drug alone. As time goes on, we may see more combination drugs. Zetia combines a statin with an absorption inhibitor. Caduet combines a statin with a blood pressure-lowering drug. Your doctor has many drug options available. He or she may try more than one to get the desired result.

YOU SHOULD KNOW—

Go easy on grapefruit juice if you take a cholesterol-lowering statin drug.

Grapefruit juice increases the level of the drug in your bloodstream and its potency, possibly causing dangerous side effects.

COUNTING CHOLESTEROL

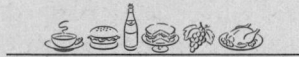

Now it's time to track your cholesterol intake for one day. Based on your blood cholesterol values and your doctor's recommendation, you should be eating less than 300 milligrams or less than 200 milligrams a day. Aim for 25 grams of fiber a day. And try to stay within your target calories range (see page 18).

Using the worksheet on the following page, write down everything you eat and drink. No one is going to look at what you wrote down, so be honest. Then use *The Cholesterol Counter* to find out how much cholesterol, fiber, and calories are in each food. You'll find information on more than 20,000 foods beginning on page 44.

Keeping track daily, or at least a few times a week, is a great way to stay on course. It will show you what to work on or reinforce how well you are doing. After a while you won't need to do this so often, because healthier eating will come naturally.

DAILY CHOLESTEROL RECORD

Cholesterol: Aim for _____ mg/day
Fiber: Aim for 25 mg/day
Target Calories: _____

	CHOLESTEROL	FIBER	CALORIES
Breakfast			
Lunch			
Snack			
Dinner			
Snack			
TOTALS:			

Did your cholesterol total less than 300 milligrams for the day? Did you get enough fiber? Did you eat the right amount of calories, based on your target weight? If not, work on making wiser choices tomorrow.

YOUR QUESTIONS, PLEASE

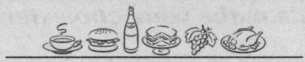

To lower my cholesterol, do I have to stop eating steak?

All foods can fit into a low-cholesterol diet, but some may need a little more negotiation than others. You can enjoy a steak every now and then. Four ounces of porterhouse has 80 milligrams of cholesterol, so make sure to keep the portion size moderate. Also, consider choices for the entire meal, balancing your high-cholesterol choice with low-cholesterol accompaniments—go easy on salad dressing, cheese, butter, and high-fat desserts. Let the steak be the splurge.

Do I have to stop eating eggs?

Eggs are a healthy food and you don't have to give them up—just eat them in moderation. A medium egg has 211 milligrams of cholesterol. So, having a scrambled egg for breakfast is no problem if you are aiming for 300 milligrams or less a day. But if you need to restrict your cholesterol to 200 milligrams a day, you'll need to make nonmeat, nondairy choices for lunch and dinner. One egg can be stretched into a larger serving by adding the white of another egg or using an egg substitute, both of which are cholesterol free. People incorrectly believe that the cholesterol in eggs is more potent than other cholesterol. This simply isn't true.

Can large meals make your cholesterol go up?

Some recent research shows that eating smaller, more frequent meals helps to lower cholesterol. The researchers think that larger meals may trigger extra cholesterol production in the body. Research subjects who ate 6 times a day had, on average, 5% lower cholesterol levels than those who ate 1 or 2 times a day. This seems like a small difference, but small changes can add up to a significant impact on your cholesterol level and your ultimate risk for heart disease.

Does drinking wine help lower cholesterol?

Alcohol in moderation, especially red wine, has been linked with higher HDL (good) cholesterol and an overall lower risk for heart disease. For those who don't drink, purple grape juice also provides a protective effect.

Does coffee raise cholesterol?

This question doesn't have a simple yes or no answer. Regularly drinking coffee made by the French-press process can increase cholesterol as much as 14%. Regular drip coffee, the preferred method in the U.S., has no effect on cholesterol levels. But when researchers looked at decaf coffee drinkers versus regular coffee drinkers, those drinking decaf had slightly higher LDL (bad) cholesterol levels. Nobody knows exactly why, though the difference may lie in the beans—robusta beans are normally used for decaf and arabica beans for regular coffee.

When it comes to coffee, it's more important to cut back on cream and whipped toppings, which add cholesterol, and other extras that pile on calories. Keep portions small, drink 4 cups or less a day, and you should be fine.

Is it true that we don't absorb all the cholesterol we eat?

Most of us think that every milligram of cholesterol we eat goes straight to our arteries, but it doesn't work like that. Not all cholesterol is bad. Some of the cholesterol you eat is used in the body to insulate nerve cells, help skin retain moisture, and produce hormones and bile. It's also part of our brains. And it's true, not all cholesterol you eat is absorbed. But absorption rates vary greatly between people. There is no way of knowing if you absorb a lot or a little, so eating moderate amounts of cholesterol is the wisest course for everyone.

How can I figure out how much cholesterol is in restaurant meals?

You will find a take-out subcategory in many categories in *The Cholesterol Counter.* This will help you estimate the cholesterol, fiber, and calories in foods you order. In Part Two, the cholesterol values for many menu items are listed for 111 restaurant chains. Beyond that, use all the knowledge you've accumulated reading this book. Does the food you are ordering have a face or was it grown in the ground? Animal foods have cholesterol; plant foods don't. You may not always know the exact amount of cholesterol, but you'll know enough to make good choices.

Can cholesterol ever be too low?

Very low cholesterol, below 100, may be a sign of mal-
nutrition, an overactive thyroid, liver damage, or some
types of cancer. When total cholesterol values fall below
180, there is an increased risk for hemorrhagic stroke,
which is when a blood vessel bursts instead of becoming
clogged with plaque. Ischemic stroke, the type in which
clogged arteries block blood flow, accounts for 80% of all
strokes. Cholesterol values between 180 and 200 may be
best to avoid both types of strokes.

USING YOUR
CHOLESTEROL COUNTER

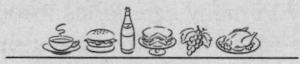

The Cholesterol Counter lists the calories, portion size, cholesterol, and fiber for more than 20,000 foods. Now you can compare the values in your favorite foods and, when necessary, choose substitutes before you go out to shop or eat. This will save you time and help you decide what to buy.

The counter section of the book is divided into two parts: Part One: Brand Name, Nonbranded (Generic), and Take-Out Foods (page 43); and Part Two: Restaurant Chains (page 585). Each part lists foods or restaurant chains alphabetically.

In Part One, for each category, you will find non-branded (generic) foods listed first in alphabetical order, followed by an alphabetical listing of brand name foods. The nonbranded listings will help you estimate the calorie, cholesterol, and fiber values when you don't see your favorite brand. They can also help you to evaluate store brands. Large categories are divided into subcategories, such as canned, fresh, frozen, and ready-to-eat, to make it easier to find what you're looking for. Some categories have *see* and *see also* references, to help you find related items.

A dash (-) appears in some entries. This means that no analysis was done for cholesterol or fiber in that food. It is not the same as a 0, which means there is no cholesterol or fiber in the food.

Because we eat out so often, more than 600 take-out foods are listed in Part One. These are found in the take-out subcategory in many categories throughout this section. Look there for foods you take-out or order in, since they are not nutrition labeled.

Most foods are listed alphabetically. In some cases, though, foods are grouped by category. For example, a tuna sandwich is found in the SANDWICH category. Other group categories include:

ASIAN FOOD   **Page 51**
> includes all types of Asian foods
> except egg rolls and sushi, which
> are found in separate categories

DELI MEATS/COLD CUTS   **Page 229**
> includes all sandwich meats
> except chicken, ham, and turkey,
> which are found in separate
> categories

DINNER   **Page 231**
> includes all by brand name,
> except pasta dinners, which are
> found in a separate category

LIQUOR/LIQUEUR   **Page 347**
> includes all alcoholic beverages
> and mixed drinks except beer,
> champagne, and wine, which are
> found in separate categories

NUTRITION SUPPLEMENTS　　**Page 377**

Includes all dieting aids, meal
replacers, and drinks, except
energy bars and energy drinks,
which are found in separate
categories

SANDWICHES　　**Page 473**

Includes popular sandwich,
calzone, and panini choices

SNACKS　　**Page 492**

Includes a variety of
miscellaneous snack items such
as trail mix, pork rinds, and
cheese puffs

SPANISH FOOD　　**Page 525**

Includes all types of Spanish
and Mexican foods except salsa
and tortillas, which are found in
separate categories

In Part Two, Restaurant Chains, 111 national and re-
gional restaurant, candy, coffee, doughnut, ice cream,
pizza, and sandwich chains are listed. Brand name foods
are required by federal law to have nutrition information
on labels, but in most areas of the country, restaurants
provide this information voluntarily.

With *The Cholesterol Counter* as your guide, you will
never again wonder how much cholesterol is in the food
you eat. You will always be able to tell if a food is high,
moderate, or low in cholesterol.

DEFINITIONS

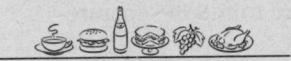

as prep (as prepared): refers to food that has been prepared according to package directions

lean and fat: describes meat with some fat on its edges that is not cut away before cooking, or poultry prepared with skin and fat as purchased

lean only: refers to lean meat that is trimmed of all visible fat, or poultry without skin

not prep (not prepared): refers to food that has not been cooked and may require the addition of other ingredients

shelf-stable: refers to prepared products found on the supermarket shelf that are ready-to-eat or are ready to be heated and do not require refrigeration

take-out: describes prepared dishes that you purchase ready-to-eat; those included serve as a guide to the calories, cholesterol, and fiber in products you may purchase.

ABBREVIATIONS

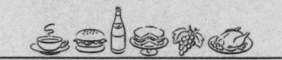

avg	=	average
diam	=	diameter
frzn	=	frozen
g	=	gram
in	=	inch
lb	=	pound
lg	=	large
med	=	medium
mg	=	milligram
oz	=	ounce
pkg	=	package
pt	=	pint
prep	=	prepared
qt	=	quart
reg	=	regular
sec	=	second
serv	=	serving
sm	=	small
sq	=	square
tbsp	=	tablespoon
tr	=	trace
tsp	=	teaspoon
w/	=	with
w/o	=	without
<	=	less than

NOTES

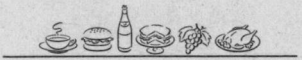

Cals = calories
Chol = cholesterol
    All cholesterol values are given in milligrams (mg)
Fiber = fiber
    All fiber values are given in grams (g)
tr (trace) = less than 1 mg of cholesterol or 1 gram of
    fiber
– (dash) indicates data was not available
0 (zero) indicates there are no calories or cholesterol or
    fiber in that food

Discrepancies in figures are due to rounding, product reformulation, and reevaluation. Labeling law allows rounding of values. Much of the data listed is analysis data, obtained directly from manufacturers, not from labels. Therefore some values here may differ slightly from labels, because they have not been rounded.

PART ONE

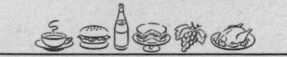

Brand Name, Nonbranded (Generic), and Take-Out Foods

YOU SHOULD KNOW—

Your goal is to pick low-cholesterol foods most of the time.

FOOD	PORTION	CALS	CHOL	FIBER
ABALONE				
breaded & fried	1 serv (3 oz)	162	80	tr
steamed	1 serv (3 oz)	127	84	0
ACEROLA				
fresh	1 (5 g)	2	0	tr
ACEROLA JUICE				
juice	1 cup	56	0	1
ADZUKI BEANS				
canned sweetened	½ cup	351	0	–
dried cooked w/o salt	½ cup	147	0	8
AKEE				
fresh	3.5 oz	223	0	–
ALCOHOL (see BEER AND ALE, CHAMPAGNE, LIQUOR/LIQUEUR, MALT, WINE)				
ALE (see BEER AND ALE)				
ALFALFA				
sprouts	½ cup	40	0	tr
ALLIGATOR				
cooked	3 oz	126	57	0
ALLSPICE				
ground	1 tsp	5	0	tr
ALMONDS				
almond butter w/o salt	2 tbsp	203	0	1
almond extract	1 tsp	38	0	0
almond paste	¼ cup	260	0	3
chocolate covered	6 pieces (0.6 oz)	102	1	2
dry roasted w/o salt	¼ cup	206	0	4
honey roasted	¼ cup	214	0	5
jordan almonds	6 (0.7 oz)	99	0	1
praline	17 pieces (1.4 oz)	210	0	3
yogurt covered	6 pieces (0.8 oz)	122	0	1
American Almond				
Marzipan	2 tbsp	130	0	1
Blue Diamond				
Almond Roca Buttercrunch	3 pieces (1.3 oz)	210	15	0

FOOD	PORTION	CALS	CHOL	FIBER
Honey Roasted	¼ cup	170	0	3
Jalapeno Smokehouse	28 pieces (1 oz)	170	0	3
Jordon Pastels	15 pieces (1.4 oz)	180	0	2
Lime 'N Chili	28 pieces (1 oz)	170	0	3
Maui Onion & Garlic	28 pieces (1 oz)	170	0	3
Milk Chocolate Covered	9 pieces (1.4 oz)	230	5	3
Salted	¼ cup	170	0	3
Smokehouse	28 pieces (1.3 oz)	170	0	3
Wasabi & Soy Sauce	28 pieces (1 oz)	170	0	3
Whole Natural	¼ cup	180	0	3
Yogurt Covered	12 pieces (1.4 oz)	210	0	0
Brach's				
Chocolate Coated	11 pieces	220	10	2
Eden				
Tamari	3 tbsp (1 oz)	160	0	4
Good Sense				
Hickory Smoked	¼ cup	180	0	2
Raw Whole	¼ cup	180	0	4
Judy's				
Sugar Free Coconut Almond Brittle	¼ piece (1 oz)	90	0	1
Kettle				
Butter Salted	2 tbsp	180	0	2
Butter Unsalted	2 tbsp	180	0	2
Love'n Bake				
Almond Paste	2 tbsp	140	0	2
Almond Schmear	2 tbsp	140	0	2
Roasted Butter	2 tbsp	180	0	3
Low Carb Creations				
Soft Almond Brittle	2 pieces (1 oz)	170	0	2
Maisie Jane's				
Almond Butter	1 oz	184	0	0
Cappuccino	9 pieces (1.4 oz)	220	5	2
Chocolate Toffee	9 pieces (1.4 oz)	210	5	2
Coffee Glazed	2 tbsp (1 oz)	150	0	3
Cowboy BBQ	2 tbsp (1 oz)	140	0	3
Mint Chocolate	9 pieces (1.4 oz)	210	0	2
Organic Honey Glazed	2 tbsp (1 oz)	160	0	4
Tamari	2 tbsp (1 oz)	160	0	4

FOOD	PORTION	CALS	CHOL	FIBER
Mama Mellace's				
Butter Rum	1 oz	150	0	2
Cinnamon Roasted	1 oz	140	0	2
Maranatha				
Almond Butter	2 tbsp	220	0	3
Raw Almond Butter	2 tbsp	190	0	4
Tamari Almonds	¼ cup	160	0	3
Odense				
Almond Paste	2 tbsp (1.4 oz)	170	5	0
Planters				
Chocolate Lovers Dark Chocolate	11 pieces (1.4 oz)	220	<5	3
Dry Roasted	23 pieces (1 oz)	160	0	3
Sweet Delights				
Almond Roasters	⅓ pkg (1 oz)	190	0	3
AMARANTH				
leaves cooked	½ cup	14	0	–
uncooked	½ cup (3.4 oz)	365	0	15
ANCHOVY				
boneless	1 oz	60	24	0
canned in oil drained	1 can (2 oz)	94	38	0
fresh	1 (4 g)	8	3	0
CANNED				
Brunswick				
Flat Fillets	1 can (2 oz)	25	10	0
ANISE				
seed	1 tsp	7	0	tr
ANTELOPE				
roasted	4 oz	215	127	0
APPLE				
CANNED				
sliced sweetened	½ cup	68	0	2
Glory				
Fried Apples	½ cup	80	0	1
DRIED				
chopped	½ cup	104	0	4
cooked w/o sugar	½ cup	73	0	3
rings	5	78	0	3

FOOD	PORTION	CALS	CHOL	FIBER
Crispy Green				
Crispy Apples	1 pkg (0.36 oz)	35	0	1
Del Monte				
Dried Apples	¼ cup	110	0	3
FRESH				
apple	1 sm	55	0	3
apple	1 med	72	0	3
apple	1 lg	110	0	5
candied	1 sm (4.9 oz)	179	0	3
candied	1 med (6.5 oz)	234	0	4
candied	1 lg (9.8 oz)	357	6	6
w/ skin sliced	1 cup	57	0	3
w/o skin sliced	1 cup	53	0	1
Chiquita				
Apple	1 med (5.4 oz)	80	0	5
Cool Cut				
Apples & Caramel Dip	1 pkg (4.25 oz)	180	5	3
Earthbound Farm				
Organic Slices	1 pkg (2 oz)	30	0	1
Rainier				
Apple	1 med (5.5 oz)	80	0	5
Sullivan				
McIntosh	1 (5.4 oz)	80	0	4
TreeTop				
Slices Red or Green	1 pkg (2 oz)	35	0	–
FROZEN				
sliced w/o sugar	½ cup	42	0	2
Roast Works				
Flame Roasted Fuji	1 serv (5 oz)	90	0	2
TAKE-OUT				
baked	1 (6 oz)	128	0	4
baked no sugar	1 (5.6 oz)	136	0	4
fried apple rings	1 serv (2.7 oz)	91	0	2
APPLE JUICE				
cider	1 cup	117	0	tr
juice + vitamin C & calcium	1 cup	117	0	tr
mulled cider	1 serv	265	0	6
unsweetened w/o vitamin C	1 cup	117	0	tr

FOOD	PORTION	CALS	CHOL	FIBER
After The Fall				
Organic	8 oz	90	0	–
Apple & Eve				
100% Juice	8 oz	110	0	–
Cider	8 oz	110	0	–
Celestial Seasonings				
Cider Apple Caramel Kiss as prep	1 cup	80	0	0
Eden				
Organic Juice	8 oz	90	0	0
Hansen's				
100% Juice	8 oz	120	0	0
Hi-C				
Sour Blast Green Apple	1 pkg	100	0	–
Hood				
100% Juice	1 cup	120	0	0
Izze				
Sparkling Apple	1 bottle (12 oz)	138	0	–
Kedem				
100% Juice	8 oz	110	0	–
Langers				
Diet Cocktail 50% Juice	8 oz	60	0	–
Harvest Apple 100% Juice	8 oz	120	0	–
Low Carb Creations				
Apple Cider as prep	1 serv	10	0	0
Minute Maid				
100% Juice	8 oz	100	0	–
Mott's				
100% Juice	8 oz	120	0	0
100% Juice	1 box (8 oz)	120	0	–
100% Natural	8 oz	120	0	0
Hot Spiced Cider All Flavors as prep	1 serv	80	0	–
Naked Juice				
Just Apple	8 oz	120	0	0
Nantucket Nectars				
100% Pressed	8 oz	100	0	–
Ocean Spray				
100% Juice	8 oz	110	0	0

FOOD	PORTION	CALS	CHOL	FIBER
Odwalla				
Spiced Harvest Cider	8 oz	130	0	0
Phat Phruit				
Green Apple	8 oz	40	0	0
Red Cheek				
100% Juice	8 oz	120	0	–
Robert & James				
100% Juice	8 oz	110	0	–
Seneca				
100% Juice	8 oz	110	0	–
Snapple				
Diet	8 oz	15	0	–
Snapple Apple	8 oz	120	0	–
Squeezit				
Green Apple	1 bottle (7 oz)	110	0	0
Swiss Miss				
Hot Apple Cider Mix	1 serv	84	0	1
Hot Apple Cider Mix Low Calorie	1 serv	14	0	0
TreeTop				
100% Juice	8 oz	120	0	–
Cider 100% Juice No Sugar Added	8 oz	120	0	–
Tropicana				
Orchard Style	1 bottle (14 oz)	200	0	0
Turkey Hill				
Herbal Cider w/ Chamomile & Lemongrass	1 cup	100	0	–
Zeigler's				
Old Fashioned Cider	8 oz	110	0	1
APPLESAUCE				
sweetened	½ cup	97	0	2
unsweetened	½ cup	52	0	2
Eden				
Organic	½ cup	60	0	2
Organic Apple Cherry	½ cup	70	0	3
Organic Apple Strawberry	½ cup	60	0	2
Organic Cinnamon	1 pkg (4 oz)	70	0	2

FOOD	PORTION	CALS	CHOL	FIBER
Jok'n'Al				
Low Carb	1 tbsp	10	0	–
Langers				
Unsweetened	½ cup	50	0	2
Mott's				
Single-Serve Cinnamon	1 pkg (4 oz)	100	0	1
Single-Serve Natural	1 pkg (4 oz)	50	0	–
Single-Serve Original	1 pkg (4 oz)	100	0	–
Musselman's				
Apple Sauce	1 pkg (4 oz)	80	0	2
Lite	1 pkg (4 oz)	50	0	2
Vermont Village				
Organic Unsweetened	½ cup	80	0	2
White House				
Apple Sauce	1 pkg (4 oz)	90	0	1

APRICOT JUICE

FOOD	PORTION	CALS	CHOL	FIBER
nectar	6 oz	106	0	1
Ceres				
Apricot	8 oz	120	0	0

APRICOTS
CANNED

FOOD	PORTION	CALS	CHOL	FIBER
heavy syrup	½ cup	91	0	3
juice pack	½ cup	59	0	2
light syrup	½ cup	80	0	2
water pack	½ cup	33	0	2
Del Monte				
Halves In Heavy Syrup	½ cup	100	0	1
Orchard Select Halves	½ cup	80	0	1
DRIED				
halves	6	51	0	2
halves cooked w/o sugar	½ cup	106	0	3
Crispy Green				
Crispy Apricots	1 pkg (0.36 oz)	40	0	tr
Sunsweet				
Apricots	6 pieces (1.4 oz)	100	0	3
FRESH				
apricots	1	17	0	1
sliced	½ cup	40	0	2

FOOD	PORTION	CALS	CHOL	FIBER
Chiquita				
Apricots	3 med (4 oz)	60	0	1
FROZEN				
sweetened	½ cup	119	0	3
ARROWHEAD				
corm boiled	1 med	9	0	–
ARROWROOT				
raw	1 root (1.2 oz)	21	0	tr
raw root sliced	1 cup	78	0	2
ARTICHOKE				
CANNED				
hearts in oil	1 serv (3 oz)	100	0	4
Progresso				
Hearts	1 piece	15	0	1
Hearts Marinated	2 pieces (1.1 oz)	170	0	0
S&W				
Marinated Hearts	2 pieces (1 oz)	20	0	1
FRESH				
cooked	1 med	60	0	7
hearts cooked	½ cup	42	0	5
FROZEN				
cooked	1 cup	42	0	5
C&W				
Hearts	12 pieces (3 oz)	40	0	5
TAKE-OUT				
stuffed	1 (8.8 oz)	397	8	10
ARUGULA				
fresh	1 cup	3	0	tr
ASIAN FOOD (*see also* DINNER, EGG ROLLS, SAUCES, SOY SAUCE, SUSHI)				
CANNED				
chow mein chicken no noodles	1 cup	194	51	2
Chun King				
Beef Pepper Oriental BiPack	1 cup (8.8 oz)	98	14	3
Chow Mein Beef BiPack	1 cup (8.6 oz)	78	6	3
Chow Mein Chicken BiPack	1 cup (8.8 oz)	98	6	3

FOOD	PORTION	CALS	CHOL	FIBER
Chow Mein Pork BiPack	1 cup (8.6 oz)	78	10	2
Hot & Spicy Chicken BiPack	1 cup (8.6 oz)	98	19	1
Sweet & Sour Chicken BiPack	1 cup (8.9 oz)	161	25	3
La Choy				
Beef Pepper Oriental BiPack	1 cup (8.8 oz)	98	14	3
Chow Mein Beef BiPack	1 cup (8.6 oz)	78	6	3
Chow Mein Chicken PiBack	1 cup (8.9 oz)	98	6	3
Chow Mein Shrimp BiPack	1 cup (8.6 oz)	52	4	3
Main Entree Chow Mein Chicken	1 cup (9.3 oz)	80	9	3
Oriental Beef w/ Noodles BiPack	1 cup (8.8 oz)	156	17	4
Oriental Chicken w/ Noodles BiPack	1 cup (8.7 oz)	154	23	2
Sweet & Sour Chicken BiPack	1 cup (8.9 oz)	161	25	3
Teriyaki Chicken BiPack	1 cup (8.6 oz)	109	20	3
FRESH				
wonton wrappers	1	23	1	–
Azumaya				
Round Wraps	10	160	10	1
Wrappers Large Square	8	160	10	1
Frieda's				
Won Ton Wrappers	4 (1 oz)	80	0	1
Nasoya				
Won Ton Wrappers	8	160	10	1
FROZEN				
Amy's				
Bowls Teriyaki	1 pkg (10 oz)	300	0	3
Skillet Meals Teriyaki Stir Fry	1 cup	320	0	4
Stir Fry Asian Noodle	1 pkg (10 oz)	240	0	6
Stir Fry Thai	1 pkg (9.5 oz)	270	0	2
Banquet				
Fried Rice w/ Chicken & Egg Rolls	1 meal (8.5 oz)	330	60	5
Contessa				
Chow Mein Chicken w/ Sauce not prep	1¾ cups	320	25	3
Curry Chicken w/ Sauce not prep	1¾ cups	240	25	2

FOOD	PORTION	CALS	CHOL	FIBER
Fried Rice Chicken w/ Sauce not prep	1¾ cups	260	100	4
General Tsao Shrimp w/ Sauce not prep	1¾ cups	270	35	4
Kung Pao Shrimp w/ Sauce not prep	1¾ cups	200	45	3
Lo Mein Shrimp w/ Sauce not prep	1¾ cups	250	35	2
Stir-Fry Beef w/ sauce not prep	1¾ cup	190	20	4
Stir-Fry Chicken w/ Sauce not prep	1¾ cups	160	25	4
Stir-Fry Shrimp w/ Sauce not prep	1¾ cups	120	40	2
Sweet & Sour Shrimp w/ Sauce not prep	1½ cups	180	50	3
Tandoori Chicken w/ Sauce not prep	1⅓ cups	200	30	3
Kahiki				
Beef & Broccoli	1 pkg (10.9 oz)	360	50	2
Chicken Fried Rice	1 pkg (10.9 oz)	460	85	2
General Tso's Chicken	1 pkg (10 oz)	400	20	2
Naturals General Tso's Chicken	1 pkg (10 oz)	330	35	3
Naturals Mandarin Orange Chicken	1 pkg (10 oz)	340	35	3
Naturals Szechuan Peppercorn Beef	1 pkg (10 oz)	350	50	3
Naturals Teriyaki Mixed Vegetables	1 pkg (10 oz)	260	0	4
Sesame Orange Chicken	1 pkg (10.9 oz)	420	25	2
Soothing Lettuce Wraps	4 tbsp (2 oz)	90	10	1
Tempura Chicken Nuggets	¾ cup (3.5 oz)	230	40	0
Tropical Sweet & Sour Chicken	1 pkg (10.9 oz)	490	25	4
La Choy				
Beef Pepper Oriental	1 cup (7.1 oz)	151	10	2
Chow Mein Vegetable	1 cup (8.9 oz)	108	0	5

FOOD	PORTION	CALS	CHOL	FIBER
Lean Cuisine				
Cafe Classics Asian Style Beef w/ Ginger & Soy	1 pkg (9.25 oz)	210	25	2
Cafe Classics Bowl Chicken Fried Rice	1 pkg (10 oz)	310	50	3
Cafe Classics Bowl Chicken Teriyaki	1 pkg (11 oz)	320	30	3
Cafe Classics Bowl Teriyaki Steak	1 pkg (10.5 oz)	340	30	4
Cafe Classics Chicken Teriyaki Stir Fry	1 pkg (10 oz)	300	30	3
Cafe Classics Hunan Beef & Broccoli	1 pkg (8.5 oz)	230	15	1
Cafe Classics Thai-Style Chicken	1 pkg (9 oz)	230	30	2
One Dish Favorites Asian Style Pot Stickers	1 pkg (9 oz)	320	20	3
One Dish Favorites Chicken Chow Mein	1 pkg (9 oz)	200	25	2
Skillet Asian Style Chicken & Vegetables	1 serv	160	20	2
Seeds Of Change				
Asian Stir-Fry Noodles	1 pkg (11 oz)	290	5	4
Spicy Peanut Noodles	1 pkg (11 oz)	370	5	4
Teriyaki Stir Fried Rice	1 pkg (11 oz)	340	5	6
MIX				
Annie Chun's				
Meal Kit Chow Mein Noodles w/ Garlic Black Bean Sauce	⅓ pkg	230	0	2
Meal Kit Chow Mein Noodles w/ Peanut Sesame Sauce	⅓ pkg	270	0	2
Meal Kit Chow Mein Noodles w/ Scallion Sauce	⅓ pkg	240	0	2
Meal Kit Chow Mein Noodles w/ Teriyaki Sauce	⅓ box	210	0	2
Meal Kit Pad Thai Noodles w/ Pad Thai Sauce	⅓ pkg	210	0	–
Meal Kit Soba Noodles w/ Soy Ginger Sauce	⅓ pkg	210	0	3

FOOD	PORTION	CALS	CHOL	FIBER
Nissin				
Chow Mein Chicken as prep	½ pkg (2 oz)	240	0	2
Chow Mein Thai Peanut as prep	½ pkg (2 oz)	270	0	tr
SHELF-STABLE				
Fantastic				
Pad Thai w/ Rice Noodles	1 pkg (7 oz)	400	0	5
Thai Lemon Grass w/ Rice Noodles	1 pkg (7.4 oz)	340	0	5
TAKE-OUT				
beef & broccoli	1 cup	221	54	3
buddha's delight w/ cellophane noodles fat choi jai	1 serv (7.6 oz)	211	tr	2
cha siu bao steamed buns w/ chicken filling	1 (2.3 oz)	160	15	tr
chow mein beef no noodles	1 cup	271	51	3
chow mein noodles	1 cup	237	0	2
chow mein pork no noodles	1 cup	284	55	3
chow mein shrimp no noodles	1 cup	154	92	2
chow mein vegetable no noodles	1 cup	224	0	4
dim sum meat filled	3 pieces (4 oz)	124	54	1
egg foo yung beef	1 patty (6 oz)	243	336	1
egg foo yung chicken	1 patty (3 oz)	121	166	1
egg foo yung pork	1 patty (3 oz)	125	166	1
egg foo yung shrimp	1 patty (3 oz)	153	184	1
filipino chicken adobo	1 serv (15 oz)	555	116	1
fried rice	1 cup	333	103	1
fried rice beef	1 cup	346	107	1
fried rice chicken	1 cup	329	105	1
fried rice pork	1 cup	335	103	1
fried rice shrimp	1 cup	323	115	1
general tsao's chicken	1 cup	296	66	1
green beans szechuan style	1 cup	176	0	6
kung pao beef	1 cup	410	62	2
kung pao chicken	1 cup	434	65	2
kung pao pork	1 cup	460	60	2
kung pao shrimp	1 cup	345	191	2

FOOD	PORTION	CALS	CHOL	FIBER
lo mein beef	1 cup	286	26	3
lo mein chicken	1 cup	262	26	3
lo mein meatless	1 cup	234	0	3
lo mein pork	1 cup	314	22	3
lo mein shrimp	1 cup	236	48	4
moo goo gai pan chicken	1 cup	272	35	3
moo shu pork w/o pancake	1 cup	512	172	1
phad thai	1 serv (9.2 oz)	232	0	1
sesame seed paste bun	1 (2.5 oz)	220	0	2
shrimp chips banh phong tom	6 med	214	21	tr
shrimp w/ lobster sauce	1 cup	298	259	1
shu mai chicken & vegetable dumplings	6 (3.6 oz)	160	35	1
sukiyaki beef	1 cup	165	130	1
sweet & sour chicken w/o rice	1 cup	670	169	2
sweet & sour pork w/ rice	1 cup	268	29	2
sweet & sour pork w/o rice	1 cup	231	38	2
sweet & sour shrimp	1 cup	480	70	1
sweet red bean bun	1 (2.5 oz)	130	0	2
szechuan chicken	1 cup	190	42	2
szechuan shrimp & vegetables	1 cup	159	94	2
tempura vegetable	8 pieces	90	36	1
tempura hawaiian fish tofu vegetable	2 cups	285	200	2
teriyaki beef	1 cup	454	149	tr
teriyaki chicken plain	¾ cup	399	92	–
teriyaki chicken w/ rice	1 serv (11 oz)	430	25	1
teriyaki shrimp	1 cup	271	269	1
wonton fried meat filled	1 (0.7 oz)	54	20	tr

ASPARAGUS
CANNED

FOOD	PORTION	CALS	CHOL	FIBER
spears	1 cup	46	0	4
spears	1	3	0	tr
Del Monte				
Cuts & Tips	½ cup	20	0	1
Spears	½ cup	20	0	1
Tips	½ cup	20	0	1

FOOD	PORTION	CALS	CHOL	FIBER
S&W				
Green	6 pieces (4.5 oz)	15	0	1
Tillen Farms				
Crispy Asparagus Pickled	3 spears	10	0	0
FRESH				
cooked	½ cup	20	0	2
cooked	4 spears	13	0	1
raw	4 spears	10	0	1
Frieda's				
White	⅔ cup	20	0	2
FROZEN				
cooked	1 pkg (10 oz)	53	0	5
cooked	4 spears	11	0	1
C&W				
Spears	7 (3 oz)	20	0	tr
Europe's Best				
Spears	7 spears	15	0	2
AVOCADO				
california mashed	¼ cup	96	0	4
california peeled & pitted	1	289	0	12
florida mashed	¼ cup	69	0	1
florida peeled & pitted	1	365	0	17
Brooks Tropical				
Lite SlimCado	1 tbsp	35	0	tr
Calavo				
Fresh	⅕ med (1 oz)	55	0	3
Chiquita				
Fresh	⅓ med (1 oz)	55	0	3
Earthbound Farm				
Organic Fresh	⅕ med (1 oz)	55	0	3
Frieda's				
Fresh Cocktail	1 (1.4 oz)	60	0	2
TAKE-OUT				
guacamole	1 serv (2.2 oz)	105	0	2
BACON				
bacon grease	1 tbsp	116	12	0
beef breakfast strips cooked	3 strips	153	40	0
pan fried	3 strips	109	16	0

FOOD	PORTION	CALS	CHOL	FIBER
Boar's Head				
Sliced Fried	2 slices	70	10	0
Health Is Wealth				
Uncured Sliced	2 slices (0.5 oz)	70	10	0
Jennie-O				
Turkey Bacon	1 slice (0.5 oz)	35	10	0
Oscar Mayer				
Center Cut cooked	2 slices (0.4 oz)	50	15	0
Cooked	2 slices (0.5 oz)	70	15	0
Wellshire				
Beef Uncured	2 oz	114	50	0
Panchetta Sliced	1 slice (0.4 oz)	60	10	0
Pork Range Sliced Dry Rubbed	2 slices	30	10	0
Uncured Turkey	1 slice (1 oz)	20	10	0

BACON SUBSTITUTES

FOOD	PORTION	CALS	CHOL	FIBER
bacon bits meatless	1 tbsp	33	0	1
meatless	1 strip	16	0	tr
Bac-Os				
Chips or Bits	1½ tbsp (7 g)	30	0	0
Lightlife				
Organic Tempeh Smokey Strips	3 slices (2 oz)	80	0	1
Smart Bacon	2 strips (0.8 oz)	45	0	1
Worthington				
Stripples	2 strips (0.5 oz)	60	0	tr

BAGEL

FOOD	PORTION	CALS	CHOL	FIBER
cinnamon raisin	1 mini	71	0	1
cinnamon raisin	1 lg (4 in)	244	0	2
egg	1 lg (4.5 in)	364	31	3
low carb	1 (4 oz)	216	10	14
mini onion	1 (1.4 oz)	100	0	1
oat bran	1 lg (4 in)	227	0	3
plain	1 sm (3 in)	190	0	2
plain	1 med (3.5 in)	289	0	2
plain	1 lg (4.5 in)	360	0	3
Alvarado Street Bakery				
Sprouted Wheat Cinnamon Raisin	1 (3.3 oz)	280	0	3

FOOD	PORTION	CALS	CHOL	FIBER
Atkins				
Cinnamon Raisin	1	200	0	11
Onion	1	190	0	11
Plain	1	190	0	11
David's				
Deli Bagels	1 (2.8 oz)	230	0	2
Natural Ovens				
Blueberry	1 (3 oz)	190	0	4
Brainy	1 (3 oz)	170	0	6
Cinnamon Raisin	1 (3 oz)	180	0	5
Golden Crunch	1 (3 oz)	190	0	8
Hearty Grains & Onion	1 (3 oz)	190	0	7
Raspberry	1 (3 oz)	180	0	5
Whole Grain	1 (3 oz)	170	0	6
Otis Spunkmeyer				
Barnstormin' Blueberry	1 (3.6 oz)	250	0	3
Barnstormin' Cinnamon Raisin	1 (3.6 oz)	230	0	3
Barnstormin' Onion	1 (3.6 oz)	230	0	3
Barnstormin' Plain	1 (3.6 oz)	240	0	3
Pepperidge Farm				
100% Whole Wheat	1	250	0	6
Mini 100% Whole Wheat	1	100	0	3
Sara Lee				
Apple Cinnamon	1 (4 oz)	310	0	3
Banana Walnut	1 (4 oz)	350	0	4
Blueberry Deluxe	1 (3.3 oz)	260	0	2
Blueberry Junior	1 (1 oz)	70	0	tr
Blueberry Toaster Size	1 (2.1 oz)	160	0	1
Cinnamon Raisin Deluxe	1 (3.3 oz)	260	0	4
Heart Healthy 100% Whole Wheat	1 (3.3 oz)	220	0	6
Heart Healthy Cinnamon Raisin	1 (3.3 oz)	250	0	7
Plain	1 (2.1 oz)	160	0	1
Sundried Tomato & Basil	1 (4 oz)	300	0	2
Whole Grain Plain	1 (3.3 oz)	240	0	3
Thomas'				
Carb Consider Plain	1	150	0	6
Carb Consider Whole Wheat	1	140	0	7

FOOD	PORTION	CALS	CHOL	FIBER
Everything	1 (3.6 oz)	300	0	3
Multi-Grain	1 (3.6 oz)	280	0	4
Plain	1 (3.6 oz)	280	0	2
Uncle B's				
Plain	1 (2.8 oz)	210	0	2
Weight Watchers				
Original	1 (2.8 oz)	190	0	10
Wonder				
Blueberry	1 (3 oz)	210	0	1
Rye	1 (3 oz)	220	0	2

BAKING POWDER

FOOD	PORTION	CALS	CHOL	FIBER
baking powder	1 tsp	2	0	0
low sodium	1 tsp	5	0	tr
Clabber Girl				
Baking Powder	1 tsp	0	0	–
Davis				
Baking Powder	1 tsp	0	0	–
Rumford				
Aluminum Free	⅛ tsp	0	0	–

BAKING SODA

FOOD	PORTION	CALS	CHOL	FIBER
baking soda	1 tsp	0	0	0

BALSAM PEAR (BITTER GOURD)

FOOD	PORTION	CALS	CHOL	FIBER
leafy tips cooked w/o salt	1 cup	20	0	1
leafy tips raw	1 cup	14	0	–
pods raw sliced	1 cup	16	0	3
pods sliced cooked w/ salt	1 cup	24	0	3

BAMBOO SHOOTS

FOOD	PORTION	CALS	CHOL	FIBER
canned sliced	½ cup	12	0	1
fresh sliced cooked w/ salt	½ cup	7	0	1
raw sliced	½ cup	20	0	2
Chun King				
Bamboo Shoots	2 tbsp (0.8 oz)	3	0	tr
La Choy				
Bamboo Shoots	2 tbsp (0.8 oz)	3	0	tr

BANANA

FOOD	PORTION	CALS	CHOL	FIBER
banana chips	1 oz	147	0	2
fresh	1 sm (6 in)	90	0	3

FOOD	PORTION	CALS	CHOL	FIBER
fresh	1 med (7 in)	105	0	3
fresh	1 lg (8 in)	121	0	4
fresh baby	1 extra sm (<6 in)	72	0	2
fresh mashed	½ cup	100	0	3
fresh sliced	1 cup	134	0	4
powder	1 tbsp	21	0	1
whole dried	1 piece (1.2 oz)	130	0	2
Chiquita				
Fresh	1 med (4.4 oz)	110	0	4
Frieda's				
Burro	1 (3 oz)	80	0	1
Dried	1 piece (1.2 oz)	130	0	2
Goodniks				
Nutty Bananas Crunchy Snack	⅔ cup	230	5	3

BARBECUE SAUCE

FOOD	PORTION	CALS	CHOL	FIBER
barbecue	2 tbsp	52	0	tr
low sodium	2 tbsp	52	0	tr
Atkins				
Barbecue Sauce	1 tbsp	15	0	0
Carb Options				
Original	2 tbsp	10	0	0
Cattlemen's				
Classic	2 tbsp	60	0	tr
Honey	2 tbsp	70	0	tr
Smokehouse	2 tbsp	60	0	tr
Consorzio				
Organic Original	1 tbsp	50	0	0
Organic Spicy	1 tbsp	50	0	0
David Burke				
Flavor Spray Memphis BBQ	2 sprays	0	0	0
Emeril's				
Original BBQ	2 tbsp	45	0	–
Hunt's				
Hickory	2 tbsp	45	0	tr
Hickory & Brown Sugar	2 tbsp	70	0	1
Honey Hickory	2 tbsp	50	0	tr
Honey Mustard	2 tbsp	50	0	1
Hot & Spicy	2 tbsp	45	0	tr

FOOD	PORTION	CALS	CHOL	FIBER
Mesquite	2 tbsp	40	0	tr
Original	2 tbsp	50	0	tr
Original Bold	2 tbsp	45	0	tr
Muir Glen				
Garlic Mesquite	2 tbsp (1.3 oz)	40	0	tr
Hot & Smoky	2 tbsp (1.2 oz)	40	0	tr
Original	2 tbsp (1.2 oz)	40	0	tr
Nando's				
Barbecue	1 tbsp	7	0	0
San-J				
Asian BBQ	2 tbsp	40	0	–
Steel's				
Sugar Free	2 tbsp	15	0	0
Wellshire				
Original	2 tbsp	39	0	0

BARLEY

FOOD	PORTION	CALS	CHOL	FIBER
flour	1 cup	511	0	15
pearled cooked	1 cup (5.5 oz)	193	0	6
pearled uncooked	¼ cup	176	0	8
Mother's				
Quick Cooking	⅓ cup	170	0	5

BARRACUDA

FOOD	PORTION	CALS	CHOL	FIBER
broiled	4 oz	239	62	0
cooked flaked	1 cup	287	75	0
poached	4 oz	227	67	0
TAKE-OUT				
breaded & fried	4 oz	282	59	tr

BASIL

FOOD	PORTION	CALS	CHOL	FIBER
fresh chopped	1 tbsp	1	0	tr
ground	1 tsp	4	0	–
leaves fresh	5	1	0	tr
Dorot				
Chopped Cube frzn	1 cube (4 g)	5	0	tr
Eden				
Shiso Leaf Powder	1 tsp	0	0	0

BASS

FOOD	PORTION	CALS	CHOL	FIBER
breaded baked	4 oz	205	129	1
pickled mero en escabeche	2 oz	156	16	tr

FOOD	PORTION	CALS	CHOL	FIBER
striped baked	3 oz	105	88	0
striped bass farm raised	4 oz	110	90	0

BAY LEAF
crumbled	1 tsp	2	0	tr

BEAN SPROUTS (see ALFALFA, SPROUTS)

BEANS (see also individual names)
CANNED
baked beans plain	½ cup	119	0	5
baked beans vegetarian	½ cup	119	0	5
baked beans w/ franks	½ cup	184	8	9
baked beans w/ pork	½ cup	134	9	7
Amy's				
Vegetarian Baked	½ cup	120	0	6
B&M				
Maple Baked	½ cup	150	0	6
Vegetarian 99% Fat Free	½ cup	150	0	6
Bush's				
Barbecue	½ cup	150	0	5
Boston Recipe	½ cup	150	0	5
Country Style	½ cup	170	0	7
Homestyle	½ cup	140	0	5
Maple Cured Bacon	½ cup	150	0	7
Onion 98% Fat Free	½ cup	140	0	5
Original	½ cup	150	0	7
Vegetarian Fat Free	½ cup	130	0	6
Campbell's				
Pork & Beans	½ cup	140	<5	7
Eden				
Organic Baked w/ Sorghum	½ cup	150	0	7
Gebhardt				
Chili	½ cup (4.6 oz)	134	0	7
Refried Jalapeno	½ cup (4.5 oz)	105	1	6
Refried No Fat	½ cup (4.5 oz)	92	0	6
Refried Traditional	½ cup (4.5 oz)	109	1	6
Refried Vegetarian	½ cup (4.5 oz)	118	tr	7
Heinz				
Vegetarian	1 cup	250	0	9

FOOD	PORTION	CALS	CHOL	FIBER
Hunt's				
Big John's Beans & Fixin's	½ cup (4.7 oz)	127	3	6
Homestyle Country Kettle	½ cup (4.6 oz)	152	1	7
Homestyle Special Recipe	½ cup (4.7 oz)	185	1	8
Mix & Serve	½ cup (4.7 oz)	125	1	8
Pork & Beans	½ cup (4.5 oz)	130	tr	4
Las Palmas				
Refried	½ cup	150	0	2
Old El Paso				
Refried Fat Free	½ cup	100	0	6
Open Range				
Ranch	½ cup (4.4 oz)	124	1	8
Ranch Style				
Original Texas	½ cup	138	0	6
Read				
3 Bean Salad	½ cup	60	0	2
Rosarita				
3 Bean Recipe Bacon & Jalapeno	½ cup (4.6 oz)	117	1	5
3 Bean Recipe Chilies & Chicken	½ cup (4.6 oz)	115	1	4
3 Bean Recipe Chilies & Chorizo	½ cup (4.6 oz)	111	1	4
3 Bean Recipe Onions & Peppers	½ cup (4.6 oz)	104	1	5
Fiesta Beans Bacon & Jalapenos	½ cup (4.6 oz)	117	1	5
Fiesta Beans Chicken & Chilies	½ cup (4.6 oz)	115	1	4
Fiesta Beans Chilies & Chorizo	½ cup (4.6 oz)	110	1	4
Fiesta Beans Onions & Peppers	½ cup (4.6 oz)	104	1	5
Refried Bacon	½ cup (4.5 oz)	116	1	8
Refried Green Chile	½ cup (4.5 oz)	110	1	7
Refried Low Fat Black	½ cup (4.5 oz)	107	0	7
Refried Nacho Cheese	½ cup (4.5 oz)	108	2	6
Refried No Fat	½ cup	90	0	5
Refried No Fat Green Chilies & Lime	½ cup (4.5 oz)	101	0	8

FOOD	PORTION	CALS	CHOL	FIBER
Refried No Fat w/ Zesty Salsa	½ cup (4.5 oz)	105	0	6
Refried Onion	½ cup (4.5 oz)	114	1	6
Refried Spicy	½ cup (4.5 oz)	118	0	6
Refried Traditional 98% Fat Free	½ cup	100	0	5
Refried Vegetarian	½ cup (4.5 oz)	237	tr	13
Van Camp's				
Baked Beans w/ Chicken	1 cup	360	20	0
Baked Fat Free	½ cup (4.6 oz)	132	0	5
Baked Original	½ cup	140	0	6
Baked Southern Style Sauteed Onion	½ cup (4.8 oz)	145	1	8
Baked Sweet Hickory & Bacon	1 can (4.8 oz)	143	tr	6
Beanee Weenee BBQ	1 cup (7.7 oz)	290	35	7
Beanee Weenee Microwave	1 cup (7.5 oz)	260	35	6
Beanee Weenee Original	1 cup (9.1 oz)	320	40	8
Beanee Weenee Zestful	1 cup (7.7 oz)	300	35	7
Brown Sugar	½ cup (4.6 oz)	170	5	6
Pork And Beans	½ cup	110	0	6
Vegetarian	½ cup (4.6 oz)	110	0	5
FROZEN				
Lean Cuisine				
Cafe Classics Sante Fe Style Rice & Beans	1 pkg (10.4 oz)	290	15	5
MIX				
Fantastic				
Instant Black Beans not prep	⅓ cup	160	0	7
Instant Refried Beans not prep	¼ cup	130	0	8
TAKE-OUT				
baked beans	½ cup	191	6	7
barbecue beans	3.5 oz	120	0	–
fijolas a la charra w/ pork tomatoes & chili peppers	1 cup	341	27	5
refried beans	½ cup	43	2	–
three bean salad	1 cup	114	0	5
BEAR				
simmered	3 oz	220	83	0

FOOD	PORTION	CALS	CHOL	FIBER
BEAVER				
roasted	4 oz	240	132	0
BEECHNUTS				
dried	1 oz	163	0	–
BEEF (see also BEEF DISHES, MEATBALLS, VEAL)				
CANNED				
corned beef	1 oz	71	24	0
Treet				
Luncheon Loaf	2 oz	130	50	0
Luncheon Loaf 50% Less Fat	2 oz	110	45	0
FRESH				
arm pot roast trim 0 fat braised	3.5 oz	297	95	0
arm pot roast trim ⅛ in fat braised	3.5 oz	302	79	0
beef crumbles 70% lean pan browned	3 oz	230	75	0
bottom round roast trim 0 in fat braised	4 oz	253	112	0
bottom round roast trim 0 in fat roasted	3.5 oz	187	86	0
bottom round roast trim ½ in fat braised	4 oz	337	109	0
bottom round roast trim ⅛ in fat braised	4 oz	280	86	0
bottom round roast trim ⅛ in fat roasted	4 oz	247	85	0
bottom sirloin butt roast trim 0 in roasted	3.5 oz	182	71	0
brisket flat half trim ⅛ in fat braised	3.5 oz	298	80	0
brisket flat trim 0 fat braised	3.5 oz	221	46	0
brisket point half trim 0 fat braised	3.5 oz	358	92	0
brisket point half trim ¼ in fat braised	3.5 oz	404	92	0
brisket point half trim ⅛ in fat braised	3.5 oz	349	92	0

FOOD	PORTION	CALS	CHOL	FIBER
chuck boston cut roast trim 0 fat roasted	3.5 oz	207	69	0
chuck boston cut roast trim ¼ in fat roasted	3.5 oz	242	75	0
chuck bottom roast trim 0 fat braised	3.5 oz	334	104	0
chuck bottom roast trim ¼ in fat braised	3.5 oz	345	104	0
chuck fillet steak trim 0 fat broiled	4 oz	181	71	0
chuck top roast trim 0 fat broiled	4 oz	245	69	0
club steak trim ½ in fat broiled	4 oz	384	91	0
corned beef brisket cooked	3 oz	213	83	0
crosscut shank trim ¼ in fat stewed	1 serv (6.8 oz)	510	155	0
delmonico steak trim ¼ in fat broiled	4 oz	409	95	0
entrecote steak trim ½ in fat broiled	4 oz	413	95	0
eye round roast trim 0 in fat roasted	4 oz	190	61	0
eye round roast trim ¼ in fat roasted	4 oz	283	82	0
eye round roast trim ⅛ in fat roasted	4 oz	236	70	0
filet mignon roast trim ¼ in fat roasted	4 oz	376	97	0
filet mignon roast trim ⅛ in fat roasted	4 oz	367	96	0
filet mignon trim 0 in fat broiled	4 oz	247	95	0
filet mignon trim ⅛ in fat broiled	4 oz	303	102	0
ground 70% lean broiled	3.5 oz	273	82	0
ground 75% lean broiled	2.5 oz	195	62	0
ground 80% lean broiled	3 oz	234	77	0
ground 85% lean pan fried	3 oz	197	73	0
ground 90% lean pan fried	3 oz	173	70	0

FOOD	PORTION	CALS	CHOL	FIBER
ground 95% lean pan fried	3 oz	139	65	0
ground 97% fat free irradiated	4 oz	160	70	0
ground lowfat w/ carrageenan raw	4 oz	160	53	–
london broil trim 0 fat broiled	3.5 oz	188	45	0
london broil trim ¼ in fat broiled	4 oz	260	95	0
new york strip steak trim 0 fat broiled	4 oz	219	66	0
oxtails cooked	6 pieces (6.3 oz)	472	191	0
porterhouse steak trim 0 in fat broiled	1 lb	1252	304	0
porterhouse steak trim ¼ in fat broiled	1 lb	1492	327	0
porterhouse steak trim ⅛ in fat broiled	1 lb	1324	322	0
porterhouse steak trim ⅛ in fat broiled	4 oz	337	80	0
rib eye roast trim ¼ in fat roasted	3.5 oz	365	85	0
rib eye steak trim ⅛ in fat broiled	4 oz	221	81	0
rib roast trim ¼ in fat roasted	4 oz	406	95	0
rib steak trim ¼ in fat broiled	4 oz	388	93	0
round tip roast trim 0 in fat roasted	4 oz	213	105	0
sandwich steaks thinly sliced	1 serv (2 oz)	173	40	0
shell steak trim ¼ in fat broiled	4 oz	366	90	0
shortribs lean & fat braised	1 serv (7.8 oz)	1060	212	0
skirt steak trim 0 fat broiled	4 oz	289	67	0
t-bone steak trim 0 fat broiled	4 oz	280	68	0
t-bone steak trim ¼ in fat broiled	1 lb	1388	295	0

FOOD	PORTION	CALS	CHOL	FIBER
t-bone steak trim ⅛ in fat broiled	1 lb	804	178	0
tip round roast trim ⅛ in fat roasted	4 oz	248	93	0
top loin steak boneless trim ⅛ in fat broiled	4 oz	299	100	0
top round roast trim 0 fat braised	4 oz	237	102	0
top round roast trim ¼ in fat braised	4 oz	281	102	0
top round roast trim ¼ in fat roasted	4 oz	265	93	0
top round steak trim ¼ in fat pan fried	4 oz	314	110	0
top sirloin steak trim ⅛ in fat broiled	4 oz	275	85	0
top sirloin steak trim ⅛ in fat pan fried	4 oz	355	111	0
tri-tip roast trim 0 fat roasted	3.5 oz	218	94	0
tri-tip steak trim 0 fat broiled	4 oz	300	77	0
Laura's Lean				
Eye Of Round Steak Or Roast	4 oz	140	50	–
Flank Steak	4 oz	140	50	–
Ground 8% Fat	4 oz	160	60	0
Ground Round 96% Lean	4 oz	140	60	–
Ribeye Steak	4 oz	145	55	–
Sirloin Steak	4 oz	140	60	–
Sirloin Tip Steak Or Roast	4 oz	120	60	–
Strip Steak	4 oz	140	55	–
Tenderloin Filet	4 oz	140	55	–
Top Round Steak Or Roast	4 oz	130	55	–
Maverick Ranch				
Filet Mignon	4 oz	120	60	0
Ground	4 oz	130	60	0
Ground Round	4 oz	130	60	0
Ground Sirloin & Chuck	4 oz	130	60	0
NY Strip Steak	4 oz	150	55	0
Rib Eye Steak	4 oz	170	50	0
Top Round Steak & Roast	4 oz	110	50	0
Top Sirloin	4 oz	160	55	0

FOOD	PORTION	CALS	CHOL	FIBER
Organic Valley				
Extra Lean Ground	3 oz	130	55	0
Extra Lean Patties	1 (3.2 oz)	130	60	0
Shady Brook				
Tri-Tip Roast Rosemary Garlic & Chardonnay	4 oz	180	50	0
Tri-Tip Roast Sizzling Ginger	4 oz	210	50	0
FROZEN				
patty broiled medium	3 oz	240	80	0
Soy Lean				
Beef Patty	1 (2.5 oz)	90	20	–
READY-TO-EAT				
dried beef smoked chopped	1 oz	37	13	0
roast beef spread	¼ cup	127	40	tr
smoked beef cooked	1 sausage (1.4 oz)	134	29	–
Alpine Lace				
Roast Beef 97% Fat Free	2 oz	70	40	0
Boar's Head				
Corned Beef Brisket	2 oz	80	40	0
Italian Style Oven Roasted Top Round	2 oz	80	40	0
Top Round Deluxe	2 oz	80	30	0
Top Round Oven Roasted No Salt Added	2 oz	90	30	0
Sara Lee				
Roast Beef Medium or Rare	2 oz	60	30	0
TAKE-OUT				
roast beef rare	2 oz	70	30	0
BEEF DISHES				
CANNED				
Hormel				
Corned Beef Hash 50% Reduced Fat	1 cup	290	60	2
Libby's				
Hash Corned Beef	1 cup	420	55	3
Lunch Bucket				
Beef Stew	1 pkg (7.5 oz)	170	25	2

FOOD	PORTION	CALS	CHOL	FIBER
FROZEN				
Banquet				
Sandwich Toppers Creamed Chipped Beef	1 pkg (4 oz)	120	25	0
Sandwich Toppers Gravy & Salisbury Steak	1 pkg (5 oz)	210	25	2
Sandwich Toppers Gravy & Sliced Beef	1 pkg (4 oz)	70	25	0
Ian's				
Italian Meatballs	3 (2.2 oz)	145	70	1
MIX				
Hamburger Helper				
BBQ Beef as prep	1 cup	320	55	1
Beef Pasta as prep	1 cup	270	50	1
Beef Romanoff as prep	1 cup	280	50	0
Beef Stew as prep	1 cup	260	50	2
Beef Taco as prep	1 cup	280	50	2
Beef Teriyaki as prep	1 cup	290	50	2
Cheddar & Broccoli as prep	1 cup	350	60	0
Cheddar Melt as prep	1 cup	310	55	1
Cheddar'n Bacon as prep	1 cup	330	65	2
Cheeseburger Macaroni as prep	1 cup	360	65	1
Cheesy Hashbrowns as prep	1 cup	400	60	2
Cheesy Italian as prep	1 cup	320	60	1
Cheesy Shells as prep	1 cup	330	60	tr
Chili Macaroni as prep	1 cup	290	55	2
Fettuccine Alfredo as prep	1 cup	300	55	0
Four Cheese Lasagne as prep	1 cup	330	55	0
Italian Parmesan w/ Rigatoni as prep	1 cup	300	50	tr
Lasagne as prep	1 cup	270	50	2
Meat Loaf as prep	1/6 loaf	270	110	0
Mushroom & Wild Rice as prep	1 cup	310	55	2
Nacho Cheese as prep	1 cup	320	55	tr
Pizza Pasta w/ Cheese Topping as prep	1 cup	280	50	2
Pizzabake as prep	1/6 pie	270	45	tr
Potatoes Au Gratin as prep	1 cup	280	55	2

FOOD	PORTION	CALS	CHOL	FIBER
Potatoes Stroganoff as prep	1 cup	250	50	2
Reduced Sodium Cheddar Spirals as prep	1 cup	300	55	0
Reduced Sodium Italian Herb as prep	1 cup	270	50	2
Reduced Sodium Southwestern Beef as prep	1 cup	300	50	2
Rice Oriental as prep	1 cup	280	50	0
Salisbury as prep	1 cup	270	50	1
Spaghetti as prep	1 cup	270	50	1
Stroganoff as prep	1 cup	320	55	0
Swedish Meatballs as prep	1 cup	290	55	2
Three Cheeses as prep	1 cup	340	55	tr
Zesty Italian as prep	1 cup	300	50	2
Zesty Mexican as prep	1 cup	280	50	2
REFRIGERATED				
Chi Chi's				
For Tacos! Ground Beef	¼ cup	90	15	0
Hormel				
Beef Roast Au Jus	1 serv (5 oz)	200	75	–
Beef Tips w/ Gravy	½ cup	170	60	1
Huxtable's				
Shepherds Pie Beef	1 pkg (10 oz)	270	35	3
Morton's Of Omaha				
Beef Pot Roast w/ Gravy	1 serv (3 oz)	160	55	0
Smithfield				
Beef Tips w/ Gravy	½ cup	170	50	tr
Tyson				
Roast Beef In Brown Gravy	1 serv + gravy (3.5 oz)	160	55	0
SHELF-STABLE				
TastyBite				
Beef Roganjosh	1 pkg (9.5 oz)	270	25	3
TAKE-OUT				
beef bourguignonne	1 cup	339	85	1
beef curry	1 cup	432	68	3
beef satay + peanut sauce	2 skewers	253	62	1
bool kogi korean marinated beef ribs	4 oz	190	55	0
bracciola	1 roll (4.7 oz)	276	76	1

FOOD	PORTION	CALS	CHOL	FIBER
bulgoghi korean grilled beef	1 serv (5.2 oz)	256	67	tr
chipped beef on toast	1 slice (5 oz)	226	22	1
goulash w/ potatoes	1 cup	298	66	2
greek moussaka	1 serv (8.5 oz)	450	179	1
meatloaf	1 lg slice (5 oz)	294	114	1
peppered steak	1 cup	317	69	1
pot roast w/ gravy	1 serv (6 oz)	320	110	0
shepherds pie	1 serv (7 oz)	282	70	2
stew w/ potatoes & vegetables	1 cup	199	30	3
stroganoff	1 cup	394	69	1
swiss steak w/ sauce	1 serv (8 oz)	234	66	1

BEEFALO

roasted	4 oz	213	66	0

BEER AND ALE

ale brown	10 oz	77	0	0
ale pale	10 oz	88	0	0
beer light	12 oz	103	0	0
beer regular	12 oz	153	0	0
black & tan	1 serv (12 oz)	146	0	1
boilermaker	1 serv	216	0	1
lager	10 oz	80	0	0
mead	1 serv	250	0	1
shandy	1 serv	125	0	1
stout	10 oz	102	0	0
Amstel				
Light	1 bottle (12 oz)	95	0	–
Anchor				
Liberty Ale	1 bottle (12 oz)	188	0	–
Porter	1 bottle (12 oz)	205	0	–
Steam	12 oz	152	0	–
Beck's				
Beer	1 bottle (12 oz)	143	0	–
Premium Light	1 bottle	64	0	–
Blue Moon				
White	1 bottle (12 oz)	171	0	–
Bud				
Ice Light	1 bottle (12 oz)	110	0	–

FOOD	PORTION	CALS	CHOL	FIBER
Budweiser				
Beer	1 bottle (12 oz)	143	0	–
Ice	1 bottle (12 oz)	148	0	–
Light	1 bottle (12 oz)	110	0	–
Busch				
Beer	1 bottle (12 oz)	133	0	–
Ice	1 bottle (12 oz)	173	0	–
Light	1 bottle (12 oz)	110	0	–
Clausthaler				
Beer	1 bottle (12 oz)	96	0	–
Colt 45				
Malt Liquor	1 bottle (12 oz)	172	0	–
Coors				
Extra Gold	1 bottle (12 oz)	147	0	–
Light	1 bottle (12 oz)	102	0	–
Nonalcoholic	1 bottle (12 oz)	73	0	–
Original	1 bottle (12 oz)	148	0	–
Corona				
Extra	1 bottle (12 oz)	148	0	–
Light	1 bottle (12 oz)	109	0	–
Deschutes				
Bachelor ESB	1 bottle (12 oz)	180	0	–
Black Butt Porter	1 bottle (12 oz)	185	0	–
Cascade Ale	1 bottle (12 oz)	140	0	–
Mirror Pond Pale	1 bottle (12 oz)	175	0	–
Edison				
Light	1 bottle	109	0	–
Genessee				
12 Horse	1 bottle (12 oz)	152	0	–
Genny Light	1 bottle (12 oz)	96	0	–
Guiness				
Draught	1 bottle (12 oz)	125	0	–
Foreign Extra Stout	1 bottle (12 oz)	176	0	–
Hamm's				
Beer	1 bottle (12 oz)	144	0	–
Light	1 bottle (12 oz)	110	0	–
Heineken				
Beer	1 bottle (12 oz)	166	0	–
I.C.				
Light	1 bottle (12 oz)	96	0	–

FOOD	PORTION	CALS	CHOL	FIBER
Icehouse				
5.0	1 bottle (12 oz)	132	0	–
5.5	1 bottle (12 oz)	149	0	–
J.W. Dundee				
Honey Brown	1 bottle (12 oz)	150	0	–
Keystone				
Light	1 bottle (12 oz)	100	0	–
Kilarney's				
Red Lager	1 bottle (12 oz)	197	0	–
Killian's				
Beer	1 bottle (12 oz)	163	0	–
Lowenbrau				
Beer	1 bottle (12 oz)	160	0	–
Michelob				
Ultra Low Carbohydrate	1 bottle (12 oz)	95	0	–
Weinhard's				
Ale	1 bottle (12 oz)	147	0	–
Amber Ale	1 bottle (12 oz)	169	0	–
Dark	1 bottle (12 oz)	150	0	–
Hefeweizen	1 bottle (12 oz)	128	0	–
BEET JUICE				
juice	7 oz	72	0	–
BEETS				
CANNED				
harvard	½ cup	90	0	3
pickled	½ cup	74	0	3
sliced	½ cup	37	0	2
Del Monte				
Pickled Sliced	½ cup	35	0	2
Sliced	½ cup	35	0	2
Greenwood				
Harvard	1 serv (4.4 oz)	100	0	1
Pickled	1 oz	25	0	0
S&W				
Julienne	½ cup (4.3 oz)	30	0	1
Pickled Sliced	1 oz	15	0	1
Pickled Whole	1 oz	15	0	1
Sliced	½ cup (4.3 oz)	30	0	1
Whole Small	½ cup (4.3 oz)	30	0	1

FOOD	PORTION	CALS	CHOL	FIBER
Veg-All				
Small Sliced	½ cup	40	0	1
FRESH				
greens cooked w/o salt	½ cup	19	0	2
sliced cooked	½ cup	37	0	2
Frieda's				
Beets	½ cup	35	0	2

BEVERAGES (see BEER AND ALE, CHAMPAGNE, COFFEE, DRINK MIXERS, ENERGY DRINKS, FRUIT DRINKS, ICED TEA, LIQUOR/LIQUEUR, MALT, MILKSHAKE, SMOOTHIES, SODA, TEA/HERBAL TEA, WATER, WINE, YOGURT DRINKS)

BISCUIT

FOOD	PORTION	CALS	CHOL	FIBER
Bisquick				
Buttermilk	½ cup	150	0	–
Cheese Garlic	½ cup	160	0	–
Cinnamon Swirl	½ cup	150	0	–
Heart Smart	⅓ cup	140	0	tr
Mix	⅓ cup (1.4 oz)	160	0	–
Jiffy				
Buttermilk as prep	1	170	<5	tr
King Arthur				
Whole Grain Buttermilk not prep	¼ cup	100	0	2
MiniCarb				
Buttery as prep	1	255	145	2
REFRIGERATED				
plain baked	1 (1 oz)	93	0	tr
Hungry Jack				
Cinnamon & Sugar	1 (1.2 oz)	110	0	tr
Flaky	1 (1.2 oz)	100	0	0
Pillsbury				
Southern Style Flaky	1 (1.2 oz)	100	0	0
TAKE-OUT				
buttermilk	1 lg (2.7 oz)	280	1	1
plain	1 sm (1.2 oz)	127	0	1
tea biscuit	1 (3 oz)	210	0	1
w/ egg	1 (4.8 oz)	373	245	1
w/ egg & bacon	1 (5.3 oz)	458	353	1
w/ egg & ham	1 (6.7 oz)	442	300	1

FOOD	PORTION	CALS	CHOL	FIBER
w/ egg & sausage	1 (6.3 oz)	581	302	1
w/ egg & steak	1 (5.2 oz)	410	272	–
w/ egg cheese & bacon	1 (5.1 oz)	477	261	–
w/ ham	1 (4 oz)	386	25	1
w/ sausage	1 (4.4 oz)	485	35	1

BITTERMELON
Frieda's
Foo Qua	1 cup	15	0	2

BLACK BEANS
dried cooked	1 cup	227	0	15

Bean Cuisine
Pasta & Beans Mediterranean Black Beans & Fusilli	1 serv	210	0	4

Progresso
Black Beans	½ cup (4.6 oz)	110	0	7

BLACKBERRIES
canned in heavy syrup	½ cup	118	0	4
fresh	½ cup	31	0	4
unsweetened frzn	½ cup	48	0	4

Oregon
In Light Syrup	½ cup	120	0	6

BLACKBERRY JUICE
canned	6 oz	65	0	tr

Clear Fruit
Blackberry Rush	8 oz	90	0	–

Everfresh
Clear Fruit Blackberry Rush	8 oz	90	0	–

Izze
Sparkling Blackberry	8 oz	140	0	–

BLACKEYE PEAS
catjang dried cooked	1 cup (2.9 oz)	200	0	–
cowpeas canned	1 cup	184	0	–
cowpeas frozen cooked	½ cup	112	0	–
cowpeas leafy tips chopped cooked	1 cup	12	0	–
cowpeas leafy tips raw chopped	1 cup	10	0	–

FOOD	PORTION	CALS	CHOL	FIBER
CANNED				
w/pork	½ cup	199	17	–
Eden				
Organic	½ cup	90	0	4
DRIED				
cooked	1 cup	198	0	16
FROZEN				
McKenzie				
Blackeye Peas	1 serv (2.8 oz)	110	0	–
TAKE-OUT				
blackeye peas & pork	1 cup	236	27	8
BLINTZE				
Cohen's & Wilton				
Cheese	1	80	13	0
Golden				
Cheese	1 (2.1 oz)	80	15	2
Potato	1	90	5	2
Vegetable	1	110	5	0
Ratner's				
Cheese	1 (2.2 oz)	90	30	tr
TAKE-OUT				
cheese	1 (2.7 oz)	160	65	tr
BLUEBERRIES				
canned in heavy syrup	½ cup	113	0	2
fresh	½ cup	41	0	2
fresh	1 pt	229	0	10
frzn unsweetened	½ cup	40	0	2
A&L Farms				
Bleuets Fresh	1 pt	80	0	5
C&W				
Ultimate	¾ cup	70	0	3
Eden				
Organic Dried Wild	¼ cup	150	0	5
Europe's Best				
Woodland frzn	¾ cup	70	0	4
Frieda's				
Dried	¼ cup (1.4 oz)	140	0	4
Hodgson Mill				
Dried Wild	¼ cup	120	0	6

FOOD	PORTION	CALS	CHOL	FIBER
Oregon				
In Light Syrup	½ cup	110	0	2
Sunsweet				
Dried	¼ cup (1.4 oz)	140	0	3
Tree of Life				
Organic	1 cup (5 oz)	80	0	2
BLUEBERRY JUICE				
Hi-C				
Blazin' Blueberry	1 box	100	0	–
Izze				
Sparkling Blueberry	8 oz	100	0	–
Van Dyk's				
100% Juice	6 oz	74	0	0
BLUEFIN				
fillet baked	4.1 oz	186	88	0
BLUEFISH				
fresh baked	3 oz	135	64	0
BONITO				
dried	1 oz	50	13	0
BORAGE				
fresh chopped	1 cup	19	0	–
BOYSENBERRIES				
frzn unsweetened	½ cup	33	0	4
in heavy syrup	½ cup	113	0	3
BRAINS				
beef pan-fried	3 oz	167	1696	0
beef simmered	3 oz	123	2635	0
lamb braised	3 oz	123	1737	0
lamb fried	3 oz	232	2128	0
pork braised	3 oz	117	2169	0
veal braised	3 oz	116	2635	0
veal fried	3 oz	181	1802	0
BRAN				
corn	1 cup (2.7 oz)	170	0	65
oat	½ cup (1.6 oz)	116	0	7
oat cooked	½ cup (3.8 oz)	44	0	3

FOOD	PORTION	CALS	CHOL	FIBER
rice	½ cup (2.1 oz)	187	0	12
wheat	½ cup (2 oz)	63	0	12

BRAZIL NUTS
dried unblanched	1 oz	186	0	–

BREAD
CANNED
boston brown	1 slice (1.6 oz)	88	0	2

FROZEN
Alexia
Baguette Garlic	2 pieces (1.6 oz)	130	10	tr

Corbi's
Chee-Zee Bread Original	½ piece (1.8 oz)	180	10	1

Marie Callender's
Cornbread & Honey Butter	1 piece + butter	210	15	1
Original Garlic	1 piece	190	<5	2
Parmesan & Romano Garlic	1 piece	200	5	2

Pepperidge Farm
Whole Grain Garlic	1 serv (2.5 in)	170	0	3
Whole Grain Garlic Texas Toast	1 slice	150	0	2

MIX
cornbread	1 piece (2 oz)	188	37	1

Atkins
Caraway Rye as prep	1 slice	150	0	5
Country White as prep	1 slice	70	0	5
Sourdough as prep	1 slice	70	0	5

Buitoni
Focaccia Italian Herb & Cheese	1 slice	110	0	0
Focaccia Rosemary & Garlic	1 piece (1 oz)	110	0	1

Carbolite
Bread Mix as prep	1 slice	45	0	–

Keto
Quick Bread All Flavors as prep	1 slice	55	0	–

MiniCarb
Country White as prep	1 slice	80	0	4

FOOD	PORTION	CALS	CHOL	FIBER
Sassafras				
12 Grain & Sunflower	1 slice (1.4 oz)	150	0	1
READY-TO-EAT				
anadama	1 (1.1 oz)	87	1	1
baguette parisian	2 oz	120	0	tr
baguette whole wheat	2 oz	140	0	1
challah	1 slice (1.4 oz)	115	20	1
cinnamon	1 slice (0.9 oz)	69	0	1
cracked wheat	1 slice (1.1 oz)	78	0	2
cuban bread	1 slice (1.1 oz)	83	0	1
french	1 slice (1.1 oz)	88	0	1
italian	1 loaf (1 lb)	1255	0	–
navajo fry	1 piece	281	6	–
oat bran	1 slice (1.1 oz)	71	0	1
oatmeal	1 slice (0.9 oz)	73	0	1
pan criollo	1 piece (0.9 oz)	69	0	tr
pannetone	1 slice (0.9 oz)	86	18	1
pita	1 sm (1 oz)	77	0	1
pita	1 lg (2 oz)	165	0	1
pita whole wheat	1 sm (1 oz)	74	0	2
pita whole wheat	1 lg (2.2 oz)	170	0	5
potato scallion	1 slice (2 oz)	120	0	0
pumpernickel	1 slice (0.9 oz)	65	0	2
raisin	1 slice (1.1 oz)	88	0	1
rye	1 slice (1.1 oz)	83	0	2
seven grain	1 slice (1.1 oz)	80	0	2
wheat berry	1 slice (0.9 oz)	65	0	1
wheat bran	1 slice (1.3 oz)	89	0	1
wheat germ	1 slice (1 oz)	73	0	1
white cubed	1 cup	93	0	1
whole wheat	1 slice (1 oz)	69	0	2
Alvarado Street Bakery				
Diabetic Lifestyle	1 (1.2 oz)	80	0	2
Arnold				
Bakery Light	1 slice	80	0	5
100% Whole Wheat				
Country Classics Buttermilk	1 slice	110	0	tr
Country Classics Wheat	1 slice	100	0	2
Raisin Cinnamon	1 slice (1 oz)	80	0	1

FOOD	PORTION	CALS	CHOL	FIBER
Smart & Healthy Omega-3 100% Whole Wheat	1 slice	80	0	2
Smart & Healthy Sugar Free 100% Whole Wheat	1 slice	80	0	2
Atkins				
Rye	1 slice	60	5	5
White	1 slice	60	5	5
Beefsteak				
Rye Soft	1 slice	70	0	0
Bread Du Jour				
French	3 in slice (2 oz)	140	0	1
Cedar's				
Wraps Whole Wheat	1 (2 oz)	180	0	4
Damascus				
Pita	1 (2 oz)	130	0	2
Pita Whole Wheat	1 (2 oz)	160	0	3
Roll-Up Flax	1 (2 oz)	110	0	9
Roll-Up Whole Wheat	1 (2 oz)	110	0	7
Wraps Honey Wheat	½ wrap (2 oz)	130	0	1
Wraps Plain	½ wrap (2 oz)	130	0	1
Wraps Spinach	1 (4 oz)	280	0	2
Earth Grains				
100% Multi Grain Extra Fiber	1 slice	110	0	5
Oat & Nut	1 slice	120	0	1
Potato	1 slice	110	0	tr
Whole Grain Honey	1 slice	110	0	2
Whole Wheat Honey	1 slice	110	0	5
Ecce Panis				
Country Wheat	1 slice (2 oz)	150	0	2
European Baguette	2 oz	150	0	1
Enjoy Life				
Rye-Less Rye	1 slice	80	0	1
Food For Life				
Brown Rice Bread Yeast Free	1 slice	100	0	1
Rice Bread Fruit & Seed Yeast Free	1 slice	140	0	0
Rice Bread Multi Seed Yeast Free	1 slice	120	0	1
White Rice Bread Yeast Free	1 slice	100	0	tr

FOOD	PORTION	CALS	CHOL	FIBER
Freihofer's				
100% Whole Wheat	1 slice	90	0	3
Whole Wheat Light	2 slices	80	0	5
French Meadow Bakery				
Health Seed	1 slice	110	0	5
Healthy Hemp	1 slice	92	0	5
Men's Bread	1 slice	89	0	4
Woman's Bread	1 slice	81	0	4
Gold Medal				
100% Whole Wheat	1 slice	70	0	2
Home Pride				
Wheat	1 slice (1 oz)	80	0	1
Kangaroo				
Bread Wraps	1 (2.6 oz)	140	0	5
Greek Pita Flat	1 (2.6 oz)	200	0	3
Greek Pita Flat Wheat	1 (2.4 oz)	145	0	3
Pita Pockets Onion	½ (1.2 oz)	90	0	1
Pita Pockets Wheat N'Honey	½ (1.2 oz)	90	0	4
Pita Pockets White	½ (1.2 oz)	90	0	1
Salad Pockets	1 (1.2 oz)	90	0	1
Sandwich Pockets Whole Grain	1 (1.2 oz)	80	0	5
La Mexicana				
Wraps Chocolate	1 (1.3 oz)	120	0	1
Wraps Southwestern Mild Chili	1 (1.3 oz)	120	0	1
Wraps Spinach	1 (1.3 oz)	120	0	1
Wraps Tomato Basil	1 (1.3 oz)	120	0	1
Matthew's				
All Natural Cinnamon Raisin	1 slice	80	0	1
Milton's				
100% Whole Wheat	1 slice	110	0	5
Buttermilk	1 slice	90	0	1
Gourmet White	1 slice	110	0	1
Original Multi-Grain	1 slice	120	0	3
Potato	1 slice	90	0	1
Whole Grain	1 slice	90	0	5
Natural Ovens				
100% Whole Grain	1 slice	60	0	5
7 Grain Herb	1 slice	70	0	4

FOOD	PORTION	CALS	CHOL	FIBER
Better White	1 slice	80	0	2
Cracked Wheat	1 slice	80	0	3
English Muffin Bread	1 slice	80	0	2
Glorious Cinnamon Raisin	1 slice	70	0	2
Happiness Raisin Pecan	1 slice	70	0	3
Health Max	1 slice	80	0	3
Hunger Filler	1 slice	60	0	4
Lo Carb Golden Crunch	1 slice	70	0	4
Lo Carb Original	1 slice	60	0	5
Mild Rye	1 slice	70	0	4
Multi-Grain Stay Slim	1 slice	60	0	5
Nutty Natural	1 slice	70	0	5
Right Wheat	1 slice	60	0	5
Soft Wheat	1 slice	70	0	3
Sunny Millet	1 slice	60	0	4
Nature's Path				
Manna Carrot Raisin	1 slice	130	0	5
Manna Millet Rice	1 slice	130	0	5
Manna SunSeed	1 slice	160	0	7
Pepperidge Farm				
Deli Rye Seedless	1 slice	80	0	1
Farmhouse Soft 100% Whole Wheat	1 slice	110	0	3
Farmhouse Soft Oatmeal	1 slice	120	0	1
Farmhouse Whole Grain White	1 slice	110	0	3
Hearty 100% Whole Wheat	1 slice	110	0	3
Hearty 15 Grain	1 slice	120	0	3
Jewish Rye Seeded	1 slice	80	0	2
Natural Whole Grain 100% Whole Wheat	1 slice	110	0	3
Natural Whole Grain 9 Grain	1 slice	110	0	3
Natural Whole Grain German Dark Wheat	1 slice	110	0	3
Natural Whole Grain Multi Grain	1 slice	120	0	3
Stoneground 100% Whole Wheat	1 slice	70	0	2
Swirl French Vanilla	1 slice	140	0	tr
Whole Grain Honey Oat	1 slice	110	0	3

FOOD	PORTION	CALS	CHOL	FIBER
Whole Grain Honey Whole Wheat	1 slice	110	0	3
Whole Grain Swirl Cinnamon	1 slice	100	0	3
Whole Grain Swirl Cinnamon Raisin	1 slice	100	0	3
Sara Lee				
100% Whole Wheat	1 slice	70	0	2
Blueberry Crumble	1 slice	180	0	4
Cinnamon Raisin	1 slice	190	0	3
Classic Wheat	1 slice	70	0	2
Delightful 100% Whole Wheat	1 slice	90	0	5
Delightful Wheat	1 slice	45	0	2
Delightful White	1 slice	90	0	4
Heart Healthy 100% Whole Wheat Essentials	1 slice	80	0	4
Heart Healthy Multigrain	1 slice	100	0	2
Honey Wheat	1 slice	70	0	1
Honey White	1 slice	100	0	tr
Multigrain	1 slice	100	0	2
White Whole Grain	1 slice	150	0	3
Stroehmann				
100% Whole Wheat	1 slice	90	0	3
Family Grains Twisted Bread	1 slice	70	0	2
Family White	1 slice (0.8 oz)	65	0	0
Honey Cracked Wheat	1 slice	90	0	1
King White	1 slice (0.8 oz)	65	0	0
New York Rye	1 slice (1 oz)	80	0	1
Potato	1 slice (1.2 oz)	100	0	tr
Ranch White	1 slice (0.8 oz)	65	0	0
Twelve Grain	1 slice (1.2 oz)	90	0	1
Super Bakery				
Athlete's Formula	1 slice (1.5 oz)	100	0	7
Fitness Formula	1 slice (1.5 oz)	90	0	7
Wrap Organic	1 (4 oz)	340	0	20
TastyBite				
Nan Kontos Massala	½ loaf (1.4 oz)	120	0	1
Nan Kontos Onion	½ loaf (1.4 oz)	120	0	1
Nan Kontos Roghani	½ loaf (1.4 oz)	125	0	1

FOOD	PORTION	CALS	CHOL	FIBER
Nan Kontos Tandoori	½ loaf (1.4 oz)	120	0	1
Roti Kontos Missy	½ loaf (1.4 oz)	125	0	2
Thomas'				
Corn	1 slice	110	0	1
Swirl Whole Grain Cinnamon Raisin	1 slice	110	0	2
Toasting Cinnamon	1 slice	130	0	1
Whole Grain Swirl Oatmeal Raisin	1 slice	110	0	2
Toufayan				
Wraps Sundried Tomato Basil	1 (2 oz)	183	0	2
Wraps Wheat	1 (2 oz)	183	0	3
TAKE-OUT				
banana	1 slice (2 oz)	196	26	1
chapatis as prep w/ fat	1 bread (1.6 oz)	95	3	3
cornbread	1 piece (2.3 oz)	183	26	2
cornstick	1 (1.4 oz)	118	17	1
focaccia onion	1 piece (4.6 oz)	282	0	2
focaccia rosemary	1 piece (3.5 oz)	251	0	2
focaccia tomato olive	1 piece (4.7 oz)	270	0	2
garlic bread	1 slice (1 oz)	96	0	1
irish soda bread	1 slice (3 oz)	247	15	2
italian garlic	1 loaf (11 oz)	990	0	8
naan	1 bread (3.5 oz)	286	46	2
paratha	1 bread (2.1 oz)	201	27	2
poori indian puffed bread	1 piece (1.3 oz)	112	0	2
zucchini	1 slice (1.4 oz)	150	26	1

BREAD COATING

Don's Chuck Wagon

Chicken Baking Mix	¼ cup	95	0	1
Fish Mix	¼ cup	95	0	1
Onion Ring Mix	¼ cup	100	0	1
Fryin' Magic				
Cornmeal	1 tbsp	30	0	0
Hodgson Mill				
Vidalia Sweet Onion Mix not prep	¼ cup	100	0	1
Luzianne				
Cajun Chicken Coating Mix	2 tbsp (1 oz)	100	0	1

FOOD	PORTION	CALS	CHOL	FIBER
BREAD MACHINE MIX				
Betty Crocker				
Harvest Wheat	1/11 loaf	140	0	2
Home-Style White	1/11 loaf	130	0	0
Carbsense				
Harvest Wheat as prep	1 slice	60	0	1
Fleischmann's				
Italian Herb	1/8 loaf	160	0	2
Stoneground Wheat	1/8 loaf	160	0	3
Keto				
Cinnamon Raisin as prep	1 slice	79	0	3
French Loaf as prep	1 slice	79	0	3
Ketogenics				
Low Carb Honey Wheat as prep	1 slice	80	0	5
Low Carb Original White as prep	1 slice	62	0	–
Low Carb Pumpernickel Rye as prep	1 slice	80	0	5
BREADCRUMBS				
dry seasoned	1/4 cup	115	0	2
fresh	1/4 cup	30	0	tr
plain	1/4 cup	107	0	1
4C				
Carb Careful Seasoned	1/3 cup	110	0	5
Salt Free Seasoned	1/3 cup	110	0	2
Arnold				
Italian	1/4 cup	110	0	1
Ian's				
Panko Italian	1/4 cup	70	0	2
Panko Original	1/4 cup	71	0	1
Panko Whole Wheat	1/4 cup	70	0	2
Progresso				
Garlic & Herb	1/4 cup (1 oz)	100	0	1
Italian Style	1/4 cup	110	0	1
Parmesan	1/4 cup (1 oz)	100	0	1
Plain	1/4 cup (1 oz)	110	0	1
Rienzi				
Italian Style	1/4 cup	120	0	2

FOOD	PORTION	CALS	CHOL	FIBER
Ronzoni				
Italian Flavored	¼ cup	120	0	2
BREADFRUIT				
fried	1 cup	379	0	9
raw	1 cup	227	0	11
BREADNUTTREE SEEDS				
dried	1 oz	104	0	–
BREADSTICKS				
plain	1 sm	21	0	tr
plain	1 lg	41	0	tr
Angonoa				
Deli Style Sesame	3 (0.5 oz)	730	0	tr
Bread Du Jour				
Original	1 (1.9 oz)	130	0	1
Sourdough	1 (1.9 oz)	130	0	1
Fattorie & Pandea				
Grissini Sesame	3	70	0	tr
John Wm Macy's				
CheeseSticks	3 (1 oz)	130	11	1
Original Cheddar				
Pepperidge Farm				
Snack Sticks Wheat	9 (1 oz)	130	0	1
Stella D'Oro				
Mini Cracked Pepper	4 (0.5 oz)	70	0	0
Original	1 (0.4 oz)	40	0	0
Sesame	1 (0.4 oz)	50	0	0

BREAKFAST BARS (*see* CEREAL BARS, ENERGY BARS)

BREAKFAST DRINKS

Carnation				
Instant Breakfast	1 serv	220	6	tr
Chocolate Malt as prep				
w/ fat free milk				
Instant Breakfast	1 serv	220	9	tr
Classic French Vanilla				
as prep w/ fat free milk				

FOOD	PORTION	CALS	CHOL	FIBER
Instant Breakfast Milk Chocolate as prep w/ fat free milk	1 serv	220	9	1
Instant Breakfast Ready-To-Drink Carb Conscious French Vanilla	1 pkg	150	10	0
Instant Breakfast Ready-To-Drink Carb Conscious Milk Chocolate	1 pkg	150	10	2
Instant Breakfast Ready-To-Drink Creamy Milk Chocolate	1 pkg	250	10	1
Instant Breakfast Ready-To-Drink French Vanilla	1 pkg	240	10	0
Instant Breakfast Ready-To-Drink Strawberry Creme	1 pkg	250	10	0
Instant Breakfast Strawberry as prep w/ fat free milk	1 serv	220	9	0
Instant Breakfast No Sugar Added Vanilla as prep w/ fat free milk	1 serv	150	9	0

BROAD BEANS

FOOD	PORTION	CALS	CHOL	FIBER
canned	½ cup	91	0	–
fava fresh cooked	½ cup	94	0	5
Progresso				
Fava Beans	½ cup (4.6 oz)	110	0	5

BROCCOFLOWER

FOOD	PORTION	CALS	CHOL	FIBER
fresh raw	½ cup (1.8 oz)	16	0	–

BROCCOLI
FRESH

FOOD	PORTION	CALS	CHOL	FIBER
chinese broccoli (gai lan) cooked	½ cup	10	0	1
raab cooked	½ cup	28	0	2
raw	1 bunch (1.3 lbs)	207	0	16
raw flower	1 piece	3	0	–
raw flowers	1 cup	20	0	–

FOOD	PORTION	CALS	CHOL	FIBER
River Ranch				
Broccoli Slaw	1 cup	25	0	2
Florets	1¼ cups	25	0	3
FROZEN				
chopped cooked	½ cup	26	0	3
spears cooked	1 pkg (10 oz)	70	0	8
spears cooked	½ cup	26	0	3
Birds Eye				
Steamfresh Cuts	1 cup	30	0	2
C&W				
Broccoli & Cheddar Cheese Sauce	1⅓ cups	70	5	2
Florets	1 cup	30	0	2
Green Giant				
Butter Sauce Low Fat	3 spears (4 oz)	40	<5	2
Health Is Wealth				
Broccoli Munchees	2 (1 oz)	60	0	1
Tree of Life				
Cuts	1 cup (3.1 oz)	25	0	2
TAKE-OUT				
batter dipped & fried	4 pieces	77	9	1
w/ cheese sauce	1 cup	242	32	5

BROWNIE
FROZEN

FOOD	PORTION	CALS	CHOL	FIBER
Otis Spunkmeyer				
Blue Yonder w/ Walnuts	1 (2 oz)	230	20	2
MIX				
plain	1 (1.2 oz)	139	9	1
plain low calorie	1 (0.8 oz)	84	0	1
Atkins				
Kitchen Fudge as prep	1 (2 in)	60	0	4
Aunt Paula's				
Low Carb Chef Fudge Brownie as prep	1 (2.5 in)	89	3	2
Betty Crocker				
Chocolate Chunk as prep	1	180	21	–
Dark Chocolate Fudge as prep	1	170	21	–

FOOD	PORTION	CALS	CHOL	FIBER
Dark Chocolate w/ Syrup as prep	1	170	21	–
Fudge as prep	1	170	21	–
German Chocolate Coconut Pecan Filling as prep	1	200	21	1
Hot Fudge as prep	1	170	21	–
Original as prep	1	180	21	–
Peanut Butter as prep	1	180	21	–
Stir'n Bake w/ Mini Kisses as prep	1 serv	220	0	1
Turtle w/ Caramel & Pecans as prep	1	170	21	–
Walnut as prep	1	180	21	–
Big Train				
Low Carb Chocolate Chip as prep	1 (2 in)	140	42	4
Jiffy				
Fudge as prep	1	160	30	1
MiniCarb				
Chocolate Brownie as prep	1	220	50	8
Nature's Path				
Organic Double Fudge	1/10 pkg	150	0	3
Organic HempPlus	1/10 pkg	140	0	3
No Pudge!				
All Flavors	1	100	0	tr
Sweet Rewards				
Low Fat Fudge as prep	1	130	0	1
Reduced Fat Supreme as prep	1	140	21	–
READY-TO-EAT				
plain	1 sm (1 oz)	115	5	1
plain	1 lg (2 oz)	227	10	1
w/ nuts	1 (1 oz)	100	14	–
Entenmann's				
Little Bites	3 (2.2 oz)	290	45	1
Ultimate Fudge	1 (1.6 oz)	220	50	2
Joseph's				
Sugar Free	1 (1.5 oz)	150	0	1
Laura's Wholesome Junk Food				
Gluten Free Better Brownie	2	120	0	2

FOOD	PORTION	CALS	CHOL	FIBER
Little Debbie				
Brownie Lights	1 (2 oz)	190	0	1
Brownie Loaves	1 (2.1 oz)	260	40	1
Fudge	1 pkg (2.1 oz)	270	15	tr
Sara Lee				
Brownie Bites Chocolate Dipped	1 (0.7 oz)	90	5	1
Tom's				
Fudge Nut	1 pkg (2.5 oz)	300	5	0
TAKE-OUT				
plain	1 2 in sq (2.1 oz)	243	10	–
BRUSSELS SPROUTS				
FRESH				
cooked	6 pieces	45	0	3
FROZEN				
cooked	1 cup	65	0	6
C&W				
Petite	10 (3 oz)	45	0	3
BUCKWHEAT				
groats roasted cooked	½ cup	323	0	2
groats roasted uncooked	½ cup	292	0	9
BUFFALO				
burger	3 oz	202	71	0
chuck braised	4 oz	205	118	0
top round steak broiled	3 oz	313	153	0
water buffalo roasted	3 oz	111	52	–
BULGUR				
cooked	½ cup	76	0	4
uncooked	½ cup	239	0	13
Fantastic				
Tabouli Mix not prep	2 tbsp	70	0	4
Sabra				
Black Bean & Wheat Pilaf	2 oz	45	0	2
Cracked Wheat Salad	2 oz	80	0	1
Tabouli	2 oz	70	0	1
TAKE-OUT				
tabbouleh	1 cup	198	0	4

FOOD	PORTION	CALS	CHOL	FIBER
BURBOT (FISH)				
fresh baked	3 oz	98	65	0
BURDOCK ROOT				
cooked w/o salt	1 root (5.8 oz)	146	0	3
cooked w/o salt	1 cup	110	0	2
Frieda's				
Gobo Root	¾ cup	60	0	3
BUTTER				
clarified butter	3.5 oz	876	256	–
ghee cow's milk	1 tbsp	126	39	0
ghee vegetable oil	1 tbsp	126	0	0
stick	1 pat (5 g)	36	11	–
stick	1 stick (4 oz)	813	248	–
whipped	1 tbsp	70	20	0
whipped	4 oz	542	165	–
whipped	1 pat (4 g)	27	8	–
Breakstone's				
Salted	1 tbsp (0.5 oz)	100	30	0
Cabot				
Salted	1 tbsp	100	30	0
Unsalted	1 tbsp	100	30	0
Corman				
Light	1 tbsp	55	5	0
Crystal Farms				
Butter	1 tbsp	100	30	0
Whipped	1 tbsp	70	20	0
Horizon Organic				
European	1 tbsp	100	30	0
Hotel Bar				
Stick	1 tbsp (0.5 oz)	100	30	0
Keller's				
European	1 tbsp (0.5 oz)	100	30	0
Land O Lakes				
Salted	1 tbsp (0.5 oz)	100	30	0
Ultra Creamy Salted	1 tbsp (0.5 oz)	110	30	0
Unsalted	1 tbsp	100	30	0
Organic Valley				
Butter	1 tbsp (0.5 oz)	100	30	0
Unsalted	1 tbsp (0.5 oz)	110	30	0

FOOD	PORTION	CALS	CHOL	FIBER
BUTTER SUBSTITUTES				
stick	1 stick	811	99	–
Butter Buds				
Granules	1 pkg (2 g)	5	0	–
Keto				
Butta	1 tsp	43	0	0
Molly McButter				
Natural Butter	1 tsp	5	0	–
Natural Cheese	1 tsp	5	0	–
Roasted Garlic	1 tsp	5	0	–
Olivio				
Spread	1 tbsp	80	0	0
Sunsweet				
Lighter Bake	1 tbsp	35	0	–
BUTTERBUR				
canned fuki chopped	1 cup	3	0	–
fresh fuki	1 cup	13	0	–
BUTTERFISH				
baked	3 oz	159	71	0
fillet baked	1 oz	47	21	0
BUTTERNUTS				
dried	1 oz	174	0	–
BUTTERSCOTCH (see also CANDY)				
Hershey's				
Chips	1 tbsp	80	0	–
Nestle				
Morsels	1 tbsp	80	0	0
CABBAGE (see also COLESLAW)				
chinese bok choy shredded cooked w/o salt	1 cup	20	0	2
chinese pe-tsai shredded cooked w/o salt	1 cup	17	0	2
green raw shredded	1 cup	19	0	2
green shredded cooked w/o salt	1 cup	34	0	3
japanese pickled	½ cup	22	0	2

FOOD	PORTION	CALS	CHOL	FIBER
red raw shredded	1 cup	22	0	2
red shredded cooked w/o salt	1 cup	44	0	4
savoy shredded cooked w/o salt	1 cup	35	0	4
Frieda's				
Baby Bok Choy	⅔ cup	10	0	1
Bok Choy	1 cup	10	0	1
Gai Choy	1 cup (3 oz)	20	0	2
Napa	1 cup (3 oz)	15	0	1
Salad Savoy	⅔ cup (3 oz)	25	0	3
Tuscan	⅔ cup (3 oz)	20	0	2
Glory				
Country Cabbage	½ cup	30	0	1
Greenwood				
Red	½ cup	100	0	0
Lohmann				
Red Cabbage Sweet & Sour	¼ cup	40	0	0
River Ranch				
Angel Hair	1½ cups	20	0	2
TAKE-OUT				
creamed	1 cup	158	6	2
kimchee	1 cup	32	0	2
stuffed cabbage w/ rice & beef	1 (3.6 oz)	117	42	1

CACTUS

napoles fresh sliced	½ cup (1.5 oz)	7	0	–
pricklypear fresh	1 cup (5.3 oz)	56	0	4
Frieda's				
Cactus Pads	¾ cup (3 oz)	20	0	1

CAKE (see also CAKE MIX)

cream puff shell	1 (2.3 oz)	239	129	–
crumpet	1 (2.3 oz)	131	0	2
sponge	1 piece (1.3 oz)	110	39	tr
sponge cake dessert shell	1 (0.8 oz)	70	20	0
Amy's				
Toaster Pops Apple	1	140	0	tr
Toaster Pops Strawberry	1	140	0	tr

FOOD	PORTION	CALS	CHOL	FIBER
Arnold				
Date Nut Loaf	1 in slice (2 oz)	190	0	2
Baby Watson				
Cheesecake	1 slice (3 oz)	260	65	tr
Boboli				
Mini Eclairs Custard Filled	4 (2.3 oz)	224	35	0
Chudleigh's				
Apple Blossoms	1 (4 oz)	350	10	2
Drake's				
Coffee Cake Low Fat	2 (2.3 oz)	210	20	1
Coffee Cakes	1 (1.2 oz)	140	5	0
Yodel's	1 (1 oz)	150	5	–
Entenmann's				
All Butter French Crumb	⅛ cake (1.8 oz)	210	50	tr
Coffee Cake Cheese Filled Crumb	1 serv (1.9 oz)	200	35	tr
Coffee Cake Crumb	1 serv (2 oz)	260	10	1
Danish Twist Raspberry	⅛ cake	220	20	tr
Fudge Iced Golden Cake	⅛ cake	290	35	1
Light Loaf Cake Fat Free	⅛ cake (1.7 oz)	120	0	0
Loaf All Butter	⅙ cake (2.4 oz)	220	70	0
Louisiana Crunch	⅑ cake (2.9 oz)	330	45	tr
Marble Loaf	⅛ cake	190	40	tr
Marshmallow Iced Devil's Food	⅛ cake	280	15	tr
Mini's Carrot Cake	1 (1.4 oz)	160	20	tr
Strawberry Cheese Buns	1 (3 oz)	320	35	1
Fillo Factory				
Apple Turnovers Vegan	5 (5 oz)	270	0	2
Goody Man				
Happy Birthday Cupcake Chocolate	1 (1.75 oz)	200	20	tr
Happy Birthday Cupcake White	1 (1.75 oz)	190	20	0
Guiltless Gourmet				
Dessert Bowl Bananas Foster Cake	1 pkg (2 oz)	200	15	tr
Dessert Bowl Black Velvet Cake	1 pkg (2 oz)	200	20	3

FOOD	PORTION	CALS	CHOL	FIBER
Hostess				
Crumb Cake Light	1 (1 oz)	100	0	0
Shortcake Dessert Cups	1 (1.1 oz)	100	25	0
Jell-O				
Dessert Delights Cheesecake	1 (1.4 oz)	160	5	tr
Dessert Delights Chocolate Fudge Pudding	1 (1.4 oz)	150	0	1
Kellogg's				
Pop-Tarts Apple Cinnamon	1 (1.8 oz)	210	0	tr
Pop-Tarts French Toast	1	220	0	tr
Pop-Tarts Frosted Cookies & Cream	1	200	0	tr
Pop-Tarts Low Fat Frosted Brown Sugar Cinnamon	1 (1.8 oz)	190	0	tr
Pop-Tarts Yogurt Blast Strawberry	1 (1.8 oz)	210	0	tr
Little Debbie				
Angel Cakes Raspberry	1 (1.6 oz)	130	0	0
Banana Nut Loaves	1 (1.9 oz)	220	10	tr
Be My Valentine Chocolate	1 (2.2 oz)	280	0	1
Be My Valentine Vanilla	1 (2.2 oz)	290	0	0
Blueberry Loaves	1 (2 oz)	220	0	tr
Chocolate Chip	1 (2.4 oz)	310	0	tr
Christmas Tree Cake	1 pkg (1.5 oz)	190	0	0
Coconut Creme	1 (1.7 oz)	210	0	0
Devil Cremes	1 (1.6 oz)	190	0	0
Devil Squares	1 (2.2 oz)	270	0	1
Easter Basket Cake Chocolate	1 (2.4 oz)	300	0	tr
Fancy Cakes	1 (2.4 oz)	300	0	0
Low Carb Creations				
Cheesecake Blueberry Swirl	1 slice (3 oz)	220	95	0
Cheesecake Chocolate	1 slice (3 oz)	250	115	0
Cheesecake Key Lime	1 slice (3 oz)	250	115	0
Cheesecake New York	1 slice (3 oz)	250	85	0
Cheesecake Pumpkin Swirl	1 slice (3 oz)	220	90	0
Marie Callender's				
Cobbler Apple	1 serv (4.25 oz)	370	0	2
Cobbler Berry	1 serv (4.25 oz)	370	<5	1
Cobbler Cherry	1 serv (4.25 oz)	380	5	0
Cobbler Peach	1 serv (4.25 oz)	380	0	0

FOOD	PORTION	CALS	CHOL	FIBER
Mrs. Smith's				
Carrot	⅙ cake (2.9 oz)	300	30	2
Nature's Path				
Organic Toaster Pastry Apple Cinnamon	1 (2 oz)	210	0	1
Organic Toaster Pastry Blueberry	1 (2 oz)	210	0	1
Organic Toaster Pastry Frosted Apple Cinnamon	1 (2 oz)	210	0	1
Organic Toaster Pastry Frosted Blueberry	1 (2 oz)	200	0	1
Organic Toaster Pastry Frosted Strawberry	1 (2 oz)	210	0	1
Philadelphia				
Snack Bars Classic Cheesecake	1 (1.5 oz)	190	15	0
Snack Bars Strawberry Cheesecake	1 (1.5 oz)	190	10	0
Sara Lee				
Cheesecake Classic French	1 piece (4.7 oz)	410	25	1
Cheesecake French Chocolate	1 piece (4.2 oz)	430	15	2
Cheesecake French Strawberry	1 piece (4.3 oz)	320	20	1
Cheesecake Strawberry Swirl	1 piece (2.9 oz)	290	60	1
Cobbler Anytime Apple	1 (4 oz)	350	10	1
Coffee Cake Butter Streusel	1 piece (2 oz)	190	35	1
Coffee Cake Crumb	1 serv (2 oz)	190	20	1
Layer Cake Coconut	1 slice (2.8 oz)	260	15	1
Layer Cake Double Chocolate	1 slice (2.8 oz)	260	10	2
Layer Cake Fudge Golden	1 slice (2.8 oz)	260	15	1
Layer Cake Vanilla	1 slice (2.8 oz)	260	15	0
Pound Cake All Butter	1 slice (0.6 oz)	240	115	1
Pound Cake Free & Light	1 slice (2.5 oz)	200	0	1
Snack & Smile				
Mini Loaf Apple Cinnamon	1 loaf (2 oz)	190	10	0
Mini Loaf Banana	1 loaf (2 oz)	200	10	0

FOOD	PORTION	CALS	CHOL	FIBER
Mini Loaf Blueberry	1 loaf (2 oz)	190	10	tr
Mini Loaf Carrot	1 loaf (2 oz)	200	10	0
SnackWell's				
Streusel Squares Apple Cinnamon	1 (1.5 oz)	150	0	tr
Streusel Squares Cherry	1 (1.5 oz)	150	0	tr
Tastykake				
Banana Creamie	1 (1.5 oz)	170	5	0
Breakfast Bun Chocolate Raisin	1 (3.2 oz)	330	0	1
Bunny Trail Treats	1 (1.3 oz)	150	30	0
Chocolate Creamie	1 (1.5 oz)	180	15	0
Cupid Kake	1 (1.3 oz)	150	30	0
Kandy Kakes Coconut	2 (2.7 oz)	330	5	2
Koffee Kakes	1 (2 oz)	210	30	tr
Koffee Kakes Cream Filled	2 (2 oz)	240	30	0
Krimpets Butterscotch Iced	2 (2 oz)	210	60	0
Kringle Kake	1 (1.3 oz)	150	30	0
Sparkle Kake	1 (1.3 oz)	150	30	0
Vanilla Creamie	1 (1.5 oz)	190	35	0
Witchy Treat	1 (1.3 oz)	150	30	0
Tom's				
Honey Bun	1 pkg (3 oz)	360	10	2
Honey Bun Jelly Filled	1 pkg (4 oz)	490	0	2
Marble Pound	1 pkg (2.5 oz)	300	50	1
Texas Cinnamon Roll	1 pkg (4 oz)	360	0	0
Weight Watchers				
Lemon w/ Lemon Icing	1 (1 oz)	80	5	2
TAKE-OUT				
angelfood	1 slice (2 oz)	143	0	tr
apple crisp	1 serv (8.6 oz)	384	0	4
baklava	1 piece (2.7 oz)	334	35	2
basbousa namoura	1 piece (1 oz)	60	0	2
bean cake	1 cake (1.1 oz)	130	0	1
black forest chocolate cherry	1 piece (2.5 oz)	187	30	1
boston cream pie	1 slice (3.2 oz)	232	34	1
carrot w/ icing	1 slice (4.7 oz)	543	80	2
cheesecake	1 slice (4.5 oz)	410	86	tr
cheesecake chocolate	1 slice (4.5 oz)	489	118	2
chinese moon cake	1 (4.8 oz)	458	69	4

FOOD	PORTION	CALS	CHOL	FIBER
coconut mochiko filipino cake	1 piece (2.7 oz)	252	0	2
coffeecake iced	1 piece (1.6 oz)	175	31	1
cream puff custard filled chocolate frosted	1 (3.9 oz)	293	142	1
dutch honey cake	1 slice (0.8 oz)	70	0	0
eclair	1 (3.5 oz)	262	127	1
french apple tart	1 (3.5 oz)	302	60	2
fruitcake	1 slice (1.5 oz)	139	2	2
funnel cake	1 (3.2 oz)	276	62	1
gingerbread	1 piece (2.4 oz)	213	24	1
jelly roll	1 slice (1.8 oz)	146	93	tr
jelly roll lemon filled	1 slice (3 oz)	210	35	tr
napoleon	1 mini (1 oz)	123	14	tr
napoleon	1 (3 oz)	348	39	1
panettone	1/12 cake (2.9 oz)	300	90	2
petit fours	2 (0.9 oz)	120	0	0
pineapple upside down	1 piece (4.2 oz)	387	27	1
pound	1 slice (1 oz)	120	32	–
pound fat free	1 slice (2 oz)	160	0	1
sacher torte	1 slice (2.2 oz)	240	50	4
strawberry shortcake	1 serv (4.1 oz)	211	109	1
strudel apple	1 piece (2.2 oz)	175	4	1
strudel cheese	1 piece (2.2 oz)	195	42	tr
strudel cherry	1 piece (2.2 oz)	179	9	1
tiramisu	1 piece (5.1 oz)	409	171	tr
tiramisu	1 cake (4.4 lbs)	5732	2395	3
torte chocolate ganache	1 slice (3.5 oz)	400	90	6
white w/ coconut icing	1 slice (3.9 oz)	399	1	1
zucchini bread	1 slice (1.4 oz)	150	26	1

CAKE ICING

FOOD	PORTION	CALS	CHOL	FIBER
chocolate	1/4 cup	269	1	1
vanilla	1/4 cup	322	0	0
Betty Crocker				
HomeStyle Mix Coconut Pecan as prep	2 tbsp	160	0	tr
HomeStyle Mix White Fluffy as prep	6 tbsp	100	0	–

FOOD	PORTION	CALS	CHOL	FIBER
Party Frosting Chocolate w/ Stars	2 tbsp (1.2 oz)	140	0	–
Rich & Creamy Butter Cream	2 tbsp (1.3 oz)	140	0	–
Rich & Creamy Cherry	2 tbsp (1.2 oz)	140	0	–
Rich & Creamy Chocolate	2 tbsp (1.2 oz)	130	0	–
Rich & Creamy Cream Cheese	2 tbsp (1.2 oz)	140	0	–
Rich & Creamy Dark Chocolate	2 tbsp (1.3 oz)	130	0	1
Rich & Creamy French Vanilla	2 tbsp (1.2 oz)	140	0	–
Rich & Creamy Milk Chocolate	2 tbsp (1.3 oz)	130	0	–
Rich & Creamy Rainbow Chip	2 tbsp (1.2 oz)	140	0	–
Rich & Creamy Vanilla	2 tbsp (1.2 oz)	140	0	–
Toppers Milk Chocolate	2 tbsp (1.2 oz)	130	0	–
Toppers Vanilla	2 tbsp (1.2 oz)	140	0	–
Jiffy				
Fudge Frosting	¼ cup	150	0	1
White Frosting	¼ cup	150	0	0
Sweet Rewards				
Ready-To-Spread Reduced Fat Chocolate	2 tbsp (1.2 oz)	120	0	–
Ready-To-Spread Reduced Fat Vanilla	2 tbsp (1.2 oz)	130	0	–

CAKE MIX
Betty Crocker

FOOD	PORTION	CALS	CHOL	FIBER
Angel Food Fat Free	1/12 cake	140	0	–
Angel Food Fat Free Confetti as prep	1/12 cake	150	0	–
Cheesecake Chocolate Chip as prep	1/8 cake	410	99	1
Cheesecake Original as prep	1/8 cake	400	102	–
Cheesecake Strawberry Swirl as prep	1/8 cake	380	96	–
Pineapple Upside Down as prep	1/6 cake	420	36	–

FOOD	PORTION	CALS	CHOL	FIBER
Quick Bread Banana	1/12 cake	170	36	-
Quick Bread Cinnamon Streusel as prep	1/14 cake	180	30	-
Quick Bread Cranberry Orange as prep	1/12 cake	170	36	-
Quick Bread Lemon Poppy Seed as prep	1/12 cake	170	36	-
Stir'n Bake Coffee Cake w/ Cinnamon Streusel as prep	1/6 cake	230	12	-
Stir'n Bake Devils Food w/ Chocolate Frosting as prep	1/6 cake	240	0	1
Stir'n Bake Yellow w/ Chocolate Frosting as prep	1/8 cake	240	9	1
SuperMoist Butter Pecan as prep	1/12 cake	240	54	-
SuperMoist Butter Yellow as prep	1/12 cake	260	75	-
SuperMoist Carrot as prep	1/10 cake	320	63	-
SuperMoist Cherry Chip	1/10 cake	300	63	-
SuperMoist Chocolate Fudge as prep	1/12 cake	270	54	1
SuperMoist Golden Vanilla as prep	1/12 cake	240	54	-
SuperMoist Lemon as prep	1/12 cake	240	54	-
SuperMoist Milk Chocolate as prep	1/12 cake	240	54	1
SuperMoist Pineapple as prep	1/12 cake	250	54	-
SuperMoist Spice as prep	1/12 cake	240	54	-
SuperMoist Strawberry as prep	1/12 cake	250	39	-
SuperMoist White as prep	1/12 cake	230	0	-
SuperMoist White Light as prep	1/10 cake	210	0	-
Bisquick				
Heart Smart	1/3 cup	140	0	tr
Mix	1/3 cup (1.4 oz)	160	0	-

FOOD	PORTION	CALS	CHOL	FIBER
Bob's Red Mills				
Gluten Free Chocolate as prep	⅙ cake	170	39	2
Carbolite				
Cheesecake Chocolate as prep	⅛ cake	260	280	–
Carbsense				
Zero Carb Baking Mix	1 oz	110	0	4
Don's Chuck Wagon				
All Purpose Batter Mix	¼ cup	100	0	1
Jiffy				
Devil's Food as prep	⅕ cake	220	42	1
Golden Yellow as prep	⅕ cake	220	36	tr
White Cake as prep	⅕ cake	210	3	tr
King Arthur				
Cinnamon Buns Kit not prep	½ cup	240	0	3
MiniCarb				
Carrot as prep	1 slice	280	45	6
Chocolate as prep	1 slice	230	60	12
Zero Carb Baking Mix not prep	½ cup	55	0	2
Sweet Rewards				
Reduced Fat White as prep	1/12 cake	180	0	–
Reduced Fat Yellow as prep	1/12 cake	200	30	–

CALZONE (see SANDWICHES)

CANADIAN BACON

FOOD	PORTION	CALS	CHOL	FIBER
grilled	2 slices (1.6 oz)	87	27	0
Boar's Head				
Canadian Bacon	2 oz	70	35	0
Celebrity				
98% Fat Free	3 slices (1.8 oz)	60	30	0
Jones				
Slices	3	70	30	0
Real Canadian Bacon				
Peameal	4 oz	130	40	–
Wellshire				
Sliced	2 oz	20	30	0

FOOD	PORTION	CALS	CHOL	FIBER
Yorkshire Farms				
Uncured	3 oz	100	44	–

CANADIAN BACON SUBSTITUTES
Yves

FOOD	PORTION	CALS	CHOL	FIBER
Canadian Veggie Bacon	1 serv (2 oz)	80	0	1

CANDY

FOOD	PORTION	CALS	CHOL	FIBER
butterscotch	1 piece (6 g)	24	1	–
candied cherries	1 (4 g)	12	0	–
candied citron	1 oz	89	0	–
candied lemon peel	1 oz	90	0	–
candied orange peel	1 oz	90	0	–
candied pineapple slice	1 slice (2 oz)	179	0	–
candy corn	1 oz	105	0	–
caramels	1 piece (8 g)	31	1	–
caramels chocolate	1 piece (6 g)	22	0	–
crisped rice bar almond	1 (1 oz)	130	0	1
crisped rice bar chocolate chip	1 (1 oz)	115	0	1
dark chocolate	1 oz	150	0	–
fondant	1 piece (0.6 oz)	57	0	–
fondant chocolate coated	1 piece (0.4 oz)	40	0	–
fondant mint	1 oz	105	0	–
fudge brown sugar w/ nuts	1 piece (0.5 oz)	56	1	–
fudge chocolate marshmallow	1 piece (0.7 oz)	84	5	–
fudge chocolate marshmallow w/ nuts	1 piece (0.8 oz)	96	5	–
fudge chocolate w/ nuts	1 piece (0.7 oz)	81	3	–
fudge peanut butter	1 piece (0.6 oz)	59	1	–
fudge vanilla w/ nuts	1 piece (0.5 oz)	62	2	–
gumdrops	10 sm (0.4 oz)	135	0	–
gumdrops	10 lg (3.8 oz)	420	0	–
hard candy	1 oz	106	0	–
jelly beans	10 sm (0.4 oz)	40	0	–
jelly beans	10 lg (1 oz)	104	0	–
lollipop	1 (6 g)	22	0	–
marzipan	1 oz	128	0	2
milk chocolate	1 bar (1.55 oz)	226	10	–

FOOD	PORTION	CALS	CHOL	FIBER
milk chocolate crisp	1 bar (1.45 oz)	203	8	–
milk chocolate w/ almonds	1 bar (1.45 oz)	215	8	–
organic dark chocolate w/ raisins & pecans	1.4 oz	220	0	3
peanut brittle	1 oz	128	4	–
peanuts chocolate covered	1 cup (5.2 oz)	773	13	–
peanuts chocolate covered	10 (1.4 oz)	208	4	–
praline	1 piece (1.4 oz)	177	0	–
sesame crunch	20 pieces (1.2 oz)	181	0	–
sweet chocolate	1 oz	143	0	–
sweet chocolate	1 bar (1.45 oz)	201	0	–
taffy	1 piece (0.5 oz)	56	1	–
toffee	1 piece (0.4 oz)	65	13	–
truffles	1 piece (0.4 oz)	59	6	–
100 Grand				
Bar	1 (1.5 oz)	200	10	tr
3 Musketeers				
Bar	1 (2.1 oz)	260	5	1
Fun Size	3 bars (1.6 oz)	190	5	1
Miniatures	7 (1.4 oz)	170	5	1
5th Avenue				
Bar	1 (0.56 oz)	80	0	–
Almond Joy				
Bar	1 (0.68 oz)	90	0	–
Altoids				
All Flavors	3 pieces	10	0	–
Anastasia				
Coco Rhum Bites	2 pieces (1 oz)	110	0	1
At Last!				
Chocolate Almond	1 bar	120	0	6
Chocolate Crisp	1 bar	110	0	6
Chocolate Mint	1 bar	110	0	7
Chocolate Peanut Butter	1 bar	120	0	5
Atkins				
Endulge Caramel Nut Chew	1 bar (1.23 oz)	140	5	tr
Endulge Chocolate Bar	1 (1.1 oz)	150	5	3
Endulge Chocolate Crunch	1 bar (1 oz)	150	<5	3
Endulge Peanut Butter Cups	3 pieces	160	0	0

FOOD	PORTION	CALS	CHOL	FIBER
Baby Ruth				
Bar	1 (2.1 oz)	270	0	2
Fun Size	1 bar (0.7 oz)	100	0	0
Bartons				
Cashew Toppers	1 (1 oz)	140	5	1
Bittyfinger				
Bars	2	170	0	tr
Body Smarts				
Chocolate Peanut Crunch	2 bars (1.8 oz)	210	<5	2
Brach's				
Bridge Mix	16 pieces	190	5	tr
Candy Corn	26 pieces	140	0	0
Caramel Clusters	3 pieces	210	5	1
Circus Peanuts	6 pieces	160	0	0
Fruit Rippers Berry Punch	1 pkg (0.5 oz)	60	0	0
Fruit Slices	3 pieces	150	0	0
Malts	15 pieces	190	10	1
Mellowcreme Pumpkins	6 pieces	130	0	0
Milk Maid Caramels	4 pieces	160	0	0
Mint Patties	3 pieces	140	0	0
Orange Slices	2 pieces	130	0	0
Peanut Butter Meltaways	3 pieces	200	0	1
Root Beer Barrels	3 pieces	70	0	0
Spearmint Leaves	5 pieces	130	0	0
Spice Drops	12 pieces	130	0	0
Sprinkles	17 pieces	200	15	1
Star Brites Butterscotch	3 pieces	60	0	0
Stars	10 pieces	200	0	0
Wild'N Fruity Gummi Bears	14 pieces	140	0	0
Breath Savers				
Sugar Free Peppermint	1 piece	5	0	–
Butterfinger				
Bar	1 (2.1 oz)	270	0	1
Crisps	1 bar (1.8 oz)	250	0	1
Crisps Minis	4 (1.5 oz)	220	0	1
Minis	4 (1.4 oz)	180	0	tr
Cadbury				
Milk Chocolate Roast Almond	10 blocks (1.4 oz)	220	10	1
Royal Dark	10 blocks (1.4 oz)	220	<5	3

FOOD	PORTION	CALS	CHOL	FIBER
Cape Cod Provisions				
Cranberry Bog Frogs	3 pieces (1.9 oz)	250	7	tr
Carbolite				
Caramel	1 bar	100	5	0
CarbAway	1 bar	100	5	0
CarboSnack	1 bar	110	5	1
Chocolate Truffle	1 bar (1 oz)	122	<5	1
Chocolate Almond	1 bar (1.75 oz)	298	7	2
Chocolate Crisp	1 bar (1.75 oz)	256	14	1
Chocolate Peanut Butter	1 bar (1.75 oz)	256	7	0
Crisy Caramel	1 bar (1 oz)	130	5	0
Milk Chocolate	1 bar (1.75 oz)	263	7	1
Peanut Butter Cup	1	170	5	1
Pecan Cluster	1 bar	120	5	1
CarbSlim				
Crunch Bites Chocolate Caramel	1 pkg	122	3	9
Crunch Bites Peanut Butter	1 pkg	171	2	9
Carmello				
Snack Size	1 (0.66 oz)	90	<5	–
Cary's Of Oregon				
English Toffee Milk Chocolate Almond	1 piece (0.75 oz)	110	10	tr
Chargers				
Chocolate Covered Expresso Beans	1 pkg (0.5 oz)	60	0	tr
ChocoSoy				
Soy Milk Chocolate	1 piece (0.4 oz)	50	0	–
Chunky				
Bar	1 (1.4 oz)	210	5	1
Classic Caramels				
Chocolate Creme Filled	3 pieces	80	<5	–
Soft & Chewy	3 pieces	80	<5	–
Cloud Nine				
Australian Orange Peel	½ bar (1.5 oz)	220	0	2
Butter Nut Toffee	½ bar (1.5 oz)	230	5	1
Cool Mint Crisp	½ bar (1.5 oz)	220	5	2
Espresso Bean Crunch	½ bar (1.5 oz)	220	0	2
Malted Milk Crunch	½ bar (1.5 oz)	230	5	1
Milk Chocolate	½ bar (1.5 oz)	230	5	1

FOOD	PORTION	CALS	CHOL	FIBER
Oregan Red Raspberry	½ bar (1.5 oz)	230	0	2
Peanut Butter Brittle	½ bar (1.5 oz)	230	5	1
Sundried Cherry	½ bar (1.5 oz)	230	5	1
Toasted Coconut Crisp	½ bar (1.5 oz)	230	5	2
Vanilla Dark	½ bar (1.5 oz)	230	0	2
CocoaVia				
Chocolate	1 bar	80	0	1
Chocolate Almond	1 bar	80	0	1
Chocolate Blueberry	1 bar	80	0	1
Chocolate Blueberry & Almond	1 bar	100	0	2
Chocolate Cherry	1 bar	80	0	1
Chocolate Covered Almonds	1 bar	140	0	3
Crispy Chocolate	1 bar	90	0	2
Original Chocolate	1 bar (0.8 oz)	100	0	2
Coffee Rio				
Coffee Candy All Flavors	4 pieces	60	5	0
Crunch				
Fun Size	4 bars	210	10	tr
Daboga				
Organic Milk Chocolate	1 bar (2 oz)	318	10	6
Del Monte				
Radical Raizins Cinnamon	1 pkg (0.7 oz)	70	0	0
Radical Raizins Rainbow	1 pkg (0.7 oz)	70	0	0
Doctor's CarbRite				
Sugar Free Dark Chocolate With Almonds	4 sq (1 oz)	132	0	4
Sugar Free Milk Chocolate With Peanuts	4 sq (1 oz)	132	4	0
Sugar Free Milk Chocolate With Soy Crisps	4 sq (1 oz)	120	4	2
Dove				
Dark Chocolate	⅓ bar	170	5	3
Dark Chocolate Covered Almonds	13 pieces	210	5	3
Dark Chocolate Miniatures	5 pieces	210	5	3
Milk Chocolate	⅓ bar	180	5	1
Milk Chocolate w/ Almonds	⅓ bar	190	5	2
Milk Chocolate Covered Almonds	13 pieces	220	5	2

FOOD	PORTION	CALS	CHOL	FIBER
Milk Chocolate Miniatures	5	220	5	1
Milk Chocolate Miniatures w/ Caramel	5 pieces	200	5	1
Eclipse				
Mints Sugarless All Flavors	3 pieces	5	0	–
Endangered Species				
Dark Chocolate w/ Espresso Beans	½ bar (1.5 oz)	200	0	5
Dark Chocolate w/ Hazelnut Toffee	½ bar (1.5 oz)	220	5	4
Milk Chocolate w/ Cherries	½ bar (1.5 oz)	230	15	1
Organic Dark Chocolate	½ bar (0.7 oz)	100	0	1
Organic Dark Chocolate w/ Tangerine	½ bar (0.7 oz)	100	0	1
Organic Milk Chocolate w/ Key Lime	½ bar (0.7 oz)	110	5	0
Estee				
Fructose Sweetened Dark Chocolate	½ bar (1.4 oz)	200	10	0
Fructose Sweetened Milk Chocolate	½ bar (1.4 oz)	230	20	0
Fructose Sweetened Milk Chocolate w/ Almonds	½ bar (1.4 oz)	230	20	0
Fructose Sweetened Milk Chocolate w/ Crisp Rice	½ bar (1.2 oz)	370	30	0
Fructose Sweetened Peanut Butter Cups	5	200	<5	1
Peanut Brittle	⅓ box (1.3 oz)	210	10	1
Sugar Free Assorted Fruit	3	15	0	14
Sugar Free Butterscotch	4	15	0	14
Sugar Free Gourmet Jelly Beans	26	70	0	0
Sugar Free Gum Drops Assorted Fruit	11	110	0	0
Sugar Free Gummy Bears Assorted Fruit	17	70	0	0
Sugar Free Peppermint	3	15	0	13
Sugar Free Sour Citrus Slices	9	60	0	0
Sugar Free Toffee	4	15	0	14
Sugar Free Tropical Fruit	3	15	0	14

FOOD	PORTION	CALS	CHOL	FIBER
Ethel's				
Truffles Assorted	4	200	15	1
Fauchon				
Assortment Truffles	3 pieces (1.3 oz)	160	<5	2
Chocolate Assortment	3 pieces (1.1 oz)	170	<5	2
Ferrero Rocher				
Candy	3 pieces (1.3 oz)	220	0	1
Figamajigs				
Fig Candy Drops Dark Chocolate Covered	1 pkg (1.4 oz)	150	0	3
Fig Candy Drops Orange & Yellow Chocolate Covered	1 pkg (1.4 oz)	150	0	2
Fruitzels				
Assorted	7 pieces	120	0	0
Godiva				
Chocolatier Dark Chocolate w/ Raspberry	1 bar (1.5 oz)	220	3	0
Chocolatier Milk Chocolate	1 bar (1.5 oz)	230	10	0
Chocolatier Milk Chocolate w/ Almonds	1 bar (1.5 oz)	230	5	0
Mochaccino Mousse	2 pieces (1.25 oz)	210	4	0
Sugar Free Chocolate	1 bar (1.5 oz)	190	5	tr
Sugar Free Chocolate w/ Almonds	1 bar (1.5 oz)	200	5	1
Sugar Free Dark Chocolate	1 bar (1.5 oz)	190	<5	4
Truffles Assorted	2 pieces (1.4 oz)	210	10	2
Goetze's				
Caramel Creams	3 pieces	130	0	tr
Cow Tales	1 pkg (1 oz)	110	tr	tr
Gol D Lite				
Milk Chocolate Crisp	1 bar	125	6	0
Seashell Truffle	1 piece	54	0	1
Goldenberg's				
Peanut Chews	3 pieces	180	0	1
Golightly				
Sugar Free Caramels	5 pieces	150	10	–
Sugar Free Doublers Chews Peach & Creme	7 pieces	150	10	tr
Sugar Free Fudgie Rolls	6 pieces	130	5	–
Sugar Free Hard Candy	4 pieces	45	0	–

FOOD	PORTION	CALS	CHOL	FIBER
Goobers				
Peanuts	1 pkg (1.38 oz)	210	5	1
Good & Plenty				
Snack Size	1 box (0.6 oz)	60	0	–
Good 'N Fruity				
Snack Size	1 box (0.6 oz)	60	0	–
Heath				
Snack Size	1 bar (0.3 oz)	50	<5	–
Hershey's				
Bites Almond Joy	8 pieces	100	<5	–
Bites Cookies 'N' Creme	8 pieces	90	0	–
Bites Milk Chocolate w/ Almond	7 pieces	90	<5	–
Bites Reese's	7 pieces	90	0	–
Bites York	9 pieces	90	0	–
Chocolate Miniatures Sugar Free	5 pieces (1.4 oz)	170	10	2
Chocolate w/ Almonds Miniatures Sugar Free	5 pieces (1.4 oz)	180	10	3
Cocoa Reserve 35% Cacao Milk Chocolate w/ Hazelnuts	3 sq (1.3 oz)	220	10	1
Cocoa Reserve 65% Cacao Extra Dark	1 bar (1.3 oz)	190	<5	4
Dark Chocolate Miniatures Sugar Free	5 pieces (1.4 oz)	190	5	3
Hugs	1 piece	25	0	–
Kisses	1	25	0	–
Kisses w/ Almonds	1 piece	25	0	–
Milk Chocolate	1 bar (1.4 oz)	210	10	1
Milk Chocolate w/ Almonds	1 bar (1.4 oz)	230	5	1
Miniature Special Dark	1 (0.3 oz)	45	0	–
Nuggets Cookies 'N' Creme	4	190	5	0
Nuggets Dark Chocolate w/ Almonds	4	220	<5	3
Nuggets Milk Chocolate	4	230	10	1
Nuggets Milk Chocolate w/ Almonds	1	60	0	–
Nuggets Milk Chocolate w/ Almonds & Toffee	1	50	<5	–

FOOD	PORTION	CALS	CHOL	FIBER
Nuggets Milk Chocolate w/ Raisins & Almonds	1	50	0	–
Pot Of Gold	3 pieces	130	<5	tr
Sweet Escapes Caramel & Peanut Butter Crispy	1	80	0	–
Sweet Escapes Crunchy Peanut Butter	1 (0.7 oz)	90	0	–
Sweet Escapes Triple Chocolate Wafer	1	80	0	–
Take 5	2 pkg (1.5 oz)	220	<5	1
Tastetations Butterscotch	3 pieces	60	<5	–
Tastetations Caramel	3 pieces	60	<5	–
Tastetations Chocolate	3 pieces	60	<5	–
Hint Mint				
All Flavors	2 pieces	10	0	–
Jelly Belly				
Jelly Beans Sugar Free	35	80	0	8
Jolly Rancher				
All Flavors	4 pieces	60	0	0
Lollipops All Flavors	1 (0.6 oz)	60	0	–
Sugar Free	4 pieces (0.6 oz)	35	0	0
Joyva				
Halvah Chocolate Covered	1 serv (2 oz)	380	0	3
Halvah Marble	1 serv (2 oz)	390	0	2
Judy's				
Sugar Free Almond Caramel Cluster	1 piece (1.5 oz)	200	<5	2
Sugar Free Cashew Caramel Cluster	1 piece (1.5 oz)	190	5	1
Sugar Free English Toffee	1 piece (1.5 oz)	220	5	3
Sugar Free Macadamia Caramel Cluster	1 piece (1.5 oz)	220	<5	2
Sugar Free Peanut Brittle	¾ cup	100	0	tr
Sugar Free Pecan Almond Cluster	1 piece (1.5 oz)	220	<5	2
Junior Mints				
Snack Size	1 box (0.7 oz)	80	0	–
Kellogg's				
Fruit Flavored Snacks Hello Kitty	10 pieces	100	0	0

FOOD	PORTION	CALS	CHOL	FIBER
Fruit Flavored Snacks Winnie The Pooh	1 pkg	80	0	0
Fruit Streamers Watermelon Madness	1 pkg (0.8 oz)	80	0	0
Fruit Twistables Triple Cherry Explosion	1 pkg (0.8 oz)	70	0	0
Gamester Rolls All Varieties	1 pkg (0.7 oz)	80	0	0
Yogos Crazy Berries	1 pkg (0.8 oz)	90	0	0
KitKat				
Bar	1 (0.5 oz)	73	tr	tr
Klein				
Sugar Free Hard Candy All Flavors	3 pieces	12	0	0
Krackel				
Bar	1 (0.6 oz)	90	0	–
Miniature	1	45	0	–
Lambertz				
Petits Soleils Chocolate Coated Gingerbread	1 piece (0.4 oz)	47	0	tr
Landies Candies				
Sugar Free Almond Clusters	2 pieces (1.5 oz)	240	<5	2
Sugar Free Bon Bons Peanut Butter	2 (1.5 oz)	240	<5	tr
Sugar Free Coconut Clusters	2 pieces (1.5 oz)	250	10	1
Sugar Free Cookies & Cream	2 pieces (1.5 oz)	240	5	tr
Sugar Free Dark Almond Bark	1 piece (1.5 oz)	230	<5	2
Sugar Free Dark Miniature Bars	7 pieces (1.5 oz)	230	<5	2
Sugar Free Milk Miniature Bars	7 pieces (1.5 oz)	240	5	tr
Sugar Free Mint Discs	7 pieces (1.5 oz)	240	5	tr
Sugar Free Peanut Clusters	2 (1.5 oz)	240	<5	2
Sugar Free White Almond Bark	1 piece (1.5 oz)	230	<5	tr
Sugar Free White Caps	6 pieces (1.5 oz)	230	5	0
Lean Protein Bites				
Milk Chocolate	1 pkg (1 oz)	120	3	0
Peanut Butter	1 pkg (1 oz)	120	1	0
White Chocolate	1 pkg (1 oz)	120	3	0

FOOD	PORTION	CALS	CHOL	FIBER
Legacy Chocolates				
Truffles Assorted	1 piece (0.5 oz)	90	tr	1
Lifesavers				
Gummi Shapes Barnum's Animals	1 pkg (0.8 oz)	70	0	–
Variety	4 pieces	60	0	–
Lindt				
Dark Chocolate 70% Cocoa	4 blocks (1.4 oz)	220	0	2
Lindor Truffles Dark Chocolate	3 pieces	220	5	0
Lindor Truffles Milk Chocolate	3 pieces	220	5	0
Low Carb Chef				
Gummi Bears	14 pieces	138	0	0
Jelly Beans	37 pieces	120	0	0
Sugar Free Caramel Marshmallow Treats	3 pieces	140	<5	0
Sugar Free Cherry Cordials	3 pieces	250	<5	tr
Sugar Free Coconut Clusters	4 pieces	210	<5	3
Sugar Free Milk Chocolate Covered Vanilla Caramels	3 pieces	160	10	0
Sugar Free Peanut Butter Cups	1 piece	200	<5	1
Sugar Free Peanut Butter Truffes	2 pieces	200	<5	1
Sugar Free Peanut Clusters	4 pieces	210	<5	2
Sugar Free Pecan Turtles	1 piece	120	5	1
Sugar Free Peppermint Patties	3 pieces	150	10	3
M&M's				
Almond	1 pkg (1.3 oz)	200	5	2
Dark Chocolate	1 pkg (1.7 oz)	240	5	2
Milk Chocolate	1 pkg (1.7 oz)	240	5	1
Minis	1 pkg (1.1 oz)	150	5	1
Peanut	1 pkg (1.7 oz)	250	5	2
Peanut Butter	1 pkg (1.6 oz)	240	5	2
Maple Grove Farms				
Maple Sugar Candy	5 pieces (1.3 oz)	140	0	–

FOOD	PORTION	CALS	CHOL	FIBER
Mauna Loa				
Macadamia Crisp Milk Chocolate	1 bar (1.8 oz)	270	10	tr
Macadamia Milk Chocolate	1 bar (1.8 oz)	280	10	1
Mentos				
Sugar Free Mixed Berries	1 piece	5	0	–
Milky Way				
Bar	1 (2 oz)	260	5	1
Fun Size	2 bars (1.2 oz)	150	5	0
Midnight	1 bar (1.8 oz)	220	5	1
Midnight Minis	5 (1.4 oz)	180	5	1
Milk Chocolate Covered Caramels	5 (1.5 oz)	200	10	0
Minis	5 (1.5 oz)	190	5	0
Mon Cheri				
Hazelnut	4 pieces	260	5	1
Mounds				
Bar	1 (0.7 oz)	90	0	–
Mr. Goodbar				
Bar	1 (1.75 oz)	270	5	2
Miniatures	1 (0.3 oz)	45	0	–
Mrs. Fields				
Decadent Chocolates	3 pieces (1.8 oz)	240	10	2
Munch				
Nut Bar	1 (1.42 oz)	220	10	2
Necco				
Bridge Mix	¼ cup (1.5 oz)	180	5	tr
Chocolate Covered Raisins	30 pieces (1.5 oz)	170	0	1
Malted Milk Balls	11 pieces (1.5 oz)	180	0	tr
Mint	1 piece	12	0	–
SkyBar	1 bar (1.5 oz)	190	5	0
Nestle				
Buncha Crunch	1 pkg (1.4 oz)	90	10	tr
Crunch	1 bar (1.55 oz)	230	10	tr
Crunch Disk	1 (1.2 oz)	180	5	tr
Crunchkins	5 pieces	190	5	tr
Jingles Milk Chocolate Butterfinger	5 pieces	180	<5	tr
Jingles Milk Chocolate Crunch	7 pieces	220	10	tr

FOOD	PORTION	CALS	CHOL	FIBER
Jingles White Crunch	7 pieces	230	10	0
Milk Chocolate	1 bar (1.45 oz)	220	10	tr
Nesteggs Milk Chocolate Butterfinger	5 pieces	210	5	tr
Nesteggs Milk Chocolate Crunch	5 pieces	190	5	tr
Nesteggs White Crunch	7 pieces	230	10	0
Pearson's Egg Nog	2 pieces	60	0	0
Toll House Brownie Bar	2 pieces (2 oz)	250	5	1
Toll House Cookie Bar	1 piece (1 oz)	130	<5	tr
Treasures Butterfinger	3 pieces	180	5	tr
Treasures Crunch	4 pieces (1.4 oz)	210	10	tr
Treasures Peanut Butter	4 pieces	250	5	1
Turtles Bite Size	1 piece (0.4 oz)	50	1	tr
Turtles Original	3 pieces	240	5	1
White Crunch	1 bar (1.4 oz)	220	10	0
Newman's Own				
Organic Chocolate Cups Dark Chocolate Peanut Butter	1 pkg (1.2 oz)	180	0	1
Organic Chocolate Cups Milk Chocolate Peanut Butter	1 pkg (1.2 oz)	180	0	1
Organic Chocolate Cups Peppermint	1 pkg (1.2 oz)	170	0	1
Organic Chocolate Sweet Dark	½ bar (¼ oz)	200	0	2
Organic Chocolate Sweet Dark Espresso	½ bar (1.4 oz)	200	0	2
Organic Chocolate Sweet Dark Orange	½ bar (1.4 oz)	200	0	2
Organic Milk Chocolate	½ bar (1.4 oz)	210	9	1
Nibs				
Licorice	9 pieces	35	0	–
Nips				
Butter Rum	2 pieces	60	0	0
Caramel	2 pieces	60	0	0
Chocolate	2 pieces	60	0	0
Chocolate Parfait	2 pieces	60	0	0

FOOD	PORTION	CALS	CHOL	FIBER
Coffee	2 pieces	50	0	0
Vanilla Almond Cafe	2 pieces	50	0	0
Nutty Ducky's				
Cashew Brittle	4 pieces (1.6 oz)	240	5	2
Cashew Brittle Dark Chocolate	2 pieces (1.5 oz)	220	5	2
Peanut Brittle	4 pieces (1.6 oz)	230	5	4
Peanut Brittle Milk Chocolate	2 pieces (1.5 oz)	220	5	2
Odense				
Marzipan	2 tbsp (1.4 oz)	170	0	0
Oh Henry!				
Bar	1 (1.8 oz)	120	<5	0
Payday				
Snack Size	1 (0.7 oz)	90	0	–
Pearson's				
Irish Cream Parfait	2 pieces	60	0	0
Mint Patties	1	30	0	tr
Pez				
Candy	1 roll (0.3 oz)	35	0	–
Candy Sugar Free	1 roll (0.3 oz)	30	0	–
Pure De-Lite				
Caramel	1 bar	120	3	1
Caramel Crisp	1 bar	120	3	1
Caramel Nougat	1 bar	110	3	1
Caramel Peanut Butter	1 bar	120	2	1
Caramel Pecan	1 bar	130	3	1
Sugar Free Dark Chocolate	1 bar	173	1	4
Sugar Free Milk Choclate w/ Mint	1 bar	187	8	1
Sugar Free Milk Chocolate	1 bar	187	8	1
Sugar Free Milk Chocolate w/ Almonds	1 bar	190	8	2
Sugar Free Milk Chocolate w/ Coconut	1 bar	190	8	1
Sugar Free Milk Chocolate w/ Orange	1 bar	187	8	1
Sugar Free Milk Chocolate w/ Peanuts	1 bar	190	9	1
Sugar Free White Chocolate	1 bar	187	26	0

FOOD	PORTION	CALS	CHOL	FIBER
Truffle Bar Caramel	1 bar	140	5	0
Truffle Bar Dark Mint	1 bar	160	5	1
Truffle Bar Hazelnut	1 bar	160	10	1
Truffle Bar Peanut Butter	1 bar	160	5	1
Raisinets				
Candy	3 pkg (1.7 oz)	200	5	1
Fun Size	3 pkg	200	5	2
Reese's				
Bites	16 pieces	220	<5	1
FastBreak	1 bar (0.7 oz)	90	0	–
Miniatures Peanut Butter Cups Sugar Free	5 pieces (1.4 oz)	170	5	5
Nutrageous	1 (0.6 oz)	95	0	1
Peanut Butter Cups Miniatures	5 (1.4 oz)	210	<5	1
Peanut Butter Cups Sugar Free	1 piece (1.5 oz)	180	5	5
Peanut Butter Eggs	1	90	0	–
Pieces	25	90	0	–
White Miniatures Peanut Butter Cups	4 pieces (1.4 oz)	210	<5	tr
White Miniatures Peanut Butter Cups Sugar Free	5 pieces (1.4 oz)	180	0	3
Ritter Sport				
Dark Chocolate Whole Hazelnuts	6 pieces (1.3 oz)	210	<2	7
Robin Eggs				
Large	2 pieces	70	0	–
Medium	4 pieces	90	0	–
Mini	10 pieces	70	0	–
Rokeach				
Cotton Candy	2 cups (1 oz)	110	0	0
Rolo				
Caramels In Milk Chocolate	3 pieces (0.64 oz)	90	<5	–
Russell Stover				
Assorted	3 pieces (1.4 oz)	170	5	1
Low Carb Pecan Delights	1 piece (1 oz)	130	0	2
Peanut Butter & Grape Jelly	1 piece (0.8 oz)	100	<5	tr

FOOD	PORTION	CALS	CHOL	FIBER
Peanut Butter & Red Raspberry	2 (1.2 oz)	140	<5	tr
Pecan Delights	1 pkg (2 oz)	280	10	tr
Pecan Roll	1 (1.75 oz)	260	<5	2
S'mores	3 (1.4 oz)	210	<5	tr
Sugar Free Peanut Butter Cups	4 pieces (1.3 oz)	200	0	2
Sugar Free Pecans & Caramel	2 pieces (1.2 oz)	170	0	0
Scharffen Berger				
Semisweet 60% Cacao	1 bar (2 oz)	320	0	tr
Sixlets				
Sixlets	3 tubes	90	0	–
Skittles				
Original Fruit	1 pkg (2.2 oz)	250	0	0
Smucker's				
Jelly Beans	25	150	0	0
Snickers				
Almond	1 (1.8 oz)	230	5	2
Bar	1 (2.07 oz)	280	5	1
Cruncher	3 fun size (1.4 oz)	230	5	1
Cruncher	1 bar (1.6 oz)	220	5	1
Minatures	4 (1.3 oz)	170	5	1
Sno Caps				
Candies	1 pkg (2.3 oz)	300	0	3
Sour Patch				
Connectors	1.5 oz	150	0	–
Kids	1.5 oz	140	0	–
Speakeasy				
Organic Mints All Flavors	4 pieces (2 g)	10	0	–
Starburst				
Baja California	1 pkg	240	0	0
Jellybeans	¼ cup	160	0	0
Original Fruit	1 pkg	240	0	0
Sour Fruit	1 pkg	240	0	0
Steel's				
Salt Water Taffy Assorted	3 pieces (1 oz)	90	0	0
Swedish Fish				
Aqua Life	1.5 oz	140	0	–
Original	20 pieces (1.5 oz)	140	0	–

FOOD	PORTION	CALS	CHOL	FIBER
Symphony				
Bar	1 (0.6 oz)	90	<5	–
Take 5				
Snack Size	2 pieces	220	<5	1
The Chocolate Traveler				
Wedges Bittersweet	4 pieces	130	0	4
Wedges Dark Chocolate Coffee	4 pieces	130	0	2
Wedges Dark Chocolate Mint	4 pieces	130	0	2
Wedges Dark Chocolate Orange	4 pieces	120	0	2
Wedges Dark Chocolate Raspberry	4 pieces	120	0	2
Wedges Dark Chocolate Tiramiso	4 pieces	120	0	2
Wedges Milk Chocolate	4 pieces	130	5	0
Wedges Milk Chocolate Dulce De Leche	4 pieces	120	5	tr
Wedges White Chocolate	4 pieces	140	5	14
Wedges White Chocolate Creme Brulee	4 pieces	140	0	0
Tobler				
Orange Dark Chocolate	5 pieces (1.5 oz)	240	<5	3
Toblerone				
Bittersweet Chocolate w/ Honey & Almond Nugget	⅓ bar (1.2 oz)	170	<5	2
Milk Chocolate w/ Honey & Almond Nougat	⅓ bar (1.76 oz)	170	10	tr
Tom's				
Cherry Sours	1 pkg (2.25 oz)	210	0	0
Jelly Beans	1 pkg (2.25 oz)	230	0	0
Tootsie Roll				
Candy	12 (1.3 oz)	130	0	–
Torras				
Sugar Free Dark Chocolate	1 oz	136	2	0
Sugar Free Milk Chocolate	1 oz	140	8	0
Sugar Free Milk Chocolate w/ Almonds	1 oz	146	6	0

FOOD	PORTION	CALS	CHOL	FIBER
Sugar Free Milk Chocolate w/ Hazelnuts	1 oz	148	6	0
Sugar Free White Chocolate	1 oz	138	6	0
Tropical Source				
Butterscotch Dream	4 pieces (0.5 oz)	60	0	0
Chocolate Dairy Free California Raisin & Currant	½ bar (1.5 oz)	230	0	1
Chocolate Dairy Free Hazelnut Espresso Crunch	½ bar (1.5 oz)	250	0	1
Chocolate Dairy Free Maple Almond Granola	½ bar (1.5 oz)	230	0	1
Chocolate Dairy Free Mint Candy Crunch	½ bar (1.5 oz)	220	0	1
Chocolate Dairy Free Red Raspberry Crush	½ bar (1.5 oz)	230	0	1
Chocolate Dairy Free Sundried Jungle Banana	½ bar (1.5 oz)	230	0	2
Chocolate Dairy Free Toasted Almond	½ bar (1.5 oz)	250	0	1
Chocolate Dairy Free Wild Rice Crisp	½ bar (1.5 oz)	230	0	1
Cool Peppermint	4 pieces (0.5 oz)	60	0	0
Lollipops All Flavors	1	24	0	0
Mango Papaya	4 pieces (0.5 oz)	60	0	0
Twix				
Peanut Butter	1 bar	280	5	2
Twizzlers				
Cherry	1 piece	30	0	–
Chocolate	1	25	0	–
Licorice	1 piece	30	0	–
Pull'N'Peel Cherry	1 piece	100	0	–
Strawberry Snack Size	3 pkgs	130	0	–
Sugar Free	4 pieces (1.5 oz)	130	0	0
Unique Origin				
Guaranda Dark Chocolate	1 piece (0.3 oz)	54	0	1
Vere				
75% Chocolate Gluten Free	1 sm bar	80	0	2
Brownie Box Coconut Gluten Free Vegan	3 pieces (1.4 oz)	210	0	5

FOOD	PORTION	CALS	CHOL	FIBER
Brownie Box Peanut Butter Gluten Free	3 pieces (1.3 oz)	180	20	3
Brownie Box Walnut Gluten Free	3 pieces (1.3 oz)	190	30	3
Clusters Chocolate Coconut Gluten Free Vegan	3 pieces (1.7 oz)	280	0	6
Clusters Chocolate Almond Gluten Free Vegan	2 pieces (1.3 oz)	210	0	4
Clusters Chocolate Rice Gluten Free Vegan	3 pieces (1.3 oz)	170	0	3
Clusters Chocolate Seed Gluten Free Vegan	2 pieces (1.3 oz)	210	0	4
Wafers Cacao Nibs Gluten Free Vegan	2 (1.1 oz)	170	0	4
Wafers Espresso Gluten Free Vegan	3 (1.6 oz)	250	0	8
Wafers Pink Peppercorn Gluten Free Vegan	3 (1.6 oz)	250	0	6
Wafers Spicy Pepita Gluten Free	2 (1.1 oz)	170	0	4
Wafers Tamari Almond Gluten Free Vegan	2 (1.2 oz)	170	0	5
Weight Watchers				
English Toffee Squares	3 pieces	160	10	6
Mint Patties	2	100	5	5
Peanut Butter Crunch	4 pieces	180	5	6
Pecan Crowns	3 pieces	150	5	8
Werther's				
Original	3 pieces (0.5 oz)	60	<5	0
Whatchamacallit				
Bar	1 (0.57 oz)	80	0	–
Whitman's				
Sampler	3 pieces (1.4 oz)	220	5	tr
Whoppers				
Malted Milk Balls	18 pieces	190	0	tr
Yamate Chocolatier				
No Sugar Almonds & Caramel	1 piece (0.6 oz)	70	0	1
York				
Peppermint Patty	3 (1.4 oz)	150	0	tr

FOOD	PORTION	CALS	CHOL	FIBER
Peppermint Patty Sugar Free	3 (1.3 oz)	110	0	1
Yummy Earth				
Organic Lollipops All Flavors	3	70	0	0
Zagnut				
Snack Size	1 piece	70	0	–
Zero				
Bar	1	70	0	–
CANTALOUPE				
dried	3.5 pieces (1.4 oz)	140	0	1
fresh cubed	1 cup	57	0	1
fresh half	½	94	0	2
Chiquita				
Wedge	¼ med (4.7 oz)	50	0	1
Del Monte				
Fresh	¼ melon (4.7 oz)	50	0	1
CARAWAY				
seed	1 tsp	7	0	–
CARDAMOM				
ground	1 tsp	6	0	–
CARDOON				
fresh shredded	½ cup	36	0	–
Frieda's				
Cardoon	1 cup	15	0	1
CARIBOU				
roasted	3 oz	142	93	0
CARISSA				
fresh	1	12	0	–
CAROB				
carob mix	3 tsp	45	0	–
carob mix as prep w/ whole milk	9 oz	195	33	–
flour	1 cup	185	0	–
flour	1 tbsp	14	0	–
Sunspire				
Carob Chips Unsweetened	13 pieces (0.5 oz)	70	0	0
Carob Chips Vegan	13 pieces (0.5 oz)	70	0	0

FOOD	PORTION	CALS	CHOL	FIBER
CARP				
fresh	3 oz	108	56	0
fresh cooked	3 oz	138	72	0
fresh cooked	1 fillet (6 oz)	276	143	–
roe raw	1 oz	37	103	–
roe salted in olive oil	2 tbsp (1 oz)	40	100	0
CARROT JUICE				
canned	6 oz	73	0	–
Bolthouse Farms				
Carrot Juice	8 oz	70	0	tr
Luvli Juices				
Zingy Carrot	1 bottle (10 oz)	145	0	2
Naked Juice				
Just Carrot	8 oz	80	0	0
CARROTS				
CANNED				
slices	½ cup	17	0	1
slices low sodium	½ cup	17	0	1
Del Monte				
Savory Sides Honey Glazed	½ cup	70	0	tr
Sliced	½ cup	35	0	3
Glory				
Seasoned Honey	½ cup	50	0	2
S&W				
Julienne	½ cup (4.3 oz)	30	0	2
Sliced	½ cup (4.3 oz)	30	0	2
Whole Small	½ cup (4.3 oz)	30	0	2
Tillen Farms				
Crispy Carrots Pickled	5 pieces (1 oz)	30	0	1
FRESH				
baby raw	1 (½ oz)	6	0	–
raw	1 (2.5 oz)	31	0	2
raw shredded	½ cup	24	0	2
slices cooked	½ cup	35	0	–
Bolthouse Farms				
Baby	1 pkg (2.25 oz)	25	0	2
Matchstix	3 oz	35	0	2
Earthbound Farm				
Organic Tops On	1 (2.7 oz)	35	0	2

FOOD	PORTION	CALS	CHOL	FIBER
Organic w/ Organic Ranch Dip	1 pkg (2.2 oz)	90	5	1
Frieda's				
Gold	⅔ cup (3 oz)	35	0	3
Grimmway				
Baby	3 oz	38	0	2
Nature's Gold				
Fresh	1 med (2.7 oz)	40	0	3
River Ranch				
Shredded	¾ cup	35	0	3
FROZEN				
slices cooked	½ cup	26	0	–
C&W				
Whole Baby	⅔ cup	35	0	2
CASABA				
cubed	1 cup	45	0	–
fresh	¹⁄₁₀	43	0	–
CASHEWS				
cashew butter w/o salt	1 tbsp	94	0	–
dry roasted salted	1 oz	163	0	–
dry roasted w/o salt	18 nuts (1 oz)	160	0	1
oil roasted salted	1 oz	163	0	–
oil roasted w/o salt	1 oz	163	0	–
Bowlby's				
Bits	½ cup	200	0	1
Frito Lay				
Salted	3 tbsp	160	0	1
Good Sense				
Jumbo Honey Roasted	¼ cup	170	0	1
Jumbo Roasted & Salted	¼ cup	190	0	1
Kettle				
Butter Creamy Unsalted	2 tbsp	160	0	1
Maranatha				
Cashew Butter	2 tbsp	190	0	2
Tamari Cashews	¼ cup	160	0	1
Planters				
Chocolate Lovers Milk Chocolate	10 pieces (1.5 oz)	230	5	tr

FOOD	PORTION	CALS	CHOL	FIBER
Dry Roasted	19 pieces (1 oz)	160	0	tr
Organic	23 pieces (1 oz)	170	0	1
Sweet Delights				
Cashew Roasters	⅓ pkg (1 oz)	170	0	2

CASSAVA

fresh	3.5 oz	120	0	–

CATFISH

channel breaded & fried	3 oz	194	69	–
channel raw	3 oz	99	49	0
wolffish atlantic baked	3 oz	105	50	0

CAULIFLOWER
FRESH

cooked	½ cup (2.2 oz)	14	0	1
flowerets cooked	3 (2 oz)	12	0	1
flowerets raw	3 (2 oz)	14	0	1
green cooked	1½ cup (3.2 oz)	29	0	3
green raw	1 head 7 in diam (18 oz)	158	0	16
green raw	1 cup (2.2 oz)	20	0	2
green raw floweret	1 (0.9 oz)	8	0	1
raw	½ cup (1.8 oz)	13	0	1
River Ranch				
Florets	1 cup	20	0	2
FROZEN				
cooked	½ cup	17	0	–
Birds Eye				
Steamfresh Garlic Cauliflower	1 cup	40	0	1
Green Giant				
Cheese Sauce	½ cup	50	<5	1

CAVIAR

black or red	2 tbsp	81	188	0

CELERIAC

raw	½ cup	31	0	–

CELERY

diced cooked	½ cup	13	0	–
fresh	1 stalk (1.3 oz)	6	0	1

FOOD	PORTION	CALS	CHOL	FIBER
raw diced	½ cup	10	0	1
seed	1 tsp	8	0	–
Dole				
Stalks	2 med (3 oz)	15	0	2
Earthbound Farm				
Organic Hearts	2 stalks (3.9 oz)	20	0	2
Frieda's				
Celery Root	¾ cup	35	0	3
River Ranch				
Sticks Fresh	4 (3 oz)	15	0	1

CELTUCE

FOOD	PORTION	CALS	CHOL	FIBER
raw	3½ oz	22	0	–

CEREAL

FOOD	PORTION	CALS	CHOL	FIBER
bran flakes	¾ cup	90	0	–
corn flakes	1¼ cup	110	0	–
farina as prep w/ water	¾ cup (6.1 oz)	88	0	2
granola	½ cup	285	0	6
oatmeal instant as prep w/ water	1 cup (8.2 oz)	138	0	4
oatmeal regular & quick as prep w/ water	¾ cup (6.1 oz)	149	0	3
oatmeal regular & quick not prep	⅓ cup (0.9 oz)	104	0	3
puffed rice	1 cup	56	0	tr
puffed wheat	1 cup	44	0	1
shredded mini wheats	1 cup	107	0	3
shredded wheat rectangular	1 biscuit (0.8 oz)	85	0	2
Albers				
Hominy Quick Grits uncooked	¼ cup	140	0	1
Alti Plano				
Hot Cereal Chai Almond	1 pkg	210	0	5
Hot Cereal Oaxacan Chocolate	1 pkg	170	0	5
Hot Cereal Orange Date	1 pkg	180	0	6
Hot Cereal Regular	1 pkg	190	0	7
Hot Cereal Spiced Apple Raisin	1 pkg	160	0	5

FOOD	PORTION	CALS	CHOL	FIBER
Alvarado Street Bakery				
Plain Grinola	½ cup	220	0	4
Atkins				
Banana Nut Harvest	⅔ cup	100	0	6
Blueberry Bounty w/ Almonds	⅔ cup	100	0	6
Crunchy Almond Crisp	⅔ cup	100	0	5
Aunt Paula's				
Hot Flax Cereal	1 serv (1.5 oz)	100	0	5
Back To Nature				
Banana Nut Multibran	¾ cup	140	0	13
Flax & Fiber Crunch	1 cup	200	0	9
Granola Apple Blueberry	½ cup	200	0	4
Granola Apple Cinnamon	½ cup	180	0	4
Granola Classic	½ cup	180	0	4
Granola French Vanilla	½ cup	220	0	4
Hi Protein Crunch	½ cup	150	0	3
Hi-Fiber Multibran	½ cup	70	0	8
Muesli	¾ cup	230	0	6
Multigrain Harvest	1 cup	210	0	9
Oat & Soy Crisp	¾ cup	180	0	3
Strawberry & Seven Grains	1 cup	210	0	5
Barbara's Bakery				
Apple Cinnamon O's	¾ cup	110	0	2
Bite Size Shredded Oats	1¼ cups (2 oz)	220	0	6
Cinnamon Puffins	1¼ cup (2 oz)	100	0	6
Cocoa Crunch Stars	1 cup (1 oz)	110	0	1
Frosted Corn Flakes	1 cup (1 oz)	110	0	4
Fruit Juice Sweetened Breakfast O's	1 cup (1 oz)	120	0	3
Fruit Juice Sweetened Brown Rice Crisps	1 cup (1 oz)	120	0	1
Fruit Juice Sweetened Corn Flakes	1 cup (1 oz)	110	0	2
GrainShop	⅔ cup (1 oz)	90	0	8
Honey Crunch Stars	1 cup (1 oz)	110	0	2
Honey Nut Toasted O's	¾ cup	120	0	2
Organic Fruity Punch	1 cup (1 oz)	110	0	0
Organic Soy Essence	¾ cup (1 oz)	100	0	5
Puffins	¾ cup (0.9 oz)	90	0	5

FOOD	PORTION	CALS	CHOL	FIBER
Shredded Spoonfuls	¾ cup	120	0	4
Shredded Wheat	2 biscuits (1.4 oz)	140	0	5
Bear Naked				
Apple Cinnamon	¼ cup	140	0	3
Banana Nut	¼ cup	140	0	3
Fruit And Nut	¼ cup	140	0	3
Peak Protein	½ cup	200	0	2
Carbsense				
Hot Cereal Country Spice not prep	½ cup	130	0	12
Hot Cereal Roasted Hazelnut not prep	½ cup	140	0	12
CoCo Wheats				
Hot Cereal	⅓ cup	200	0	2
Country Choice Naturals				
Instant Oatmeal Apples 'N' Cinnamon	1 pkg	140	0	3
Instant Oatmeal Maple Syrup	1 pkg	170	0	4
Instant Oatmeal Organic Plus French Vanilla	1 pkg	180	0	3
Instant Oatmeal Organic Plus Golden Brown Sugar	1 pkg	180	0	3
Instant Oatmeal Regular	1 pkg	110	0	3
Oatmeal Steel Cut not prep	½ cup	150	0	4
Oats Old Fashioned not prep	½ cup	150	0	4
Oats Quick not prep	½ cup	150	0	4
Organic Multi Grain Hot Cereal not prep	½ cup	130	0	5
Deliciously Slim				
Granola Cranberry Cashew	¾ cup	230	0	12
Granola Strawberry Almond	¾ cup	230	0	12
Earthbound Farm				
Organic Granola Maple Almond	½ cup	260	0	4
Enjoy Life				
Cinnamon Crunch Nut & Gluten Free	¾ cup	160	0	5
EnviroKidz				
Organic Orangutan O's	¾ cup	120	0	2

FOOD	PORTION	CALS	CHOL	FIBER
Erewhon				
Apple Stroodles	¾ cup	110	0	1
Aztec	1 cup	110	0	1
Banana O's	¾ cup	110	0	2
Brown Rice Cream	¼ cup	170	0	1
Corn Flakes	1¼ cups	210	0	3
Crispy Brown Rice	1 cup	110	0	1
Crispy Brown Rice No Salt Added	1 cup	110	0	1
Fruit'n Wheat	¾ cup	170	0	5
Kamut Flakes	⅔ cup	110	0	4
Raisin Bran	1 cup	170	0	6
Rice Twice	¾ cup	120	0	0
Whole Wheat Flakes	1 cup	180	0	6
Expert Foods				
Low Carb Hot Cereal Sub	½ cup	24	0	–
Fantastic				
Oatmeal Big Cup Apple Cinnamon	1 pkg	270	0	6
Oatmeal Big Cup Maple Raisin 3 Grain	1 pkg	270	0	8
General Mills				
Basic 4	1 cup (1.9 oz)	200	0	3
Boo Berry	1 cup (1 oz)	120	0	–
Cheerios	1 cup	110	0	3
Cheerios Apple Cinnamon	¾ cup	120	0	1
Cheerios Frosted	1 cup (1 oz)	120	0	1
Cheerios Honey Nut	1 cup (1 oz)	120	0	2
Cheerios Yogurt Burst Strawberry	¾ cup	120	0	2
Cheerios Yogurt Burst Vanilla	¾ cup	120	0	2
Chex Corn	1 cup (1 oz)	110	0	0
Chex Honey Nut	¾ cup	120	0	–
Chex Morning Mix Cinnamon	1 pkg (1.1 oz)	130	0	1
Chex Morning Mix Fruit & Nut	1 pkg (1.1 oz)	180	0	1
Chex Morning Mix Honey Nut	1 pkg (1.1 oz)	130	0	1
Chex Multi-Bran	1 cup (2 oz)	200	0	8

FOOD	PORTION	CALS	CHOL	FIBER
Chex Rice	1¼ cup (1.1 oz)	120	0	0
Cinnamon Grahams	¾ cup (1 oz)	120	0	1
Cinnamon Toast Crunch	¾ cup (1 oz)	130	1	1
Cocoa Puffs	1 cup (1 oz)	120	0	–
Cookie Crisp	1 cup (1 oz)	120	0	0
Count Chocula	1 cup (1 oz)	120	0	0
Country Corn Flakes	1 cup (1 oz)	120	0	–
Fiber One	½ cup (1 oz)	60	0	14
Fiber One Honey Clusters	1¼ cup	170	0	14
Franken Berry	1 cup (1 oz)	120	0	–
French Toast Crunch	¾ cup (1 oz)	120	0	0
Gold Medal Raisin Bran	1⅓ cups (1.9 oz)	170	0	6
Golden Grahams	¾ cup (1 oz)	120	0	1
Harmony	1¼ cups (1.9 oz)	200	0	2
Honey Nut Clusters	1 cup (1.9 oz)	210	0	3
Kix	1⅓ cup (1 oz)	120	0	1
Kix Berry Berry	¾ cup (1 oz)	120	0	0
Lucky Charms	1 cup (1 oz)	120	0	1
Nature Valley Low Fat Fruit Granola	⅔ cup (1.9 oz)	210	0	3
Newquick	¾ cup (1 oz)	120	0	–
Oatmeal Crisp Almond	1 cup (1.9 oz)	220	0	4
Oatmeal Crisp Apple Cinnamon	1 cup (1.9 oz)	210	0	4
Oatmeal Crisp Raisin	1 cup (1.9 oz)	210	0	4
Para Su Familia Cinnamon Stars	1 cup (1 oz)	120	0	–
Para Su Familia Fruitis	1 cup (1 oz)	120	0	–
Para Su Familia Raisin Bran	1¼ cups (2 oz)	170	0	6
Raisin Nut Bran	¾ cup (1.9 oz)	200	0	4
Reese's Puffs	¾ cup	130	0	0
Snack'N Dash Cinnamon Toast Crunch	1 pkg (1.2 oz)	140	0	1
Snack'N Dash Honey Nut Cheerios	1 pkg (1 oz)	110	0	2
Snack'N Dash Lucky Charms	1 pkg (1 oz)	110	0	1
Sunrise Organic	¾ cup (1 oz)	110	0	1
Total Brown Sugar & Oat	¾ cup (1 oz)	110	0	1
Total Honey Clusters	¾ cup	170	0	3
Total Protein	¾ cup	120	0	3

FOOD	PORTION	CALS	CHOL	FIBER
Total Raisin Bran	1 cup	170	0	5
Total Whole Grain	¾ cup (1 oz)	100	0	3
Trix	1 cup (1 oz)	120	0	1
Wheaties	1 cup (1 oz)	110	0	3
Wheaties Energy Crunch	1 cup (1.9 oz)	210	0	4
Wheaties Frosted	¾ cup (1 oz)	110	0	–
Wheaties Raisin Bran	1 cup (1.9 oz)	180	0	5
Gram's Gourmet				
Cream Of Flax not prep	½ cup	142	0	8
Crunch Granolas All Flavors	½ cup	349	2	6
Grandy Oats				
Organic Granola Classic	½ cup	252	0	5
Organic Granola Low Fat Cranberry Chew	½ cup	191	0	3
Organic Granola Mainely Maple	½ cup	204	0	4
Hansen's				
Orange & Chocolate	½ cup	230	0	4
Strawberry & Yogurt	½ cup	230	0	6
Toasted Nut Crunch	½ cup	230	0	7
Tropical Cluster	½ cup	210	0	6
Hi-Lo				
Low Carb Cereal	½ cup	90	0	6
Hodgson Mill				
Hot Cereal Bulgur Wheat w/ Soy not prep	¼ cup	115	0	3
Hot Cereal Oat Bran not prep	¼ cup	120	0	6
Kashi				
7 Whole Grain Flakes	1 cup	180	0	6
7 Whole Grain Honey Puffs	1 cup	120	0	2
7 Whole Grain Nuggets	½ cup	210	0	7
7 Whole Grain Pilaf as prep	½ cup	170	0	6
7 Whole Grain Puffs	1 cup	70	0	1
GoLean	1 cup	140	0	10
GoLean Crunch!	1 cup	190	0	8
GoLean Crunch Honey Almond Flax	1 cup	200	0	8
GoLean Instant Hot Cereal Creamy Truly Vanilla	1 pkg	150	0	7

FOOD	PORTION	CALS	CHOL	FIBER
GoLean Instant Hot Cereal Hearty Honey & Cinnamon	1 pkg	150	0	5
Good Friends	1 cup	170	0	12
Heart To Heart Instant Oatmeal Golden Brown Maple	1 pkg	160	0	5
Heart To Heart Instant Oatmeal Raisin Spice	1 pkg	150	0	4
Heart To Heart Oat Flakes & Blueberry Clusters	1¼ cups	200	0	4
Heart To Heart Toasted Oat	¾ cup	110	0	5
Mighty Bites All Flavors	1 cup	110	0	3
Organic Promise Autumn Wheat	1 cup	190	0	6
Organic Promise Cinnamon Harvest	1 cup	190	0	5
Organic Promise Strawberry Fields	1 cup	120	0	1
Vive	1¼ cups	170	0	12
Kellogg's				
All-Bran	½ cup	80	0	10
All-Bran Extra Fiber	½ cup	50	0	13
Apple Jacks	1 cup	130	0	1
Caramel Nut Crunch	1 cup	210	0	1
Cocoa Krispies	¾ cup	120	0	1
Complete Oat Bran Flakes	¾ cup	110	0	1
Corn Flakes	1 cup	100	0	1
Corn Pops	1 cup	120	0	tr
Cracklin' Oat Bran	¾ cup	200	0	6
Crispix	1 cup	110	0	1
Frosted Flakes	¾ cup	120	0	1
Frosted Flakes ⅓ Less Sugar	1 cup	120	0	tr
Fruit Harvest	¾ cup	120	0	1
Fruit Loops	1 cup	120	0	1
Fruit Loops ⅓ Less Sugar	1¼ cups	120	0	1
Granola Low Fat w/ Raisins	⅔ cup	230	0	3
Honey Smacks	¾ cup	100	0	1
Mini-Wheat Frosted	5 (1.8 oz)	180	0	5

FOOD	PORTION	CALS	CHOL	FIBER
Mueslix Raisins Dates & Almonds	⅔ cup	200	0	4
Organic Mini Wheats Frosted	24 pieces	190	0	5
Organic Raisin Bran	1 cup	190	0	8
Organic Rice Krispies	1¼ cups	120	0	0
Product 19	1 cup	100	0	1
Raisin Bran	1 cup	190	0	7
Rice Krispies	1¼ cup	120	0	0
Smart Start Antioxidants	1 cup	190	0	3
Smart Start Healthy Heart	1¼ cups	230	0	5
Smorz	1 cup	120	0	tr
Special K	1 cup	110	0	tr
Special K Fruit & Yogurt	¾ cup	120	0	1
Special K Low Carb Lifestyle Protein Plus	¾ cup	100	0	5
Special K Red Berries	1 cup	110	0	1
Special K Vanilla Almond	¾ cup	110	0	1
Keto				
Cocoa Crisp	½ cup	110	0	1
Frosted Flakes All Flavors	¾ cup	110	0	2
Hot Cereal Apple Cinnamon	2 scoops	150	0	9
Hot Cereal Strawberry & Creme	2 scoops	150	0	9
Oatmeal Old Fashioned	2 scoops	150	0	9
Liquid Cereal				
Apple & Cinnamon	1 can (11 oz)	160	5	1
Chocolate	1 can (11 oz)	170	5	1
Fruit	1 can (11 oz)	150	5	tr
Peanut Butter	1 can (11 oz)	170	5	1
Lundberg				
Purely Organic Hot'n Creamy Rice	⅓ cup	190	0	3
McCann's				
Irish Oatmeal Instant Apples & Cinnamon	1 pkg (1 oz)	130	0	2
Irish Oatmeal Instant Maple & Brown Sugar	1 pkg (1 oz)	160	0	3
Irish Oatmeal Instant Regular	1 pkg (1 oz)	100	0	3

FOOD	PORTION	CALS	CHOL	FIBER
MiniCarb				
Milk Chocolate Hot Cereal not prep	½ cup	140	10	13
Mother's				
Cinnamon Oat Crunch	1 cup	230	0	5
Cocoa Bumpers	1 cup	120	0	1
Groovy Grahams	¾ cup	100	0	1
Honey Round-Ups	¾ cups	110	0	1
Multigrain Hot Cereal	½ cup	130	0	5
Oat Bran Hot Cereal	½ cup	150	0	6
Oatmeal Instant	½ cup	150	0	4
Peanut Butter Bumpers	1 cup	130	0	1
Rolled Oats	½ cup	150	0	4
Toasted Oat Bran	¾ cup	120	0	3
Whole Wheat Hot Cereal	½ cup	130	0	4
Natural Ovens				
Great Granola	¼ cup	110	0	5
Paul's Oatmeal not prep	⅓ cup	120	0	3
Nature's Path				
Optimum Organic ReBound	¾ cup	190	0	6
Organic Zen Instant Oatmeal Cranberry Ginger	1 pkg	150	0	3
Perky's				
Nutty Flax	¾ cup	230	0	7
PerkyO's Original	¾ cup	120	0	3
Post				
Alpha-Bits Marshmallow	1 cup (1 oz)	120	0	0
Grape-Nuts	½ cup	200	0	6
Great Grains Raisins Dates Pecans	½ cup	210	0	4
Honey Bunches Of Oats	¾ cup	120	0	2
Honey Bunches Of Oats Strawberry	¾ cup	120	0	2
Raisin Bran	1 cup (2 oz)	190	0	8
Selects Blueberry Morning	¾ cup (1.3 oz)	140	0	2
Shredded Wheat Original	2 biscuits (1.6 oz)	160	0	6
Shredded Wheat Spoon Size	1 cup	170	0	6
Quaker				
Instant Oatmeal Apples & Cinnamon	1 pkg	130	0	3

FOOD	PORTION	CALS	CHOL	FIBER
Instant Oatmeal Cinnamon & Spice	1 pkg	170	0	3
Instant Oatmeal Cinnamon Roll	1 pkg	160	0	3
Instant Oatmeal Lower Sugar Apples & Cinnamon	1 pkg	110	0	3
Instant Oatmeal Lower Sugar Maple & Brown Sugar	1 pkg	120	0	3
Instant Oatmeal Maple & Brown Sugar	1 pkg	160	0	3
Instant Oatmeal Nutrition For Women Golden Brown Sugar	1 pkg	170	0	3
Instant Oatmeal Nutrition For Women Vanilla Cinnamon	1 pkg	160	0	3
Instant Oatmeal Peaches & Cream	1 pkg	130	0	3
Instant Oatmeal Raisin & Spice	1 pkg	150	0	3
Instant Oatmeal Regular	1 pkg	100	0	3
Instant Oatmeal Strawberries & Cream	1 pkg	130	0	3
Instant Oatmeal Take Heart Blueberry	1 pkg	160	0	6
Instant Oatmeal Take Heart Golden Maple	1 pkg	160	0	5
Instant Oatmeal Weight Control Banana Bread	1 pkg	160	0	6
Instant Oatmeal Weight Control Cinnamon	1 pkg	160	0	6
Life	¾ cup	120	0	2
Life Cinnamon	¾ cup	120	0	2
Life Honey Graham	¾ cup	120	0	2
Life Vanilla Yogurt Crunch	1¼ cup	210	0	4
Old Fashioned Oats not prep	½ cup	150	0	4
Ralston				
100% Hot Wheat	⅓ cup	150	0	5
Apple Dapples	1 cup	120	0	tr

FOOD	PORTION	CALS	CHOL	FIBER
Cocoa Crumbles	1 cup	120	0	0
Confruity Crisp	¾ cup	110	0	0
Corn Biscuits	1 cup	110	0	tr
Corn Flakes	1 cup	100	0	tr
Crisp Crunch	¾ cup	120	0	tr
Crisp Crunch Berry Treats	1 cup	120	0	tr
Crisp Rice	1¼ cups	120	0	0
Enriched Bran Flakes	¾ cup	90	0	5
Farina	3 tbsp	120	0	1
Freaky Fruits	1 cup	120	0	0
Frosted Flakes	¾ cup	120	0	tr
Fruit Rings	1 cup	120	0	0
Grits	¼ cup	140	0	1
Instant Oats Bananas & Cream	1 pkg	130	0	2
Magic Stars	¾ cup	120	0	1
Oats & More W/ Almonds	¾ cup	130	0	1
Oats Instant	1 pkg	100	0	3
Oats Instant Apples & Cinnamon	1 pkg	130	0	3
Oats Instant Blueberries & Cream	1 pkg	130	0	2
Oats Instant Cinnamon & Spice	1 pkg	170	0	3
Oats Instant For Kids Cinnawow	1 pkg	140	0	3
Oats Instant For Kids Maplicious & Brown Sugar	1 pkg	150	0	3
Oats Instant For Kids Roarin' Raspberry	1 pkg	150	0	3
Oats Instant For Kids Strawberries & Stars	1 pkg	140	0	3
Oats Instant Maple Brown Sugar	1 pkg	160	0	3
Oats Instant Peaches & Cream	1 pkg	130	0	2
Oats Instant Raisins & Spice	1 pkg	150	0	3
Oats Instant Strawberries & Cream	1 pkg	140	0	2
Oats Old Fashioned	½ cup	150	0	4

FOOD	PORTION	CALS	CHOL	FIBER
Oats Quick	½ cup	140	0	4
Raisin Bran	1 cup	200	0	8
Rice Biscuits	1¼ cups	120	0	0
Shredded Wheat Frosted Bite Size	1¼ cups	200	0	5
Silly Spheres	1½ cups	110	0	0
Tasteeos	1 cup	110	0	3
Tasteeos Apple Cinnamon	¾ cup	120	0	1
Tasteeos Honey Nut	1 cup	120	0	2
South Beach Diet				
Toasted Wheats	1¼ cups (2 oz)	210	0	8
Whole Grain Crunch	¾ cup (1 oz)	110	0	4
Stark Sisters				
Granola Lo-Fat Raspberry Blueberry	½ cup	230	0	4
Granola Nutty Maple	½ cup	250	0	4
Granola Original Maple Almond	½ cup	240	0	5
Sunbelt				
Granola Low Fat Cinnamon & Raisis	½ cup	250	0	3
Uncle Sam				
Cereal	1 cup (1.9 oz)	190	0	10
Wheatena				
Cereal	⅓ cup (1.4 oz)	150	0	5
Zoe's				
Granola Cinnamon Raisin	½ cup	190	0	7
Granola Cranberries Currants	½ cup	190	0	7
Granola Honey Almond	½ cup	190	0	7
O's Cinnamon	¾ cup	120	0	5
O's Honey	¾ cup	120	0	5
O's Natural	¾ cup	120	0	tr

CEREAL BARS (see also ENERGY BARS)
Barbara's Bakery

FOOD	PORTION	CALS	CHOL	FIBER
Nature's Choice Apple Cinnamon	1 (1.3 oz)	120	0	2
Nature's Choice Blueberry	1 (1.3 oz)	120	0	2
Nature's Choice Cherry	1 (1.3 oz)	120	0	2

FOOD	PORTION	CALS	CHOL	FIBER
Nature's Choice Granola Carob Chip	1 (0.7 oz)	80	0	2
Nature's Choice Granola Cinnamon & Raisin	1 (0.7 oz)	80	0	3
Nature's Choice Granola Oats 'N Honey	1 (0.7 oz)	80	0	2
Nature's Choice Granola Peanut Butter	1 (0.7 oz)	80	0	2
Nature's Choice Raspberry	1 (1.3 oz)	120	0	2
Nature's Choice Strawberry	1 (1.3 oz)	120	0	2
Nature's Choice Triple Berry	1 (1.3 oz)	120	0	2
Enjoy Life				
Caramel Apple Nut & Gluten Free	1 (1 oz)	110	0	2
Entenmann's				
Apple Cinnamon	1 (1.3 oz)	140	0	tr
Multi-Grain Chocolate Chip	1	140	0	2
Multi-Grain Rainbow Chip	1	180	5	tr
Multi-Grain Real Strawberry	1 (1.3 oz)	140	0	tr
Oatmeal Apple Cinnamon	1 (1.3 oz)	140	0	1
Oatmeal Apple Raisin	1 (1.3 oz)	140	0	1
EnviroKidz				
Crispy Rice Panda Peanut Butter	1 (1 oz)	110	0	tr
Estee				
Rice Crunchy Chocolate	1	60	0	tr
Rice Crunchy Chocolate Chip	1	70	0	0
Rice Crunchy Vanilla	1	70	0	tr
General Mills				
Milk 'N Cereal Bars Chex	1 (1.6 oz)	160	0	–
Milk 'N Cereal Bars Cinnamon Toast Crunch	1 (1.6 oz)	180	0	1
Team Cheerios Strawberry	1	160	0	2
Trix	1	160	0	2
Glenny's				
Organic Muesli Raisins & Dates	1 (1.6 oz)	170	0	3
Organic Museli Chocolate Chip	1 (1.6 oz)	170	0	3

FOOD	PORTION	CALS	CHOL	FIBER
Hershey's				
Crispy Rice Peanut Butter	1 (0.5 oz)	60	0	–
Kashi				
TLC Chewy Granola Honey Almond Flax	1 (1.2 oz)	140	0	4
TLC Chewy Granola Peanut Peanut Butter	1 (1.2 oz)	140	0	4
TLC Chewy Trail Mix	1 (1.2 oz)	140	0	4
Kellogg's				
All-Bran Brown Sugar Cinnamon	1	130	0	5
All-Bran Honey Oat	1	130	0	5
All-Bran Oatmeal Raisin	1	120	0	5
Crunchy Nut Sweet & Salty Chocolatey Almond	1 (1.1 oz)	160	0	2
Nutri-Grain Apple Cinnamon	1	140	0	1
Nutri-Grain Banana Muffin	1	170	0	1
Nutri-Grain Chewy Granola Chocolatey Chunk	1	110	0	tr
Nutri-Grain Cinnamon Raisin Muffin	1	170	0	1
Nutri-Grain Yogurt Vanilla	1	140	0	tr
Smart Start Healthy Heart Cinnamon	1 (1.4 oz)	150	0	2
Snack Bites	1 pkg (0.8 oz)	90	0	tr
Special K Chocolatey Drizzle	1 (0.8 oz)	90	0	tr
Special K Meal Bar Chocolate Peanut Butter	1 (1.6 oz)	190	5	2
Special K Snack Bar Chocolate Peanut	1 (0.9 oz)	110	0	1
Special K Strawberry	1 (0.8 oz)	90	0	tr
Special K Vanilla Crisp	1 (0.8 oz)	90	0	tr
Kudos				
Granola Chocolate Chip	1	120	0	1
Granola Peanut Butter	1	130	0	1
Granola w/ M&M's	1	100	0	1
Granola w/ Snickers	1	100	0	1
Natural Ovens				
Great Granola Chocolate Almond	1	150	0	3

FOOD	PORTION	CALS	CHOL	FIBER
Great Granola Fruit & Lemon	1	130	0	3
Great Granola Mixed Fruit	1	130	0	3
Nature Valley				
Chewy Granola Blueberry Yogurt	1	140	0	1
Chewy Granola Lemon Yogurt	1	140	0	1
Chewy Granola Vanilla Yogurt	1	140	0	1
Chewy Trail Mix Granola Apple Cinnamon	1	140	0	1
Chewy Trail Mix Granola Fruit & Nut	1	140	0	2
Chewy Trail Mix Granola Mixed Berry	1	140	0	1
Crunchy Granola Apple Crisp	1	140	0	1
Crunchy Granola Apple Crisp	1	104	0	1
Crunchy Granola Banana Nut	2	190	0	2
Crunchy Granola Maple Brown Sugar	2	180	0	2
Crunchy Granola Peanut Butter	2	160	0	2
Crunchy Granola Roasted Almond	2	190	0	2
Healthy Heart Granola Oatmeal Raisin	1	150	0	3
Heart Healthy Chewy Granola Honey Nut	1	160	0	3
Sweet & Salty Granola Almond	1	160	0	2
Sweet & Salty Granola Peanut	1	170	0	2
Nutri-Grain				
Nutri-Grain Blueberry	1	140	0	tr
Nutri-Grain Mixed Berry	1	140	0	tr

FOOD	PORTION	CALS	CHOL	FIBER
Post				
Honey Bunches Of Oats Cranberry Almond	1 (1.2 oz)	140	0	1
Quaker				
Breakfast Graham Strawberry	1 (1 oz)	120	0	1
Breakfast Bar Apple Crisp	1 (1.3 oz)	130	0	1
Breakfast Bar Iced Raspberry	1 (1.3 oz)	130	0	1
Breakfast Bites Iced Raspberry	1 pkg (1.3 oz)	130	0	3
Breakfast Bites Strawberry	1 pkg (1.3 oz)	130	0	2
Chewy Chocolate Chip	1 (0.8 oz)	100	0	1
Chewy Cookies & Cream	1 (0.8 oz)	90	0	2
Chewy 90 Calorie Cinnamon Sugar	1 (1 oz)	90	0	1
Chewy 90 Calorie Honey Nut	1 (0.8 oz)	90	0	1
Chewy Low Fat Maple Brown Sugar	1 (1 oz)	110	0	1
Chewy Low Fat S'mores	1 (1 oz)	110	0	1
Crunch Granola Oats & Berries	1 (1 oz)	130	0	1
Oatmeal To Go Brown Sugar Cinnamon	1 (2.1 oz)	220	15	5
Q-Smart Cranberry Vanilla Almond	1 (1 oz)	120	0	2
Trail Mix Cranberry Raisin & Almond	1 (1.2 oz)	150	0	1
Rice Krispies				
Treats Original	1 (0.8 oz)	90	0	0
Skippy				
Peanut Butter	1	180	0	1
Peanut Butter & Fudge	1	190	0	1
Peanut Butter & Marshmallow	1	140	0	1
Peanut Butter & Strawberry	1	170	0	1
SnackWell's				
Fat Free Blueberry	1 (1.3 oz)	120	0	1
Fat Free Strawberry	1 (1.3 oz)	120	0	1
Hearty Fruit'n Grain Crisp Autumn Apple	1 (1.3 oz)	130	0	1

FOOD	PORTION	CALS	CHOL	FIBER
Hearty Fruit'n Grain Mixed Berry	1 (1.3 oz)	120	0	1
South Beach Diet				
100 Calorie Chocolate Delight	1 (1 oz)	100	0	3
100 Calorie Peanut Butter Chocolate Chip	1 (1 oz)	100	0	3
100 Calorie Snack Bar Mixed Berry	1 (1 oz)	100	0	3
High Protein Chocolate	1 (1.2 oz)	140	0	3
High Protein Cinnamon Raisin	1 (1.2 oz)	140	5	3
High Protein Cranberry Almond	1 (1.2 oz)	140	0	3
High Protein Maple Nut	1 (1.2 oz)	140	5	3
High Protein Peanut Butter	1 (1.2 oz)	140	0	3

CHAMPAGNE

mimosa	1 serv	117	0	tr
punch	1 serv	113	0	0
sekt german champagne	3.5 oz	84	0	–

CHAYOTE

fresh cooked	1 cup	38	0	–
raw	1 (7 oz)	49	0	–
raw cut up	1 cup	32	0	–

CHEESE (see also CHEESE DISHES, CHEESE SUBSTITUTES, COTTAGE CHEESE, CREAM CHEESE, NEUFCHATEL)

american	1 oz	93	18	–
beaufort	1 oz	115	34	0
blue	1 oz	100	21	–
blue crumbled	1 cup (4.7 oz)	477	102	–
bocconcini smoked	1 oz	90	25	0
brick	1 oz	105	27	–
brie	1 oz	95	28	–
cacio di roma sheep's milk cheese	1 oz	130	30	0
camembert	1 oz	85	20	–
cantal	1 oz	105	26	0
chabichou	1 oz	95	23	0
chaource	1 oz	83	20	0

FOOD	PORTION	CALS	CHOL	FIBER
cheddar	1 oz	114	30	–
cheddar low fat	1 oz	49	6	–
cheddar low sodium	1 oz	113	28	–
cheddar shredded	1 cup	455	119	–
cheshire	1 oz	110	29	–
colby	1 oz	112	27	–
colby low fat	1 oz	49	6	–
colby low sodium	1 oz	113	28	–
comte	1 oz	114	34	0
coulommiers	1 oz	88	23	0
crottin	1 oz	105	23	0
edam	1 oz	101	25	–
emmentaler	1 oz	115	26	–
feta	1 oz	75	25	–
fontina	1 oz	110	33	–
goat fresh	1 oz	23	5	0
goat hard	1 oz	128	30	–
gouda	1 oz	101	32	–
grana padano parmesan shaved	1 tbsp	20	5	0
gruyere	1 oz	117	31	–
limburger	1 oz	93	26	–
maroilles	1 oz	97	26	0
morbier	1 oz	99	23	0
mozzarella	1 oz	80	22	–
mozzarella fresh	1 oz	80	20	0
mozzarella part skim	1 oz	72	16	–
muenster	1 oz	104	27	–
parmesan grated	1 tbsp (5 g)	23	4	–
parmesan hard	1 oz	111	19	–
picodon	1 oz	99	23	0
pimento	1 oz	106	27	–
pont l'eveque	1 oz	86	20	0
port du salut	1 oz	100	35	–
provolone	1 oz	100	20	–
pyrenees	1 oz	101	26	0
quark 20% fat	1 oz	33	5	–
quark 40% fat	1 oz	48	11	–
quark made w/ skim milk	1 oz	22	tr	–
queso anego	1 oz	106	30	–

FOOD	PORTION	CALS	CHOL	FIBER
queso asadero	1 oz	101	30	–
queso chichuahua	1 oz	106	30	–
queso manchego	1 oz	107	27	0
raclette	1 oz	102	26	0
reblochon	1 oz	88	23	0
ricotta part skim	½ cup (4.4 oz)	171	38	–
ricotta whole milk	½ cup (4.4 oz)	216	63	–
romano	1 oz	110	29	–
roquefort	1 oz	105	26	–
rouy	1 oz	95	23	0
saint marcellin	1 oz	94	23	0
saint nectaire	1 oz	97	23	0
saint paulin	1 oz	85	20	0
sainte maure	1 oz	99	23	0
selles sur cher	1 oz	93	20	0
swiss	1 oz	107	26	–
swiss processed	1 oz	95	24	–
tilsit	1 oz	96	29	–
tome	1 oz	92	23	0
triple creme	1 oz	113	34	0
vacherin	1 oz	92	23	0
yogurt cheese	1 oz	80	15	0
Alouette				
Garlic & Herbs	2 tbsp (0.8 oz)	70	30	0
Alpine Lace				
American Jalapeno Peppers	1 slice (1 oz)	80	20	0
American Less Fat Less Sodium White	1 slice (1 oz)	50	20	0
American Less Fat Less Sodium Yellow	1 slice (1 oz)	80	20	0
Cheddar Reduced Fat	1 slice (1 oz)	70	15	0
Colby Reduced Fat	1 slice (1 oz)	80	15	0
Fat Free Parmesan	2 tsp (5 g)	10	0	0
Feta Reduced Fat	1 oz	50	10	0
Feta Reduced Fat Sun Dried Tomato & Basil	1 oz	50	10	0
Goat Reduced Fat	1 oz	40	5	0
Mozzarella Reduced Fat	1 oz	70	10	0
Muenster Reduced Sodium	1 slice (1 oz)	100	25	0

FOOD	PORTION	CALS	CHOL	FIBER
Provolone Smoked Reduced Fat	1 slice (1 oz)	70	15	0
Swiss Reduced Fat	1 slice (1 oz)	90	20	0
Athenos				
Blue	1 oz	100	30	0
Feta	1 oz (1 in cube)	80	20	0
Feta Crumbled	¼ cup	90	20	tr
Feta Reduced Fat	1 in cube (1 oz)	60	10	0
Gorgonzola Crumbled	3 tbsp	110	30	tr
Back To Nature				
Organic American Slices	1 slice (0.7 oz)	80	20	0
Organic Cheddar Cubes	8 pieces (1.1 oz)	130	30	0
Organic Cheddar Shredded	¼ cup	110	30	0
Organic Cream Cheese	⅛ pkg (1 oz)	100	30	0
Organic Mozzarella Shredded	¼ cup	80	15	0
Organic White Cheddar Slices Reduced Fat	1 slice (0.7 oz)	60	10	0
Boar's Head				
American	1 oz	100	25	0
American 25% Lower Sodium 25% Lower Fat	1 oz	90	20	0
ButterKase	1 oz	100	30	0
Cheddar Sharp	1 oz	110	30	0
Colby Jack	1 oz	110	25	0
Cream Havarti	1 oz	110	35	0
Creamy Blue	1 oz	90	30	0
Double Glouster Yellow	1 oz	110	35	0
Edam	1 oz	90	20	0
Feta	1 oz	60	10	0
Gouda	1 oz	110	30	0
Lacey Swiss	1 oz	90	15	0
Longhorn Colby	1 oz	110	30	0
Monterey Jack	1 oz	100	25	0
Mozzarella	1 oz	90	20	0
Muenster	1 oz	100	25	0
Muenster Low Sodium	1 oz	100	20	0
Provolone 42% Lower Sodium	1 oz	100	20	0

FOOD	PORTION	CALS	CHOL	FIBER
Provolone Picante Sharp	1 oz	100	25	0
Swiss No Salt Added	1 oz	110	25	0
Boursin				
Garlic & Fine Herbs	2 tbsp	120	35	–
Cabot				
American	1 slice (0.7 oz)	80	20	0
Cheddar	1 oz	110	30	0
Cheddar Smoked	1 oz	110	30	0
Cheddar Light 50% Reduced Fat	1 oz	70	15	0
Cheddar Light 50% Reduce Fat Jalapeno	1 oz	70	15	0
Cheddar Light 75% Reduced Fat	1 oz	60	10	0
Cheddar Shake	2 tsp	25	5	0
Colby Jack	1 oz	110	30	0
Fancy Blend Shredded	¼ cup	100	20	0
Monterey Jack	1 oz	110	30	0
Mozzarella Shredded	¼ cup	80	15	0
Pepper Jack	1 oz	110	30	0
Swiss Slices	1 slice (1 oz)	110	30	0
Cantare				
Baked Brie En Croute	1 oz	100	30	0
Cedar Grove				
Marble Colby	1 oz	110	30	0
Organic Tomato Basil Cheddar	1 oz	110	30	0
Chavrie				
Goat's Milk	2 tbsp	50	20	0
Connoisseur				
Asiago Spread	1 tbsp	90	20	0
Cracker Barrel				
Sharp Cheddar 2% Milk	1 oz	90	20	0
Crystal Farms				
American Singles	1 slice (0.7 oz)	70	15	0
American Singles 2%	1 slice (0.7 oz)	50	10	0
American Singles Fat Free	1 slice (0.7 oz)	30	<5	0
Blue Crumbled	2 tbsp	100	25	0
Cheese Curds	8 pieces (1 oz)	110	15	0
Cheezoids Sticks	1 piece (0.8 oz)	70	15	0

FOOD	PORTION	CALS	CHOL	FIBER
Danish Havarti	1 oz	110	25	0
Deli Slices Muenster	1 slice (0.8 oz)	80	16	0
Deli Slices Swiss	1 slice (0.7 oz)	80	20	0
Feta Crumbled	¼ cup	90	20	tr
Gorganzola Crumbled	2 tbsp	100	25	0
It's So Cheesy Cheddar Aerosol	2 tbsp	90	15	0
Little Chunks To Go	1 pkg (0.7 oz)	80	20	0
Marble Jack	1 oz	110	30	0
Parmesan Grated	2 tsp	25	<5	0
Pepper Jack	1 oz	110	30	0
Ricotta	¼ cup	90	30	0
Shredded Mexican 4 Cheese	¼ cup	100	25	0
Shredded Mozzarella	¼ cup	80	20	0
Shredded Pizza Blend	¼ cup	100	25	0
Shredded Sharp Cheddar	¼ cup	110	30	0
Smoked Gouda	1 oz	100	25	0
String	1 piece (1 oz)	80	15	0
Fage				
Feta	1 oz	80	4	0
Finlandia				
Muenster	1 slice (1.1 oz)	120	30	0
Formaggio				
Fresh Mozzarella	1 oz	90	20	0
Friendship				
Farmer	2 tbsp (1 oz)	50	10	0
Handi-Snacks				
Ritz Crackers 'n Cheese	1 pkg (0.9 oz)	100	<5	0
Heluva Good Cheese				
Cheddar Extra Sharp	1 oz	110	30	0
Hollow Road Farms				
Sheep's Milk	1 oz	45	15	–
Horizon Organic				
American	1 slice (0.7 oz)	60	15	0
Cheddar	1 oz	110	30	0
Monterey Jack	1 oz	100	30	0
Shred Mexican	¼ cup	110	30	0
Shred Parmesan	1 tbsp	20	5	0
Slice Provolone	1 slice (0.7 oz)	70	15	0

FOOD	PORTION	CALS	CHOL	FIBER
Sticks Colby	1 (1 oz)	110	30	0
String Mozzarella	1 stick (1 oz)	80	15	0
J.L. Kraft				
Spreadable Feta & Spinach	2 tbsp	80	25	0
Jordan's				
Provolone	1 slice (1 oz)	100	20	0
Kraft				
Cheddar Extra Sharp	1 oz	120	30	0
Singles American 2%	1 (0.7 oz)	50	10	0
Land O Lakes				
American	1 slice (0.7 oz)	80	20	0
American Jalapeno	1 slice (0.6 oz)	70	15	0
American Light	1 oz	70	20	0
American Reduced Salt	1 oz	110	30	0
American Sharp	2 slices (1 oz)	100	30	0
American & Swiss	1 slice (0.6 oz)	70	15	0
Baby Swiss	1 oz	110	25	0
Chedarella	1 oz	100	25	0
Cheddar	1 oz	100	30	0
Cheddar Extra Sharp	1 oz	110	30	0
Cheddar Mild	1 slice (1 oz)	110	30	0
Cheese Spread Golden Velvet	1 oz	80	20	0
Co-Jack	1 slice (1 oz)	110	25	0
Colby	1 oz	110	30	0
Jalapeno Light	1 oz	70	15	0
Monterey Jack	1 oz	110	30	0
Mozzarella	1 oz	80	15	0
Muenster	1 oz	100	25	0
Parmesan Grated	1 tbsp	35	10	0
Provolone	1 oz	100	20	0
Swiss	1 slice (1 oz)	110	30	0
Swiss Light	1 oz	80	15	0
Laughing Cow				
Cheese Bites Light	6 pieces (0.8 oz)	35	10	0
Creamy French Onion Light	1 wedge	35	10	0
Creamy Garlic & Herb Light	1 wedge (0.7 oz)	35	10	0
Creamy Swiss Light Original	1 wedge (0.7 oz)	35	10	0
Creamy Swiss Original	1 wedge (0.7 oz)	50	15	0
Mini Babybel Bonbel	1 piece (0.7 oz)	70	20	0
Mini Babybel Gouda	1 piece (0.7 oz)	80	20	0

FOOD	PORTION	CALS	CHOL	FIBER
Mini Babybel Light Original	1 piece (0.7 oz)	50	15	0
Mini Babybel Mild Cheddar	1 piece (0.7 oz)	70	20	0
Mini Babybel Original	1 piece (0.7 oz)	70	20	0
Meza				
Baked Brie In Pastry w/ Cranberries & Spiced Almonds	1 oz	110	30	tr
Miller's				
Mozzarella	1 slice (1 oz)	81	20	0
Mont Chevre				
Assorted Crottins	1 oz	70	10	0
Mt Vikos				
Feta Sheep & Goat Milk	1 oz	80	19	0
Northfield				
Naturally Slender	1 oz	90	10	–
Organic Valley				
Aged Swiss Unpasteurized	1 oz	100	25	0
Farmer Reduced Fat	1 oz	90	15	0
Mozzarella Part Skim	1 oz	80	16	0
Polly-O				
Mozzarella Shredded	¼ cup	90	20	0
Mozzerella Part Skim	1 oz	70	15	0
Ricotta Part Skim	¼ cup	90	20	0
Ricotta Lite	¼ cup	70	10	0
String-Ums	1 stick (1 oz)	80	20	0
President				
Feta	1 in cube (1 oz)	90	15	0
Sargento				
Cheddar Extra Sharp	1 oz	110	30	0
Fancy 6 Cheese Italian Shredded	¼ cup	90	20	0
Muenster Deli Style	1 slice (0.7 oz)	80	20	0
Provolone Deli Style	1 slice (0.7 oz)	70	15	0
Reduced Fat 4 Cheese Mexican Shredded	¼ cup (1 oz)	80	20	0
String	1 piece (0.8 oz)	70	15	0
Smart Balance				
Cheddar Shredded	1 oz	80	5	0
Mozzarella Shredded	1 oz	80	5	0

FOOD	PORTION	CALS	CHOL	FIBER
Sorrento				
Mozzarella Fresh	1 oz	90	30	0
Mozzarella w/ Tomato & Basil Shredded	¼ cup	80	15	0
Pizza Cheese Shredded	¼ cup	90	20	0
Stringsters	1 stick (1 oz)	80	15	0
Suisse Delicat				
Healthy Swiss	1 oz	90	25	0
Tree of Life				
Cheddar 33% Reduced Fat Organic Milk	1 oz	90	15	–
Colby	1 oz	110	30	–
Colby Organic Milk	1 oz	120	30	–
Farmer Part-Skim Organic Milk	1 oz	90	15	–
Jalapeno Organic Milk	1 oz	110	20	–
Monterey Jack 35% Reduced Fat Organic Milk	1 oz	80	15	–
Monterey Jack Organic Milk	1 oz	100	20	–
Mozzarella Organic Milk	1 oz	80	16	–
Muenster Organic Milk	1 oz	100	25	–
Provolone	1 oz	100	20	–

CHEESE DISHES
FROZEN

FOOD	PORTION	CALS	CHOL	FIBER
Alexia				
Mozzarella Stix	2 pieces	120	15	tr
Banquet				
Mozzeralla Nuggets	6	260	40	1
Fillo Factory				
Tyropita Cheese Fillo Appetizers	5 (5 oz)	340	30	2
Health Is Wealth				
Mozzarella Stick	2 (1.3 oz)	120	15	0
TAKE-OUT				
fondue	½ cup (3.8 oz)	247	49	–
fried mozzarella sticks	3 (4.6 oz)	503	107	1
souffle	1 serv (7 oz)	504	370	1

FOOD	PORTION	CALS	CHOL	FIBER
CHEESE SUBSTITUTES				
mozzarella	1 oz	70	0	–
Yves				
Good Slice American	1 slice (0.7 oz)	35	0	0
Good Slice Cheddar	1 slice (0.7 oz)	35	0	1
Good Slice Jalapeno Jack	1 slice (0.7 oz)	35	0	0
Good Slice Mozzarella	1 slice (0.7 oz)	30	0	0
Good Slice Swiss	1 slice (0.7 oz)	35	0	0
CHERIMOYA				
fresh	1	515	0	–
CHERRIES				
CANNED				
sour in heavy syrup	½ cup	232	0	–
sour in light syrup	½ cup	189	0	–
sour water packed	1 cup	87	0	–
sweet in heavy syrup	½ cup	107	0	–
sweet in light syrup	½ cup	85	0	–
sweet juice pack	½ cup	68	0	–
sweet water pack	½ cup	57	0	–
Del Monte				
Sweet Dark Pitted In Heavy Syrup	½ cup	100	0	tr
DRIED				
bing unsulfured	¼ cup	130	0	2
montmorency tart pitted	⅓ cup	160	0	2
rainier unsulfured	⅓ cup	140	0	2
yogurt covered	¼ cup	170	0	5
Eden				
Montmorency	¼ cup	140	0	3
Frieda's				
Bing	¼ cup (1.4 oz)	120	0	3
Tart	⅓ cup (1.4 oz)	150	0	2
Good Sense				
Cherries	⅓ cup	145	0	2
Sunsweet				
Tart & Sweet	¼ cup (1.4 oz)	100	0	2
FRESH				
sour	1 cup	51	0	–
sweet	10	49	0	–

FOOD	PORTION	CALS	CHOL	FIBER
Chiquita				
Cherries	21	90	0	9
Rainier				
Sweet Premium Northwest	1 cup	90	0	3
Super Cherry				
Rainier	21	90	0	3
FROZEN				
dark sweet unsweetened	1 cup	110	0	3
sour unsweetened	1 cup	72	0	–
sweet sweetened	1 cup	232	0	–
CHERRY JUICE				
Eden				
Organic Montmorency	8 oz	140	0	0
Hi-C				
Sour Blast Wild Cherry	1 pkg	110	0	–
Wild Cherry	1 box	100	0	–
Juicy Juice				
Drink	1 box (4.23 oz)	70	0	0
Drink	1 box (8.5 oz)	140	0	0
L&A				
Black Cherry 100% Juice	8 oz	180	0	–
Minute Maid				
Coolers Clear Cherry	1 pouch (7 oz)	100	0	–
Mott's				
Cherry	1 box (8 oz)	120	0	–
Ocean Spray				
Black Cherry	8 oz	140	0	0
Squeezit				
Cherry Cola	1 bottle (7 oz)	110	0	0
CHERVIL				
seed	1 tsp	1	0	–
CHESTNUTS				
chinese steamed	3 (1 oz)	43	0	–
creme de marrons	1 oz	73	0	1
japanese roasted	1 oz	57	0	–
ready-to-eat vacuum packed	5 (1 oz)	40	0	0
roasted	3 (1 oz)	70	0	1

FOOD	PORTION	CALS	CHOL	FIBER
CHEWING GUM				
bubble gum	1 block (8 g)	27	0	–
stick	1 (3 g)	10	0	–
Aquafresh				
Peppermint	2 pieces	5	0	–
Bazooka				
Bubble Gum	1 piece (4 g)	15	0	–
Big Red				
Gum	1 piece	10	0	–
Brach's				
Abra Cabubble	1 piece	45	0	0
CareFree				
Koolerz Lemonaide	1 piece	5	0	0
Dentyne				
Ice Peppermint	2 pieces (3 g)	5	0	–
Doublemint				
Gum	1 piece	10	0	–
Eclipse				
Flash All Flavors	1 piece	0	0	–
Sugarless All Flavors	2 pieces	5	0	–
Extra				
Sugar Free All Flavors	1 piece	5	0	–
Sugar Free Bubble Gum	1 piece	5	0	–
Glee Gum				
Peppermint	2 pieces (2.5 g)	5	0	–
Hubba Bubba				
Bubble Gum Cola	1 piece	23	0	–
Bubble Gum Sugarfree Grape	1 piece	13	0	–
Bubble Gum Sugarfree Original	1 piece	14	0	–
Original	1 piece	23	0	–
Strawberry Grape Raspberry	1 piece	23	0	–
Juicy Fruit				
Gum	2 pieces	10	0	–
Orbit				
All Flavors	1 piece	5	0	0
Sugarless All Flavors	2 pieces	5	0	–

FOOD	PORTION	CALS	CHOL	FIBER
Skittles				
Bubble Gum	2 pieces	10	0	–
Speakeasy				
Natural Rainforest All Flavors	2 pieces	10	0	–
SteviaDent				
Gum	2 pieces	3	0	0
Stride				
All Flavors	1 piece	<5	0	–
Winterfresh				
Gum	1 stick	10	0	–
Thin Ice Mountain Rush	1 piece	0	0	–
Wrigley's				
Spearmint	1 stick	10	0	–
Xylichew				
Licorice	2 pieces	4	0	0

CHIA SEEDS

dried	1 oz	134	0	–

CHICKEN (see also CHICKEN DISHES, CHICKEN SUBSTITUTES, DINNER, HOT DOGS)

FOOD	PORTION	CALS	CHOL	FIBER
CANNED				
breast meat in water	2 oz	70	25	0
Valley Fresh				
Chunk White	2 oz	70	25	0
FRESH				
broiler/fryer breast w/ skin batter dipped & fried	½ breast (4.9 oz)	364	119	–
broiler/fryer breast w/ skin roasted	½ breast (3.4 oz)	193	83	0
broiler/fryer breast w/ skin stewed	½ breast (3.9 oz)	202	83	0
broiler/fryer breast w/o skin fried	½ breast (3 oz)	161	78	–
broiler/fryer breast w/o skin roasted	½ breast (3 oz)	142	73	0
broiler/fryer drumstick w/ skin batter dipped & fried	1 (2.6 oz)	193	62	–
broiler/fryer drumstick w/ skin floured & fried	1 (1.7 oz)	120	44	–

FOOD	PORTION	CALS	CHOL	FIBER
broiler/fryer drumstick w/ skin roasted	1 (1.8 oz)	112	48	0
broiler/fryer drumstick w/ skin stewed	1 (2 oz)	116	48	0
broiler/fryer drumstick w/o skin fried	1 (1.5 oz)	82	40	0
broiler/fryer drumstick w/o skin roasted	1 (1.5 oz)	76	41	0
broiler/fryer drumstick w/o skin stewed	1 (1.6 oz)	78	40	0
broiler/fryer leg w/ skin batter dipped & fried	1 (5.5 oz)	431	142	–
broiler/fryer leg w/ skin floured & fried	1 (3.9 oz)	285	105	–
broiler/fryer leg w/ skin roasted	1 (4 oz)	265	105	0
broiler/fryer leg w/ skin stewed	1 (4.4 oz)	275	105	0
broiler/fryer leg w/o skin fried	1 (3.3 oz)	195	93	–
broiler/fryer leg w/o skin roasted	1 (3.3 oz)	182	89	0
broiler/fryer leg w/o skin stewed	1 (3.5 oz)	187	90	0
broiler/fryer neck w/ skin stewed	1 (1.3 oz)	94	27	0
broiler/fryer neck w/o skin stewed	1 (.6 oz)	32	14	0
broiler/fryer skin floured & fried	from ½ chicken (2 oz)	281	41	–
broiler/fryer skin roasted	from ½ chicken (2 oz)	254	46	0
broiler/fryer skin stewed	from ½ chicken (2.5 oz)	261	45	0
broiler/fryer thigh w/ skin batter dipped & fried	1 (3 oz)	238	80	–
broiler/fryer thigh w/ skin floured & fried	1 (2.2 oz)	162	60	–
broiler/fryer thigh w/ skin roasted	1 (2.2 oz)	153	58	0

FOOD	PORTION	CALS	CHOL	FIBER
broiler/fryer thigh w/ skin stewed	1 (2.4 oz)	158	57	0
broiler/fryer thigh w/o skin fried	1 (1.8 oz)	113	53	–
broiler/fryer thigh w/o skin roasted	1 (1.8 oz)	109	49	0
broiler/fryer thigh w/o skin stewed	1 (1.9 oz)	107	49	0
broiler/fryer w/ skin floured & fried	½ chicken (11 oz)	844	283	–
broiler/fryer w/ skin fried	½ chicken (16.4 oz)	1347	404	–
broiler/fryer w/ skin roasted	½ chicken (10.5 oz)	715	263	0
broiler/fryer w/ skin stewed	½ chicken (11.7 oz)	730	262	0
broiler/fryer w/ skin neck & giblets batter dipped & fried	1 chicken (2.3 lbs)	2987	1054	–
broiler/fryer w/ skin neck & giblets roasted	1 chicken (1.5 lbs)	1598	730	–
broiler/fryer w/ skin neck & giblets stewed	1 chicken (1.6 lbs)	1625	726	–
broiler/fryer w/o skin fried	1 cup	307	131	–
broiler/fryer w/o skin roasted	1 cup (5 oz)	266	125	0
broiler/fryer w/o skin stewed	1 cup (5 oz)	248	116	0
broiler/fryer wing w/ skin batter dipped & fried	1 (1.7 oz)	159	39	–
broiler/fryer wing w/ skin floured & fried	1 (1.1 oz)	103	26	–
broiler/fryer wing w/ skin roasted	1 (1.2 oz)	99	29	0
broiler/fryer wing w/ skin stewed	1 (1.4 oz)	100	28	0
capon w/ skin neck & giblets roasted	1 chicken (3.1 lbs)	3211	1458	–
cornish hen w/ skin roasted	1 hen (8 oz)	595	299	0
cornish hen w/o skin & bone roasted	1 hen (3.8 oz)	144	113	–
cornish hen w/o skin & bone roasted	½ hen (2 oz)	72	57	–

FOOD	PORTION	CALS	CHOL	FIBER
cornish hen w/skin roasted	½ hen (4 oz)	296	149	–
roaster dark meat w/o skin roasted	1 cup (5 oz)	250	104	–
roaster light meat w/o skin roasted	1 cup (5 oz)	214	105	–
roaster w/ skin neck & giblets roasted	1 chicken (2.4 lbs)	2363	1003	–
roaster w/ skin roasted	½ chicken (1.1 lbs)	1071	365	0
roaster w/o skin roasted	1 cup (5 oz)	469	160	0
stewing dark meat w/o skin stewed	1 cup (5 oz)	361	132	–
stewing w/ skin neck & giblets stewed	1 chicken (1.3 lbs)	1636	603	–
stewing w/ skin stewed	½ chicken (9.2 oz)	744	205	0
Amish Select				
Boneless Skinless Breast w/ Honey Dijon Mustard	1 serv (4 oz)	130	60	0
Murray's				
Breast Boneless & Skinless	4 oz	110	70	0
Ground	3 oz	130	90	0
Whole Lean	4 oz	170	90	0
Perdue				
Boneless Skinless Breasts Cooked	3 oz	110	70	0
Boneless Breast Roasted Garlic Herb	1 piece (3 oz)	90	50	–
Breaded Breast Strips Barbecue	3 oz	120	30	–
Breaded Breast Strips Hot & Spicy	3 oz	110	30	–
Breaded Breast Strips Original	3 oz	120	35	–
Burger Cooked	1 (3 oz)	160	110	–
Chicken Breast Seasoned Italian Cooked	1 piece (3 oz)	90	50	–
Chicken Breast Seasoned Teriyaki Cooked	1 piece (3 oz)	90	50	–
Ground Cooked	3 oz	170	125	–
Ground Breast Cooked	3 oz	80	55	0
Honey Rotisserie Dark Meat	3 oz	200	80	–

FOOD	PORTION	CALS	CHOL	FIBER
Honey Rotisserie White Meat	3 oz	140	70	–
Oven Stuffer Dark Meat Roasted	3 oz	210	100	0
Oven Stuffer Drumstick Roasted	1 (3.6 oz)	190	120	0
Oven Stuffer White Meat Roasted	3 oz	170	80	0
Oven Stuffer Wingette Roasted	3 (3.4 oz)	220	120	0
Ovenables Breast Lemon Pepper Cooked	1 piece (3 oz)	90	50	–
Seasoned Roasting Chicken Toasted Garlic Dark Meat	3 oz	190	100	–
Seasoned Roasting Chicken Toasted Garlic White Meat	3 oz	160	75	–
Seasoned Strips Parmesan Garlic cooked	3 oz	100	55	–
Seasoned Strips Savory Classic cooked	3 oz	90	55	–
Seasoned Strips Spicy Fiesta cooked	3 oz	140	75	–
Split Breast Cooked	1 piece (6.8 oz)	370	180	0
Thin Sliced Breast Rosemary Garlic Thyme	1 piece (3 oz)	90	60	–
Thin Sliced Breast Tomato Herb	1 piece (3 oz)	90	60	–
Whole Dark Meat cooked	3 oz	150	110	0
Whole White Meat Cooked	3 oz	170	85	0
Wings Roasted	2 (3.2 oz)	210	115	0
Wampler				
Breast Tenders	4 oz	130	70	0
FROZEN				
Banquet				
Breast Nuggets	7	280	40	1
Breast Patties Grilled Honey BBQ	1	110	40	0
Breast Patties Grilled Honey Mustard	1	120	25	0
Breast Tenders Our Original	3	250	40	tr
Breast Tenders Southern	3 pieces	260	40	1

FOOD	PORTION	CALS	CHOL	FIBER
Country Fried	1 serv (3 oz)	270	65	1
Fat Free Baked Breast Patties	1	100	20	1
Fried Our Original	1 serv (3 oz)	280	65	1
Honey BBQ Skinless Fried	1 serv (3 oz)	230	55	1
Hot 'n Spicy Fried	1 serv (3 oz)	260	65	1
Nuggets Our Original	6	270	35	1
Nuggets Southern Fried	5	270	35	2
Patties Our Orignal	1	190	30	1
Patties Southern Fried	1	190	25	tr
Skinless Fried	1 serv (3 oz)	220	65	2
Smokehouse Big Wings	2	200	70	0
Southern Fried	1 serv (3 oz)	280	65	1
Wings Firehouse Big	2	190	70	0
Wings Honey BBQ	4	380	70	1
Wings Hot & Spicy	4 pieces	280	90	tr
Bell & Evans				
Breaded Breast Nuggets	1 serv (4 oz)	190	45	1
Breaded Whole Breast Tenders	1 (4 oz)	190	45	1
Burgers	1 (3 oz)	120	85	0
Chicken Sandwich Steaks	1 serv (2 oz)	60	40	0
Country Skillet				
Bites	5	270	20	1
Breast Tenders	3	240	25	1
Chunks	5	270	20	1
Fried	3 oz	270	65	1
Nuggets	10	280	25	1
Patties	1	190	20	1
Southern Fried Chunks	5	270	20	1
Southern Fried Patties	1	190	20	1
Health Is Wealth				
Nuggets	4 (3 oz)	150	40	0
Patties	1 (3 oz)	150	40	0
Tenders	3 (3 oz)	130	35	0
Ian's				
Fingers	3 pieces	190	40	0
Nuggets	5 pieces	190	40	0
Nuggets Allergy Free	5 pieces	190	40	0
Patties	1 (3.4 oz)	220	40	0

FOOD	PORTION	CALS	CHOL	FIBER
Weaver				
Breast Strips	3 pieces	230	35	1
Breast Tenders	5 pieces	240	35	0
Buffalo Popcorn Chicken	7 pieces	230	35	1
Crispy Breast Strips	2 pieces	220	20	2
Crispy Mini Drums	5 pieces	250	40	1
Croquettes	2 + gravy	230	30	0
Honey Batter Breast Tenders	5 pieces	220	30	2
Hot Wings Buffalo Style	3 pieces	190	95	0
Nuggets	4 pieces	210	35	1
Patties Italian	1	210	20	1
Patties Breast	1	170	20	1
Patties Original	1	180	30	1
Wings Honey BBQ BB	3	200	95	–
Wellshire				
Chicken Bites Dinosaur Shaped Gluten Free	5 pieces	160	30	2
READY-TO-EAT				
chicken salad sandwich spread	¼ cup	104	16	0
Banquet				
Fat Free Baked Breast Tenders	3	120	30	2
Boar's Head				
Breast Hickory Smoked	2 oz	60	35	0
Breast Oven Roasted	2 oz	60	35	0
Butterball				
Crispy Baked Breasts Italian Style Herb	1 piece (0.5 oz)	190	55	1
Crispy Baked Breasts Lemon Pepper	1 piece (0.5 oz)	200	50	tr
Crispy Baked Breasts Original	1 piece (0.5 oz)	180	45	1
Crispy Baked Breasts Parmesan	1 piece (0.5 oz)	200	55	tr
Crispy Baked Breasts Southwestern	1 piece (0.5 oz)	170	35	2
Tenders Baked Breast	3 pieces	170	35	1

FOOD	PORTION	CALS	CHOL	FIBER
Tenders Hickory Smoked Grilled	4 pieces + sauce	160	50	1
Tenders Oriental Grilled	4 pieces + sauce	160	45	1
Carl Buddig				
Chicken Sliced	1 pkg (2.5 oz)	110	40	–
Lean Slices Honey Smoked Breast	1 pkg (2.5 oz)	70	30	–
Lean Slices Roasted Breast	1 pkg (2.5 oz)	60	30	–
Hillshire Farm				
Smoked Breast	6 slices (2 oz)	60	25	0
Perdue				
Breast Cutlets Homestyle	1 (2.9 oz)	110	35	–
Breast Cutlets Italian Style	1 (2.9 oz)	120	40	–
Breast Filets In Barbecue Sauce	1 piece + 3 tbsp sauce (5.9 oz)	200	70	–
Breast Strips In Garlic & Herb Sauce	1 serv (5 oz)	100	50	2
Breast Strips In Marinara Sauce	1 serv (5 oz)	120	50	–
Breast Strips In Teriyaki Sauce	1 serv (5 oz)	190	50	–
Carved Breast Honey Roasted	½ cup (2.5 oz)	100	45	–
Carved Breast Original Roasted	½ cup (2.5 oz)	90	50	–
Cutlets Cooked	1 (3.5 oz)	220	55	–
Nuggets	5 (3.4 oz)	210	50	–
Nuggets Chicken & Cheese	5 (3.4 oz)	230	55	–
Short Cuts Chicken Strips Fajita Style	½ cup	90	35	–
Short Cuts Grilled Chicken Breast	½ cup (2.5 oz)	90	40	–
Short Cuts Grilled Italian	½ cup	90	35	–
Short Cuts Grilled Lemon Pepper	½ cup (2.5 oz)	80	40	–
Sara Lee				
Breast Oven Roasted	2 slices (1.6 oz)	45	15	0
Tyson				
Grilled Breast Strips	1 serv (3 oz)	120	60	0

FOOD	PORTION	CALS	CHOL	FIBER
Roasted Whole Chicken w/ Skin	1 serv (3 oz)	160	75	0
TAKE-OUT				
oven roasted breast of chicken	2 oz	60	25	0

CHICKEN DISHES
CANNED
Lunch Bucket

Dumplings'n Chicken	1 pkg (7.5 oz)	140	10	1

FROZEN
Maple Leaf Farms

Chicken Breast Stuffed Broccoli & Cheese	1 serv (6 oz)	340	40	0

MIX
Chicken Skillet Helper

Stir-Fried Chicken as prep	1 cup	270	105	1

Hamburger Helper

Reduced Sodium Cheddar Spirals Chicken Recipe as prep	1 cup	240	40	0
Reduced Sodium Italian Herb Chicken Recipe as prep	1 cup	200	35	2
Reduced Sodium Southwestern Beef Chicken Recipe as prep	1 cup	220	35	2

REFRIGERATED

salad low fat	⅓ cup	90	20	–

Lloyd's

Barbecue Shredded Chicken	¼ cup (2 oz)	90	15	–

Old El Paso

For Tacos Shredded Chicken	¼ cup	60	25	1

Oscar Mayer

Lunchables Chicken Wraps	1 pkg	440	40	3

Tyson

Chicken Breast Medallions In Tomato & Herb Sauce	1 serv (5 oz)	120	40	0

Wellshire

Shredded Chicken In BBQ Sauce	¼ cup	70	20	0

FOOD	PORTION	CALS	CHOL	FIBER
SHELF-STABLE				
TastyBite				
Chicken Moglai	1 pkg (9.5 oz)	300	45	3
TAKE-OUT				
boneless breast w/ apple stuffing	1 serv (5 oz)	260	80	1
breast & wing breaded & fried	2 pieces (5.7 oz)	494	149	–
chicken & dumplings	¾ cup	256	109	tr
chicken & noodles	1 cup	365	103	–
chicken a la king	1 cup	470	221	–
chicken cacciatore	¾ cup	394	99	2
chicken paprikash	1½ cups	296	90	–
chicken cordon bleu	1 serv (5 oz)	280	70	0
chicken curry	1 serv (½ breast)	160	45	1
chicken curry boneless	1 serv (6.2 oz)	219	62	2
chicken curry leg & thigh	1 serv	180	51	1
chicken satay + peanut sauce	2 skewers	239	64	1
drumstick breaded & fried	2 pieces (5.2 oz)	430	165	–
grilled breast strips	4 strips (3 oz)	100	50	0
groundnut stew hkatenkwan	1 serv (15.7 oz)	576	116	4
jamaican jerk wings	4 wings (9.9 oz)	709	172	tr
kobete turkish chicken w/ pastry	1 serv	513	71	–
sancocho de pollo dominican chicken stew	1 serv	702	195	1
thigh breaded & fried	2 pieces (5.2 oz)	430	165	–

CHICKEN SUBSTITUTES

FOOD	PORTION	CALS	CHOL	FIBER
Boca				
Chik'n Nuggets	1 serv (3 oz)	180	0	3
Chik'n Patties	1 (2.5 oz)	160	0	2
Health Is Wealth				
Buffalo Wings	3 pieces (2.2 oz)	100	0	3
Chicken-Free Nuggets	3 pieces (2.25 oz)	90	0	2
Chicken-Free Patties	1 (3 oz)	120	0	2
Lightlife				
Smart Cutlet Seasoned Chicken	1 (4 oz)	180	0	4

FOOD	PORTION	CALS	CHOL	FIBER
Smart Menu Chick'n Nuggets	4 pieces	220	0	2
Smart Menu Chick'n Patties	1 patty	160	0	2
Smart Menu Chick'n Strips	1 serv (3 oz)	80	0	3
Loma Linda				
Fried Chik'n w/ Gravy	2 pieces (2.8 oz)	150	0	2
Morningstar Farms				
Chik'n Roasted Herb	1 pattie (2.2 oz)	110	0	2
Meal Starters Chik'n Strips	12 pieces (3 oz)	140	0	1
Quorn				
Cutlets	1 (3.5 oz)	200	0	4
Gruyere Cutlet	1 (4 oz)	260	20	3
Naked Cutlet	1 (2.4 oz)	80	5	2
Nuggets	3-4 pieces (3 oz)	180	0	3
Patties	1 patty (2.6 oz)	160	0	3
Tenders	1 cup (3 oz)	90	0	3
Viana				
Veggie Chickin Fillets	1 (3.7 oz)	260	0	4
Veggie Chickin Nuggets	3 pieces (2.6 oz)	200	0	2
Worthington				
FriChik Original	2 pieces (3.2 oz)	140	0	1
Meatless Chicken Style	1 slice (2 oz)	90	0	1
Yves				
Veggie Chicken Burgers	1 (3 oz)	120	0	3

CHICKPEAS
CANNED
chickpeas	1 cup	285	0	–
Eden				
Organic Garbanzo	½ cup	130	0	5
Progresso				
Chick Peas	½ cup (4.6 oz)	120	0	5
Garbanzo	½ cup (4.4 oz)	110	0	5

DRIED
cooked	1 cup	269	0	–

REFRIGERATED
Sabra
Balela Vinaigrette	2 oz	100	0	3
Spicy Armenian Salad	2 oz	50	0	1

CHICORY
endive fresh chopped	½ cup	4	0	–

FOOD	PORTION	CALS	CHOL	FIBER
greens raw chopped	½ cup	21	0	–
root raw	1 (2.1 oz)	44	0	–
roots raw cut up	½ cup (1.6 oz)	33	0	–
witloof head raw	1 (1.9 oz)	9	0	–
witloof raw	½ cup (1.6 oz)	8	0	–
Frieda's				
Belgian Endive	2 cups	115	0	3

CHILI

FOOD	PORTION	CALS	CHOL	FIBER
chili w/ beans	1 cup	286	43	–
powder	1 tsp	8	0	–
Amy's				
Chili & Cornbread	1 pkg (10.5 oz)	320	10	8
Organic Black Bean	1 cup	200	0	15
Organic Medium	1 cup	190	0	7
Organic Medium w/ Vegetables	1 cup	190	0	8
Boca				
Chili w/ Ground Burger	1 pkg (9.4 oz)	150	0	12
Bush's				
ChiliMagic Chili Starter as prep	1 cup	250	55	4
Original No Beans	1 cup	240	25	3
Carroll Shelby's				
Original Texas Chili Kit	2 tbsp	60	0	0
Chef Boyardee				
Chili Mac	½ can (7 oz)	260	30	3
Del Monte				
Sauce	1 tbsp	20	0	0
Fantastic				
3 Bean	1 pkg (8 oz)	180	0	5
Vegetarian Mix not prep	¼ cup	100	0	4
Gebhardt				
Chili Powder	¼ tsp (0.3 g)	1	0	tr
Chili Quik Seasoning	1 tbsp (0.3 oz)	43	0	2
Plain	1 cup (9.4 oz)	232	0	3
With Beans	1 cup (9.4 oz)	322	29	15
Gringo Billy's				
Chili Mix	1 tbsp	24	0	2

FOOD	PORTION	CALS	CHOL	FIBER
Hunt's				
Chili Beans	½ cup (4.5 oz)	87	0	6
Family Favorites Chili	¼ cup (2.2 oz)	25	0	1
Instant India				
Chili Ginger Paste	2 tbsp (1 oz)	90	0	0
Just Rite				
With Beans	1 cup (9 oz)	379	35	13
Lean Cuisine				
Cafe Classics Three Bean Chili	1 pkg (10 oz)	260	10	8
Lightlife				
Smart Chili	1 pkg	200	0	12
Lunch Bucket				
Chili With Beans	1 pkg (7.5 oz)	260	25	8
Marie Callender's				
Chili & Cornbread	1 meal (16 oz)	560	60	7
McCormick				
Mexican Style Chili Powder	¼ tsp	0	0	0
Original Chili Seasoning	1⅓ tbsp (9 g)	30	0	2
Nature's Entree				
Texas Chili	1 pkg (12 oz)	320	15	11
Open Range				
Plain	1 cup (8.8 oz)	353	48	6
With Beans	1 cup (9 oz)	281	26	10
Pacific Foods				
Beef Steak w/ Beans	1 cup	250	35	8
Ro-Tel				
Chili Fixin's	½ cup	35	0	3
Soy7				
Chili Mix as prep	1 cup	150	0	7
Stagg				
Chunkero w/ Beans	1 cup	300	45	5
Classic w/ Beans	1 cup	310	35	6
Country Blend	1 cup	330	40	6
Country Blend w/ Beans	1 cup	33	40	6
Ranch House Chicken w/ Beans	1 cup	290	50	6
Silverado Beef w/ Beans	1 cup	230	45	6
Turkey Ranchero w/ Beans	1 cup	240	35	6
Vegetable Garden Four Bean	1 cup	200	0	7

FOOD	PORTION	CALS	CHOL	FIBER
Van Camp's				
Beanee Weenee Chilee	1 cup (7.7 oz)	240	35	9
Chili With Beans	1 cup (8.9 oz)	350	45	7
Mexican Style Chili Beans	½ cup (4.6 oz)	110	0	8
Wick Fowler's				
2 Alarm Chili Kit	3 tbsp	60	0	0
False Alarm Chili Kit	2 tbsp	50	0	0
Worthington				
Vegetarian	1 cup	280	0	8
Yves				
Veggie Chili	1 pkg (10.5 oz)	230	0	14
TAKE-OUT				
chiles rellenos cheese filled	1 (5 oz)	365	167	1

CHILI PEPPER (see PEPPERS)

CHINESE FOOD (see ASIAN FOOD)

CHINESE PRESERVING MELON

cooked	½ cup	11	0	–

CHIPS (see also SNACKS)

apple chips	10	101	0	2
corn	1 oz	153	0	1
corn cones	1 oz	145	0	–
potato	1 oz	152	0	–
potato light	1 oz	134	0	–
potato sticks	1 pkg (1 oz)	148	0	–
potato sticks	½ cup (0.6 oz)	94	0	1
taro	10 (0.8 oz)	115	0	–
tortilla	1 oz	142	0	2
tortilla nacho	1 oz	141	0	2
tortilla nacho light	1 oz	126	0	–
tortilla ranch	1 oz	139	0	–
Atkins				
Crunchers Barbeque	1 pkg (1 oz)	100	0	4
Crunchers Nacho Cheese	1 pkg (1 oz)	100	0	3
Crunchers Original	1 pkg (1 oz)	90	0	4
Crunchers Sour Cream & Onion	1 pkg (1 oz)	100	5	3

FOOD	PORTION	CALS	CHOL	FIBER
Bachman				
Potato Golden Crisp	1 pkg (1 oz)	150	0	0
Barbara's Bakery				
Potato	1¼ cup (1 oz)	150	0	1
Potato No Salt Added	1¼ cups (1 oz)	150	0	1
Potato Ripple	1¼ cup (1 oz)	150	0	1
Potato Yogurt & Green Onion	1¼ cup (1 oz)	150	0	1
Tortilla Blue Corn	15 (1 oz)	140	0	1
Tortilla Blue Corn No Salt	15 (1 oz)	140	0	1
Tortilla Pinta Salsa	15 (1 oz)	130	0	2
Bravos!				
Tortilla Nacho Cheese	1 oz	150	0	1
Bruno & Luigi's				
Pasta Chips Garlic & Herb	1 oz	117	0	1
Cape Cod				
Potato 40% Reduced Fat	19	130	0	1
Potato Beachside BBQ	19	150	0	1
Potato Classic	19	150	0	1
Potato Fresh Garden Herb Reduced Fat	19	130	0	1
Potato Jalapeno & Cheddar	19	140	0	3
Potato No Salt	19	150	0	tr
Potato Robust Russet	19	150	0	1
Potato Salt & Vinegar	19	150	0	1
Potato Sea Salt & Cracked Pepper	19	140	0	1
Tortilla Reduced Carb	10	140	0	2
Tortilla Veggie	12	140	0	1
Corazonas				
Tortilla Jalapeno Jack	1 oz	140	0	3
Tortilla Original	1 oz	140	0	3
Tortilla Salsa Picante	1 oz	140	0	3
Deliciously Slim				
Tortilla Black Bean & Sour Cream	1 oz	140	0	5
Tortilla Lightly Salted	1 oz	140	0	5
Tortilla Ranch	1 oz	140	0	5
Doritos				
Baked Cooler Ranch	15 (1 oz)	120	0	2
Baked Nacho Cheesier	15	120	0	2

FOOD	PORTION	CALS	CHOL	FIBER
Cooler Ranch	12	140	0	1
Four Cheese	12	140	0	1
Guacamole	12	150	0	1
Light Nacho Cheesier	11	90	0	1
Natural White Nacho Cheese	11	150	0	1
Ranchero	12	150	0	1
Rollitos Cooler Ranch	17	140	0	1
Rollitos Zesty Taco	17	150	0	1
Toasted Corn	13	140	0	1
Durangos				
Tortilla	15 (1 oz)	150	0	2
Eatsmart				
Cafe Fries Malt Vinegar & Sea Salt	1 oz	150	0	–
Cafe Fries Tangy Tomato & Spices	1 oz	150	0	–
CheddAirs	1 oz	135	0	–
Soy Crisps Parmesan Garlic & Olive Oil	1 oz	160	0	–
Soy Crisps Tomato Romano & Olive Oil	1 oz	160	0	–
Veggie Crisps	1 oz	140	0	–
Veggie Crisps Cheddar & Jalapeno	1 oz	130	0	–
Veggie Crisps Sundried Tomato & Pesto	1 oz	140	0	–
Eden				
Brown Rice Chips	25	150	0	0
Sea Vegetable Chips	25	140	0	0
Vegetable	25	130	0	0
Wasabi	25	130	0	0
French's				
Potato Sticks Barbecue	¾ cup	160	0	1
Potato Sticks Cheddar	¾ cup	170	0	tr
Potato Sticks Original	¾ cup	190	0	1
Fritos				
Corn Chips King Size	12	160	0	1
Original	32	160	0	1
Scoops	10	160	0	1
Twists	23	150	0	1

FOOD	PORTION	CALS	CHOL	FIBER
Garden Of Eatin'				
Organic Pita Baked Brown Sugar & Cinnamon	8	120	0	1
Organic Tortilla Blue Corn	7	140	0	2
Organic Tortilla Blue No Salt Added	16	140	0	2
Organic Tortilla White Corn	7	140	0	2
GeniSoy				
Soy Crisps	1 oz	110	0	2
Soy Crisps Apple Cinnamon Crunch	1 oz	120	0	2
Soy Crisps Creamy Ranch	1 oz	110	0	2
Soy Crisps Deep Sea Salt	1 oz	110	0	2
Soy Crisps Rich Cheddar Cheese	1 oz	110	0	2
Soy Crisps Roasted Garlic & Onion	1 oz	100	0	2
Soy Crisps Zesty Barbeque	1 oz	110	0	2
Glenny's				
Soy Crisps Caramel	½ pkg (1.3 oz)	70	0	1
Veggie Fries	½ pkg (0.6 oz)	70	0	0
Zen Health Tortilla Crisps Original	1 oz	110	0	tr
Guiltless Gourmet				
Potato Au Gratin	1 oz	100	0	3
Potato Pico De Gallo	1 oz	100	0	3
Potato Sea Salt	1 oz	90	0	3
Tortilla Chili Lime	18 (1 oz)	110	0	2
Tortilla Chili Verde	18 (1 oz)	120	0	2
Tortilla Chipotle	18 (1 oz)	120	0	2
Tortilla Red Corn	18 (1 oz)	110	0	2
Tortilla Spicy Black Bean	18 (1 oz)	110	0	2
Tortilla Sweet White Corn	18 (1 oz)	110	0	2
Tortilla Yellow Corn Unsalted	18 (1 oz)	110	0	2
Herr's				
Potato	1 oz	140	0	1
Husman's				
Deli Style Tortilla	11	150	0	1
Potato	18 (1 oz)	160	0	1

FOOD	PORTION	CALS	CHOL	FIBER
Potato Sour Cream & Onion	18 (1 oz)	150	0	1
Potato Sweet N'Sassy	18 (1 oz)	155	0	1
Keto				
Low Carb Tortilla All Flavors	1 oz	150	0	4
Kettle				
Bakes Potato Aged White Cheddar	1 oz	120	0	2
Bakes Potato Hickory Honey Barbeque	1 oz	120	0	2
Bakes Potato Lightly Salted	1 oz	120	0	2
Krinkle Cut Potato Barbeque	1 oz	150	0	2
Krinkle Cut Potato Dill & Sour Cream	1 oz	150	0	2
Krinkle Cut Potato Lightly Salted	1 oz	150	0	2
Krinkle Cut Potato Salt & Fresh Ground Pepper	1 oz	150	0	2
Organic Tortilla Blue Corn	1 oz	140	0	2
Organic Tortilla Brown Rice & Black Bean w/ Garlic & Onions	1 oz	120	0	2
Organic Tortilla Fire Roasted Chili	1 oz	140	0	2
Organic Tortilla Five Grain Yellow Corn	1 oz	140	0	2
Organic Tortilla Lightly Salted Yellow Corn	1 oz	140	0	2
Organic Tortilla Little Dippers	1 oz	140	0	2
Organic Tortilla Sesame Blue Moons	1 oz	150	0	2
Potato Cheddar Beer	1 oz	150	0	1
Potato Honey Dijon	1 oz	150	0	1
Potato Sea Salt & Vinegar	1 oz	150	0	1
Potato Spicy Thai	1 oz	150	0	1
Potato Unsalted	1 oz	150	0	2
Potato Yogurt & Green Onion	1 oz	150	0	1
Lay's				
Baked KC Masterpiece	11 (1 oz)	120	0	2
Baked Sour Cream & Onion	12 (1 oz)	120	0	2
Chile Limon	1 oz	150	0	1

FOOD	PORTION	CALS	CHOL	FIBER
Classic	1 pkg (1 oz)	150	0	1
Deli Style Original	17 (1 oz)	150	0	1
Dill Pickle	20 (1 oz)	160	0	1
Flamin' Hot	17 (1 oz)	160	0	1
KC Masterpiece BBQ	15 (1 oz)	150	0	1
Kettle Cooked Jalapeno	15 (1 oz)	140	0	1
Kettle Cooked Mesquite BBQ	18 (1 oz)	140	0	tr
Kettle Cooked Original	22 (1 oz)	150	0	1
Kettle Cooked Sea Salt & Vinegar	18 (1 oz)	140	0	1
Light Fat Free KC Masterpiece	20 (1 oz)	75	0	1
Light Fat Free Original	20 (1 oz)	75	0	1
Limon	17 (1 oz)	150	0	1
Natural Country BBQ	14 (1 oz)	150	0	1
Natural Sea Salt & Vinegar	16 (1 oz)	150	0	tr
Natural Sea Salted	16 (1 oz)	150	0	tr
Original Baked	11 (1 oz)	110	0	2
Salt & Vinegar	17 (1 oz)	150	0	1
Sour Cream & Onion	17 (1 oz)	160	<5	1
Stax	13 (1 oz)	160	0	1
Wavy	11 (1 oz)	150	0	1
Wavy Au Gratin	13 (1 oz)	150	<5	1
Wavy Hickory Barbecue	13 (1 oz)	150	0	1
Wavy Ranch	12 (1 oz)	150	0	1
Madhouse Munchies				
Potato Creamy French Onion	16	150	0	1
Potato Sea Salted	16	150	0	1
Tortilla White	9	140	0	1
Manny's				
Organic Tortilla Blues	1 oz	150	0	3
Tortilla No Salt Added	1 oz	150	0	3
Maui				
Shrimp Chips	17	140	0	tr
Met-Rx				
Pro Chips Bar-B-Que	1 pkg (2 oz)	260	0	0
Pro Chips Nacho	1 pkg (2 oz)	260	0	0
Moore's				
Corn Chips	1 oz	160	0	1

FOOD	PORTION	CALS	CHOL	FIBER
New York Deli				
Potato Kettle Cooked	1 oz	150	0	1
Old Dutch Foods				
Potato	12-15 (1 oz)	150	0	1
Potato BBQ	12-15 (1 oz)	150	0	1
Potato BBQ Ripple	12-15 (1 oz)	150	0	tr
Potato Cajun Ripple	12-15 (1 oz)	150	0	1
Potato Cheddar & Sour Cream Ripple	12-15 (1 oz)	160	0	1
Potato Dill	12-15 (1 oz)	140	0	1
Potato Dutch Crunch	15-20 (1 oz)	130	0	2
Potato French Onion Ripple	12-15 (1 oz)	150	0	1
Potato Jalapeno & Cheddar Dutch Crunch	15-20 (1 oz)	130	0	1
Potato Jalapeno Cheese	12-15 (1 oz)	150	0	1
Potato Mesquite BBQ Dutch Crunch	15-20 (1 oz)	130	0	2
Potato Onion & Garlic	12-15 (1 oz)	140	0	1
Potato Outback Spicy BBQ	12-15 (1 oz)	150	0	1
Potato Ripples	12-15 (1 oz)	150	0	1
Potato Salt & Vinegar Dutch Crunch	15-20 (1 oz)	130	0	1
Potato Sour Cream & Onion	12-15 (1 oz)	150	0	1
Tortilla Bite Size White Corn	20 (1 oz)	150	0	1
Tortilla Nacho Cheese	15 (1 oz)	150	0	1
Tortilla Restaurant Style White	9 (1 oz)	140	0	2
Tostados White Corn	11 (1 oz)	140	0	2
Tostados Yellow	11 (1 oz)	140	0	1
Pita-Snax				
Cheddar Cheese	34 (1 oz)	110	0	tr
Chili & Lime	34 (1 oz)	120	0	tr
Cinnamon	34 (1 oz)	120	0	tr
Dill Ranch	34 (1 oz)	120	0	tr
Garlic	34 (1 oz)	120	0	tr
Lightly Salted	34 (1 oz)	110	0	tr
Pringles				
Jalapeno	15 (1 oz)	150	0	tr
Loaded Baked Potato	15 (1 oz)	150	0	tr
Minis Cheddar Cheese	1 pkg	120	0	tr

FOOD	PORTION	CALS	CHOL	FIBER
Minis Original	1 pkg	120	0	tr
Original	14 (1 oz)	160	0	tr
Pizza	15 (1 oz)	150	0	tr
Select Cinnamon Sweet Potato	28 (1 oz)	150	0	1
Select Parmesan Garlic	28 (1 oz)	140	0	tr
Snack Stacks Original	1 pkg	140	0	tr
Racquet				
Wheat Chips All Flavors	6 chips	30	0	0
Revival				
Baked Soy Pasta Chips Lightly Salted Sunshine	1 bag (0.9 oz)	100	0	0
Baked Soy Pasta Chips Naturally Nice	1 bag (0.9 oz)	80	0	0
Baked Soy Pasta Chips Rev It Up Ranch	1 bag (0.9 oz)	105	0	0
Ruffles				
Baked Original	10	120	0	2
Cheddar & Sour Cream	11	160	0	1
KC Masterpiece Mesquite BBQ	11	150	0	1
Light Cheddar & Sour Cream	15	75	0	1
Light Original	17	70	0	1
Original	12	160	0	1
Potato Crisps	16	160	0	1
Reduced Fat Sea Salted	15	140	0	1
Sour Cream & Onion	11	160	0	1
Santitas				
White Corn	9	130	0	1
Yellow Corn	9	130	0	1
Skinny				
BBQ	1½ cups	90	0	1
Corn	1½ cups	90	0	1
Nacho Cheese	1½ cups	90	0	1
Sour Cream & Onion	1½ cups	90	0	1
Sticks Garden Veggie	1 oz	140	0	1
Sticks Island Lime Chili	1 oz	140	0	1
Sticks Maui Wowie	1 oz	140	0	1
Sticks Original Spud	1 oz	140	0	1

FOOD	PORTION	CALS	CHOL	FIBER
Snyder's Of Hanover				
Barbeque Corn	1.5 oz	230	0	2
BBQ Rib	1 oz	140	0	tr
Cheddar Bacon	1 oz	150	0	3
Corn Chips	1.5 oz	230	0	2
Grilled Steak & Onion	1 oz	140	0	4
Hot Buffalo	1 oz	150	0	4
Kosher Dill	1 oz	140	0	3
No Salt	1 oz	140	0	3
Potato	1 oz	140	0	3
Ripple	1 oz	140	0	4
Salt & Vinegar	1 oz	140	0	4
Sausage Pizza	1 oz	150	0	4
Sour Cream & Onion	1 oz	150	0	4
Tasty Veggie Potato Chips	1 oz	150	0	4
Tortilla Nacho	1 oz	140	0	1
Tortilla No Salt Yellow Corn	1 oz	140	0	1
Tortilla White Corn	1 oz	140	0	1
Tortilla Yellow Corn	1 oz	140	0	1
Tortilla Yellow Corn Mini	1 oz	160	0	1
Veggie Crisps	1 pkg (1.5 oz)	190	0	2
Solea				
Polenta Corn	1 oz	120	0	0
Potato Olive Oil Sea Salt	1 oz	120	0	1
Soya King				
Soy Mongolian BBQ	23 (1 oz)	140	0	3
Soy Original	23 (1 oz)	140	0	3
Soy Sour Cream & Onion	23 (1 oz)	140	0	3
Soy Taco	23 (1 oz)	140	0	3
Stacy's				
Pita Chips Multigrain	1 pkg	140	0	2
Pita Chips Parmesan Garlic & Herb	1 oz	140	0	2
Pita Chips Texarkana Hot	1 oz	130	0	2
Soy Thin Chips Sticky Bun	18 (1 oz)	130	0	3
Soy Thin Crisps Simply Cheese	18 (1 oz)	130	0	3
Sunchips				
French Onion	10	140	0	2
Harvest Cheddar	10	140	0	2

FOOD	PORTION	CALS	CHOL	FIBER
Tastee				
Potato Yukon Gold	1 oz	130	0	1
Terra				
Parsnip Chips	12	150	0	5
Potato Unsalted Au Natural	18	150	0	2
Potato Unsalted Hickory BBQ	16	150	0	1
Potato Unsalted Lemon Pepper	16	150	0	1
Spiced Sweet Potato	1 pkg (0.5 oz)	190	0	3
Torengos				
Chips	13 (1 oz)	140	0	1
Tostitos				
Blue Corn	6	140	0	1
Crispy Rounds	13	140	0	1
Gold	6	140	0	1
Light Restaurant Style	6	90	0	1
Original Bite Size	20	110	0	2
Restaurant Style	6	130	0	1
Santa Fe	7	140	0	1
Scoops	13	140	0	1
Yellow Corn	6	140	0	1
Utz				
Baked Crisps	12 (1 oz)	110	0	2
No Salt Added	20 (1 oz)	150	0	1
Tortilla Low Fat Baked	10 (1 oz)	120	0	2
Wavy	20 (1 oz)	150	0	1
Wise				
Dipsy Doodles Corn Chips	1 oz	160	0	1
Potato	1 pkg (1 oz)	150	0	1
Potato Lightly Salted	1 oz	150	0	1
Potato Ridgies	1 oz	150	0	1
Potato Unsalted	1 oz	150	0	1
CHITTERLINGS				
pork cooked	3 oz	258	122	0
CHIVES				
freeze-dried	1 tbsp	1	0	–
fresh chopped	1 tbsp	1	0	–
fresh chopped	1 tsp	0	0	–

FOOD	PORTION	CALS	CHOL	FIBER

CHOCOLATE (see also CANDY, CHOCOLATE SPREAD, CHOCOLATE SYRUP, COCOA, HOT COCOA, ICE CREAM TOPPINGS, MILK DRINKS)

BAKING

FOOD	PORTION	CALS	CHOL	FIBER
baking	1 oz	145	0	–
grated unsweetened	¼ cup	165	0	6
liquid unsweetened	1 oz	134	0	5
mexican	1 sq (0.7 oz)	85	0	1
squares unsweetened	1 sq (1 oz)	145	0	5
Love'n Bake				
Chocolate Schmear	2 tbsp	140	0	2
Nestle				
Choco Bake	0.5 oz	80	0	2
Premier White Bar	0.5 oz	80	<5	0
Premier White Morsels	1 tbsp	80	0	0
Semi-Sweet Bar	0.5 oz	70	0	tr
Unsweetened Bar	0.5 oz	80	0	2
CHIPS				
milk chocolate	1 cup (6 oz)	862	38	–
semisweet	60 pieces (1 oz)	136	0	–
Baker's				
Chocolate Chunks	13 pices (0.5 oz)	70	0	tr
Cloud Nine				
Double Dark Chocolate	13 pieces (0.5 oz)	80	5	0
Ghirardelli				
Semi-Sweet	33 pieces (0.5 oz)	70	0	tr
Hershey's				
Holiday Baking Bits	1 tbsp	70	0	–
Milk Chocolate	1 tbsp	80	<5	–
Mini Milk Chocolate	1 tbsp	80	0	–
Mini Kisses For Baking	11 pieces	80	<5	–
Premier White Milk Chips	1 tbsp	80	0	–
Raspberry Chips	1 tbsp	80	0	–
Semi-Sweet	1 tbsp	80	0	–
Semi-Sweet Mini	1 tbsp	80	0	–
Skor English Toffee Baking Bits	1 tbsp	70	10	–
M&M's				
Baking Bits Milk Chocolate	1 tbsp	70	5	0
Baking Bits Semi-Sweet Chocolate	1 tbsp	70	0	1

FOOD	PORTION	CALS	CHOL	FIBER
Nestle				
Crunch Baking Pieces	1½ tbsp	80	0	0
Milk Chocolate Morsels	1 tbsp	70	<5	0
Morsels Semi-Sweet	1 tbsp	70	0	tr
Semi-Sweet Mega Morsels	1 tbsp	70	0	tr
Semi-Sweet Mini Morsels	1 tbsp	70	0	tr
Sunspire				
Chocolate Sundrops	47 pieces (1.4 oz)	190	0	1
Dark Chocolate Grain Sweetened	13 pieces (0.5 oz)	70	0	1
Organic	13 pieces (0.5 oz)	70	0	0
Tropical Source				
Espresso Roast Dairy Free	13 pieces (1.5 oz)	70	0	1
Semi-Sweet Dairy Free	13 pieces (1.5 oz)	80	5	0
MIX				
powder	2-3 heaping tsp	75	0	–
powder as prep w/ whole milk	9 oz	226	33	–
Quik				
Chocolate Powder	2 tbsp (0.8 oz)	90	0	1
Chocolate Powder No Sugar	2 tbsp (0.4 oz)	40	0	2

CHOCOLATE MILK (see MILK DRINKS)

CHOCOLATE SPREAD

FOOD	PORTION	CALS	CHOL	FIBER
Twist				
Sugar Free Chocolate Spread	2 tbsp	170	0	0

CHOCOLATE SYRUP

FOOD	PORTION	CALS	CHOL	FIBER
syrup	1 cup	653	0	–
syrup as prep w/ whole milk	9 oz	232	33	–
Ah!Laska				
Organic	2 tbsp	85	0	–
Colac				
Chocolate Topping	1 tbsp	37	0	0
DaVinci Gourmet				
Sugar Free	2 tbsp	15	0	1
Hershey's				
Chocolate Fudge	1 tbsp	70	<5	–
Double Chocolate	1 tbsp	50	0	–

FOOD	PORTION	CALS	CHOL	FIBER
Lite	2 tbsp	50	0	–
Syrup	2 tbsp	100	0	–
Nesquik				
Calcium Fortified	2 tbsp	100	0	1
Quik				
Chocolate	2 tbsp (1.3 oz)	100	0	tr
Smucker's				
Sundae Syrup Chocolate	2 tbsp	110	0	1
Toll House				
Mint Chocolate	2 tbsp (1.5 oz)	130	0	1
Semi-Sweet	2 tbsp (1.5 oz)	130	0	1
Walden Farms				
Sugar Free	2 tbsp	0	0	0
Whoppers				
Chocolate Malt	2 tbsp	100	0	–
CHUTNEY				
coconut	¼ cup	74	0	2
mango	1 tbsp	54	0	tr
tomato	1 tbsp	32	0	tr
Patak's				
Major Grey	1 tbsp	60	0	0
Mango Hot	1 tbsp	60	0	0
Mango Sweet	1 tbsp	60	0	0
Wild Thyme Farms				
Apricot Cranberry Walnut	1 tbsp	15	0	–
Pineapple Peach Lime	1 tbsp	14	0	–
CILANTRO				
Dorot				
Chopped Cube frzn	1 cube (4 g)	5	0	tr
CINNAMON				
cinnamon sugar	1 tsp	16	0	tr
ground	1 tsp	6	0	–
Gringo Billy's				
Cinnamon Sweetener	½ tsp	0	0	0
CISCO				
smoked	1 oz	50	9	0

FOOD	PORTION	CALS	CHOL	FIBER
CLAMS				
CANNED				
meat only	3 oz	126	57	–
meat only	1 cup	236	107	–
Brunswick				
Baby	2 oz	50	25	0
Bumble Bee				
Baby	¼ cup	50	40	0
Chopped Or Minced	¼ cup	25	10	0
Smoked	¼ cup	130	40	0
Chicken Of The Sea				
Chopped	¼ cup	30	12	0
Minced	¼ cup	30	12	–
Whole Baby	¼ cup	30	10	0
Orleans				
Clam Juice	1 tbsp	0	0	0
Progresso				
Creamy Clam Sauce	½ cup (4.2 oz)	110	10	0
Minced	¼ cup (2.1 oz)	25	10	0
Red Clam Sauce	½ cup (4.4 oz)	60	10	1
White Clam Sauce	½ cup (4.4 oz)	150	20	0
FRESH				
cooked	3 oz	126	57	–
cooked	20 sm	133	60	–
raw	20 sm (6.3 oz)	133	60	–
raw	9 lg (6.3 oz)	133	60	–
raw	3 oz	63	29	–
TAKE-OUT				
breaded & fried	20 sm	379	115	–
CLEMENTINE JUICE				
Izze				
Sparkling Clementine	8 oz	100	0	–
CLEMENTINES				
Haddon House				
In Light Syrup	½ cup	80	0	1
Sunkist				
Fresh	2	80	0	4
Tina				
Fresh	1	50	0	3

FOOD	PORTION	CALS	CHOL	FIBER
CLOVES				
ground	1 tsp	7	0	–
COCOA (see also HOT COCOA)				
powder unsweetened	1 cup (3 oz)	197	0	29
powder unsweetened	1 tbsp (5 g)	11	0	2
Ah!Laska				
Organic	2 tbsp	100	0	5
Organic Bakers Cocoa	1 tbsp	20	0	1
Hershey's				
Cocoa	1 tbsp	20	0	–
European Cocoa	1 tbsp	20	0	–
Nestle				
Cocoa	1 tbsp	15	0	1
COCONUT				
dried sweetened flaked	1 cup	351	0	–
dried sweetened flaked canned	1 cup	341	0	–
dried sweetened shredded	1 cup	466	0	–
dried toasted	1 oz	168	0	–
dried unsweetened	1 oz	187	0	–
fresh	1 piece (1.5 oz)	159	0	4
fresh shredded	1 cup	283	0	7
Frieda's				
White	¼ cup (1.4 oz)	140	0	4
COCONUT JUICE				
coconut water fresh	1 cup	552	0	5
milk canned	1 cup	445	0	–
milk frozen	1 cup	485	0	–
A Taste Of Thai				
Coconut Milk	⅓ cup	140	0	0
Lite Coconut Milk	⅓ cup	45	0	0
Amy & Brian				
Juice	8 oz	76	0	–
Goya				
Coconut Water	1 can (11.8 oz)	120	0	tr
O.N.E.				
Natural Coconut Water	1 box (11 oz)	60	0	0

FOOD	PORTION	CALS	CHOL	FIBER
Thai Kitchen				
Milk	2 oz	124	0	0
Vita Coco				
Coconut Water	1 box (11 oz)	65	0	–
Coconut Water w/ Fruit Juice All Flavors	1 box (11 oz)	110	0	5
Zico				
Coconut Water Mango	11 oz	60	0	0
Coconut Water Natural	11 oz	60	0	0
Coconut Water Passion Fruit + Orange Peel	11 oz	60	0	0
COD				
atlantic canned	3 oz	89	47	0
atlantic canned	1 can (11 oz)	327	171	0
atlantic dried	3 oz	246	129	0
atlantic fresh cooked	3 oz	89	47	0
atlantic fresh cooked	1 fillet (6.3 oz)	189	99	0
atlantic fresh raw	3 oz	70	37	–
pacific fresh baked	3 oz	95	43	0
COFFEE (*see also* COFFEE BEVERAGES, COFFEE SUBSTITUTES)				
INSTANT				
decaffeinated as prep	8 oz	2	0	0
decaffeinated powder	1 rounded tsp	4	0	0
powder	1 rounded tsp	4	0	0
Nescafe				
Decafe	1 tsp (2 g)	0	0	0
Decafe w/ Chicory	1 tsp (2 g)	0	0	0
French Vanilla	1 tsp (2 g)	5	0	0
French Vanilla Decaf	1 tsp (2 g)	5	0	0
Hazelnut	1 tsp (2 g)	5	0	0
Irish Creme	1 tsp (2 g)	5	0	0
Regular	1 tsp (2 g)	0	0	0
With Chicory	1 tsp (2 g)	5	0	0
REGULAR				
brewed	8 oz	2	0	0
Flavia				
English Breakfast	1 bag	0	0	0
Espresso Roast	1 bag	0	0	0

FOOD	PORTION	CALS	CHOL	FIBER
French Roast	1 bag	0	0	0
French Vanilla	1 bag	0	0	0
Nescafe				
Cafe Mocha	1 can (10 oz)	140	10	1
Caffe Latte	1 can (10 oz)	130	15	1
Caffe Latte Decaffeinated	1 can (10 oz)	130	15	0
Espresso	1 tsp (2 g)	0	0	0
Espresso Cafe Latte	1 pkg (0.6 oz)	70	10	0
Espresso Cafe Mocha	1 pkg (1 oz)	110	10	1
Espresso Cappuccino	1 pkg (0.6 oz)	80	10	0
Espresso Roast	1 can (10 oz)	90	<5	0
French Vanilla	1 can (10 oz)	150	15	2
Hazelnut	1 can (10 oz)	130	15	0
Roasted Ground as prep	1 cup (6 oz)	0	0	0
Roasted Ground Decaffeinated as prep	1 cup (6 oz)	0	0	0
Revival				
Soy Caramal Corn	1 cup (8 oz)	0	0	0
Soy Hazelnut	1 cup (8 oz)	0	0	0
Soy Original Roast	1 cup (8 oz)	0	0	0
Soy Java				
All Flavors	1 tbsp	20	0	0

COFFEE BEVERAGES

FOOD	PORTION	CALS	CHOL	FIBER
AchievONE				
All Flavors	1 bottle (9.5 oz)	120	20	–
America's Best Brew				
Iced Coffee All Flavors	8 oz	110	0	–
Big Train				
Low Carb Blended Ice Mocha as prep	1 serv (16 oz)	90	0	1
Cafe Sepia				
House Blend	1 bottle (6.2 oz)	80	5	0
Mocha	1 bottle (6.2 oz)	70	0	0
Chock full o'Nuts				
New York Cappuccino French Vanilla	1 pkg (0.9 oz)	90	0	0
New York Cappuccino Hazelnut	1 pkg. (0.9 oz)	90	0	0

FOOD	PORTION	CALS	CHOL	FIBER
Cinnabon				
Latte Caramel Nut	1 can (8 oz)	170	15	1
Latte Cinnamon Vanilla	1 can (8 oz)	170	15	1
Lattes All Flavors	1 can (9.5 oz)	190	15	1
Coffee House USA				
All Flavors	1 bottle (9.5 oz)	100	15	tr
Cool Java				
Cappuccino Dark Roast	1 bottle (11 oz)	190	15	0
Cappuccino French Vanilla	1 bottle (11 oz)	190	15	0
Cappuccino Mocha	1 bottle (11 oz)	190	15	0
Double Bean Elixir				
Coffee Soda All Flavors	8 oz	90	0	–
Double Hit				
Maximum Energy Coffee Drink	1 can (12 oz)	80	0	–
Flavour Creations				
Coffee Flavoring Tablets All Flavors	1 tablet	0	0	0
Frappio				
Iced Coffee Energy Drink	1 can (15 oz)	260	30	0
Froid				
Original or French Vanilla	1 bottle (11 oz)	180	10	1
General Foods				
International Coffees Cafe Francais	1 serv	60	0	–
International Coffees Cafe Vienna	1 serv	70	0	–
International Coffees Cafe Vienna Sugar Free	1 serv	30	0	–
International Coffees French Vanilla Cafe	1 serv	60	0	–
International Coffees French Vanilla Sugar & Fat Free Decaffeinated	1 serv	30	0	–
International Coffees French Vanilla Sugar Free	1 serv	30	0	–
International Coffees Italian Cappuccino	1 serv	50	0	–

FOOD	PORTION	CALS	CHOL	FIBER
International Coffees Orange Cappuccino	1 serv	70	0	–
International Coffees Suisse Mocha	1 serv	60	0	–
International Coffees Suisse Mocha Decaffeinated Sugar Free	1 serv	30	0	–
International Coffees Suisse Mocha Sugar Free	1 serv	30	0	–
International Coffees Swiss White Chocolate	1 serv	70	0	–
International Coffees Vanilla Creme Decaffeinated Sugar Free	1 serv	35	0	–
International Coffees Vanilla Creme Decaffeinated	1 serv	60	0	–
International Coffees Viennese Chocolate Cafe	1 serv	50	0	–
Godiva				
Latte French Vanilla	1 bottle (12 oz)	200	15	0
Mocha Dark Chocolate	1 bottle (16 oz)	200	15	1
Iced 'Spresso				
Ultra Light American Vanilla	1 bottle (9.5 oz)	90	10	0
Ultra Light Expresso Latte	1 bottle (9.5 oz)	70	0	0
Jakada				
Latte Mocha	1 bottle (10.5 oz)	180	10	0
Latte Vanilla	1 bottle (10.5 oz)	180	10	0
Loco-Joe				
Iced Coffee	1 box (8.25 oz)	160	15	0
Low Carb Creations				
Cappuccino	1 cup	30	0	0
Shock				
Latte	8 oz	150	7	tr
Silk				
Coffee Soylatte	1 bottle (11 oz)	220	0	0
Sipper Sweets				
Sugar Free Low Carb Cappuccino	1 serv	50	0	0

FOOD	PORTION	CALS	CHOL	FIBER
Starbucks				
DoubleShot	1 (6.5 oz)	140	20	–
Frappuccino	1 bottle (9.5 oz)	190	12	0
Frappuccino Mocha	1 bottle (9.5 oz)	190	12	0
Frappuccino Vanilla	1 bottle (9.5 oz)	190	12	0
Stomping Grounds				
Latte Caramel not prep	⅓ cup	70	0	0
Latte Espresso not prep	⅓ cup	35	0	0
Latte Mocha not prep	⅓ cup	60	0	0
Latte Vanilla not prep	⅓ cup	60	0	0
Tully's Coffee				
Bellaccino All Flavors	1 bottle (9.5 oz)	210	20	0
Wolfgang Puck				
Gourmet Heated Lattes All Flavors	1 can (10 oz)	100	25	0
TAKE-OUT				
cafe amaretto w/ alcohol	1 serv	192	33	0
cafe au lait	1 cup (8 oz)	77	17	–
cafe brulot	1 cup	48	0	–
cafe brulot w/ alcohol	1 serv	130	0	3
cappuccino	1 cup (8 oz)	77	17	–
coffee con leche	1 cup (6 oz)	104	10	0 .
espresso	1 cup (4 oz)	2	0	0
irish coffee	1 serv (8 oz)	209	38	0
latte w/ skim milk	1 serv (13 oz)	88	4	0
latte w/ whole milk	1 serv (14 oz)	143	20	0
mocha	1 serv (17 oz)	403	29	2
turkish	1 cup (4 oz)	50	0	0

COFFEE SUBSTITUTES
Teecinno
Herbal Coffee All Flavors	1 cup	15	0	1

COFFEE WHITENERS
Coffee-Mate
Half & Half Original	2 tbsp	40	15	–
Half & Half Vanilla	2 tbsp	60	15	–
Latte Classic	2 tbsp	100	0	–
Latte Mocha	2 tbsp	90	0	–
Latte Vanilla	2 tbsp	90	0	–
Liquid All Flavors	1 tbsp	40	0	–

FOOD	PORTION	CALS	CHOL	FIBER
Liquid French Vanilla Fat Free	1 tbsp	10	5	–
Liquid Original	1 tbsp	20	0	–
Liquid Original Fat Free	1 tbsp	10	0	–
Liquid Original Low Fat	1 tbsp	10	0	–
Original Powder	1 tsp	10	0	–
Original Lite Powder	1 tsp	10	0	–
Sugar Free All Flavors	1 tbsp	15	0	–
Farmland				
Nondairy Creamer	2 tbsp	40	15	0
Hood				
Country Creamer Non Dairy	1 tbsp	20	0	0
N-Rich				
Coffee Creamer	1 tsp (2 g)	10	0	0
Silk				
Creamer	1 tbsp	15	0	0
Creamer French Vanilla	1 tbsp	20	0	0
Creamer Hazelnut	1 tbsp	15	0	0

COLESLAW
Dole
Classic Cole Slaw	1½ cups (3 oz)	25	0	2
Fresh Express				
3 Color Deli	1½ cups	20	0	2
Cole Slaw Kit as prep	2 cups	120	5	2
River Ranch				
Country Homestyle Kit	1 cup	140	6	2
Honey Dijon Peppercorn Kit	1 cup	120	9	2
Mix	1¼ cups	25	0	2
TAKE-OUT				
coleslaw w/ dressing	¾ cup	147	5	–
vinegar & oil coleslaw	3.5 oz	150	0	–

COLLARDS
fresh cooked	½ cup	17	0	–
frzn chopped cooked	½ cup	31	0	–
raw chopped	½ cup	6	0	–
Allens				
Seasoned Southern Style	½ cup	35	0	1
Glory				
Green Fresh	2 cups	25	0	3

FOOD	PORTION	CALS	CHOL	FIBER
Seasoned canned	½ cup	35	0	2
Sensibly Seasoned canned	½ cup	20	0	2

COOKIES
MIX

FOOD	PORTION	CALS	CHOL	FIBER
chocolate chip	1 (0.56 oz)	79	7	–
oatmeal	1 (0.6 oz)	74	7	tr
oatmeal raisin	1 (0.6 oz)	74	7	tr
Aunt Paula's				
Low Carb Chef Chocolate Chip as prep	1	66	2	1
Low Carb Chef Peanut Butter as prep	1	66	2	1
Betty Crocker				
Chocolate Peanut Butter as prep	1	180	18	–
Date Bar as prep	1	150	0	1
Oatmeal as prep	2	150	12	1
Big Train				
Low Carb Chocolate Chip as prep	2	140	42	4
Low Carb Peanut Butter as prep	2	140	24	4
Bob's Red Mill				
Gluten Free Chocolate Chip as prep	2	260	39	2
GoldnBrown				
Fat Free	1 (1.1 oz)	120	0	0
King Arthur				
Chocolate Chip Whole Grain not prep	2 tbsp	90	0	1
MiniCarb				
All Flavors as prep	1	110	5	5
Nature's Path				
Organic Chocolate Chip	1/10 pkg	150	0	3
READY-TO-EAT				
animal crackers	1 box (2.4 oz)	299	11	–
australian anzac biscuit	1	98	0	1
chocolate chip	1 box (1.9 oz)	233	12	–
chocolate chip low fat	1 (0.25 oz)	45	0	–

FOOD	PORTION	CALS	CHOL	FIBER
chocolate chip low sugar low sodium	1 (0.24 oz)	31	0	–
chocolate chip soft-type	1 (0.5 oz)	69	0	tr
chocolate wafer	1 (0.2 oz)	26	0	–
cream cheese	1 (1.1 oz)	141	25	tr
gingersnaps	1 (0.24 oz)	29	0	–
graham	1 sq (0.24 oz)	30	0	–
graham chocolate covered	1 (0.49 oz)	68	0	–
graham honey	1 (0.24 oz)	30	0	tr
hermits	1 (1 oz)	117	23	1
jumbles coconut	1 (1 oz)	121	26	1
ladyfingers	1 (0.38 oz)	40	40	–
macaroons	1 (0.8 oz)	97	0	–
madeleines	1 (0.8 oz)	86	46	tr
meringue	1 (0.3 oz)	20	0	0
molasses	1 (0.5 oz)	65	0	–
oatmeal	1 (0.6 oz)	81	0	1
oatmeal raisin	1 (0.6 oz)	81	0	1
oatmeal raisin low sugar no sodium	1 (0.24 oz)	31	0	–
peanut butter sandwich	1 (0.5 oz)	67	0	–
peanut butter soft-type	1 (0.5 oz)	69	0	tr
pinenut cookies	1 (1.1 oz)	134	0	1
raisin soft-type	1 (0.5 oz)	60	0	–
reginette queen's biscuit	1 (0.8 oz)	86	tr	tr
shortbread	1 (0.28 oz)	40	2	–
shortbread pecan	1 (0.49 oz)	79	5	tr
spritz	1 (0.4 oz)	42	6	tr
sugar	1 (0.52 oz)	72	8	–
sugar low sugar sodium free	1 (0.24 oz)	30	0	–
sugar wafers w/ creme filling	1 (0.12 oz)	18	0	–
sugar wafers w/ creme filling sugar free sodium free	1 (0.14 oz)	20	0	–
toll house original	1 (0.8 oz)	105	15	tr
vanilla sandwich	1 (0.35 oz)	48	0	tr
zeppole	1 (0.8 oz)	78	24	tr
Alex & Dani's				
Original Hazelnut	3 (1 oz)	130	25	1

FOOD	PORTION	CALS	CHOL	FIBER
Alternative Baking				
Vegan Chocolate Chip	1 serv (2.5 oz)	280	0	1
Vegan Expresso Chocolate Chip	1 serv (2 oz)	230	0	1
Vegan Lemon	1 serv (2.25 oz)	250	0	1
Vegan Oatmeal	1 serv (2.25 oz)	250	0	2
Vegan Peanut Butter	1 serv (2.25 oz)	270	0	1
Vegan Pumpkin	1 serv (2 oz)	200	0	1
Vegan Wheat Free Choco Cherry Chunk	1 serv (1.75 oz)	190	0	1
Vegan Wheat Free Hula Nut	1 serv (1.75 oz)	190	0	2
Vegan Wheat Free P-nut Fudge Fusion	1 serv (1.75 oz)	190	0	1
Vegan Wheat Free Snickerdoodle	1 serv (1.75 oz)	170	0	1
Amay's				
Chinese Style Almond	1 (0.5 oz)	80	4	0
Annie's Homegrown				
Bunny Grahams All Flavors	26	130	0	tr
Archway				
Fruit Filled Apricot	1 (0.8 oz)	90	<5	0
Fruit Filled Raspberry	1 (0.8 oz)	90	<5	0
Oatmeal Raisin	1	120	<5	tr
Windmill	1	90	0	0
Arico				
Gluten Free Casein Free	1 bar	150	0	3
Gluten Free Casein Free Almond Cranberry	1 bar	150	25	3
Gluten Free Casein Free Double Chocolate	1 bar	150	20	3
Arnott's				
Raspberry Tartlets	2	100	0	tr
Atkins				
Endulge Wafer Bars Chocolate Creme	2 (1 oz)	120	0	3
Endulge Wafer Bars Mint	2 (1 oz)	120	0	3
Endulge Wafer Bars Peanut Butter	2 (1 oz)	120	0	3

FOOD	PORTION	CALS	CHOL	FIBER
Back To Nature				
Chocolate Chunk	2	130	0	tr
Crispy Oatmeal	2	120	0	tr
Sandwich Chocolate & Mint Creme	2	130	0	tr
Sandwich Classic Creme	2	130	0	tr
Bahlsen				
Afrika	8 (1.1 oz)	170	5	2
Butter Leaves	7 (1 oz)	140	15	tr
Choco Leibniz	2 (1 oz)	140	5	tr
Choco Star Dark Chocolate	3 (1.1 oz)	170	0	1
Choco Star Milk Chocolate	3 (1.1 oz)	180	<5	1
Chocolate Hearts	4 (1 oz)	160	5	1
Delice	6 (1 oz)	140	0	tr
Deloba	4 (0.9 oz)	130	0	tr
Hanover Waffelin	5 (1 oz)	160	0	0
Hit Chocolate Vanilla Filled	2 (1 oz)	140	0	tr
Hit Vanilla Chocolate Filled	2 (1 oz)	140	0	tr
Leibniz	6 (1 oz)	130	10	1
Nuss Dessert	3 (1.1 oz)	170	10	0
Probiers	6 (1.1 oz)	150	0	tr
Twingo	6 (1.1 oz)	170	0	1
Waffeletten	4 (1 oz)	160	<5	1
Baker's Breakfast Cookie				
Apple Pie	1 (3 oz)	204	0	6
Banana Walnut	1 (3 oz)	274	0	5
Chocolate Chunk Raisin	1 (3 oz)	260	0	5
Double Chocolate Chunk	1 (3 oz)	250	0	5
Fruit & Nut	1 (3 oz)	270	0	5
Lemon Poppy Seed	1 (3 oz)	230	0	5
Mocha Chocolate Chunk	1 (3 oz)	250	0	5
Oatmeal Raisin	1 (3 oz)	250	0	5
Peanut Butter	1 (3 oz)	290	0	6
Peanut Butter & Jelly	1 (3 oz)	320	0	6
Pumpkin Spice	1 (3 oz)	230	0	5
Vegan Chocolate Chunk	1 (3 oz)	260	0	5
Vegan Peanut Butter Chocolate Chunk	1 (3 oz)	310	0	6
Baker's Harvest				
Cinnamon Grahams Low Fat	2 (0.9 oz)	110	0	1

FOOD	PORTION	CALS	CHOL	FIBER
Graham Low Fat	2 (0.9 oz)	110	0	1
Iced Oatmeal	1 (0.6 oz)	70	0	0
Pecan Shortbread	1 (0.5 oz)	80	<5	0
Barbara's Bakery				
Apple Cinnamon Bars Fat Free Whole Wheat	1 (0.7 oz)	60	0	2
Chocolate Chip	1 (0.6 oz)	80	5	1
Double Dutch Chocolate	1 (0.6 oz)	80	5	1
Fig Bars Fat Free Wheat Free	1 (0.7 oz)	60	0	1
Fig Bars Fat Free Whole Wheat	1 (0.7 oz)	60	0	2
Nature's Choice Coconut Almond	1 bar (1 oz)	120	0	1
Nature's Choice Espresso Bean	1 bar (1 oz)	120	0	1
Nature's Choice Lemon Yogurt	1 bar (1 oz)	120	0	1
Nature's Choice Roasted Peanut	1 bar (1 oz)	130	0	1
Old Fashioned Oatmeal	1 (0.6 oz)	70	5	1
Raspberry Bars Fat Free Wheat Free Raspberry	1 (0.7 oz)	60	0	1
Snackimals Chocolate Chip	8 (1 oz)	120	0	1
Snackimals Oatmeal Wheat Free	8 (1 oz)	120	0	2
Snackimals Vanilla	8 (1 oz)	120	0	1
Traditional Blueberry Low Fat	1 (0.7 oz)	60	0	1
Traditional Fig Low Fat	1 (0.7 oz)	60	0	1
Traditional Shortbread	1 (0.6 oz)	80	10	1
Bed & Breakfast				
Cranberry Orange Oatmeal	1 (0.8 oz)	110	10	1
Enrobed Shortbread	2 (1.4 oz)	190	15	1
Fruit Center Key Lime	2 (1.1 oz)	140	<5	0
Fruit Center Raspberry	2 (1.1 oz)	140	<5	0
BP Gourmet				
Dreams Chocolate	7 (1 oz)	120	0	0
Dreams Fat Free Chocolate Fudge	13 (1 oz)	100	0	0

FOOD	PORTION	CALS	CHOL	FIBER
Breaktime				
Chocolate Chip	1 (0.3 oz)	37	0	tr
Coconut	1 (0.3 oz)	35	0	tr
Ginger	1 (0.3 oz)	34	0	–
Oatmeal	1 (0.3 oz)	35	0	tr
Sprinkles	1 (0.3 oz)	36	0	–
Brent & Sam's				
Toffee Pecan	2 (0.5 oz)	80	5	0
Bud's Best				
Cacoa Creme	7 (1 oz)	140	0	2
Chocolate Chip	6 (1 oz)	140	0	1
French Vanilla	7 (1 oz)	150	0	2
Oatmeal	6 (1 oz)	130	0	tr
Cafe				
Twists Cinnamony	1 (0.3 oz)	40	0	0
Carbolite				
Chocolate Chip	1 (1 oz)	120	11	4
Peanut Butter	1 (1 oz)	120	11	4
Shortbread	1 (1 oz)	180	2	5
Cookie Lover's				
Chocolate Chip	1 (0.8 oz)	90	10	0
Creme Supremes	2 (0.9 oz)	120	0	1
Creme Supremes Mint	2 (0.9 oz)	120	0	1
Grahams	2 (1 oz)	100	0	1
Grahams Cinnamon	2 (1 oz)	110	0	1
Peanut Butter	1 (0.8 oz)	100	15	0
Shortbread	1 (0.8 oz)	120	15	0
Country Choice Naturals				
Chocolate Chip Walnut	1	100	5	tr
Double Fugde Brownie	1 (0.8 oz)	90	5	tr
Ginger	1	90	5	tr
Ginger Snaps	5	120	0	2
Lemon	1	90	5	tr
Oatmeal Chocolate Chip	1 (0.8 oz)	100	5	1
Oatmeal Raisin	1 (0.8 oz)	100	5	1
Old Fashioned Oatmeal	1 (0.8 oz)	100	5	1
Peanut Butter	1	100	5	tr
Sandwich Cremes Chocolate	1	130	0	0
Sandwich Cremes Duplex	2	130	0	0

FOOD	PORTION	CALS	CHOL	FIBER
Sandwich Cremes Ginger Lemon	2	130	0	0
Sandwich Cremes Mint Creme	2	130	0	0
Sandwich Cremes Vanilla	2	130	0	0
Vanilla Wafers	7	120	5	2
Crummy				
Organic Chocolate Chip	1 (2 oz)	240	30	0
Organic Lavender Chocolate Chip	1 (2 oz)	240	30	0
Dare				
Blueberry Cheesecake	1 (0.6 oz)	90	4	tr
Butter Shortbread	1 (0.5 oz)	63	6	tr
Butter Creme	1 (0.6 oz)	85	2	1
Carrot Cake	1 (0.6 oz)	92	3	tr
Chocolate Chip	1 (0.5 oz)	77	2	tr
Chocolate Fudge	1 (0.7 oz)	97	1	1
Cinnamon Danish	1 (0.4 oz)	47	2	tr
Coconut Creme	1 (0.7 oz)	99	1	tr
French Creme	1 (0.5 oz)	80	1	tr
Harvest From The Rain Forest	1 (0.5 oz)	70	2	tr
Key Lime Creme	1 (0.6 oz)	86	0	tr
Lemon Creme	1 (0.7 oz)	95	1	tr
Maple Leaf Creme	1 (0.6 oz)	83	0	tr
Maple Walnut Fudge	1 (0.7 oz)	99	0	tr
Milk Chocolate Fudge	1 (0.7 oz)	99	1	tr
Oatmeal Raisin	1 (0.4 oz)	59	4	tr
Social Tea	1 (0.2 oz)	26	0	tr
Sun Maid Raisin Oatmeal	1 (0.5 oz)	52	5	tr
David's				
Hamantash Raspberry	1 (0.7 oz)	85	7	7
De Beukelaer				
Pirouline	8 (1 oz)	130	15	tr
Delarce				
Chocosprits	1 (0.6 oz)	90	9	tr
Marquisettes	3 (0.9 oz)	140	5	1
Roules d'Or	4 (1 oz)	180	0	0
DiCamillo				
Biscotti DiPrato	5 (1 oz)	130	15	tr

FOOD	PORTION	CALS	CHOL	FIBER
Doritos				
Barras De Coco	5	120	0	tr
Dove				
Beyond Chocolate Chunk	1 (0.7 oz)	110	10	1
Chocolate Walnut Rendezvous	1 (0.7 oz)	110	10	1
Milk Chocolate Moment	3 (1.1 oz)	160	5	1
Mint Chocolate Serenade	3 (1.1 oz)	160	0	1
Dunkaroos				
Chocolate Graham	1 pkg	120	0	–
Cinnamon Graham	1 pkg	130	0	–
Honey Graham	1 pkg	120	0	tr
Earthbound Farm				
Organic Ginger Snaps	2	120	20	0
Elite				
Tea Biscuits Chocolate	4	80	0	0
English Bay				
Strawberry Fruit Bar	1 (1.2 oz)	120	5	1
Enjoy Life				
Gingerbread Spice Nut & Gluten Free	2 (1 oz)	100	0	1
No-Oat Oatmeal Nut & Gluten Free	2 (1 oz)	110	0	1
Snickerdoodle Nut & Gluten Free	2 (1 oz)	130	0	1
Entenmann's				
Little Bites Chocolate Chip	8 (1.8 oz)	240	10	1
Original Chocolate Chip	3	140	<5	tr
Soft Baked Chocolate Chunk	1 (1.3 oz)	190	15	0
Soft Baked White Chocolate Macadamia Nut	1 (0.7 oz)	100	10	tr
Soft Baked Light Chocolatey Chip	2 (1 oz)	120	0	tr
Soft Baked Light Oatmeal Raisin	2 (1 oz)	100	0	1
Estee				
Fructose Sweetened Chocolate Chip	4	160	0	1
Fructose Sweetened Lemon	4	160	0	2

FOOD	PORTION	CALS	CHOL	FIBER
Fructose Sweetened Sandwich Chocolate	3	170	0	tr
Fructose Sweetened Sandwich Original	3	170	0	0
Fructose Sweetened Sandwich Peanut Butter	3	190	0	tr
Fructose Sweetened Vanilla	4	160	0	1
Fructose Sweetened Vanilla Sandwich	3	170	0	0
Sugar Free Chocolate Chip	3	110	0	1
Sugar Free Lemon	3	110	0	1
Sugar Free Wafer Chocolate Creme	4	150	0	0
Sugar Free Wafer Lemon Creme	4	150	0	0
Sugar Free Wafer Peanut Butter Creme	4	150	0	0
Sugar Free Wafer Strawberry Creme	4	150	0	0
Sugar Free Wafer Vanilla Creme	4	150	0	0
Falcone's				
Sorrentini	1 (1 oz)	100	10	2
Fauchon				
Assorted Chocolate	4 (2 oz)	330	55	5
Frieda's				
Asian Almond	2 (1 oz)	170	0	0
Frookie				
Double Chocolate Wheat & Gluten Free	3 (1.1 oz)	130	0	1
Lemon Wafers	8 (1 oz)	110	0	tr
Sandwich Chocolate	2 (0.7 oz)	100	0	1
Sandwich Lemon	2 (0.7 oz)	100	0	1
Sandwich Peanut Butter	2 (0.7 oz)	100	0	1
Sandwich Vanilla	2 (0.7 oz)	100	0	1
Vanilla Wafers	8 (1 oz)	110	0	0
Gamesa				
Animalitos	14	110	0	tr
Arcoiris Marshmallow	2	120	0	tr

FOOD	PORTION	CALS	CHOL	FIBER
Arcoiris Merengue	6	200	0	1
Emperador Chocolate	2	120	0	tr
Emperador Fresa	2	120	<5	tr
Emperador Limon	6	270	0	1
Emperador Vanilla	2	120	<5	0
Hawaianas	3	130	0	tr
Marias	8	120	0	tr
Ricanelas	8	140	0	2
Roscas	3	130	0	1
Sugar Wafers Chocolate	3	160	0	0
Sugar Wafers Strawberry	3	160	0	0
Sugar Wafers Vanilla	3	160	0	0
General Henry				
Fruit Bars Apple	1 (0.6 oz)	60	0	tr
Fruit Bars Blueberry	1 (0.6 oz)	60	0	tr
Fruit Bars Fig	1 (0.6 oz)	60	0	tr
Girl Scout				
Cafe Cookies	5	150	0	1
Lemon Cooler Reduced Fat	5	130	0	0
Samoas	2	150	0	tr
Tagalongs	2	130	0	1
Thin Mints	4	140	0	tr
Trefoils	4	130	0	0
Godiva				
Biscotti Dipped In Milk Chocolate	1 (0.9 oz)	120	20	0
Gol D Lite				
Low Carb Pizzelle	1 (0.3 oz)	46	0	1
Golden Grahams Treats				
Honey Graham	1 bar (0.8 oz)	90	0	0
King Size Chocolate Chunk	1 bar (1.6 oz)	190	0	1
King Size Honey Graham	1 bar (1.6 oz)	180	0	1
Golightly				
Fabulous Tastes Caramel Dulce De Leche	4	100	0	5
Goody Man				
Marshmallow Crispy Squares	1 (1.17 oz)	130	0	0
Grandma's				
Homestyle Big Chocolate Chip	1 (1.4 oz)	190	0	tr

FOOD	PORTION	CALS	CHOL	FIBER
Homestyle Big Fudge Chocolate Chip	1 (1.4 oz)	170	10	1
Homestyle Big Oatmeal Raisin	1 (1.4 oz)	180	10	1
Homestyle Big Peanut Butter	1 (1.4 oz)	200	10	1
Mini Vanilla Creme	9	150	<5	tr
Peanut Butter Sandwich	5	210	0	1
Rich N'Chewy Chocolate Chip	1 pkg	270	10	2
Vanilla Creme Sandwich	5	210	5	tr
Granny Oats				
Low Carb Oatmeal	4	98	25	3
Healthy Handfuls				
Organic Crocodile Cookies	1 pkg (1 oz)	130	0	7
Organic Koala Krackers	1 pkg (1 oz)	120	5	2
Heavenly				
Meringues All Flavors Sugar Free Fat Free	1	0	0	0
Hellema				
Almond	1 pkg (0.6 oz)	90	0	tr
Hershey's				
Cripsy Rice Snacks Peanut Butter	1 (0.6 oz)	70	0	tr
Jacques Gourmet				
Palmier Cinnamon	3 (1 oz)	140	0	0
Palmier Vanilla	3 (1 oz)	140	0	0
Joseph's				
Almond Sugar Free	4	100	0	1
Chocolate Chip Sugar Free	4	100	0	1
Lemon Sugar Free	4	95	0	0
Oatmeal Chocolate Chip w/ Pecans Sugar Free	4	100	0	1
Peanut Butter Sugar Free	4	95	0	0
Karen's				
Fabulous Tastes Heavenly Chocolate Chip	4	90	0	5
Fabulous Tastes Luscious Raspberry Almond	4	110	0	5

FOOD	PORTION	CALS	CHOL	FIBER
Fabulous Tastes Pecan Vanilla Pralines	4	120	0	6
Kashi				
TLC Happy Trail Mix	1 (1 oz)	130	0	4
TLC Oatmeal Raisin Flax	1 (1 oz)	130	0	4
TLC Oatmeal Dark Chocolate	1 (1 oz)	130	0	3
Kedem				
Tea Biscuits Chocolate	2	32	0	tr
Tea Biscuits Orange	2	32	0	tr
Keebler				
Butter	5 (1.1 oz)	150	10	tr
Chips Deluxe	1 (0.5 oz)	80	0	tr
Droxies	3 (1.1 oz)	140	0	tr
Fudge Shoppe Double Fudge 'n Caramel	2 (1 oz)	140	0	tr
Ginger Snaps	5 (1.1 oz)	150	0	0
Golden Fruit Cranberry	1 (0.7 oz)	80	0	tr
Golden Fruit Raisin	1 (0.7 oz)	80	0	tr
Graham Honey	8 (1.1 oz)	140	0	0
Lemon Coolers	5 (1 oz)	140	0	tr
Oatmeal Country Style	2 (0.8 oz)	120	0	tr
Sandies Fruit Delights Lemon	1 (0.6 oz)	80	<5	0
Sandies Strawberry Shortcake	1 (0.6 oz)	80	<5	0
Snack Size Chips Deluxe	1 pkg (2 oz)	300	5	tr
Snack Size Chips Deluxe Chocolate Lovers	1 pkg (2 oz)	280	20	1
Snack Size Mini Fudge Stripes	1 pkg (2 oz)	280	0	2
Snackin' Grahams Cinnamon	21 (1 oz)	130	0	1
Snackin' Grahams Honey	23 (1 oz)	130	0	tr
Soft Batch Chocolate Chip	1 (0.6 oz)	80	0	tr
Soft Batch Oatmeal Raisin	1 (0.5 oz)	70	0	tr
Sugar Wafers Creme	3 (0.9 oz)	130	0	tr
Sugar Wafers Peanut Butter	4 (1.1 oz)	170	0	1
Keto				
Low Carb Biscotti Chocolate	1 (1.2 oz)	157	200	3

FOOD	PORTION	CALS	CHOL	FIBER
Low Carb Biscotti Lemon Nut	1 (1.2 oz)	157	200	3
Low Carb Biscotti Vanilla Almond	1 (1.2 oz)	157	200	3
Knott's Berry Farm				
Shortbread Apricot	3 (1 oz)	120	4	0
Shortbread Boysenberry	3 (1 oz)	120	4	0
Shortbread Raspberry	3 (1 oz)	120	4	0
La Choy				
Fortune	4 (1 oz)	112	0	1
La Dolce Vita				
Biscotti Chocolate Passion	1 (1.2 oz)	130	45	1
Landies Candies				
Sugar Free Dark Royal Pecan Shortbread	2	167	0	1
Sugar Free Milk Chocolate Chip	2	173	<5	tr
Sugar Free Milk Chocolate Peanut Butter	2	171	<5	tr
Sugar Free White Chocolate Lemon	2	177	<5	0
Laura's Wholesome Junk Food				
Anna Banana Split	1	105	0	1
Gluten Free Charlotte's Chocolate Chip	2	120	0	1
Gluten Free Sally's Raisin	2	110	0	tr
Lemon Vanilla	2	120	0	1
Oatmeal Chocolate Chip	2	110	0	1
Oatmeal Raisin	2	100	0	1
Wheat Free X-Treme Chocolate Fudge	2	110	0	2
Lee's				
Dreamy Mallows	2	150	0	0
Leibniz				
Butter Biscuits	6	130	10	1
Linden's				
Lemon	1 (1 oz)	120	10	–
Little Debbie				
Apple Flips	1 (1.2 oz)	150	5	tr

FOOD	PORTION	CALS	CHOL	FIBER
Cherry Cordials	1 (1.3 oz)	170	0	tr
Coconut Rounds	1 (1.2 oz)	150	0	tr
Easter Puffs	1 (1.2 oz)	140	0	0
Marshmallow Crispy Bar	1 (1.3 oz)	140	0	0
Yo-Yo's	1 (1.2 oz)	130	0	tr
Low Carb Creations				
Chocolate Chip	1 (1 oz)	140	25	1
Coconut	1 (1 oz)	140	30	1
Lemon	1 (1 oz)	140	30	1
Snickerdoodle	1 (1 oz)	140	30	1
LU				
Chocolatier	3 (1 oz)	150	0	1
Le Bastogne	2 (0.8 oz)	120	0	0
Le Dore	4 (1 oz)	140	<5	0
Le Fondant	4 (1.1 oz)	170	0	1
Le Petit Beurre	4 (1.2 oz)	150	10	tr
Le Petit Ecolier Dark Chocolate	2 (0.9 oz)	130	<5	1
Le Petit Ecolier Extra Dark Chocolate	2	120	<5	2
Le Petit Ecolier Hazelnut Milk Chocolate	2 (0.9 oz)	130	5	0
Le Petit Ecolier Milk Chocolate	2 (0.9 oz)	130	5	tr
Le Petit Fruit Strawberry	5 (1.2 oz)	110	30	0
Le Raisin Dore	4 (1.2 oz)	160	20	tr
Le Truffe Coconut	4 (1.2 oz)	190	0	1
Pim's Orange	2 (0.9 oz)	90	10	tr
Pim's Raspberry	2 (0.9 oz)	90	5	tr
Pim's Sensation Bar Chocolate	1	110	0	tr
Pim's Sensation Bar Hazelnut	1	110	0	tr
Shortbread	2	140	25	tr
Mamma Says'				
Biscotti Almond Pistachio	1 (0.5 oz)	50	7	1
Biscotti Chocolate Macadamia	1 (0.5 oz)	45	10	1
Biscotti Orange Citrine	1 (0.5 oz)	60	10	1

FOOD	PORTION	CALS	CHOL	FIBER
Mauna Loa				
Macadamia Nut Chocolate Chip	2	130	5	1
Macadamia Nut Hawaiian Crunch	2	150	10	1
Macadamia Nut White Chocolate Chip	2	130	6	1
Miss Meringue				
Chocolatette Strawberry Vanilla	4	130	0	1
Chocolettes Crunchy Chocolate	4	110	4	21
Classiques Cappuccino	4	110	0	0
Classiques Chocolate Chip	4	120	0	1
Classiques Dulce De Leche Artisan	4	110	0	0
Macaroons Traditional	1 (1.3 oz)	180	0	1
Madeleines Traditional	2 (1.2 oz)	160	55	0
Minis Vanilla	13 (1.1 oz)	110	0	0
Minis Vanilla Sugar Free	13	35	0	3
MoonPie				
Chocolate	1 (2.75 oz)	330	0	0
Mother's				
Chocolate Chip Parade	4	130	0	1
Circus Animals	6	140	0	0
Cocadas	5	150	5	2
Cookie Parade	4	140	0	2
Marias	3	170	5	1
Oatmeal Chocolate Chip	2	120	0	1
Oatmeal Raisin	5	150	5	2
Oatmeal Walnut Chocolate Chip	2	130	0	1
Wallops Honey Graham Fig	1	80	0	1
Zoo Pals	14	140	0	1
Mrs. Alison's				
Coconut Bar	2 (1 oz)	130	0	0
Creme Wafers	5 (1.1 oz)	170	0	tr
Fudge Fingers	3 (1 oz)	160	0	0
Ginger Snaps	4 (1 oz)	130	<2	tr
Jelly Tops	5 (1 oz)	140	0	0

FOOD	PORTION	CALS	CHOL	FIBER
Lemon Creme	3 (1 oz)	130	0	0
Macaroons	2 (1 oz)	140	0	tr
Pecan	2 (1 oz)	140	0	0
Shortbread	5 (1 oz)	120	0	0
Nabisco				
Barnum's Animal Crackers	10 (1 oz)	130	0	tr
Biscos Sugar Wafers	8 (1 oz)	140	0	0
Cafe Cremes Cappuccino	2 (1.1 oz)	160	0	0
Cafe Cremes Vanilla	2 (1.1 oz)	160	0	0
Cafe Cremes Vanilla Fudge	2 (1.1 oz)	200	0	tr
ChocoStix Nutter Butter	1 pkg (1 oz)	140	0	1
Honey Maid Cinnamon Sticks	1 pkg (1 oz)	120	0	tr
Honey Maid Honey Grahams Low Fat	8	120	0	tr
Lorna Doone	4 (1 oz)	140	0	0
Mallomars	2	120	0	tr
Oreo Mini	1 pkg (1.2 oz)	160	0	1
Social Tea	6	140	0	1
Teddy Grahams Honey	2 pkg (1 oz)	120	0	tr
Natural Ovens				
Carob Chip	1	90	0	3
Chocolate Raspberry	1	120	0	3
Oatmeal Raisin	1	90	0	3
Nature's Path				
Organic Signature Lemon Poppyseed	4	130	0	tr
Organic Animal Vanilla	9	120	0	tr
Nestle				
Flipz Crunchy Graham White Fudge Chocolate	8 (1 oz)	140	0	0
Newman's Own				
Organic Champion Chip Chocolate Chip	4	160	0	1
Organic Champion Chip Chocolate Chocolate Chip	4	160	0	1
Organic Champion Chip Double Chocolate Mint Chip	4	160	0	1
Organic Champion Chip Expresso Chocolate Chip	4	150	0	1

FOOD	PORTION	CALS	CHOL	FIBER
Organic Champion Chip Orange Chocolate Chip	4	160	0	1
Organic Champion Chip Wheat Free Dairy Free	4	160	0	0
Organic Fig Newmans Low Fat	2	140	0	1
Organic Fig Newmans Wheat Free Dairy Free	2	120	0	1
Organic Fig Newman's Fat Free	2	120	0	1
Organic Newman-O's Chocolate Creme	2	130	0	1
Organic Newman-O's Ginger-O's	2	120	0	0
Organic Newman-O's Mint Creme	2	130	0	1
Organic Newman-O's Original	2	130	0	1
Organic Newman-O's Tops & Bottoms	6	120	0	1
Organic Newman-O's Wheat Free Dairy Free	2	130	0	0
Nonni's				
Biscotti Decadence	1 (1.1 oz)	130	25	1
Biscotti Original	1 (1 oz)	100	25	1
Olde World				
Pizzelle Almond	3 (1 oz)	90	45	0
Pizzelle Anise	3 (1 oz)	90	45	0
Pizzelle Chocolate	3 (1 oz)	100	45	0
Pizzelle Lemon	3 (1 oz)	90	45	0
Pizzelle Vanilla	3 (1 oz)	90	45	0
Otis Spunkmeyer				
Butter Sugar	1 med (1.3 oz)	160	15	tr
Butter Sugar	1 (2 oz)	250	20	1
Carnival	1 med (1.3 oz)	170	10	0
Chocolate Chip	1 bite size (0.75 oz)	100	5	0
Chocolate Chip	1 med (1.3 oz)	170	10	0
Chocolate Chip	1 (2 oz)	250	15	tr
Chocolate Chip Pecan	1 med (1.3 oz)	170	10	tr
Chocolate Chip Walnut	1 bite size (0.75 oz)	100	5	0

FOOD	PORTION	CALS	CHOL	FIBER
Chocolate Chip Walnut	1 med (1.3 oz)	180	10	tr
Chocolate Chip Walnut	1 (2 oz)	270	15	tr
Double Chocolate Chip	1 bite size (0.75 oz)	100	5	1
Double Chocolate Chip	1 med (1.3 oz)	180	10	tr
Oatmeal Raisin	1 bite size (0.75 oz)	90	5	tr
Oatmeal Raisin	1 med (1.3 oz)	160	10	1
Otis Express Chocolate Chunk	1 (2 oz)	280	20	1
Otis Express Double Chocolate Chip	1 (2 oz)	270	15	1
Otis Express Oatmeal Raisin	1 (2 oz)	240	15	2
Otis Express Peanut Butter	1 (2 oz)	270	15	2
Peanut Butter	1 med (1.3 oz)	180	10	1
Pinnacle Checkpoint Chocolate Almond Coconut	1 (2.4 oz)	320	25	2
Pinnacle Mach One Mocha Chocolate Chunk	1 (2.4 oz)	300	20	1
Pinnacle Passport Peanut Butter Chocolate Chunk	1 (2.4 oz)	300	25	1
Pinnacle Ripcord Rocky Road	1 (2.4 oz)	310	15	2
Pinnacle Takeoff Triple Chocolate	1 (2.4 oz)	310	20	tr
Pinnacle Transatlantic Turtle	1 (2.4 oz)	300	20	2
Travel Lite Low Fat Apple Cinnamon	1 (1.3 oz)	130	0	tr
Travel Lite Low Fat Chocolate Chip	1 (1.3 oz)	130	0	tr
Travel Lite Low Fat Ginger Spice	1 (1.3 oz)	130	0	tr
Travel Lite Low Fat Oatmeal Rum Raisin	1 (1.3 oz)	130	0	1
White Chocolate Macadamia Nut	1 med (1.3 oz)	180	10	tr
White Chocolate Macadamia Nut	1 (2 oz)	280	20	tr
Pally				
Carnival	5 (1 oz)	130	0	1
Peek Freans				
Petit Beret Creme Caramel	2 (0.8 oz)	110	0	tr

FOOD	PORTION	CALS	CHOL	FIBER
Petit Beret Fudge Truffle	2 (0.8 oz)	110	0	tr
Traditional Oatmeal	1 (0.7 oz)	90	0	tr
Pepperidge Farm				
Brussels	2	100	<5	tr
Chantilly Raspberry	2 (1 oz)	120	0	tr
Chessman	3	120	20	tr
Chocolate Chunk Chesapeake	1 (0.7 oz)	140	10	0
Chocolate Chunk Minis Nantauket	1 pkg (1.75 oz)	260	10	0
Chocolate Chunk Minis Sausalito	4 (1 oz)	160	10	0
Chocolate Chunk Montauk	1 (0.9 oz)	130	10	0
Chocolate Chunk Sausalito	1 (0.7 oz)	140	10	0
Chocolate Chunk Tahoe	1 (0.9 oz)	130	10	0
Ginger Man	4 (1 oz)	130	10	tr
Goldfish Grahams Cinnamon	1 pkg (1.75 oz)	240	5	2
Milano Double Chocolate	2 (0.7 oz)	140	10	tr
Pirouettes Chocolate Laced	5 (1.1 oz)	180	5	tr
Soft Baked Chocolate Chunk Dark Chocolate	1	140	10	0
Soft Baked Chocolate Chunk Milk Chocolate Caramel	1	140	5	tr
Soft Baked Sugar	1	140	10	0
Spritzers Cool Key Lime	6 (1.1 oz)	140	<5	0
Spritzers Ripe Red Raspberry	5 (1.1 oz)	140	<5	0
Spritzers Zesty Lemon	5 (1.1 oz)	140	<5	0
Verona Strawberry	3 (1.1 oz)	140	10	tr
Whims Chocolate Cashew	9 (1 oz)	150	<5	tr
Pure De-Lite				
High Protein Chocolate Fudge	1 (2.2 oz)	210	10	5
High Protein Peanut Butter Crunch	1 (2.2 oz)	210	5	5
Quaker				
Breakfast Cookie Oatmeal Raisin	1	180	0	5
Ralston				
Cinnamon Grahams Low Fat	2 (0.9 oz)	110	0	1

FOOD	PORTION	CALS	CHOL	FIBER
Reko				
Pizzelle Maple	5 (1 oz)	150	15	0
Right Direction				
Chocolate Chip	1	60	10	5
Royal				
Apple Bars	1 (1.1 oz)	100	0	1
Apple Cake	1 (1.1 oz)	110	0	1
Brownie Rounds	1 (1.1 oz)	130	0	0
Chocolate Chip	1 (1.1 oz)	140	0	1
Devilfood	1 (1 oz)	110	0	0
Fig Bars	1 (1.1 oz)	100	0	1
Oatmeal	1 (1.1 oz)	130	0	1
Raisin	1 (1 oz)	110	0	0
Strawberry Bars	1 (1.1 oz)	100	0	1
Savion				
Tea Biscuits	5 (1 oz)	120	0	0
Tea Biscuits Vanilla	5 (1 oz)	120	0	0
Scotto's				
Biscotti Fat Free French Vanilla	4 (1 oz)	80	0	0
Simple Pleasures				
Almond	1 (0.3 oz)	37	0	tr
Cinnamon Snaps	1 (0.2 oz)	31	0	tr
Digestive	1 (0.3 oz)	46	0	tr
Encore Tea Cookie	1 (0.2 oz)	29	0	tr
Lemon Social Tea	1 (0.2 oz)	29	0	tr
Oatmeal	1 (0.5 oz)	74	0	1
Spice Snaps	1 (0.3 oz)	34	0	tr
Sugar	1 (0.4 oz)	45	3	tr
SnackWell's				
Creme Sandwich	1 pkg (1.7 oz)	210	0	tr
Mint Creme	2	110	0	tr
Sugar Free Chocolate Chip	3 (1.2 oz)	150	<5	tr
Sugar Free Oatmeal	1 (0.8 oz)	90	0	tr
South Beach Diet				
Oatmeal Chocolate Chip	1 pkg	100	0	3
Peanut Butter	1 pkg	100	0	4
Soybite				
All Flavors	1	79	0	1

FOOD	PORTION	CALS	CHOL	FIBER
Stella D'Oro				
Lady Stella	3	130	5	tr
Streit's				
Wafers	3 (1 oz)	160	0	1
Sweetzels				
Chocolate Chip	7 (1 oz)	160	5	0
Ginger Snaps	4 (1.2 oz)	140	0	tr
Vanilla Wafers	7 (1.1 oz)	137	0	0
Tom's				
Animal Crackers	½ pkg (1 oz)	120	0	tr
Big Cookie Chocolate Chip	1 pkg (2.75 oz)	340	0	1
Big Cookie Peanut Butter Chocolate Chip	1 pkg (2 oz)	280	0	1
Chocolate Chip	1 pkg (2 oz)	280	0	1
Confetti Chip	1 pkg (2 oz)	300	0	tr
Fat Free Apple Bar	1 pkg (1.75 oz)	160	0	1
Fat Free Fig Bar	1 pkg (1.75 oz)	160	0	2
Vanilla Wafers	½ pkg (1 oz)	130	0	tr
Tree of Life				
Fat Free Almond Butter	1 (0.8 oz)	60	0	1
Fat Free Carrot Cake	1 (0.8 oz)	60	0	1
Fat Free Devil's Food Chocolate	1 (0.8 oz)	70	0	1
Fat Free Oatmeal Raisin	1 (0.8 oz)	70	0	1
Fruit Bars Fat Free Fig	1 (0.8 oz)	70	0	2
Fruit Bars Fat Free Peach Apricot	1 (0.8 oz)	70	0	1
Fruit Bars Fat Free Wildberry	1 (0.8 oz)	70	0	2
Monster Carob Chip	1 (4.7 oz)	700	10	5
Monster Granola	1 (4.7 oz)	700	10	5
Monster Macaroon	1 (4.7 oz)	750	10	5
Monster Peanut Butter	1 (4.7 oz)	700	20	5
Monster Fat Free Carrot Cake	1 cookie (3.8 oz)	240	0	4
Monster Fat Free Devil's Food Chocolate	1 cookie (3.8 oz)	320	0	8
Monster Fat Free Gingerbread	1 cookie (3.8 oz)	320	0	8
Monster Fat Free Maple Pecan	1 cookie (3.8 oz)	360	0	8

FOOD	PORTION	CALS	CHOL	FIBER
Oatmeal	1 (0.8 oz)	100	15	0
Sandwich Royal Vanilla	2 (0.9 oz)	120	0	1
Wheat Free Carob	1 (0.8 oz)	100	0	6
Wheat Free Maple Walnut	1 (0.8 oz)	100	0	6
Wheat Free Oatmeal	1 (0.8 oz)	90	0	1
Wheat Free Peanut Butter	1 (0.8 oz)	109	0	1
Voortman				
Turnovers Blueberry	1 (0.9 oz)	100	<5	0
Turnovers Strawberry	1 (0.9 oz)	100	<5	0
REFRIGERATED				
chocolate chip	1 (0.42 oz)	59	3	–
chocolate chip unbaked	1 oz	126	7	–
oatmeal	1 (0.4 oz)	56	3	–
oatmeal raisin	1 (0.4 oz)	56	3	–
peanut butter	1 (0.4 oz)	60	4	–
peanut butter dough	1 oz	130	8	–
sugar	1 (0.42 oz)	58	4	–
sugar dough	1 oz	124	8	–
Pillsbury				
Bunny	2	130	<5	0
Chocolate Chunk	1 (1 oz)	130	<5	tr
Christmas Tree	2	130	<5	0
Double Chocolate	1 (1 oz)	130	<5	tr
Flag	2	130	<5	0
Frosty	2	130	<5	0
M&M's	1 (1 oz)	130	<5	tr
One Step Pan Chocolate Chip	⅛ pan (1 oz)	130	<5	tr
One Step Pan M&M's	⅛ pan (1 oz)	130	<5	tr
Pumpkin	2	130	<5	0
Reeses	1 (1 oz)	130	<5	tr
Shamrock	2	130	<5	0
Sugar Holiday Red & Green	2	130	<5	0
Valentine	2	130	<5	0
White Chocolate Chunk	1 (1 oz)	130	<5	0
TAKE-OUT				
biscotti w/ nuts chocolate dipped	1 (1.3 oz)	117	18	1
black & white	1 lg (3 oz)	302	58	1
finikia	1 (1.2 oz)	171	27	1

FOOD	PORTION	CALS	CHOL	FIBER
koulourakia butter cookie twist	1 (0.9 oz)	113	32	tr
linzer tart	1 (2.4 oz)	280	40	0

CORIANDER

FOOD	PORTION	CALS	CHOL	FIBER
cilantro fresh	1 tsp (2 g)	tr	0	tr
cilantro fresh	1 cup (1.6 oz)	11	0	1
leaf dried	1 tsp	2	0	–
leaf fresh	¼ cup	1	0	–
seed	1 tsp	5	0	–
Instant India				
Tomato Coriander Paste	2 tbsp (1 oz)	90	0	0

CORN
CANNED

FOOD	PORTION	CALS	CHOL	FIBER
cream style	½ cup	93	0	–
w/ red & green peppers	½ cup	86	0	–
white	½ cup	66	0	–
yellow	½ cup	66	0	1
Del Monte				
Cream Style	½ cup	60	0	2
Cream Style No Salt Added	½ cup	60	0	2
Fiesta	½ cup	50	0	2
Gold & White	½ cup	80	0	2
Savory Sides In Butter Sauce	½ cup	90	5	tr
Savory Sides Santa Fe	½ cup	70	0	1
Summer Crisp	½ cup	70	0	3
White	½ cup	60	0	3
Green Giant				
Mexicorn	⅓ cup	70	0	1
Yellow & White	⅓ cup	60	0	1
S&W				
Cream Style	½ cup (4.4 oz)	60	0	2
Whole Kernel	⅓ cup (3 oz)	70	0	2
Veg-All				
Whole Kernel	½ cup	80	0	2
FRESH				
white cooked	½ cup	89	0	–
white raw	½ cup	66	0	–
yellow cooked	1 ear (2.7 oz)	83	0	–
yellow cooked	½ cup	89	0	–

FOOD	PORTION	CALS	CHOL	FIBER
yellow raw	½ cup	66	0	–
FROZEN				
cooked	½ cup	67	0	–
Birds Eye				
Steamfresh Southwestern	⅔ cup	90	0	1
Steamfresh Super Sweet	⅔ cup	70	0	2
Steamfresh Sweet Mini Corn On The Cob	1	90	0	1
C&W				
Cheddar Bacon	½ cup	130	10	3
Early Harvest Supersweet Petite	⅔ cup	70	0	2
Salsa Corn	1 cup	90	0	3
Europe's Best				
Baby Sweet	⅔ cup	50	0	2
Glory				
Savory Accents Fried Corn	½ cup	110	0	2
Green Giant				
Niblets & Butter Sauce Low Fat	⅔ cup	110	<5	2
Pictsweet				
Cut Corn	⅔ cup	100	0	1
Roast Works				
Flame Roasted Cob Corn	1 cob (3 oz)	130	0	4
Tree Of Life				
Corn	⅔ cup (3.2 oz)	80	0	1
TAKE-OUT				
fritters	1 (1 oz)	62	12	1
on-the-cob w/ butter cooked	1 ear	155	6	–
scalloped	1 cup	257	152	3

CORNISH HEN (see CHICKEN)

CORNMEAL

cornmeal mush as prep w/ water	1 cup	223	0	5
cornmeal yellow	1 cup	505	0	10
harina de maize con leche	1 cup	295	25	7
Albers				
White	3 tbsp	110	0	tr
Yellow	3 tbsp	110	0	tr

FOOD	PORTION	CALS	CHOL	FIBER
Expert Foods				
Low Carb Grits Mix	1½ tsp	15	0	2
Indian Head				
Stone Ground	¼ cup	100	0	2
McKenzie's				
Hush Puppies	1 serv (1.9 oz)	190	0	2
Quaker				
Quick Grits not prep	¼ cup	130	0	2
Yellow	3 tbsp (1 oz)	90	0	2
TAKE-OUT				
corn pone	1 piece (2.1 oz)	128	0	2
fritter puerto rican style	1 (1.4 oz)	109	8	1
harina de maiz con coco	½ cup	383	0	4
hush puppies	1 (0.8 oz)	74	10	1
johnnycake	1 piece (1.7 oz)	134	35	2

CORNSTARCH

cornstarch	1 cup (4.5 oz)	488	0	1
Argo				
Cornstarch	1 tbsp	30	0	–
Kingsford's				
Cornstarch	1 tbsp	30	0	–

COTTAGE CHEESE

creamed	4 oz	117	17	–
creamed	1 cup (7.4 oz)	217	31	–
creamed w/ fruit	4 oz	140	13	–
dry curd	1 cup (5.1 oz)	123	10	–
dry curd	4 oz	96	8	–
lowfat 1%	4 oz	82	5	–
lowfat 1%	1 cup (7.9 oz)	164	10	–
lowfat 2%	4 oz	101	9	–
lowfat 2%	1 cup (7.9 oz)	203	19	–
Breakstone's				
Cottage Doubles Peach	1 pkg (5.5 oz)	140	15	tr
Fat Free	½ cup	80	10	0
Cabot				
Cottage Cheese	½ cup	100	15	0
No Fat	½ cup	70	5	0
Hood				
4% Fat w/ Pineapple	½ cup	130	20	0

FOOD	PORTION	CALS	CHOL	FIBER
Fat Free	½ cup	80	10	0
Low Fat	½ cup	90	15	0
Low Fat No Salt Added	½ cup	90	15	0
Low Fat w/ Peaches	½ cup	110	10	0
Horizon Organic				
Cottage Cheese	½ cup (3.9 oz)	110	15	0
Lowfat	½ cup	100	15	0
Regular	½ cup	120	20	0
Light N'Lively				
Lowfat	½ cup	80	10	0

COTTONSEED

kernels roasted	1 tbsp	51	0	–

COUSCOUS

cooked	1 cup (5.5 oz)	176	0	2
dry	1 cup (6.1 oz)	650	0	9
Hodgson Mill				
Whole Wheat not prep	⅓ cup	210	0	5
Marrakesh Express				
Mango Salsa as prep	1 cup	190	0	1
Mushroom as prep	1 cup	190	0	1
Plain as prep	1 cup	270	0	2
Near East				
Broccoli & Cheese as prep	1 cup	230	9	3
Curry as prep	1 cup	220	0	3
Herbed Chicken as prep	1 cup	220	0	3
Original as prep	1 cup	230	0	2
Parmesan as prep	1 cup	220	9	2
Roasted Garlic Olive Oil as prep	1 cup	230	0	2
Toasted Pine Nut as prep	1 cup	230	27	2
Tomato Lentil as prep	1 cup	220	0	3
Wild Mushroom Herb as prep	1 cup	230	9	3
Rice Select				
All Varieties not prep	¼ cup	150	0	–

CRAB
CANNED

blue	½ cup	67	60	0
blue drained	1 can (6.5 oz)	124	111	0

FOOD	PORTION	CALS	CHOL	FIBER
Brunswick				
Crabmeat 15% Leg	2 oz	40	50	0
Fancy Lump	2 oz	45	50	0
Bumble Bee				
Lump	¼ cup	40	50	0
Pink	¼ cup	35	50	0
White	¼ cup	40	50	0
Chicken Of The Sea				
Fancy	½ can (2 oz)	40	50	0
Lump	½ can (2 oz)	35	50	0
Madam				
Crab Meat	½ cup	40	55	0
Terry's				
Crabmeat	¼ cup	40	50	0
FRESH				
alaska king meat only steamed	3 oz	82	45	0
blue cooked flaked	1 cup (4 oz)	120	118	0
dungeness steamed	3 oz	94	65	0
queen steamed	3 oz	98	60	0
FROZEN				
Margaritaville				
Coral Reef Cakes + Sauce	1	200	71	0
Phillips Seafood				
Crab Cakes	1 (3 oz)	160	85	–
Crab Meat Stuffing	1 serv (3.5 oz)	170	85	–
Mini Cakes	4	160	85	–
Slammers	2	150	40	–
TAKE-OUT				
alaska king leg steamed	1 leg (4.7 oz)	130	71	0
baked	1 (3.8 oz)	160	184	–
cakes	2 (4.2 oz)	186	180	0
crab imperial	1 crab (6.8 oz)	289	242	0
crab salad	1 serv (5.5 oz)	285	109	1
crab thermidor	1 serv (6.4 oz)	456	313	tr
deviled	1 serv (4.5 oz)	254	126	1
dungeness steamed	1 crab (4.5 oz)	140	97	0
empanada de jueyes	1 (4.4 oz)	341	45	2

FOOD	PORTION	CALS	CHOL	FIBER
fried crab puffs	4 (3.2 oz)	323	85	1
salmorejo d jueyes (in tomato sauce)	1 serv (4.5 oz)	215	99	tr
soft-shell breaded & fried	1 med (2.3 oz)	216	79	1
taco de jueye	1 (4.2 oz)	266	79	2

CRACKER CRUMBS

cracker meal	1 cup	440	0	3
graham cracker crumbs	1 cup	355	0	2
Baker's Harvest				
Graham	⅓ cup (1 oz)	130	0	1
Kellogg's				
Corn Flake Crumbs	6 tbsp (1.2 oz)	120	0	tr

CRACKERS

melba toast round	1	12	0	tr
oyster cracker	¼ cup	48	0	tr
saltines	1	13	0	tr
American Vintage				
Wine Biscuits All Flavors	5	140	1	tr
Andre's				
CarboSave Crackerbread All Flavors	1 oz	140	0	4
Annie's Homegrown				
Cheddar Bunnies BBQ	50	130	0	2
Cheddar Bunnies Original	50	150	<5	1
Cheddar Bunnies Ranch	50	130	0	2
Cheddar Bunnies Whole Wheat	50	130	0	2
Austin				
Cracker Sandwich Cheese On Cheese	6 (1.3 oz)	170	0	tr
Cracker Sandwich Cheese Peanut Butter	6 (1.3 oz)	170	0	1
Cracker Sandwich Toasty Peanut Butter	6 (1.3 oz)	170	0	1
Cracker Sandwich Whole Wheat Cheese	6 (1.3 oz)	170	0	tr
Back To Nature				
Classic Rounds	5	70	0	0

FOOD	PORTION	CALS	CHOL	FIBER
Crispy Wheats	17	130	0	1
Rice Thin Sesame Ginger	16	120	0	0
Rice Thin White Cheddar	16	120	0	0
Baker's Harvest				
Cheese	23 (1 oz)	150	0	tr
Cheese Reduced Fat	29 (1 oz)	130	0	tr
Barbara's Bakery				
Cheese Bites	26 (1 oz)	120	0	1
Right Lite Rounds Original	5 (0.5 oz)	55	0	0
Rite Lite Rounds Savory Poppy	5 (0.5 oz)	70	0	0
Rite Lite Rounds Tamari Sesame	5 (0.5 oz)	70	0	0
Wheatines All Flavors	1 lg sq (0.5 oz)	50	0	1
Blue Diamond				
Nut Thins Almond	16 (1 oz)	130	0	tr
Nut Thins Hazelnut	16 (1 oz)	120	0	1
Nut Thins Pecan	16 (1 oz)	130	0	tr
Nut-Thins Almond	16	130	0	1
Nut-Thins Hazelnut	16	130	0	tr
Nut-Thins Pecan	16	130	0	tr
Bran-A-Crisp				
Low Carb Wheat Bran	1	20	0	2
Breton				
Cabaret	3 (5 g)	70	0	0
Garden Vegetable	3	60	0	1
Light	1 (5 g)	20	0	tr
Minis	20 (0.6 oz)	89	0	tr
Minis Cheddar Cheese	20 (0.6 oz)	87	3	–
Minis Garden Vegetable	20 (0.6 oz)	87	0	1
Multigrain	3 (0.5 oz)	80	0	1
Original	3	60	0	0
Reduced Fat & Sodium	3	60	0	tr
Sesame	3	60	0	tr
Cheeters				
Low Carb All Flavors	1 pkg (1 oz)	104	0	2
Cheetos				
Cheddar	1 pkg	240	5	1
Cheez It				
Hot & Spicy	26 (1 oz)	150	0	tr

FOOD	PORTION	CALS	CHOL	FIBER
Reduced Fat	29 (1 oz)	140	0	tr
White Cheddar	26 (1 oz)	150	<5	tr
Courtney's				
Sun-Dried Tomato Organic	4 (0.5 oz)	60	0	0
Dare				
Cabaret	3	70	0	0
Vinta	1 (6 g)	30	0	1
Doritos				
Jalapeno Chesse	1 pkg	230	<5	1
Nacho Cheesier	1 pkg	240	<5	1
Dr. Kracker				
Flatbread Klassic 100% Whole Wheat 3 Seed	1	90	<5	5
Flatbread Klassic Seed	1	100	0	3
Flatbread Pumpkin Seed	1	100	<5	3
Flatbread Seeded Spelt	1	110	0	3
Flatbread Seedlander	1	100	0	2
Flatbread Spelt Sunflower Cheese	1	100	<5	3
Kribbons Krispy Graham	5	120	5	3
Kribbons Muesli	5	120	0	5
Eden				
Brown Rice	8 (1.1 oz)	120	0	2
Nori Nori Rice	15 (1 oz)	110	0	2
Foods Alive				
Golden Flax Maple & Cinnamon	5	150	0	8
Golden Flax Mexican Harvest	5	150	0	9
Golden Flax Onion Garlic	5	140	0	9
Golden Flax Organic Hemp	5	130	0	11
Golden Flax Regular	5	150	0	11
Frookie				
Cheddar	17 (1 oz)	140	0	1
Cracked Pepper	8 (0.7 oz)	70	0	1
Garden Vegetable	13 (1 oz)	130	0	2
Garlic & Herb	8 (0.7 oz)	70	0	1
Pizza	17 (1 oz)	130	0	1
Snack & Party	10 (1 oz)	140	0	1
Water Crackers	8 (0.7 oz)	70	0	1

FOOD	PORTION	CALS	CHOL	FIBER
Wheat & Onion	12 (1 oz)	120	0	2
Wheat & Rye	13 (1 oz)	120	0	3
Gamesa				
Sabrisas	11	150	0	0
Gold'n Krackle				
Cheese	½ oz	65	2	0
Cheese & Oregano	½ oz	65	2	0
Hot & Spicy	½ oz	58	0	0
Onion & Garlic	½ oz	58	0	0
Plain	½ oz	58	0	0
Healthy Handfuls				
Lucky Duckies Cheddar Cheese	1 pkg (1 oz)	100	0	1
Heavenly				
All Flavors Cholesterol Free Sugar Free	1	16	0	0
Kashi				
TLC Country Cheddar	18 (1 oz)	130	0	tr
TLC Honey Sesame	15 (1 oz)	130	0	2
TLC Natural Ranch	15 (1 oz)	130	0	2
TLC Original 7 Grain	15 (1 oz)	130	0	2
Keebler				
Elfin	23 (1 oz)	130	0	tr
Export Soda	3 (0.5 oz)	60	0	tr
Harvest Bakery Multigrain	2 (0.6 oz)	70	0	tr
Munch'ems Cheddar	30 (1 oz)	130	0	tr
Munch'ems Cheddar	39 (1 oz)	140	0	1
Munch'ems Chili Cheese	28 (1.1 oz)	130	0	1
Munch'ems Mexquite BBQ	40 (1 oz)	140	0	1
Munch'ems Ranch	33 (1 oz)	130	0	tr
Munch'ems Ranch	40 (1 oz)	140	0	1
Munch'ems Salsa	28 (1.1 oz)	130	0	1
Munch'ems Sour Cream & Onion	39 (1 oz)	140	0	1
Munch'ems Sour Cream & Onion 55% Reduced Fat	33 (1 oz)	130	0	0
Sandwich Cracker Wheat & Cheddar	1 pkg	200	<5	tr
Toasteds Buttercrisp	9 (1 oz)	140	<5	tr

FOOD	PORTION	CALS	CHOL	FIBER
Toasteds Buttercrisp	5 (0.6 oz)	80	0	0
Toasteds Sesame	9 (1 oz)	140	0	tr
Toasteds Sesame	5 (0.6 oz)	80	0	tr
Toasteds Sesame Reduced Fat	10 (1 oz)	120	0	2
Toasteds Wheat	9 (1 oz)	140	0	tr
Toasteds Wheat	5 (0.6 oz)	80	0	tr
Toasteds Wheat Reduced Fat	10 (1 oz)	120	0	1
Toasteds Wheat Reduced Fat	5 (0.5 oz)	60	0	tr
Town House	5 (0.6 oz)	80	0	tr
Town House 50% Reduced Sodium	5 (0.6 oz)	80	0	tr
Town House Reduced Fat	6 (0.6 oz)	70	0	tr
Town House Wheat	5 (0.6 oz)	80	0	tr
Wheatables Honey Wheat	12 (1 oz)	140	0	1
Wheatables Seven Grain	12 (1 oz)	140	0	1
Kitchen Table Bakers				
Aged Paramesan	3	80	15	0
Caraway Cheese	3	80	15	1
Sesame Cheese	3	80	15	1
Little Debbie				
Cheese Crackers With Peanut Butter	1 (0.9 oz)	140	0	tr
Milton's				
Multi-Grain	2	70	0	0
Nabisco				
Vegetable	4	90	0	tr
Water Original	4	60	0	0
Water Pepper & Poppy	4	60	0	tr
Wheat	4	90	0	tr
Nature's Path				
Signature Tamari Flax	15	110	0	tr
New York Style				
Panetini Garlic Parmesan	5	130	0	1
No-Carb Kitchen				
Cheese	1	25	5	0
No-No				
Flatbreads Tortilla Corn Low Fat Sugar Free Everything	3 (1 oz)	95	0	1

FOOD	PORTION	CALS	CHOL	FIBER
Old London				
Mediterranean Toast	3	60	0	0
Pepperidge Farm				
Giant Goldfish Peanut Butter Sandwich	1 pkg (1.4 oz)	190	<5	1
Giant Goldfish Wheat	14	140	0	1
Goldfish Cheddar	55	140	<5	tr
Goldfish Colors On The Go	1 pkg	170	5	1
Goldfish Original	55	140	0	tr
Goldfish Pizza	55 (1 oz)	140	0	tr
Goldfish Pretzel	43	130	0	tr
Goldfish w/ Whole Grain	55	140	<5	2
Peter Pan				
Peanut Butter Cheese	1 pkg	210	0	1
Peanut Butter Toast	1 pkg	210	0	1
Premium				
Saltine Fat Free	5	60	0	0
Saltine Unsalted Tops	5	60	0	0
Ralston				
Cheese	23 (1 oz)	150	0	tr
Cheese Reduced Fat	29 (1 oz)	130	0	tr
Saltines Fat Free	5 (0.5 oz)	60	0	–
RedOval Farms				
Stoned Wheat Thins Cracked Pepper	4 (0.6 oz)	70	0	tr
Ritz				
Reduced Fat	5	70	0	0
Rykrisp				
Seasoned	2	60	0	3
Sara Lee				
Cracked Pepper Trio	7	130	0	tr
English Water	7	130	0	tr
Harvest Vegetable	6	140	0	tr
SnackWell's				
Cracked Pepper	5	60	0	0
South Beach Diet				
Whole Wheat	1 pkg	100	0	3
Sunshine				
Hi Ho Reduced Fat	5 (0.5 oz)	70	0	tr
Krispy Fat Free	5 (0.5 oz)	50	0	0

FOOD	PORTION	CALS	CHOL	FIBER
Krispy Soup & Oyster	17 (0.5 oz)	60	0	tr
Krispy Whole Wheat	5 (0.5 oz)	60	0	tr
Tree Of Life				
Bite Size Fat Free Cracked Pepper	12 (0.5)	55	0	0
Bite Size Fat Free Garden Vegetable	12 (0.5 oz)	55	0	0
Bite Size Fat Free Garlic & Herb	12 (0.5 oz)	55	0	0
Bite Size Fat Free Toasted Onion	12 (0.5 oz)	55	0	0
Oyster	40 (0.5 oz)	60	0	0
Saltine Cracked Pepper Fat Free	4 (0.5 oz)	60	0	1
Saltine Fat Free	4 (0.5 oz)	50	0	0
Wasa				
Crisp'N Light 7 Grain	3	60	0	2
Fiber Rye	1	30	0	2
Hearty Rye	1	45	0	2
Oats	1	60	0	2
Sourdough Rye	1	35	0	2
Wheat Thins				
Harvest Crisps Five-Grain	13	140	0	1
Wheatsworth				
Crackers	5	80	0	tr
Wisecrackers				
Low Fat Roasted Garlic	10	110	0	tr
Wortz				
Cheese	23 (1 oz)	150	0	tr
Saltines Fat Free	5 (0.5 oz)	60	0	–

CRANBERRIES

FOOD	PORTION	CALS	CHOL	FIBER
cranberry sauce sweetened	½ cup	209	0	–
dried organic	⅓ cup	120	0	2
fresh chopped	1 cup	54	0	–
Earthbound Farm				
Organic Dried	⅓ cup	130	0	2
Eden				
Organic Dried	⅓ cup	140	0	2

FOOD	PORTION	CALS	CHOL	FIBER
Frieda's				
Dried	⅓ cup (1.4 oz)	110	0	2
Good Sense				
Cranberries 'N More	¼ cup	170	0	2
Dried Sweetened	½ cup	130	0	4
Jok'n'Al				
Cranberry Sauce	1 tbsp	8	0	–
Lollipop Tree				
Cranberry Curd	1 tbsp	50	15	–
Newman's Own				
Organic Dried	¼ cup	130	0	2
Ocean Spray				
Craisins	⅓ cup	130	0	2
Cranberry Sauce Jellied	¼ cup	110	0	tr
Cranorange	¼ cup	120	0	1
Whole Berry Sauce	¼ cup	110	0	1
Steel's				
Spiced Cranberry Sauce	⅓ cup	20	0	1
Sunsweet				
Dried	⅓ cup (1.5 oz)	140	0	2
Wild Thyme Farms				
Cranberry Sauce	1 tbsp	19	0	–
CRANBERRY BEANS				
canned	½ cup	108	0	8
dried cooked w/o salt	½ cup	120	0	9
CRANBERRY JUICE				
cranberry juice cocktail	6 oz	108	0	–
cranberry juice cocktail low calorie	6 oz	33	0	–
cranberry juice cocktail frzn	12 oz can	821	0	–
cranberry juice cocktail frzn as prep	6 oz	102	0	–
Keto				
Kooler	½ tsp	0	0	0
Langers				
Cranberry 100	8 oz	140	0	–
Mott's				
Cocktail	8 oz	150	0	–

FOOD	PORTION	CALS	CHOL	FIBER
Nantucket Nectars				
Big Cran	8 oz	140	0	0
Northland				
100% Juice	8 oz	130	0	–
Ocean Spray				
Cocktail	8 oz	140	0	0
Cocktail Reduced Calorie	8 oz	50	0	0
Cocktail Light Low Calorie	8 oz	40	0	0
Cranberry Spritzer	8 oz	160	0	–
Cranberry Drink	8 oz	130	0	–
Crantastic	8 oz	100	0	0
White Cranberry	8 oz	120	0	–
White Cranberry Peach	8 oz	120	0	–
White Cranberry Strawberry	8 oz	120	0	–

CRAYFISH

FOOD	PORTION	CALS	CHOL	FIBER
cooked	3 oz	97	151	0
raw	8	24	37	0
raw	3 oz	76	118	0

CREAM (see also WHIPPED TOPPINGS)

FOOD	PORTION	CALS	CHOL	FIBER
clotted cream	2 tbsp (1 oz)	164	48	0
creme fraiche	2 tbsp (1 oz)	100	40	0
half & half	1 tbsp (0.5 oz)	20	6	–
half & half	1 cup (8.5 oz)	315	89	–
heavy whipping	1 tbsp (0.5 oz)	52	21	–
heavy whipping whipped	1 cup (4.1 oz)	411	163	–
light coffee	1 tbsp (0.5 oz)	29	10	–
light coffee	1 cup (8.4 oz)	496	159	–
light whipping	1 tbsp (0.5 oz)	44	17	–
light whipping cream whipped	1 cup (4.2 oz)	345	132	–
Cabot				
Whipped	2 tbsp	30	10	0
Coffee-Mate				
Half & Half Fat Free	2 tbsp	20	0	–
Hood				
Half & Half	2 tbsp	40	15	0
Light	1 tbsp	30	10	0

FOOD	PORTION	CALS	CHOL	FIBER
Simply Smart Fat Free Half & Half	2 tbsp	15	<5	0
Whipping Cream	1 tbsp	45	20	0
Horizon Organic				
Half & Half	2 tbsp	35	10	0
Heavy Whipping	1 tbsp	50	20	0
Land O Lakes				
Fat Free Half & Half	2 tbsp (1 oz)	20	0	0
Half & Half	2 tbsp (1 oz)	40	15	0
Heavy Whipping	1 tbsp (0.5 oz)	50	20	0
CREAM CHEESE				
cream cheese	1 oz	99	31	–
cream cheese	1 pkg (3 oz)	297	93	–
Alpine Lace				
Reduced Fat Roasted Garlic & Herbs	1 tbsp (1 oz)	60	10	0
Reduced Fat Sundried Tomato & Basil	2 tbsp (1 oz)	70	15	0
Boar's Head				
Cream Cheese	2 tbsp (1 oz)	100	30	0
Crystal Farms				
Regular	1 oz	90	30	0
Tub	2 tbsp	100	25	0
Whipped	2 tbsp	70	20	0
Horizon Organic				
Reduced Fat	2 tbsp	70	25	0
Spreadable	2 tbsp	110	30	0
Organic Valley				
Cream Cheese	1 oz	100	30	0
Philadelphia				
⅓ Less Fat	1 oz	70	20	0
Fat Free	1 oz	30	5	0
CREAM CHEESE SUBSTITUTE				
WholeSoy & Co.				
Soy Cream Organic Original & Flavored	2 tbsp	70	0	1
CREAM OF TARTAR				
cream of tartar	1 tsp	8	0	0

FOOD	PORTION	CALS	CHOL	FIBER
CREAM SUBSTITUTES				
ExpertExtras				
RealCream	1 tsp	14	6	–
CREPES				
basic crepe unfilled	1 (7 in)	112	78	tr
Frieda's				
Ready-To-Use	1 (0.5 oz)	30	5	0
CROAKER				
atlantic breaded & fried	3 oz	188	71	–
atlantic raw	3 oz	89	52	0
CROISSANT				
Sara Lee				
Croissant	1 (1.5 oz)	170	5	1
Petite	2 (2 oz)	230	5	1
TAKE-OUT				
w/ egg & cheese	1 (4.5 oz)	368	216	–
w/ egg cheese & bacon	1 (4.5 oz)	413	215	–
w/ egg cheese & ham	1 (5.3 oz)	474	213	–
w/ egg cheese & sausage	1 (5.6 oz)	523	216	–
CROUTONS				
plain	1 cup (1 oz)	122	0	2
Cardini's				
Italian	2 tbsp	30	0	0
Pepperidge Farm				
Whole Grain Caesar	6	35	0	0
Whole Grain Seasoned	6	30	0	tr
Rothbury Farms				
Seasoned	2 tbsp	30	0	0
Up Country Naturals				
Organic Whole Wheat Garlic & Herb	¼ cup (0.3 oz)	35	0	tr
CUCUMBER				
fresh peeled	1 med (7 oz)	24	0	1
fresh sliced	1 cup	14	0	1
fresh w/ peel sliced	½ cup	34	0	tr
Chiquita				
Cucumber	⅓ med (3.5 oz)	15	0	1

FOOD	PORTION	CALS	CHOL	FIBER
Frieda's				
Japanese	⅔ cup	10	0	1
Seedless Hothouse	⅔ cup	110	0	1
TAKE-OUT				
cucumber & onion salad w/ vinegar	1 cup	52	0	1
cucumber salad w/ oil & vinegar	1 cup	183	0	1
cucumber salad w/ sour cream dressing	1 cup	68	12	1
kimchee	½ cup (1.8 oz)	36	0	tr
tzatziki	½ cup (3.4 oz)	72	5	1
CUMIN				
seed	1 tsp	8	0	–
CURRANT JUICE				
CurrantC				
Black Currant Juice	8 oz	130	0	0
CURRANTS				
black fresh	½ cup	36	0	–
zante dried	½ cup	204	0	–
Sun-Maid				
Zante	¼ cup	130	0	2
CURRY				
curry powder	1 tsp	7	0	1
A Taste Of Thai				
Curry Paste Green	1 tsp	15	0	1
Curry Paste Panang	1 tsp	25	0	0
Curry Paste Red	1 tsp	20	0	0
Curry Paste Yellow	1 tsp	30	0	1
Instant India				
Curry Paste Cilantro Garlic	2 tbsp (1 oz)	110	0	0
Curry Paste Ginger Garlic	2 tbsp (1 oz)	90	0	0
Patak's				
Curry Paste Biryani	2 tbsp	180	0	3
Garam Masala Paste	2 tbsp	130	0	0
Tandoori Paste	2 tbsp	30	0	1
Vandaloo Paste	2 tbsp	160	0	0

FOOD	PORTION	CALS	CHOL	FIBER
CUSK				
fillet baked	3 oz	106	50	0
CUSTARD				
MIX				
as prep w/ 2% milk	½ cup (4.7 oz)	148	74	–
flan as prep w/ 2% milk	½ cup (4.7 oz)	135	9	–
flan as prep w/ whole milk	½ cup (4.7 oz)	150	17	–
Betty Crocker				
Flan w/ Caramel Sauce as prep	1 serv	330	24	–
READY-TO-EAT				
Kozy Shack				
Flan	1 pkg (4 oz)	145	40	0
Swiss Miss				
Egg Custard	1 pkg (4 oz)	153	4	0
TAKE-OUT				
baked	½ cup (5 oz)	148	123	–
flan	½ cup (5.4 oz)	220	140	–
flan de calabaza	1 piece (3.5 oz)	225	112	tr
tocino del cielo heaven's delight	1 cup	856	967	0
zabaione	½ cup (57.2 g)	135	213	0
CUTTLEFISH				
steamed	3 oz	134	190	–
DANDELION GREENS				
fresh cooked	½ cup	17	0	–
raw chopped	½ cup	13	0	–
Frieda's				
Dandelion Greens	2 cups	40	0	3
DANISH PASTRY				
FROZEN				
Morton				
Honey Buns	1 (2.28 oz)	270	0	1
Honey Buns Mini	1 (1.3 oz)	160	0	1
READY-TO-EAT				
Entenmann's				
Danish Ring Walnut	⅙ ring (2 oz)	260	25	2

FOOD	PORTION	CALS	CHOL	FIBER
Tastykake				
Cheese	1 (3 oz)	290	20	tr
Lemon	1 (3 oz)	290	20	1
Raspberry	1 (3 oz)	290	20	1
TAKE-OUT				
cheese	1 (2.5 oz)	266	11	1
cinnamon	1 (5 oz)	572	30	2
fruit	1 (5 oz)	527	162	3
lemon	1 (2.5 oz)	263	28	1
raisin nut	1 (2.3 oz)	280	30	1
DATES				
deglet noor dried	10	240	0	–
dried chopped	1 cup	489	0	–
dried whole	10	228	0	–
jujube fresh	1 oz	30	0	–
medjool	2-3 (1.4 oz)	120	0	3
Calavo				
Dried Pitted	5-6 (1.4 oz)	120	0	3
Earthbound Farm				
Organic Dried	6 (1.4 oz)	120	0	3
Frieda's				
Medjool	2 to 3 (1.4 oz)	120	0	3
SunDate				
Fancy Medjool	3	120	0	3
Sunsweet				
California Pitted	5 to 6 (1.4 oz)	120	0	3
DELI MEATS/COLD CUTS (*see also* BEEF, CHICKEN, HAM, MEAT SUBSTITUTES, TURKEY)				
barbecue loaf pork & beef	1 slice (0.8 oz)	40	9	0
beerwurst beef	2 oz	155	35	1
berliner pork & beef	1 slice (0.8 oz)	53	11	0
blood sausage	1 slice (0.9 oz)	95	30	0
bologna beef	1 slice (1 oz)	88	16	0
bologna beef low fat	1 slice (1 oz)	57	12	0
bologna beef reduced sodium	1 slice (1 oz)	88	16	0
bologna beef & pork	1 slice (1 oz)	87	17	0
bologna beef & pork low fat	1 slice (1 oz)	64	11	0
braunschweiger pork	1 slice (1 oz)	92	50	0

FOOD	PORTION	CALS	CHOL	FIBER
dutch brand loaf pork & beef	1 slice (1.3 oz)	104	23	tr
headcheese pork	1 slice (1.6 oz)	71	31	0
honey loaf pork & beef	1 slice (1 oz)	35	10	0
lebanon bologna beef	2 slices (1 oz)	105	31	0
mortadella beef & pork	1 slice (0.5 oz)	47	8	0
olive loaf pork	2 slice (2 oz)	134	22	0
pastrami beef	1 slice (1 oz)	41	19	tr
peppered loaf pork & beef	1 slice (1 oz)	41	13	0
pepperoni pork & beef	15 slices (1 oz)	135	34	tr
picnic loaf pork & beef	1 slice (1 oz)	65	11	0
salami cooked beef & pork	1 slice (0.8 oz)	58	15	0
salami hard pork	3 slices (0.9 oz)	14	27	0
salami hard pork & beef less sodium	1 slice (1 oz)	113	26	tr
sandwich spread pork & beef	¼ cup	141	23	tr
summer sausage thuringer cervelat	2 oz	203	41	0
Boar's Head				
Abruzzese Hot & Sweet	1 oz	100	25	0
Bologna 25% Lowered Sodium	2 oz	150	30	0
Bologna Beef	2 oz	150	35	0
Bologna Garlic	2 oz	150	35	0
Bologna Lebanon	2 oz	100	40	0
Bologna Pork & Beef	2 oz	150	35	0
Braunschweiger Lite	2 oz	120	50	0
Capocollo Hot & Sweet	1 oz	80	25	0
Dutch Loaf	2 oz	150	25	0
Liverwurst Smoked	2 oz	170	45	0
Mortadella	2 oz	160	30	0
Olive Loaf	2 oz	130	20	0
Pastrami	2 oz	70	30	0
Pickle & Pepper Loaf	2 oz	150	30	0
Prosciutto	1 oz	60	15	0
Salami Beef	2 oz	120	25	0
Salami Cooked	2 oz	130	40	0
Salami Hard	1 oz	110	30	0
Sopressata Hot & Sweet	1 oz	100	25	0
Spiced Ham	2 oz	120	30	0

FOOD	PORTION	CALS	CHOL	FIBER
Carl Buddig				
Beef	1 pkg (2.5 oz)	100	50	–
Corned Beef	1 pkg (2.5 oz)	100	50	–
Pastrami	1 pkg (2.5 oz)	100	50	–
Hebrew National				
Bologna Beef	1 slice (1 oz)	80	15	0
Bologna Lean Beef	4 slices (2 oz)	90	20	–
Salami Beef	3 slices (2 oz)	150	35	0
Salami Lean Beef	4 slices (2 oz)	90	25	–
Hormel				
Pepperoni Sliced	16 slices (1 oz)	140	25	–
Russer				
Turkey Breast Honey Roasted	1 slice (1 oz)	25	10	0
Sara Lee				
Corned Beef	1 slice (2 oz)	50	25	0
Pastrami	2 slices (1.6 oz)	60	25	0
Salami Genoa	4 slices (1 oz)	110	35	0
Salami Hard	4 slices (1 oz)	120	40	0
Wellshire				
Salami Genoa	1 oz	100	30	0
Salami Hard	1 oz	100	30	0
Sopressata Sliced	1 oz	100	30	0
TAKE-OUT				
corned beef brisket	2 oz	90	35	0
DILL				
seed	1 tsp	6	0	–
sprigs fresh	5	0	0	–
weed dry	1 tsp	3	0	–
DINNER (*see also* ASIAN FOOD, PASTA DINNERS, POT PIES, SPANISH FOOD)				
Amy's				
Country Dinner Vegetable Salisbury Steak	1 pkg (11 oz)	380	15	9
Banquet				
Beef Patty w/ Country Style Vegetables	1 meal (9.5 oz)	310	40	2
Boneless Pork Rib	1 meal (10 oz)	400	45	4
Boneless White Fried Chicken	1 meal (8.25 oz)	540	60	3

FOOD	PORTION	CALS	CHOL	FIBER
Chicken Parmigiana	1 meal (9.5 oz)	320	50	3
Chicken Fingers Meal	1 meal (7.1 oz)	740	70	6
Chicken Fried Beef Steak	1 pkg (10 oz)	420	35	4
Chicken Nuggets Meal	1 meal (6.75 oz)	430	50	4
Extra Helping Boneless Pork Riblet	1 meal (15.25 oz)	720	80	7
Extra Helping Fried Beef Steak	1 meal (16 oz)	820	70	6
Extra Helping Fried Chicken	1 meal (14.7 oz)	910	160	5
Extra Helping Meatloaf	1 meal (16 oz)	610	110	6
Extra Helping Salisbury Steak	1 meal (16.5 oz)	740	130	7
Extra Helping Turkey & Gravy w/ Dressing	1 meal (17 oz)	620	80	10
Extra Helping White Fried Chicken	1 meal (13 oz)	690	70	8
Extra Helping Yankee Pot Roast	1 meal (14.5 oz)	410	50	3
Family Size Brown Gravy & Salisbury Steak	1 serv	240	40	1
Family Size Brown Gravy & Sliced Beef	1 serv	140	40	tr
Family Size Chicken & Broccoli Alfredo	1 serv	270	40	3
Family Size Country Style Chicken & Dumplings	1 serv	290	40	7
Family Size Creamy Broccoli Chicken Cheese & Rice	1 serv	280	45	2
Family Size Hearty Beef Stew	1 cup	170	30	4
Family Size Homestyle Gravy & Sliced Turkey	2 slices	140	40	1
Family Size Mushroom Gravy & Charbroiled Beef Patties	1 patty	250	35	2
Family Size Potato Ham & Broccoli Au Gratin	2/3 cup	210	30	2
Family Size Savory Gravy & Meatloaf	1 slice	120	35	1
Fish Sticks	1 meal (6.6 oz)	290	30	4
Grilled Chicken	1 meal (9.9 oz)	330	50	2

FOOD	PORTION	CALS	CHOL	FIBER
Honey Roast Turkey Breast	1 meal (9 oz)	270	30	4
Meatloaf	1 meal (9.5 oz)	280	60	3
Our Original Fried Chicken	1 meal (9 oz)	470	90	2
Pork Cutlet Meal	1 meal (10.25 oz)	420	35	4
Sliced Beef	1 meal (9 oz)	270	70	4
Turkey Meal	1 meal (9.25 oz)	290	35	6
Veal Parmagiana	1 meal (8.75 oz)	330	20	2
Western Style Beef Patty	1 meal (9.5 oz)	360	40	3
White Meat Fried Chicken	1 meal (8.75 oz)	460	100	2
Yankee Pot Roast	1 meal (9.4 oz)	230	60	4
Birds Eye				
Voila! Pasta Primavera w/ Chicken	1²/₃ cups	250	10	7
Voila! Shrimp Scampi	1¾ cups	190	60	3
Voila! Southwestern Chicken	2 cups	250	30	2
Boston Market				
Glazed Rotisserie Chicken w/ Mashed Potatoes Gravy Vegetables	1 pkg (16 oz)	390	75	4
Meatloaf w/ Mashed Potatoes & Gravy	1 pkg (16 oz)	880	100	3
C&W				
Stir Fry Feast Pot Sticker + Sauce	2 cups	200	15	4
Stir Fry Feast Ultimate + Sauce	1½ cups	190	30	3
Contessa				
Beef Goulash not prep	1¾ cups	210	50	3
Chicken Cacciatore not prep	1¾ cups	230	35	6
Chicken Alfredo not prep	1¾ cups	330	70	2
Fantastic				
Ginger Shitake w/ Rice Noodles	1 pkg (7.4 oz)	340	0	4
Fillo Factory				
Fillo Pie Broccoli & Cheese	¼ pie (4 oz)	350	20	3
Fillo Pie Spinach & Cheese	⅕ pie (4.8 oz)	210	15	2
Glory				
Savory Singles Chicken & Dumplings	1 pkg	290	75	6

FOOD	PORTION	CALS	CHOL	FIBER
Savory Singles Chicken Smoked Sausage & Rice Casserole	1 pkg	440	60	1
Savory Singles Ham & Sausage Jambalaya	1 pkg	400	50	2
Savory Singles Turkey & Gravy w/ Cornbread Stuffing	1 pkg	440	30	2
Golden Cuisine				
Beef Stew	1 pkg	350	61	9
Boneless Pork Patty	1 pkg	504	57	13
Breaded Baked Fish w/ Rice Pilaf	1 pkg	300	27	6
Chicken Cacciatore	1 pkg	417	48	10
Chicken & Noodles	1 pkg	331	54	8
Chicken Parmesan	1 pkg	430	30	14
Chicken w/ Marinara Sauce	1 pkg	329	44	15
Meatloaf Patty & Gravy	1 pkg	340	48	7
Mesquite Chicken	1 pkg	320	30	10
Pot Roast w/ Gravy	1 pkg	343	50	10
Salisbury Steak & Mushroom Sauce	1 pkg	350	38	7
Swedish Meatballs	1 pkg	440	48	9
Turkey Tetrazzini	1 pkg	304	58	11
Healthy Choice				
Beef Merlot	1 pkg	240	40	6
Beef Pot Roast	1 pkg	320	45	6
Beef Stroganoff	1 pkg	320	65	6
Beef Teriyaki	1 pkg	310	40	5
Beef Tips Portabello	1 pkg	280	50	3
Blackened Chicken	1 pkg	300	35	5
Boneless Beef Ribs w/ Classic BBQ Sauce	1 pkg	360	55	8
Charbroiled Beef Patty	1 pkg	310	40	6
Cheesy Rice & Chicken	1 pkg	250	50	4
Chicken Carbonara	1 pkg	290	45	2
Chicken Margherita	1 pkg	340	50	6
Chicken Parmigiana	1 pkg	320	20	6
Chicken Breat & Vegetables	1 pkg	260	45	6
Chicken Broccoli Alfredo	1 pkg	300	50	2

FOOD	PORTION	CALS	CHOL	FIBER
Chicken Piccata	1 pkg	260	40	2
Chicken Teriyaki	1 pkg	270	40	6
Chicken Tuscany	1 pkg	340	40	4
Country Breaded Chicken	1 pkg	370	45	5
Country Glazed Chicken	1 pkg	230	45	3
Country Herb Chicken	1 pkg	280	40	5
Creamy Herb Roasted Chicken	1 pkg	240	60	5
Grilled Basil Chicken	1 pkg	330	40	5
Grilled Chicken Breast & Pasta	1 pkg	250	40	4
Grilled Chicken Breast w/ Mashed Potatoes	1 pkg	190	50	3
Grilled Chicken Caesar	1 pkg	300	35	5
Grilled Chicken Marinara	1 pkg	270	35	5
Grilled Steak w/ Roasted Garlic Sauce	1 pkg	220	35	5
Grilled Turkey Breast	1 pkg	250	35	5
Grilled Whiskey Steak	1 pkg	280	40	6
Herb Baked Fish	1 pkg	360	35	6
Homestyle Chicken & Pasta	1 pkg	250	40	5
Honey Glazed Chicken	1 pkg	320	40	6
Lemon Pepper Fish	1 pkg	280	20	4
Mandarin Chicken	1 pkg	250	40	4
Mesquite Chicken BBQ	1 pkg	300	45	5
Mixed Grills Chicken Honey BBQ w/ Dipping Sauce	1 pkg	380	25	8
Mixed Grills Chicken Honey Mustard w/ Dipping Sauce	1 pkg	360	25	10
Mixed Grills Chicken Teriyaki w/ Dipping Sauce	1 pkg	340	35	9
Mixed Grills Chicken Tomato Garlic w/ Dipping Sauce	1 pkg	370	30	10
Mixed Grills Steak BBQ Sauce	1 pkg	420	45	7
Mixed Grills Steak Teriyaki w/ Dipping Sauce	1 pkg	350	30	11
Mixed Grills Steak w/ Zesty Steak Sauce	1 pkg	350	40	8
Oriental Style Beef	1 pkg	310	35	5
Oriental Style Chicken	1 pkg	240	35	4

FOOD	PORTION	CALS	CHOL	FIBER
Oven Roasted Beef	1 pkg	280	60	5
Princess Chicken	1 pkg	310	60	5
Roast Turkey Breast	1 pkg	220	40	3
Roasted Chicken Breast	1 pkg	280	45	7
Roasted Chicken Chardonnay	1 pkg	290	40	4
Salisbury Steak	1 pkg	360	45	5
Salisbury Steak w/ Red Skin Mashed Potatoes	1 pkg	200	40	4
Sesame Chicken	1 pkg	260	35	4
Slow Roasted Turkey Breast w/ Mashed Potatoes	1 pkg	210	45	4
Sweet & Sour Chicken	1 pkg	340	25	3
Traditional Meatloaf	1 pkg	300	40	6
Tradtional Turkey Breast	1 pkg	330	35	4
Tuna Casserole	1 pkg	270	30	5
Ian's				
Chicken Finger Meal Allergen Free	1 pkg (7 oz)	368	40	3
Chicken Nugget Meal	1 pkg (8 oz)	440	50	2
Fish Stick Meal	1 pkg (8.4 oz)	480	25	4
Hamburger Meal	1 pkg (7 oz)	296	25	3
Pizza Meal	1 pkg (6.7 oz)	340	25	4
Popcorn Turkey Dog Meal Allergen Free	1 pkg (7 oz)	442	21	1
Kashi				
Black Bean Mango	1 pkg (10 oz)	340	0	7
Lemon Rosemary Chicken	1 pkg (10 oz)	330	15	5
Lime Cilantro Shrimp	1 pkg (10 oz)	250	0	6
Southwest Style Chicken	1 pkg (10 oz)	240	30	6
Sweet & Sour Chicken	1 pkg (10 oz)	320	35	6
Kid Cuisine				
All American Fried Chicken	1 meal	500	80	4
All Star Chicken Breast Nuggets	1 meal	460	25	8
Bug Safari Chicken Breast Nuggets	1 meal	450	25	6
Carnival Corn Dog	1 meal	430	30	7
Deep Sea Adventure Fish Sticks	1 meal	400	20	4

FOOD	PORTION	CALS	CHOL	FIBER
Fiesta Beef Taco Dippers	1 meal	370	18	4
Pop Star Popcorn Chicken	1 meal	410	15	6
Lean Cuisine				
Cafe Classics Baked Chicken Florentine	1 pkg (8 oz)	200	40	3
Cafe Classics Baked Lemon Pepper Fish	1 pkg (9 oz)	220	65	7
Cafe Classics Beef Peppercorn	1 pkg (8.75 oz)	220	25	3
Cafe Classics Beef Portabello	1 pkg (9 oz)	200	30	2
Cafe Classics Beef Pot Roast	1 pkg (9 oz)	190	25	2
Cafe Classics Bowl Creamy Basil Chicken	1 pkg (10.5 oz)	310	35	3
Cafe Classics Bowl Grilled Chicken Caesar	1 pkg (9 oz)	270	35	3
Cafe Classics Chicken Carbonara	1 pkg (9 oz)	280	30	2
Cafe Classics Chicken & Vegetables	1 pkg (10.5 oz)	240	30	2
Cafe Classics Chicken L'Orange	1 pkg (9 oz)	230	35	2
Cafe Classics Chicken Marsala	1 pkg (8.1 oz)	140	35	3
Cafe Classics Chicken Parmesan	1 pkg (10.9 oz)	280	40	3
Cafe Classics Chicken Tuscan	1 pkg (12 oz)	300	45	5
Cafe Classics Chicken w/ Almonds	1 pkg (8.5 oz)	260	30	3
Cafe Classics Chicken w/ Basil Cream Sauce	1 pkg (8.5 oz)	270	30	2
Cafe Classics Fiesta Grilled Chicken	1 pkg (9.5 oz)	250	40	3
Cafe Classics Garlic Beef & Broccoli	1 pkg (9 oz)	170	30	3
Cafe Classics Glazed Chicken	1 pkg (8.5 oz)	220	35	2
Cafe Classics Glazed Turkey Tenderloins	1 pkg (9 oz)	260	20	4
Cafe Classics Grilled Chicken	1 pkg (9.4 oz)	160	35	4

FOOD	PORTION	CALS	CHOL	FIBER
Cafe Classics Grilled Chicken w/ Teriyaki Glaze	1 pkg (10 oz)	270	40	0
Cafe Classics Herb Roasted Chicken	1 pkg (8 oz)	190	30	3
Cafe Classics Honey Dijon Grilled Chicken	1 pkg (8 oz)	220	50	2
Cafe Classics Honey Mustard Chicken	1 pkg (8 oz)	250	30	1
Cafe Classics Honey Roasted Pork	1 serv (9.5 oz)	230	50	5
Cafe Classics Mandarin Chicken	1 pkg (9 oz)	270	30	2
Cafe Classics Meatloaf w/ Gravy & Whipped Potatoes	1 pkg (9.4 oz)	280	45	3
Cafe Classics Orange Peel Chicken	1 pkg (12 oz)	390	25	3
Cafe Classics Oven Roasted Beef	1 pkg (9.25 oz)	210	35	2
Cafe Classics Roasted Garlic Chicken	1 pkg (8.8 oz)	200	40	2
Cafe Classics Roasted Turkey & Vegetables	1 pkg (8 oz)	150	25	3
Cafe Classics Roasted Turkey Breast	1 pkg (12 oz)	280	30	4
Cafe Classics Roasted Turkey Breast w/ Dressing	1 pkg (9.75 oz)	270	20	3
Cafe Classics Salisbury Steak	1 pkg (12.5 oz)	310	50	8
Cafe Classics Salisbury Steak w/ Mac & Cheese	1 pkg (9.5 oz)	280	50	3
Cafe Classics Sesame Chicken	1 pkg (9 oz)	330	20	2
Cafe Classics Southern Beef Tips	1 pkg (8.75 oz)	250	25	3
Cafe Classics Steak Tips Dijon	1 pkg (12 oz)	320	35	5
Cafe Classics Steak Tips Portobello	1 pkg (7.5 oz)	180	40	3
Cafe Classics Stuffed Cabbage	1 pkg (9.5 oz)	200	15	4

FOOD	PORTION	CALS	CHOL	FIBER
Cafe Classics Swedish Meatballs	1 pkg (9.1 oz)	290	50	2
Cafe Classics Sweet & Sour Chicken	1 pkg (10 oz)	290	25	1
Cafe Classics Three Cheese Chicken	1 pkg (8 oz)	230	45	2
Comfort Classics Baked Chicken	1 pkg (8.6 oz)	230	30	2
Dinnertime Selects Balsamic Glazed Chicken	1 pkg (12 oz)	400	40	4
Dinnertime Selects Chicken Florentine	1 pkg (13.25 oz)	420	45	6
Dinnertime Selects Chicken Portabello	1 pkg (12 oz)	370	40	3
Dinnertime Selects Lemon Garlic Shrimp	1 pkg (12 oz)	350	75	5
Skillet Beef Teriyaki & Rice	1 serv	190	15	2
Spa Cuisine Chicken Mediterranean	1 pkg (10.5 oz)	240	20	6
Spa Cuisine Chicken In Peanut Sauce	1 pkg (9 oz)	280	25	2
Spa Cuisine Chicken Pecan	1 pkg (9 oz)	260	30	4
Spa Cuisine Lemon Chicken	1 pkg (9 oz)	290	25	1
Spa Cuisine Lemongrass Chicken	1 pkg (9.4 oz)	240	30	4
Spa Cuisine Pork w/ Cherry Sauce	1 pkg (8.25 oz)	260	35	4
Spa Cuisine Rosemary Chicken	1 pkg (8.25 oz)	230	35	3
Spa Cuisine Salmon w/ Beef	1 pkg (9.5 oz)	360	30	5
Luzianne				
Cajun Creole Dirty Rice	1 serv	160	0	0
Cajun Creole Etouffee	1 serv	200	0	1
Cajun Creole Gumbo	1 serv	160	0	1
Cajun Creole Jambalaya	1 serv	200	0	1
Marie Callender's				
Beef Stroganoff w/ Noodles	1 meal (13 oz)	600	70	4
Beef Tips In Mushroom Sauce	1 meal (13 oz)	430	50	6

FOOD	PORTION	CALS	CHOL	FIBER
Breaded Chicken Parmigiana	1 meal (16 oz)	860	50	5
Breaded Fish w/ Mac & Cheese	1 meal (12 oz)	550	60	3
Cheesy Rice w/ Chicken & Broccoli	1 meal (12 oz)	390	55	6
Chicken & Dumplings	1 meal (14 oz)	390	130	4
Chicken & Noodles	1 meal (13 oz)	520	80	5
Chicken Cordon Bleu	1 meal (13 oz)	610	75	6
Chicken Fried Beef Steak & Gravy	1 meal (15 oz)	650	50	7
Chicken Teriyaki	1 meal (13 oz)	510	55	2
Country Fried Chicken & Gravy	1 meal (16 oz)	620	75	6
Country Fried Pork Chop	1 meal (15 oz)	540	65	8
Escalloped Noodles & Chicken	1 meal (13 oz)	740	90	5
Glazed Chicken	1 meal (13 oz)	490	90	1
Grilled Southwestern Style Chicken	1 meal (14 oz)	410	80	6
Grilled Chicken & Mashed Potatoes	1 meal (10 oz)	340	90	1
Grilled Chicken Breast & Rice Pilaf	1 meal (11.75 oz)	360	40	4
Grilled Chicken In Mushroom Sauce	1 meal (14 oz)	480	65	7
Grilled Turkey Breast & Rice Pilaf	1 meal (11.75 oz)	310	40	4
Herb Roasted Chicken & Mashed Potatoes	1 meal (14 oz)	580	205	7
Homestyle Turkey & Noodles	1 meal (12 oz)	600	90	5
Honey Roasted Chicken	1 meal (14 oz)	440	140	7
Honey Smoked Ham Steak w/ Macaroni & Cheese	1 meal (14 oz)	490	80	5
Meatloaf & Gravy w/ Mashed Potatoes	1 meal (14 oz)	540	95	5
Old Fashioned Beef Pot Roast & Gravy	1 meal (15 oz)	500	110	3
Roast Beef	1 meal (14.5 oz)	390	70	11
Sirloin Salisbury Steak & Gravy	1 meal (14 oz)	550	85	6

FOOD	PORTION	CALS	CHOL	FIBER
Skillet Meal Au Gratin Potatoes	⅔ cup (5 oz)	190	30	2
Skillet Meal Beef Pot Roast	½ pkg	290	60	5
Skillet Meal Beef Stroganoff	½ pkg	310	60	5
Skillet Meal Chicken & Rice w/ Broccoli & Cheese	½ pkg	440	70	8
Skillet Meal Chicken Teriyaki	½ pkg	340	30	5
Skillet Meal Herb Chicken	½ pkg	290	35	5
Skillet Meal Roasted Chicken & Vegetables	½ pkg	260	40	7
Skillet Meal White & Wild Rice In Cheese Sauce	1 cup	300	35	2
Swedish Meatballs	1 meal (12.5 oz)	520	65	3
Sweet & Sour Chicken	1 meal (14 oz)	570	40	7
Turkey w/ Gravy & Dressing	1 meal (14 oz)	500	80	4
Morton				
Breaded Chicken Pattie	1 meal (6.75 oz)	290	35	4
Chicken Nuggets	1 meal (7 oz)	340	30	2
Chili Gravy w/ Beef Enchilada & Tamale	1 meal (10 oz)	270	10	7
Fried Chicken	1 meal (9 oz)	470	90	3
Gravy & Charbroiled Beef Patty	1 meal (9 oz)	310	20	5
Gravy & Salisbury Steak	1 meal (9 oz)	310	30	3
Gravy & Turkey w/ Stuffing	1 meal (9 oz)	240	40	4
Tomato Sauce w/ Meat Loaf	1 meal (9 oz)	250	20	3
Veal Parmagiana w/ Tomato Sauce	1 meal (8.75 oz)	290	25	4
Nature's Choice				
Broccoli Parmesan Alfredo	1 pkg (12 oz)	270	10	5
Nature's Entree				
Hearty Stew	1 pkg (12 oz)	290	10	3
Tuscany White Bean	1 pkg (12 oz)	330	5	4
Pacific Foods				
Beef Steak Stew	1 cup	250	35	8
Chicken Stew	1 cup	200	40	2
Patak's				
Vegetable Curry w/ Rice Creamy Coconut	1 pkg	400	10	5

FOOD	PORTION	CALS	CHOL	FIBER
Vegetable Curry w/ Rice Rich Tomato & Onion	1 pkg (10.5 oz)	290	0	5
Vegetable Curry w/ Rice Tangy Lemon & Cilantro	1 pkg	300	0	5
Patio				
Ranchera	1 pkg (13 oz)	470	35	9
Quorn				
Meat Free Simply Saute Indian	½ pkg	240	15	9
Meat Free Simply Saute Mexican	½ pkg	340	15	7
Meat Free Simply Saute Thai	½ pkg	240	15	8
Savvy Faire				
Baja Jack Scramble	1 pkg (8.2 oz)	370	50	2
Braised Beef	1 pkg (9.4 oz)	320	60	3
Herb Crusted Chicken	1 pkg (9.7 oz)	430	75	6
Seeds Of Change				
Chicken Teriyaki	1 pkg (10 oz)	300	30	4
Mushroom Wild Pilaf	1 pkg (11 oz)	350	45	5
Seven Grain Pilaf	1 pkg (11 oz)	390	20	10
Shady Brook				
Roasted Carved Turkey	1 pkg (18.6 oz)	550	55	4
South Beach Diet				
Beef & Broccoli & Asian Style Noodles	1 pkg	320	45	9
Caprese Style Chicken w/ Cauliflower & Broccoli	1 pkg	250	95	3
Cashew Chicken w/ Sugar Snap Peas	1 pkg	360	55	8
Chicken Alfredo A La Roma	1 pkg	270	65	8
Chicken Basilico w/ Rotini	1 pkg	280	50	7
Garlic Herb Chicken w/ Green Beans Almondine	1 pkg	250	70	4
Garlic Parmesan Chicken w/ Penne	1 pkg	290	55	8
Garlic Sesame Beef w/ Cauliflower Sugar Snap Peas & Peppers	1 pkg	250	65	4

FOOD	PORTION	CALS	CHOL	FIBER
Kung Pao Chicken Breast Strips w/ Peppers & Broccoli	1 pkg	300	80	5
Orange Beef Slices & Brown Rice In Sauce w/ Broccoli & Carrots	1 pkg	260	55	4
Savory Beef w/ Cheesy Broccoli	1 pkg	240	70	3
Savory Pork w/ Pecans & Green Beans	1 pkg	260	65	4
Szechwan Pork & Asian Noodles In Sauce	1 pkg	270	40	9
Swanson				
Beef Pot Roast	1 pkg (14 oz)	320	35	4
Chicken Parmigiana w/ Spaghetti	1 pkg (11 oz)	380	25	5
Turkey Breast & Stuffing Dinner	1 pkg (11.7 oz)	350	35	4
Tamarind Tree				
Alu Chole	1 pkg (9.25 oz)	320	0	7
Channa Dal Masala	1 pkg (9.25 oz)	290	0	90
Dal Makhani	1 pkg (9.25 oz)	350	10	11
Navratan Korma	1 pkg (9.25 oz)	370	10	7
Palak Paneer	1 pkg (9.25 oz)	350	25	8
Saag Chole	1 pkg (9.25 oz)	330	0	9
Vegetable Jalfrazi	1 pkg (9.25 oz)	280	0	7
Weight Watchers				
Smart Ones Lemon Herb Chicken Piccata	1 pkg (8.5 oz)	190	25	3
Smart Ones Swedish Meatballs	1 pkg (9 oz)	280	30	3
Yves				
Veggie Country Stew	1 pkg (10.5 oz)	170	0	7

DIP

FOOD	PORTION	CALS	CHOL	FIBER
spinach sour cream	¼ cup	155	13	1
Bravos!				
Salsa	2 tbsp	15	0	0
Salsa Con Queso	1 tbsp	25	0	0

FOOD	PORTION	CALS	CHOL	FIBER
Cabot				
Bac'n Horseradish	2 tbsp	50	15	0
Clam	2 tbsp	50	15	0
French Onion	2 tbsp	50	15	0
Ranch	1 tbsp	50	15	0
Salsa Grande	2 tbsp	50	15	0
Veggie	2 tbsp	50	15	0
Eatsmart				
Flame Roasted Salsa Con Queso	2 tbsp	35	0	–
Garden Style Sweet Salsa	2 tbsp	20	0	–
Jalapeno & Lime Tres Bean	2 tbsp	25	0	–
Fritos				
Bean	2 tbsp	40	0	1
Chili Cheese	2 tbsp	45	<5	0
Hot Bean	2 tbsp	40	0	1
Jalapeno Cheddar Cheese	2 tbsp	50	5	0
Mild Cheddar	2 tbsp	60	5	0
Gringo Billy's				
Guacamole Mix	1 tsp	10	0	1
Guiltless Gourmet				
Black Bean Mild	2 tbsp	30	0	2
Roasted Red Pepper Salsa	2 tbsp	15	0	0
Southwestern Grill Salsa	2 tbsp	15	0	0
Marzetti				
Veggie Fat Free Ranch	2 tbsp	35	0	0
Veggie Dip Light Veggie	1 pkg (3.25 oz)	170	15	0
Phillips Seafood				
Crab & Spinach	2 tbsp	50	15	–
Maryland Crab	2 tbsp	70	30	–
Racquet				
Hot Cheddar Jalapeno	2 tbsp	30	0	0
Ruffles				
French Onion	¼ cup	200	0	2
Ranch	2 tbsp	60	<5	tr
Snyder's Of Hanover				
Microwavable Hot Nacho Cheese	2 tbsp	48	3	0
Microwavable Mild Cheese	2 tbsp	45	5	0

FOOD	PORTION	CALS	CHOL	FIBER
Mustard Pretzel	2 tbsp	60	0	0
Sour Cream & Onion	2 tbsp	60	15	0
Utz				
Fat Free Sour Cream & Onion	2 tbsp (1.1 oz)	30	0	0
Jalapeno & Cheddar	2 tbsp (1 oz)	30	0	0
Low Fat Desert Garden	2 tbsp (1.1 oz)	40	0	0
Low Fat Salsa Con Queso	2 tbsp (1 oz)	40	0	0
Mild Cheddar	2 tbsp (1 oz)	45	5	0
Sour Cream & Onion	2 tbsp (1 oz)	60	15	0
Walden Farms				
Low Carb Bruschetta	2 tbsp	35	0	0
Low Carb Pesto Bruschetta	1 tsp	10	0	0
Wise				
French Onion	2 tbsp	60	0	0
Nacho Cheese	2 tbsp	50	0	0

DOCK

FOOD	PORTION	CALS	CHOL	FIBER
fresh cooked	3½ oz	20	0	–
raw chopped	½ cup	15	0	–

DOUGHNUTS

FOOD	PORTION	CALS	CHOL	FIBER
cake type unsugared	1 (1.6 oz)	198	18	1
creme filled	1 (3 oz)	307	20	–
french cruller glazed	1 (1.4 oz)	169	5	–
honey bun	1 (2.1 oz)	242	4	1
jelly	1 (3 oz)	289	22	–
old fashioned	1 (1.6 oz)	198	18	1
sugared	1 (1.6 oz)	192	14	1
wheat glazed	1 (1.6 oz)	162	9	–
wheat sugared	1 (1.6 oz)	162	9	–
yeast glazed	1 (2.1 oz)	242	4	1
Entenmann's				
Crumb	1	260	10	tr
Frosted Devil's Food	1	310	10	2
Glazed	1	260	15	tr
Glazed Popems	4	220	0	0
Mini Frosted	1 (1 oz)	150	<5	tr
Plain Old Fashion	1	230	15	tr
Rich Chocolate Frosted	1	280	10	1

FOOD	PORTION	CALS	CHOL	FIBER
Little Debbie				
Donut Sticks	1 (1.6 oz)	210	10	0
Snack & Smile				
Mini Donuts Chocolate	6	370	10	2
Mini Donuts Glazed	6	340	20	tr
Mini Donuts Powdered Sugar	6	320	10	1
Super Bakery				
Daily Donut	1 (2.2 oz)	250	10	tr
Proballs Slam Powdered Baseballs	1 (1.3 oz)	130	5	0
Tom's				
Chocolate Gem	1 pkg (2.5 oz)	320	10	1
Dunkin' Sticks	1 pkg (2.5 oz)	370	10	tr
Powdered Gems	1 pkg (2.5 oz)	320	10	1
DRINK MIXERS				
whiskey sour mix not prep	1 pkg (0.6 oz)	64	0	–
whiskey sour mix	2 oz	55	0	0
Baja Bob's				
Bloody Mary Mix Lean & Mean	4 oz	20	0	0
Pina Colada	4 oz	30	0	1
Sugar Free Margarita Mix	4 oz	10	0	–
Sugar Free Margarita Mix Desert Lime	4 oz	10	0	0
Sugar Free Margarita Mix Wild Strawberry	4 oz	10	0	–
Sweet-n-Sour Mix	4 oz	10	0	–
Daily's				
Bloody Mary Original	1 serv (6 oz)	50	0	–
Margarita Daiquiri Strawberry	1 serv (4 oz)	180	0	2
Margarita Green Demon	1 serv (3 oz)	80	0	–
Pina Colada	1 serv (3 oz)	160	0	1
Ocean Spray				
Bloody Mary Mix	4 oz	40	0	–
Margarita Mix	4 oz	160	0	–
Sour Mix	4 oz	140	0	–

FOOD	PORTION	CALS	CHOL	FIBER
DRUM				
freshwater fillet baked	5.4 oz	236	126	0
freshwater baked	3 oz	130	70	0
DUCK				
w/ skin roasted	1 cup (4.9 oz)	472	118	0
w/ skin w/ bone leg roasted	3 oz	184	97	0
w/ skin w/o bone breast roasted	3 oz	172	116	0
w/o skin roasted	1 cup (4.9 oz)	281	125	0
w/o skin w/ bone leg braised	1 cup (6.1 oz)	310	183	0
w/o skin w/o bone breast broiled	1 cup (6.1 oz)	244	249	0
wild w/ skin raw	½ duck (9.5 oz)	571	216	0
Grimaud Farms				
Muscovy Duck Confit	1 serv (3 oz)	170	95	–
Maple Leaf Farms				
Breast Filet	4 oz	360	60	0
Leg Quarters	4 oz	420	90	0
Orange Breast Filet	4 oz	320	75	–
DUMPLING				
Health Is Wealth				
Potstickers Chicken Free	2 (1.6 oz)	80	0	1
Potstickers Pork Free	2 (1.6 oz)	80	0	1
Potstickers Vegetable	2 (1.6 oz)	90	0	5
Steamed Dumpling	2 (1.6 oz)	50	0	1
Kahiki				
Potstickers Chicken	5 (3.3 oz)	230	10	1
Samosas Coconut Curry Chicken	4 (2.8 oz)	170	15	1
Traveling Chef				
Potstickers Chicken + Dipping Sauce	5 pieces + 1 tbsp sauce	285	20	1
DURIAN				
fresh	3.5 oz	141	0	–
EEL				
fresh cooked	3 oz	200	137	0
fresh cooked	1 fillet (5.6 oz)	375	257	0
raw	3 oz	156	107	0

FOOD	PORTION	CALS	CHOL	FIBER
EGG (see also EGG DISHES, EGG SUBSTITUTES)				
CHICKEN				
hard or soft cooked	1	77	211	0
pickled	1	72	198	0
poached	1	73	210	0
scrambled plain	2	199	400	0
sunny side up	2	155	365	0
white cooked	1	17	0	0
yolk cooked	1	55	209	0
Crystal Farms				
In Shell Pasteurized	1	70	215	0
Peeled Hard Cooked	1	70	190	0
Egg-Land's Best				
Large	1	70	180	0
Organic Brown	1	70	180	0
Eggology				
100% Organic Egg Whites	¼ cup	30	0	0
Gold Circle Farms				
Cage Free	1 large	70	215	–
Horizon Organic				
Jumbo	1 (2.2 oz)	90	270	0
Land O Lakes				
Brown Extra Large	1 (2 oz)	80	240	–
Organic Valley				
Brown Extra Large	1 (2.2 oz)	90	225	–
Brown Large	1 (2 oz)	80	200	–
Brown Medium	1 (1.8 oz)	70	175	–
Sunny Fresh				
Eggs ASAP!	2	140	380	0
OTHER POULTRY				
duck 100 year old	1 (1 oz)	49	173	–
duck cooked	1 (2.5 oz)	129	616	0
duck preserved hard core	1 (1.8 oz)	80	220	0
duck preserved soft core	1 (1.8 oz)	80	220	0
duck salted	1 (1 oz)	54	184	–
goose cooked	1 (5 oz)	265	1223	0
quail canned	1 (0.3 oz)	14	75	0
turkey raw	1 (2.8 oz)	135	737	0

FOOD	PORTION	CALS	CHOL	FIBER
EGG DISHES				
TAKE-OUT				
deviled	1 half	62	121	0
eggs benedict	2	825	784	2
omelet cheese	3 eggs	387	588	0
omelet mushroom	3 eggs	251	511	1
omelet mushroom & onion	3 eggs	294	600	1
omelet plain	3 eggs	338	736	0
omelet spanish	3 eggs	496	626	3
omelet spinach	3 eggs	279	568	1
omelet western	3 eggs	355	537	tr
salad	½ cup	353	344	0
tortilla de amarillo omelet w/ plantain	3 eggs	536	467	3
EGG ROLLS				
egg roll wrapper fresh	1	83	3	–
Chun King				
Chicken Mini	6	210	15	2
Chicken Restaurant Style	1 (3 oz)	190	20	2
Pork & Shrimp Mini	6	210	15	2
Shrimp Mini	6	190	10	2
Shrimp Restaurant Style	1 (3 oz)	180	15	2
Frieda's				
Egg Roll Wrappers	2 (1.6 oz)	130	0	1
Health Is Wealth				
Broccoli	1 (3 oz)	150	5	2
Oriental Vegetable	1 (3 oz)	160	0	2
Oriental Chicken Free	1 (3 oz)	120	0	2
Pizza	1 (3 oz)	200	0	3
Spinach	1 (3 oz)	180	0	3
Spring Rolls	1 (1.6 oz)	70	0	5
Veggie	1 (3 oz)	130	0	3
Kahiki				
Chicken	1 (3 oz)	160	10	1
Chipotle Lime Chicken	1 (3 oz)	170	10	2
Lemongrass Chicken Stix	3 (2.6 oz)	100	20	tr
Pork & Shrimp	1 (3 oz)	140	30	1
Vegetable	1 (3 oz)	90	0	1

FOOD	PORTION	CALS	CHOL	FIBER
La Choy				
Chicken Mini	6	210	15	2
Chicken Restaurant Style	1 (3 oz)	210	15	2
Pork Restaurant Style	1 (3 oz)	220	10	2
Pork & Shrimp Bite Size	12	210	10	2
Pork & Shrimp Mini	6	210	15	2
Shrimp Mini	6	190	10	2
Shrimp Restaurant Style	1 (3 oz)	180	15	2
Sweet & Sour Chicken Restaurant Style	1 (3 oz)	220	15	2
Vegetable w/ Lobster Mini	6	190	5	2
Lean Cuisine				
Cafe Classics Vegetable	1 pkg (9 oz)	310	5	3
Loompya				
Lumpia Chicken & Vegetables	2	170	10	2
Nasoya				
Egg Roll Wrapper	3	170	10	1
Pagoda				
Sweet & Sour Chicken	1 (2.7 oz)	170	5	2
Phillips				
Spring Rolls Crab & Shrimp w/ Sauce	3 (3.75 oz)	220	60	–
TAKE-OUT				
chicken	1 (3 oz)	140	15	4
lobster	1 (4.8 oz)	270	0	6
lumpia vegetable & shrimp	2 (3 oz)	120	10	2
meat & shrimp	1 (4.8 oz)	320	10	4
pork & shrimp	1 (5 oz)	300	15	7
shrimp	1 (3 oz)	170	<5	5
spicy pork	1 (3 oz)	200	5	3
vegetable	1 (3 oz)	170	0	4
EGG SUBSTITUTES				
Better'n Eggs				
All Whites	¼ cup	30	0	0
Ham & Cheese	¼ cup	45	5	0
Original	¼ cup (2 oz)	30	0	0
Plus	¼ cup	35	0	0
Three Cheese	¼ cup	45	5	0

FOOD	PORTION	CALS	CHOL	FIBER
Egg Beaters				
Original	¼ cup	30	0	0
Fantastic				
Tofu Scrambler not prep	1 tbsp	35	0	1
Horizon Organic				
Liquid Egg	¼ cup	35	0	0
Land O Lakes				
Liquid Egg	¼ cup	30	0	0
Quick Eggs				
Fat Free Cholesterol Free	¼ cup	30	0	0
EGGNOG				
eggnog	1 qt	1368	596	–
eggnog	1 cup	342	149	–
eggnog flavor mix as prep w/ milk	9 oz	260	33	–
Farmland				
Egg Nog	½ cup	180	50	0
Hood				
Fat Free Sugar Free	1 cup	110	<5	0
Golden	½ cup	180	65	0
Light	½ cup	140	45	0
Horizon Organic				
Lowfat	½ cup	140	45	0
Oberweis				
Egg Nog	½ cup	240	40	0
TAKE-OUT				
eggnog	1 cup	306	63	0
EGGNOG SUBSTITUTES				
Silk				
Nog	½ cup	90	0	0
EGGPLANT				
cubed cooked w/ oil	1 cup	133	0	5
pickled	½ cup	33	0	2
slices grilled	1 (2 oz)	36	0	1
Celentano				
Eggplant Parmigiana	1 serv (7 oz)	330	25	5
Frieda's				
Chinese	⅔ cup (3 oz)	20	0	2
Japanese Nasu	⅔ cup (3 oz)	20	0	2

FOOD	PORTION	CALS	CHOL	FIBER
Peloponnese				
Baba Ganoush	2 tbsp	40	0	1
Progresso				
Caponata	2 tbsp (1 oz)	25	0	2
Sabra				
Baba Ghanoush	2 oz	50	0	1
TastyBite				
Punjab Eggplant	½ pkg (5 oz)	130	0	4
TAKE-OUT				
baba ghannouj	¼ cup	55	0	–
caponata	2 tbsp (1 oz)	30	0	–
iman bayildi eggplant w/ onion & tomato	1 serv (15.6 oz)	345	0	2
indian eggplant runi	1 serv	180	0	1
moussaka	1 serv (9 oz)	372	54	5
papoutsakis little shoes	1 serv (15.5 oz)	245	40	1

ELDERBERRIES

FOOD	PORTION	CALS	CHOL	FIBER
fresh	1 cup	105	0	–

ELDERBERRY JUICE

FOOD	PORTION	CALS	CHOL	FIBER
elderberry	7 oz	76	0	–

ELK

FOOD	PORTION	CALS	CHOL	FIBER
roasted	4 oz	215	127	0

EMU

FOOD	PORTION	CALS	CHOL	FIBER
cooked	3 oz	130	111	–

ENERGY BARS (*see also* CEREAL BARS, NUTRITION SUPPLEMENTS)

FOOD	PORTION	CALS	CHOL	FIBER
Activex				
Organic All Flavors	1 (1.6 oz)	200	0	2
All In One				
All Flavors	1 (1.8 oz)	180	<5	5
AllGoode Organics				
Amazin' Peanut Raisin	1	210	0	3
Banana Nut Nirvana	1	190	0	3
Cashew Almond Passion	1	210	0	3
Chocolate Peanut Pleasure	1	200	5	3
Honey Nut Harvest	1	210	0	3
Nutty Chocolate Apricot	1	200	5	5

FOOD	PORTION	CALS	CHOL	FIBER
Atkins				
Advantage Almond Brownie	1 (1.6 oz)	220	5	7
Advantage Chocolate Coconut	1 (1.6 oz)	230	2	9
Advantage Chocolate Decadence	1 (1.6 oz)	220	2	11
Advantage Chocolate Mocha Crunch	1 (1.6 oz)	220	2	10
Advantage Chocolate Peanut Butter	1 (1.6 oz)	240	2	10
Advantage Cookies 'N Creme	1 (1.6 oz)	220	2	11
Advantage S'mores	1 (1.6 oz)	220	0	11
Balance				
Big Bar Honey Peanut	1	310	5	tr
Chocolate Banana + Antioxidants	1	200	5	1
Chocolate Mint + Antioxidants	1	200	<5	0
Gold Caramel Nut Blast	1	210	0	tr
Gold Chocolate Peanut Butter	1	210	0	tr
Gold Rocky Road	1	210	0	1
Gold Triple Chocolate Chaos	1	200	0	tr
Gold Crunch Chocolate Chocolate	1	210	0	tr
Gold Crunch Chocolate Mint Cookie	1	210	0	tr
Gold Crunch S'mores	1	210	0	0
Honey Peanut + Ginseng	1	200	<5	tr
Lemon Meringue + Calcium	1	190	0	0
Original Almond Brownie	1	200	<5	2
Original Chocolate	1	200	<5	tr
Original Chocolate Raspberry Fudge	1	200	0	1
Original Honey Peanut	1	200	<5	tr
Original Mocha Chip	1	200	0	tr
Original Peanut Butter	1	200	<5	1
Original Yogurt Honey Peanut	1	200	<5	tr

FOOD	PORTION	CALS	CHOL	FIBER
Outdoor Chocolate Crisp	1	200	<5	3
Outdoor Crunchy Peanut	1	200	<5	2
Outdoor Honey Almond	1	200	<5	3
Outdoor Nut Berry	1	200	<5	2
Satisfaction Apple Cinnamon Oatmeal	1	280	0	6
Satisfaction Chocolate Crisp	1	280	0	6
Satisfaction Chocolate Peanut	1	280	0	6
Satisfaction Peanut Butter Crisp	1	280	0	6
Yogurt Berry + Antioxidants	1	200	5	0
Be Natural				
Almond & Apricot	1	218	0	4
Almond & Coconut	1	248	0	1
Banana & Wheat Bran	1	201	0	4
Fruit & Nut Delight	1	225	0	3
Macadamia & Apricot	1	224	0	3
Nut Delight	1	266	0	3
Sesame Nut Split	1	256	0	2
Walnut & Date	1	147	0	1
Yogurt Coated Almond & Apricot	1	233	0	2
Yogurt Coated Fruit & Nut	1	190	0	1
Belly-bar				
Baby Needs Chocolate	1	170	0	2
Berry Nutty Cravings	1	170	0	2
Mellow Oat	1	180	0	2
Better Bar				
Chocolate Coated Caramel Pecan	1 (1.8 oz)	180	0	0
Chocolate Coated Peanut	1 (1.8 oz)	180	0	0
Yogurt Coated Raspberry	1 (1.8 oz)	180	0	0
Boomi Bar				
Almond Protein Plus	1	270	15	4
Cashew Almond Delicacy	1	260	0	1
Cranberry Apple	1	210	0	4
Merry Macadamia	1	220	0	3
Pistachio Pineapple	1	200	0	3

FOOD	PORTION	CALS	CHOL	FIBER
Boost				
Chocolate Crunch	1 (1.5 oz)	190	<5	tr
Carb Options				
Chocolate Chip	1	200	<5	tr
Chocolate Peanut	1	200	<5	tr
Cinnamon Delight	1	200	<5	0
Carbolite				
Chocolate Peanut Butter Sugar Free	1 (1 oz)	144	4	0
CarbWise				
Chocolate S'Mores Crunch	1	240	0	1
Centrum				
Energy Chocolate Nougat	1 (1.98 oz)	220	0	tr
Energy Chocolate Peanut Butter	1 (1.98 oz)	220	0	tr
Choice				
Berry Almond Crispy	1	50	0	0
Fudge Brownie	1	140	<5	3
Peanut Butter Crispy	1	60	0	tr
Peanutty Chocolate	1	140	<5	3
Clif				
Banana Nut Bread	1 (2.4 oz)	250	0	5
Builders Chocolate Mint	1 (2.4 oz)	270	0	4
Builders Peanut Butter	1 (2.4 oz)	270	0	4
Carrot Cake	1 (2.4 oz)	240	0	5
Chocolate Brownie	1 (2.4 oz)	240	0	5
Chocolate Chip	1 (2.4 oz)	250	0	5
Cool Mint Chocolate	1 (2.4 oz)	250	0	5
Crunchy Peanut Butter	1 (2.4 oz)	250	0	5
Mojo Mixed Nuts	1 (1.6 oz)	220	0	3
Mojo Mountain Mix	1 (1.6 oz)	200	0	2
Nectar Cinnamon Pecan	1 (1.6 oz)	170	0	6
Nectar Lemon Vanilla Cashew	1 (1.6 oz)	180	0	6
Oatmeal Raisin Walnut	1 (2.4 oz)	240	0	5
ZBar Peanut Butter	1 (1.3 oz)	140	0	3
Deliciously Slim				
Chocolate Fudge Cake	1 (2.1 oz)	200	0	tr
DrSoy				
Double Chocolate	1 (1.76 oz)	180	0	1

FOOD	PORTION	CALS	CHOL	FIBER
Ensure				
All Flavors	1 (2.1 oz)	230	<5	1
Fast Fuel Up				
Natural Chocolate Espresso	1 (2.3 oz)	300	0	3
Natural Chocolate Crunch	1 (2.3 oz)	300	0	3
Organic Chocolate Espresso	1 (1.8 oz)	230	0	2
Organic Chocolate Crunch	1 (1.8 oz)	230	0	2
Gatorade				
All Flavors	1 (2.3 oz)	260	0	2
GeniSoy				
Soy Protein Artic Frost Crispy Chocolate Mint	1 (2.2 oz)	230	0	2
Soy Protein Dutch Crunch Sour Apple Crisp	1 (2.2 oz)	230	0	1
Soy Protein Fair Trade Arabica Cafe Mocha Fudge	1 (2.2 oz)	220	0	1
Soy Protein New York Style Blueberry Cheesecake	1 (2.2 oz)	220	0	1
Soy Protein Obsession Fudge Cookies & Cream	1 (2.2 oz)	230	0	2
Soy Protein Pure Golden Honey Creamy Peanut Yogurt	1 (2.2 oz)	230	0	1
Soy Protein Southern Style Chunky Peanut Butter Fudge	1 (2.2 oz)	240	0	1
Soy Protein Ultimate Chocolate Fudge Brownie	1 (2.2 oz)	230	0	2
Xtreme Carrot Cake Quake	1 (1.6 oz)	190	0	1
Xtreme Peanut Butter Fix	1 (1.6 oz)	200	0	2
Xtreme Raspberry Rush	1 (1.6 oz)	190	0	2
Xtreme Rocky Roadtrip	1 (1.6 oz)	190	0	2
Glucerna				
All Flavors	1 (1.3 oz)	140	<5	4
Hansen's				
Chocolate Banana Crunch	1	180	0	2
Chocolate Orchard Crunch	1	170	0	2
Natural Bar Tropical Fruit Crunch	1	170	0	1

FOOD	PORTION	CALS	CHOL	FIBER
Natural Bar Yogurt Strawberry Crunch	1	190	0	1
Hi-Lo				
Chocolate Caramel	1 (1.76 oz)	200	<5	0
Chocolate Mint	1 (2.1 oz)	200	0	tr
Chocolate Peanut Butter	1 (2.1 oz)	210	0	0
Chocolate Raspberry	1 (2.1 oz)	200	0	tr
Hooah!				
Chocolate Crisp	1 (2.29 oz)	280	<5	2
Ideal				
Mixed Berry Tart	1 (1.7 oz)	200	0	0
Jenny Craig				
Meal Bar Chocolate Peanut	1 (2 oz)	220	0	1
Meal Bar Lemon Meringue	1 (2 oz)	210	0	0
Meal Bar Milk Chocolate	1 (2 oz)	210	0	1
Meal Bar Oatmeal Raisin	1 (1.97 oz)	210	0	3
Meal Bar Yogurt Peanut	1 (2 oz)	220	0	0
Kashi				
GoLean Chocolate Almond Toffee	1 (2.7 oz)	290	0	6
GoLean Cookies 'N Cream	1 (2.7 oz)	290	0	6
GoLean Crunchy Chocolate Peanut	1 (1.8 oz)	180	0	6
GoLean Malted Chocolate Chip	1 (2.7 oz)	290	0	6
GoLean Oatmeal Raisin Cookie	1 (2.7 oz)	280	0	6
GoLean Peanut Butter & Chocolate	1 (2.7 oz)	290	0	6
GoLean Roll Caramel Peanut	1 (1.9 oz)	200	0	6
TLC Chewy Granola Cherry Dark Chocolate	1 (1.2 oz)	120	0	4
TLC Crunchy Granola Honey Toasted 7 Grain	1 (1.4 oz)	180	0	4
TLC Crunchy Granola Pumpkin Spice	1 (1.4 oz)	180	0	4
TLC Crunchy Granola Roasted Almond	1 (1.4 oz)	180	0	4
LaraBar				
Apple Pie	1	190	0	4

FOOD	PORTION	CALS	CHOL	FIBER
Banana Cookie	1	210	0	5
Cashew Cookie	1	230	0	3
Cherry Pie	1	190	0	4
Chocolate Coconut Chew	1	220	0	5
Cocoa Mule	1	200	0	5
Ginger Snap	1	220	0	5
Lean Body For Her				
Chocolate Honey Peanut	1 (1.76 oz)	190	0	tr
Luna				
Caramel Nut Brownie	1 (1.7 oz)	190	0	4
Chai Tea	1 (1.7 oz)	180	0	3
Dulce De Leche	1 (1.7 oz)	180	0	3
Iced Oatmeal Raisin	1 (1.7 oz)	180	0	3
Key Lime Pie	1 (1.7 oz)	180	0	2
LemonZest	1 (1.7 oz)	180	0	3
Nutz Over Chocolate	1 (1.7 oz)	180	0	3
Met-Rx				
Big 100 Gram Bar Peanut Butter	1 (3.5 oz)	340	15	2
Source/One Chocolate Cheesecake	1 (2.1 oz)	160	5	tr
Momentum				
Chocolate Caramel Nut	1	150	0	3
Chocolate Peanut Butter	1	150	0	2
Double Chocolate	1	150	0	2
Mommy Munchies				
Chocolate Mint	1 (1.8 oz)	180	5	5
Cinnamon Bun	1 (1.8 oz)	180	0	5
Moto Bar				
Bodacious Banana Split	1	300	0	6
Charming Cherry Almond	1 (2.9 oz)	300	0	3
Cozy Pumpkin Pie	1	300	0	6
Jazzy Peanut Butter & Jelly	1	300	0	4
Kooky Cappuccino	1	300	0	8
Luscious Lemon Blueberry	1	300	0	4
Saucy Apple Cinnamon	1	280	0	6
Zany Cranberry Orange	1	300	0	4

FOOD	PORTION	CALS	CHOL	FIBER
Nature's Path				
Optimum Blueberry Flax & Soy	1 (2 oz)	200	0	5
Optimum Cranberry Ginger & Soy	1 (2 oz)	200	0	5
Optimum Peanut Butter	1 (2 oz)	230	0	4
Optimum ReBound	1 (2 oz)	190	0	4
New You				
Chocolate Crisp	1 (1.65 oz)	180	0	3
NuGo				
Banana Chocolate Protein	1	190	0	3
Blue Berry Boom	1	180	0	3
Chocolate Blast	1	180	0	3
Coffee Break	1	180	0	3
Orange Smoothie Protein	1	190	0	1
Peanut Butter Pleaser	1	180	0	3
Nutiva				
Organic Flax & Raisin	1 (1.4 oz)	200	0	4
Organic Flaxseed Flax Chocolate	1 (1.4 oz)	200	0	5
Original Organic Hempseed	1 (1.4 oz)	210	0	5
Nutribar				
Chocolate Covered Chocolate Fudge	1 (2.3 oz)	267	5	2
Odwalla Bar!				
Peanut Crunch	1 (2.2 oz)	260	0	3
Oh Mama!				
Chocolate Peanut Butter	1 (1.8 oz)	190	0	3
Frosted White Lemon	1 (1.8 oz)	180	0	3
Frosted White Raspberry	1 (1.8 oz)	180	0	3
Peacekeeper				
Nuts About Peace All Flavors	1 (1.4 oz)	180	0	2
Perfect 10				
Bliss Apricot	1 (1.8 oz)	215	2	5
Bliss Cranberry	1 (1.8 oz)	215	2	4
Natural Apricot	1 (1.8 oz)	205	0	4
Natural Cranberry	1 (1.8 oz)	164	0	4
Natural Lemon	1 (1.8 oz)	210	0	5

FOOD	PORTION	CALS	CHOL	FIBER
PermaLean				
Protein Crunch Chocoholic Chocolate	1 (1.8 oz)	170	0	tr
Protein Crunch Chocolate Raspberry	1 (1.8 oz)	180	10	0
Protein Crunch Stark Raving Peanutz	1 (1.8 oz)	180	0	0
PowerBar				
Harvest Apple Cinnamon Crisp	1 (2.3 oz)	240	0	4
Harvest Chunky Cherry Crunch	1 (2.3 oz)	240	0	4
Harvest Peanut Butter Chocolate Chip	1 (2.3 oz)	240	0	4
Harvest Strawberry Crunch	1 (2.3 oz)	230	0	4
Harvest Dipped Double Chocolate Crisp	1 (2.3 oz)	250	0	3
Harvest Dipped Oatmeal Raisin Cookie	1 (2.3 oz)	250	0	3
Harvest Dipped Toffee Chocolate Chip	1 (2.3 oz)	250	0	3
Performance Apple Cinnamon	1 (2.3 oz)	230	0	3
Performance Banana	1 (2.3 oz)	230	0	3
Performance Cappuccino	1 (2.3 oz)	230	0	3
Performance Chocolate	1 (2.3 oz)	230	0	3
Performance Chocolate Peanut Butter	1 (2.3 oz)	240	0	3
Performance Cookies & Cream	1 (2.3 oz)	240	0	2
Performance Malt Nut	1 (2.3 oz)	230	0	3
Performance Oatmeal Raisin	1 (2.3 oz)	230	0	3
Performance Peanut Butter	1 (2.3 oz)	230	0	3
Performance Strawberry Cream	1 (2.3 oz)	230	0	2
Performance Vanilla Crisp	1 (2.3 oz)	230	0	3
Performance Wild Berry	1 (2.3 oz)	230	0	3
Protein Plus Carb Select Chocolate	1 (2.5 oz)	260	5	1

FOOD	PORTION	CALS	CHOL	FIBER
Protein Plus Carb Select Chocolate Caramel Crunch	1 (2.6 oz)	270	5	2
Protein Plus Carb Select Chocolate Peanut Butter	1 (2.5 oz)	270	5	2
Protein Plus Carb Select Peanut Caramel	1 (2.6 oz)	270	5	1
Protein Plus Chocolate Fudge Brownie	1 (2.7 oz)	270	0	2
Protein Plus Chocolate Peanut Butter	1 (2.7 oz)	290	0	1
Protein Plus Cookies & Cream	1 (2.7 oz)	290	0	1
Protein Plus Vanilla Yogurt	1 (2.7 oz)	290	0	1
Triple Treat Caramel Peanut Crisp	1 (1.9 oz)	220	0	4
Triple Treat Caramel Peanut Fusion	1 (1.9 oz)	230	5	4
Triple Treat Chocolate Caramel Fusion	1 (1.9 oz)	230	0	4
Triple Treat Chocolate Peanut Butter Crisp	1 (1.9 oz)	220	0	4
Prana Bar				
Apricot Goji	1 (1.7 oz)	220	0	3
Coconut Acai	1 (1.7 oz)	220	0	3
Pear Ginseng	1 (1.7 oz)	220	0	4
Pria				
Carb Select Caramel Nut Brownie	1 (1.7 oz)	170	5	2
Carb Select Chocolate Mocha Crisp	1 (1.7 oz)	130	0	4
Carb Select Chocolate Peanut Butter Crisp	1 (1.7 oz)	130	0	4
Carb Select Cookies N' Caramel	1 (1.7 oz)	170	5	2
Carb Select Peanut Butter Caramel Nut	1 (1.7 oz)	170	5	2
Chocolate Peanut Crunch	1 (1 oz)	110	0	1
Complete Nutrition Chocolate Mint Crisp	1 (1.6 oz)	170	0	5

FOOD	PORTION	CALS	CHOL	FIBER
Complete Nutrition Chocolate Peanut Butter Crisp	1 (1.6 oz)	170	0	5
Complete Nutrition French Vanilla Crisp	1 (1.6 oz)	170	0	5
Creme Carmel Crisp	1 (1 oz)	110	0	1
Double Chocolate Cookie	1 (1 oz)	110	0	1
Mint Chocolate Cookie	1 (1 oz)	110	0	1
Strawberry Shortcake	1 (1 oz)	110	0	1
Pure Protein				
Blueberry Cheesecake	1	190	5	0
PureFit				
Almond Crunch	1 (2 oz)	230	0	3
Peanut Butter Crunch	1 (2 oz)	240	0	2
Revival				
Soy Apple Cinnamon Celebration	1	200	0	1
Soy Autumn Frost Low Carb	1	200	0	1
Soy Chocolate Raspberry Zing Low Carb	1	200	0	2
Soy Chocolate Temptation	1	220	0	tr
Soy Marshmallow Krunch	1	220	0	tr
Soy Peanut Butter Chocolate Pal	1	240	0	1
Soy Peanut Butter Pal	1	240	0	tr
Sharkies				
Organic Energy Fruit Chews All Flavors	1 pkg (1.8 oz)	170	0	1
Slim-Fast				
Classic Meal Bar Chocolate Cookie Dough	1	220	<5	2
Classic Meal Bar Milk Chocolate Peanut	1	220	<5	2
High Protein Granola Bar Peanut	1	200	0	2
High Protien Granola Bar Chocolate Chip	1	190	<5	2
Low Carb Breakfast Bar Apple Cobbler	1	180	<5	3
Low Carb Breakfast Bar Peanut Butter	1	190	<5	3

FOOD	PORTION	CALS	CHOL	FIBER
Low Carb Snack Bar Caramel Nut	1	120	<5	1
Low Carb Snack Bar Coconut Almond	1	120	<5	2
Low Carb Snack Bar Peanut Butter Crunch	1	120	<5	1
Optima Meal Bar Apple Crisp	1	180	0	3
Optima Meal Bar Caramel Crispy Peanut	1	220	<5	2
Optima Meal Bar Chewy Granola Trail Mix	1	210	<5	2
Optima Snack Bar Banana Nut Muffin	1	150	<5	1
Optima Snack Bar Blueberry Muffin	1	140	<5	1
Optima Snack Bar Chocolate Peanut Nougat	1	120	<5	1
Optima Snack Bar Oatmeal Raisin Cookie	1	120	0	1
Snickers Marathon				
Chewy Chocolate Peanut	1 (1.9 oz)	210	0	5
SoBe				
Milk Chocolate	1 (1.75 oz)	240	15	tr
Solo GI				
Berry Bliss	1 (1.6 oz)	190	0	3
Chocolate Charger	1 (1.6 oz)	190	5	4
Mint Mania	1 (1.6 oz)	190	5	4
Peanut Power	1 (1.6 oz)	200	0	3
South Beach Diet				
Meal Replacement Chocolate Crisp	1	210	0	5
Meal Replacement Chocolate Peanut Butter	1	210	0	6
Meal Replacement Cinnamon & Creme	1	220	0	5
Meal Replacement Peanut Crisp	1	210	0	5
Meal Replacement Vanilla Creme	1	210	0	5

FOOD	PORTION	CALS	CHOL	FIBER
Balance				
Chocolate as prep w/ 2% milk	1 serv	310	25	2
Vanilla as prep w/ 2% milk	1 serv	310	25	2
Bally Blast				
Energy Drink	1 can (8.3 oz)	120	0	–
Sugar Free	1 can (8.3 oz)	10	0	–
Banzai				
Energy Drink	8 oz	120	0	–
Bawls				
Guarana	1 bottle (10 oz)	120	0	–
Guaranexx Sugar Free	1 bottle (10 oz)	0	0	0
Beaver Buzz				
Cirus	1 can	140	0	–
Black Hole				
Blueberry	8 oz	100	0	–
Citrus	8 oz	110	0	–
Bliss				
Energy Drink	1 can (8.4 oz)	110	0	–
Low Carb	1 can (8.4 oz)	26	0	–
Blox				
Black Cherry	8 oz	86	0	–
Orange Rush	8 oz	103	0	–
Original	8 oz	105	0	–
Blu Fuel				
Energy Drink	1 can (10 oz)	133	0	–
BooKoo				
Energy Drink	8 oz	110	0	–
Shot All Flavors	1 can (5.57 oz)	80	0	–
Zero Carb	8 oz	0	0	0
Boost				
High Protein Vanilla	8 oz	240	10	0
Bossa Nova				
Acai Juice Mango	1 bottle (10 oz)	132	0	1
Brain Twist				
Flu & Cold Defense All Flavors	8 oz	70	0	–
Caballo Negro				
Double Kick	8 oz	120	0	–
Energy Drink	1 can (8.4 oz)	120	0	–

FOOD	PORTION	CALS	CHOL	FIBER
Cascabel				
Energy Drink	1 can (8.4 oz)	110	0	–
Sugar Free	1 can (8.4 oz)	10	0	–
Cheetah				
Energy Drink	1 can (12 oz)	80	0	–
Choice				
Chocolate	1 can (8 oz)	220	0	3
Chocolate Fudge Sugar Free	1 pkg (11 oz)	125	<5	9
French Vanllia Sugar Free	1 pkg (11 oz)	100	<5	6
Strawberries'n Cream Sugar Free	1 pkg (11 oz)	100	<5	6
Vanilla	1 can (8 oz)	220	0	3
Crunk				
Energy Drink	1 can	120	0	–
Cytomax				
Sport Drinks All Flavors	1 bottle (20 oz)	130	0	tr
Defcon3				
Healthy Energy Soda	1 can (12 oz)	45	0	2
Defense				
Effervescent Supplement	1 can	150	0	–
Diablo				
Energy Drink	1 can (8.7 oz)	151	0	–
Double Hit				
Maximun Energy Coffee Drink Sugar Free	1 can (12 oz)	0	0	0
Energy 69				
Energy Drink	1 can	110	0	–
Sugar Free	1 can	0	0	0
Everlast				
High Energy Citrus Blast	1 can (8.3 oz)	140	0	–
Freedom				
Energy Drink	1 can (12 oz)	160	0	–
Full Throttle				
Energy Drink	8 oz	100	0	–
Fury	8 oz	110	0	–
Fuze				
Energize Blackberry Grape	8 oz	100	0	–
Energize Exotic Punch	8 oz	100	0	–
Energize Mojo Mango	8 oz	100	0	–

FOOD	PORTION	CALS	CHOL	FIBER
Essential Cranberry Grapefruit	8 oz	90	0	–
Focus Orange Carrot	8 oz	90	0	–
Refresh Banana Colada	8 oz	90	0	–
Refresh Mixed Berry	8 oz	90	0	–
Refresh Peach Mango	8 oz	90	0	–
Replenish Agave Cactus	8 oz	90	0	–
Stamina Grape & Aronia Punch	8 oz	80	0	–
Vitaboost Citrus Starfruit Punch	8 oz	90	0	–
Gatorade				
All Flavors	1 cup (8 oz)	50	0	–
Lemonade All Flavors	8 oz	50	0	–
Nutrition Shake All Flavors	1 can (11 oz)	370	0	1
Rain All Flavors	8 oz	50	0	–
X-Factor All Flavors	8 oz	50	0	–
GeniSoy				
Soy Protein Shake Chocolate	1 scoop (1.2 oz)	120	0	2
Soy Protein Shake Vanilla	1 scoop (1.2 oz)	130	0	0
Soy Protein Shake Strawberry Banana	1 scoop	130	0	1
Gleukos				
Preformance All Flavors	8 oz	70	0	0
Go Fast				
Energy Drink	1 can (8.4 oz)	90	0	–
Light	1 can (8.4 oz)	20	0	–
Sportsman's	1 can (8.4 oz)	90	0	–
Guaraviton				
Energy Drink	8 oz	98	0	–
Guru				
Energy Drink	1 can (8.3 oz)	100	0	–
Lite	1 can (8.3 oz)	5	0	–
Hansen's				
Energy Kiwi Strawberry	8 oz	120	0	–
Energy Peach	8 oz	130	0	–
Energy Punch	8 oz	120	0	–
Healthy Start Carrot Orange Antioxidant Blend	8 oz	130	0	–

FOOD	PORTION	CALS	CHOL	FIBER
Healthy Start Citrus Punch Focus Blend	8 oz	130	0	–
Healthy Start Cranberry Grape Defense Blend	8 oz	110	0	–
Healthy Start Tropical Orange Vitamix Blend	8 oz	110	0	–
Happy Bunny				
Spaz Juice	1 can (8.4 oz)	110	0	0
Healthy Pleasures				
Chocolate Irish Cream	1 bottle (10.5 oz)	260	6	0
Her Energy				
Pink Lemonade	1 can (8.4 oz)	130	0	0
Pink Lemonade Sugar Free	1 can (8.4 oz)	0	0	0
Hiball				
All Flavors	1 bottle (10 oz)	10	0	0
High Voltage				
Sugar Free	8 oz	5	0	–
Hooah!				
Soldier Fuel All Flavors	1 can (12 oz)	160	0	–
Hydrive				
All Flavors	1 bottle (11.2 oz)	25	0	–
Hype				
Classic Energy	1 can (8.3 oz)	110	0	–
Impulse				
Energy Drink	1 can (8.3 oz)	110	0	–
Sugar Free	1 can (8.3 oz)	5	0	–
Invigor8				
Energy Boost	1 can	110	0	1
Nutrition Boost	1 can	110	0	1
Iron Energy				
All Flavors	8 oz	90	0	–
Jet Set				
Club Soda	1 can (12 oz)	0	0	0
Ginger Ale	1 can (12 oz)	150	0	0
Original	1 can (12 oz)	105	0	0
Tonic Water	1 can (12 oz)	150	0	0
Jones Soda				
Big Energy	8 oz	120	0	–
Lemon Lime Energy	1 can (8.4 oz)	140	0	0
Mixed Berry Energy	1 can (8.4 oz)	140	0	0

FOOD	PORTION	CALS	CHOL	FIBER
Orange Energy	1 can (8.4 oz)	140	0	0
Sugar Free Energy	1 can (8.4 oz)	10	0	–
Jugular				
Energy Drink	1 can (8.3 oz)	49	0	–
Kabbalah				
Original	1 can (12 oz)	174	0	–
Sugar Free	1 can (12 oz)	<3	0	–
KaBoom				
All Flavors	8 oz	105	0	0
Krank'd				
All Flavors	1 bottle (16 oz)	80	0	–
Liv Natural				
Hydrate Restore	8 oz	70	0	0
Lolli's Pop				
Cheery Energy Drink	1 bottle	170	0	–
Passion Stimulating Elixir	1 bottle	140	0	–
Mr. Re				
Restorative	1 can (11 oz)	80	0	0
Nantucket Nectars				
Super Nectars Ginkgo Mango	8 oz	150	0	–
Super Nectars Green Angel	8 oz	140	0	–
Super Nectars Protein Smoothie	8 oz	170	0	–
Super Nectars Red Guarana Tea	8 oz	110	0	–
Super Nectars Vital C	8 oz	130	0	–
Natural Ovens				
Ultra Omega Balance	1 tbsp	75	3	4
Zesty Flax Energy Mix	1 tbsp	40	0	3
New York Minute				
Energy Drink	1 can (8.4 oz)	130	0	–
Nexcite				
Herbal Fizz	1 bottle	72	0	–
Nitro2Go				
High Energy	1 can	110	0	–
High Energy Lite	1 can	20	0	0
NOS				
High Performance	8 oz	110	0	–

FOOD	PORTION	CALS	CHOL	FIBER
Odwalla				
C Monster	8 oz	150	0	2
Femme Vitale	8 oz	130	0	1
Glorious Morning	8 oz	130	0	3
Mango Tango	8 oz	150	0	0
Mo Beta	8 oz	140	0	1
Serious Energy	8 oz	150	0	1
Strawberry C Monster	8 oz	150	0	tr
Super Protein	8 oz	170	0	2
Superfood	8 oz	140	0	2
Wellness	8 oz	150	0	1
Orange County Choppers				
High Octane Fuel	1 can (8.4 oz)	110	0	–
Peep One				
Erotic Drink	1 can (8.3)	109	0	–
Pickle Juice				
Dill	8 oz	0	0	–
Sport	8 oz	7	0	–
Pimp Juice				
Energy Drink	1 can (8 oz)	140	0	–
Tight	1 can (8 oz)	140	0	–
Pink				
Diet	1 can	10	0	–
Piranha				
Phunky Fruit Punch	1 can (8.4 oz)	140	0	0
Pit Bull				
Energy Drink	1 can (8.4 oz)	110	0	–
Sugar Free	1 can (8.4 oz)	0	0	0
Pounds Off				
Dark Chocolate Ecstasy	1 can (11 oz)	200	0	6
French Vanilla	1 can (11 oz)	220	0	5
Power Trip				
Xtreme	1 can (10.5 oz)	140	0	–
Powerade				
Arctic Shatter	8 oz	64	0	–
Flava 23	8 oz	63	0	–
Fruit Punch	8 oz	65	0	–
Green Squall	8 oz	64	0	–
Jagged Ice	8 oz	65	0	–
NASCAR Grape	8 oz	64	0	–

FOOD	PORTION	CALS	CHOL	FIBER
Olympic Citrus	8 oz	63	0	–
Option All Flavors	8 oz	10	0	–
PowerBar				
Endurance Sport Drink	1 pkg (0.6 oz)	70	0	–
Performance Recovery Drink	1 pkg (0.8 oz)	90	0	–
Pure Power				
Energy Drink	1 can (8.4 oz)	110	0	–
Shotz	1 can (5.75 oz)	80	0	0
Raw Dawg				
Energy Drink	8 oz	110	0	–
Sugar Free	8 oz	0	0	0
Rawlings EX2				
Sustained Energy	1 can (8.4 oz)	132	0	–
Red Bull				
Energy Drink	1 can (8.3 oz)	110	0	–
Sugar Free	1 can	10	0	–
Red Eye				
Classic	1 bottle (12 oz)	208	0	–
Extreme	1 bottle (12 oz)	140	0	–
Gold	1 bottle (12 oz)	208	0	–
Passion	1 bottle (12 oz)	149	0	–
Platnum	1 bottle (12 oz)	149	0	–
Rehab				
Recovery Supplement	1 can (12 oz)	150	0	–
RESQ				
Energy Drink	1 can (8 oz)	126	0	–
Resurrect				
Daily Detox & Anti-Hangover Elixir	1 can (12 oz)	5	0	–
Rip It				
Citrus X	8 oz	130	0	–
Citrus X Sugar Free	8 oz	0	0	0
Energy Fuel	8 oz	130	0	–
Energy Lite	8 oz	0	0	–
Rockstar				
Energy Cola	8 oz	120	0	–
Energy Drink	8 oz	110	0	–
Juiced	8 oz	90	0	0

FOOD	PORTION	CALS	CHOL	FIBER
Ronin				
Diet	1 can (16 oz)	15	0	–
Original	1 can (16 oz)	180	0	–
Rox				
Energy Drink	1 can	110	0	–
Zero	1 can	10	0	–
Rumba				
Energy Juice	8 oz	120	0	–
Slim-Fast				
Classic Ready-To-Drink Creamy Milk Chocolate	1 can	220	5	5
Classic Ready-To-Drink French Vanilla	1 can	220	5	5
High Protein Ready-to-Drink All Flavors	1 can	190	10	5
Low Carb Diet Ready To Drink All Flavors	1 can	190	15	4
Snapple A Day				
Meal Replacement All Flavors	1 bottle (11.5 oz)	210	0	5
SoBe				
Adrenaline Rush	1 can (8.3 oz)	140	0	–
Black & Blue Berry Brew	8 oz	120	0	–
Courage Cherry Citrus	8 oz	110	0	–
Drive	8 oz	120	0	–
Elixir Cranberry Grapefruit	8 oz	110	0	–
Elixir Orange Carrot 3C	8 oz	90	0	–
Elixir Pomegranate Cranberry	8 oz	100	0	–
Energy	8 oz	120	0	–
Fuerte	8 oz	130	0	–
Karma	8 oz	120	0	–
Lean Diet Citrus	8 oz	5	0	–
Long John Lizard's Grape Grog	8 oz	120	0	–
Power	8 oz	120	0	–
Synergy All Flavors	1 can (11.5 oz)	120	0	–
Tsunami	8 oz	110	0	–
Wisdom	8.5 oz	110	0	–
Zen Blend	8.5 oz	90	0	–

FOOD	PORTION	CALS	CHOL	FIBER
Sol Mate				
All Flavors	1 bottle	90	0	–
Source Burn				
2	8 oz	130	0	–
Energy Drink	8 oz	140	0	–
Sugar Free	8 oz	10	0	0
Speed Zone				
Energy Drink	1 can (8.4 oz)	110	0	–
Stevita				
All Flavors	2 tsp	0	0	0
Stewie's				
Domination Serum	1 can (8.45 oz)	110	0	–
Mind Erase Elixir	1 can (8.45 oz)	100	0	–
Stinger				
All Flavors	1 can (8.4 oz)	130	0	0
Sugar Free All Flavors	1 can (8.4 oz)	0	0	0
Sum Poosie				
Energy Drink	1 bottle (12 oz)	170	0	–
Sweet Success				
Creamy Milk Chocolate	1 can	200	4	3
Creamy Milk Chocolate as prep w/ skim milk	1 serv	180	6	6
Swing Juice				
Energy Drink	8 oz	60	0	–
Tab				
Energy Drink	1 can (10.5 oz)	5	0	0
Tantra				
Erotic	1 can (8.4 oz)	130	0	–
The Beast				
Energy Drink	1 can (8.3 oz)	120	0	–
Tornado				
Energy Drink	8 oz	110	0	–
TwinLab				
Hydra Fuel	16 oz	132	0	–
Nitro Fuel	16 oz	460	0	–
Ultra Fuel	16 oz	400	0	–
Vault				
Energy Drink	8 oz	120	0	–
Zero	8 oz	0	0	–

FOOD	PORTION	CALS	CHOL	FIBER
Vida				
Energy Drink	8 oz	120	0	–
Vipa				
Energy Drink	1 can (12 oz)	0	0	0
Who's Your Daddy				
Original	8 oz	110	0	–
Sugar Free	8 oz	0	0	0
Wide Open Performance				
Energy Drink	1 can (8.3 oz)	120	0	–
Wired				
Energy Drink	8 oz	110	0	–
Sugar Free	8 oz	5	0	–
X 3000 Taurine	8 oz	110	0	–
Xcyto				
Sugar Free	1 can (12.5 oz)	10	0	0
XL				
Diet	1 can (8.8 oz)	10	0	–
Energy Drink	1 can (8.8 oz)	113	0	–
XO				
Balance	8 oz	50	0	–
Berry	1 bottle	90	0	–
Citrus	1 bottle	90	0	–
Defense	8 oz	40	0	–
Diet	1 bottle	15	0	–
Endurance	8 oz	50	0	–
Energy	8 oz	40	0	–
Essential	8 oz	40	0	–
Focus	8 oz	40	0	–
Grape	1 Bottle	90	0	–
Multi-V	8 oz	40	0	–
Original	1 bottle	110	0	–
Peach	1 bottle	90	0	–
Power-C	8 oz	40	0	–
Rescue	8 oz	40	0	–
Revive	8 oz	50	0	–
Stress-B	8 oz	40	0	–
Vanilla	1 bottle	90	0	–
XS Energy				
Citrus Blast	1 can (8.4 oz)	8	0	0
Cranberry Grape	1 can (8.4 oz)	8	0	0

FOOD	PORTION	CALS	CHOL	FIBER
Electric Lemon Blast	1 can (8.4 oz)	16	0	–
Tropical Blast	1 can (8.4 oz)	8	0	0
Xtazy				
All Flavors	1 can	160	0	–
YET				
Your Energy Drink	1 can	8	0	–

ENGLISH MUFFIN
READY-TO-EAT

FOOD	PORTION	CALS	CHOL	FIBER
apple cinnamon	1	138	0	–
crumpets	1 (1.5 oz)	80	0	tr
granola	1	155	0	–
mixed grain	1	155	0	–
plain	1	134	0	–
plain toasted	1	133	0	–
raisin cinnamon	1	138	0	–
sourdough	1	134	0	–
wheat	1	127	0	–
whole wheat	1	134	0	4
Crystal Farms				
English Muffin	1	130	0	1
Food For Life				
7 Sprouted Grains	1	160	0	6
Ezekiel 4:9 Cinnamon Raisin	1	160	0	4
Ezekiel 4:9 Sprouted Grain	1	160	0	6
Genesis 1:29 Original	1	180	0	6
Pepperidge Farm				
100% Whole Wheat	1	140	0	3
7 Grain	1	130	0	3
Sara Lee				
Heart Healthy Wheat w/ Honey	1	140	0	2
Original w/ Whole Grain	1	140	0	2
Thomas'				
Blueberry	1	140	0	1
Carb Consider	1	100	<5	9
Corn	1	150	0	2
Hearty Grains 100% Whole Wheat	1	120	0	3
Hearty Grains Honey Wheat	1	130	0	2

FOOD	PORTION	CALS	CHOL	FIBER
Original	1	120	0	1
Raisin Bran	1	150	0	2
Raisin Cinnamon	1	140	0	1
Sourdough	1	120	0	1
Super Size	1	190	0	2
Super Size Multi Grain	1	240	0	3
Wonder				
Cinnamon Raisin	1 (2.1 oz)	140	0	2
Original	1 (2 oz)	130	0	1
Sourdough	1 (2 oz)	130	0	1
TAKE-OUT				
w/ butter	1 (2.2 oz)	189	13	–
w/ cheese & sausage	1 (4 oz)	393	59	–
w/ egg cheese & canadian bacon	1 (4.8 oz)	289	234	2
w/ egg cheese & sausage	1 (5.8 oz)	487	274	–

EPAZOTE

fresh	1 tbsp (1 g)	tr	0	tr
fresh sprig	1 (2 g)	1	0	tr

EPPAW

raw	½ cup	75	0	–

FALAFEL
Near East

Falafel as prep	2½ patties	230	0	5
Sabra				
Burger	1 (1.8 oz)	90	0	3
VeggieLand				
FalafelBurger	1 (4 oz)	190	0	8
TAKE-OUT				
falafel	1 (1.2 oz)	57	0	–

FAT (see also BUTTER, BUTTER SUBSTITUTES, MARGARINE, OIL)

bacon grease	1 tbsp	116	12	0
beef shortening	1 tbsp	115	13	0
beef suet	1 oz	242	19	0
chicken	1 cup	1846	174	0
chicken	1 tbsp	115	11	0
cocoa butter	1 tbsp	120	0	0
duck	1 tbsp (13 g)	115	13	0

FOOD	PORTION	CALS	CHOL	FIBER
goose	1 tbsp	115	13	0
lamb new zealand	1 oz	182	25	–
lard	1 cup (205 g)	1849	195	0
lard	1 tbsp (13 g)	115	12	0
meat pan drippings	½ tbsp	124	14	0
pork raw	1 oz	230	16	0
salt pork	1 cube (1 oz)	215	26	0
shortening	1 cup	1812	0	0
shortening	1 tbsp	113	0	0
turkey	1 tbsp	115	13	0
Nebraska Land				
Pork Fatback	½ oz	110	5	0
Smart Balance				
Shortening	1 tbsp	110	0	0
Spectrum				
Organic Shortening	1 tbsp	110	0	0
FEIJOA				
fresh	1 (1.75 oz)	25	0	–
puree	1 cup	119	0	–
FENNEL				
fresh bulb	1 (8.2 oz)	72	0	–
fresh sliced	1 cup	27	0	–
seed	1 tsp	7	0	–
FENUGREEK				
seed	1 tsp	12	0	–
FIBER				
apple fiber	0.5 oz	40	0	7
Apple Fiber				
Pure	2 tbsp (7 g)	16	0	4
Benefiber				
Supplement	1 pkg (4 g)	20	0	3
Choice				
Fiber Burst Lemon Lime	3 pieces	45	0	3
Fiber Burst Tropical Fruit	3 pieces	45	0	3
Metamucil				
Fiber Wafers Apple Crisp	2	120	0	6
Natural Fiber Regular Flavor	1 rounded tsp (7 g)	25	0	3

FOOD	PORTION	CALS	CHOL	FIBER
ND Labs				
Pure Apple Fiber	1 tbsp (7 g)	16	0	4
FIDDLEHEAD FERNS				
fresh	3.5 oz	34	0	–
FIGS				
calimyrna	3 (5.4 oz)	120	0	4
canned in heavy syrup	3	75	0	–
canned in light syrup	3	58	0	–
canned water pack	3	42	0	–
dried california	½ cup (3.5 oz)	200	0	17
dried cooked	½ cup	140	0	–
dried whole	10	477	0	17
fresh	1 med	50	0	–
Blue Ribbon				
California Figs	1 pkg (1.5 oz)	120	0	5
Figamajigs				
Chocolate Covered Bar	1 (1.4 oz)	130	0	5
Chocolate Covered Bar w/ Almonds	1 (1.4 oz)	150	0	4
Jenny				
Sundried Kalamata	4	120	0	5
Trucco				
Kalamata	2	100	0	4
FIREWEED				
leaves chopped	1 cup (0.8 oz)	24	0	2

FISH (*see also individual names,* FISH SUBSTITUTES, SUSHI)
CANNED

FOOD	PORTION	CALS	CHOL	FIBER
Beach Cliff				
Fish Steak In Louisiana Hot Sauce	1 can (3.7 oz)	160	75	0
Fish Steaks In Mustard Sauce	1 can (3.7 oz)	160	80	0
Fish Steaks In Soybean Oil	1 can (3.7 oz)	200	80	0
Fish Steaks w/ Hot Green Chilies	1 can (3.7 oz)	160	65	0
Fish Steaks w/ Jalapeno Peppers	1 can (3.7 oz)	130	80	0

FOOD	PORTION	CALS	CHOL	FIBER
Brunswick				
Fish Steak In Louisiana Hot Sauce	1 can (3.7 oz)	160	75	0
Fish Steaks In Mustard Sauce	1 can (3.7 oz)	160	80	0
Fish Steaks In Soybean Oil	1 can (3.7 oz)	200	80	0
Fish Steaks In Spring Water	1 can (3.7 oz)	150	115	0
Fish Steaks w/ Hot Tabasco Peppers	1 can (3.7 oz)	220	80	0
Seafood Snacks Golden Smoked	1 can (3.2 oz)	170	55	0
Seafood Snacks In Lemon & Cracked Pepper	1 can (3.2 oz)	160	55	0
Seafood Snacks In Louisiana Hot Sauce	1 can (3.2 oz)	140	70	0
Seafood Snacks In Teriyaki Sauce	1 can (3.2 oz)	160	70	0
Seafood Snacks In Tomato & Basil Sauce	1 can (3.2 oz)	140	70	0
Seafood Snacks Kippered	1 can (3.2 oz)	160	55	0
Chicken Of The Sea				
Fish Steaks	½ can (2 oz)	70	50	1
FROZEN				
breaded fillet	1 (2 oz)	155	64	–
sticks	1 stick (1 oz)	76	31	–
Gorton's				
Baked Au Gratin	1 piece (4.6 oz)	130	50	–
Baked Broccoli Cheddar	1 piece (4.6 oz)	130	50	–
Baked Primavera	1 piece (4.6 oz)	120	50	–
Batter Dipped Portions	1 piece (2.5 oz)	170	20	–
Crunchy Golden Fillets Breaded	2 (3.8 oz)	250	35	–
Crunchy Golden Sticks	6 (3.8 oz)	250	30	–
Garlic & Herb	2 pieces (3.6 oz)	220	30	–
Garlic Butter Crumb	1 piece (4.6 oz)	170	55	–
Grilled Cajun Blackened	1 piece (3.8 oz)	120	60	–
Grilled Garlic Butter	1 piece (3.8 oz)	100	60	–
Grilled Italian Herb	1 piece (3.8 oz)	100	60	–
Grilled Lemon Butter	1 piece (3.8 oz)	120	60	–
Grilled Lemon Pepper	1 piece (3.8 oz)	120	60	–
Parmesan	2 pieces (3.6 oz)	260	30	–

FOOD	PORTION	CALS	CHOL	FIBER
Ranch	1 piece (3.6 oz)	240	30	–
Southern Fried Country Style	2 pieces (3.6 oz)	230	30	–
Tenders	3.5 pieces (4 oz)	250	30	–
Tenders Extra Crunchy	3.5 pieces (4 oz)	270	30	–
Ian's				
Fillets	1 (3.4 oz)	260	20	2
Fish Stick Allergy Free	5 pieces	190	15	1
Fish Sticks	5 pieces	190	15	1
TAKE-OUT				
jamaican brown fish stew	1 serv	426	84	2
taramasalata	2 tbsp	124	10	–
FISH OIL				
cod liver	1 tbsp	123	78	0
herring	1 tbsp	123	104	0
menhaden	1 tbsp	123	71	0
salmon	1 tbsp	123	66	0
sardine	1 tbsp	123	97	0
Cormega				
Omega-E Orange	1 pkg	20	8	0
Spectrum				
Cod Liver Oil w/ Lemon	1 tsp	40	25	0
FLAXSEED				
Arrowhead				
Organic Flax Seeds	¼ cup	140	0	6
Bite Me				
Flax Bar	1 (1.8 oz)	242	0	12
Bob's Red Mill				
Flax Seed Meal	2 tbsp	60	0	4
Cracker Flax				
Organic Apple Raisin	1 oz	130	5	9
Hodgson Mill				
Milled	2 tbsp	60	0	4
FLOUNDER				
FRESH				
cooked	1 fillet (4.5 oz)	148	86	0
cooked	3 oz	99	58	0

FOOD	PORTION	CALS	CHOL	FIBER
TAKE-OUT				
breaded & fried	3.2 oz	211	31	–
stuffed w/ crab	1 piece (7.6 oz)	332	160	1
FLOUR				
arrowhead	1 cup	457	0	4
buckwheat whole groat	1 cup	402	0	12
corn masa	1 cup (4 oz)	416	0	11
cottonseed lowfat	1 oz	94	0	–
peanut defatted	1 cup	196	0	–
peanut lowfat	1 cup	257	0	–
potato	1 cup (6.3 oz)	628	0	–
rice brown	1 cup (5.5 oz)	574	0	7
rice white	1 cup (5.5 oz)	578	0	4
rye dark	1 cup (4.5 oz)	415	0	29
rye light	1 cup (3.6 oz)	374	0	15
rye medium	1 cup (3.6 oz)	361	0	15
sesame lowfat	1 oz	95	0	–
triticale whole grain	1 cup (4.6 oz)	439	0	19
white all-purpose	1 cup (4.4 oz)	455	0	2
white bread	1 cup (4.8 oz)	495	0	3
white cake unsifted	1 cup (4.8 oz)	496	0	2
white self-rising	1 cup (4.4 oz)	443	0	3
white unbleached	1 cup (4.4 oz)	455	0	3
whole wheat	1 cup (4.2 oz)	407	0	15
Arrowhead				
Whole Grain Oat	⅓ cup	120	0	3
Bob's Red Mill				
Flour	⅓ cup	130	0	5
Gold Medal				
All Purpose	¼ cup (1 oz)	100	0	tr
Better For Bread	¼ cup (1 oz)	100	0	tr
Organic All Purpose	¼ cup (1 oz)	100	0	tr
Self Rising	¼ cup (1 oz)	100	0	tr
Unbleached	¼ cup (1 oz)	100	0	tr
Wondra	¼ cup	100	0	tr
Heckers				
All Purpose Unbleached	¼ cup	100	0	tr
Whole Wheat	¼ cup	100	0	3

FOOD	PORTION	CALS	CHOL	FIBER
Hodgson Mill				
Best For Bread	¼ cup	100	0	1
Buckwheat	¼ cup	100	0	3
Oat Bran Flour	¼ cup	110	0	3
Kentucky Kernel				
Seasoned Flour	4 tsp	36	0	0
King Arthur				
All Purpose Unbleached	¼ cup	110	0	1
Organic White Whole Wheat	¼ cup	100	0	3
Organic Whole Wheat	½ cup	110	0	4
Organic Artisan	¼ cup	110	0	tr
Self-Rising	¼ cup	120	0	1
White Whole Wheat	¼ cup	100	0	3
La Pina				
Flour	¼ cup (1 oz)	100	0	1
Red Band				
All Purpose	¼ cup (1 oz)	100	0	tr
Self-Rising	¼ cup (1 oz)	100	0	tr
Robin Hood				
Whole Wheat	¼ cup (1 oz)	90	0	3

FOOD COLORS

FOOD	PORTION	CALS	CHOL	FIBER
blue	1 tsp	0	0	–
orange	1 tsp	0	0	0
red	1 tsp	tr	0	0
yellow	1 tsp	tr	0	–

FRENCH BEANS

dried cooked	1 cup	228	0	17

FRENCH FRIES (see POTATOES)

FRENCH TOAST
FROZEN

french toast	1 slice (2 oz)	126	48	2
Eggo				
Toaster Sticks Original	2	220	20	1
Ian's				
Sticks	5 (3.2 oz)	250	5	6
TAKE-OUT				
plain	1 slice	151	75	–

FOOD	PORTION	CALS	CHOL	FIBER
sticks	5 (4.9 oz)	513	75	3
w/ butter	2 slices	356	116	–

FROG LEGS
frog legs	3 oz	175	1	–

TAKE-OUT
as prep w/ seasoned flour & fried	1 (0.8)	70	12	–

FRUCTOSE
Estee
Fructose	1 tsp	15	0	0
Packet	1 pkg	10	0	0

FRUIT DRINKS (see also individual names, SMOOTHIES, YOGURT DRINKS)
MIX
Crystal Light
Sugar Free All Flavors as prep	1 serv	5	0	0

Tang
Orange Strawberry as prep	1 serv (8 oz)	110	0	0
Orange Pineapple as prep	1 serv (8 oz)	100	0	0

READY-TO-DRINK
fruit punch	6 oz	87	0	–

After The Fall
Banana Casablanca	8 oz	150	0	–
Mango Montage	8 oz	150	0	–

Apple & Eve
Apple Cranberry	8 oz	120	0	–

Bolthouse Farms
Berry Blast	8 oz	110	0	4
Green Goodess	8 oz	140	0	1
Passion Fruit Apple Carrot Juice	8 oz	120	0	2

Capri Sun
Fruit Punch	1 pkg (7 oz)	90	0	–

Ceres
Cranberry & Kiwi	8 oz	110	0	0
Medley	8 oz	130	0	2
Youngberry	8 oz	120	0	0

FOOD	PORTION	CALS	CHOL	FIBER
Champion Lyte				
All Flavors	1 bottle	0	0	0
Citrus Squeeze				
California Punch	8 oz	130	0	–
Florida Punch	8 oz	120	0	–
Crystal Light				
Strawberry Kiwi Sugar Free	8 oz	5	0	0
Del Monte				
Peach Raspberry	5.5 oz	160	0	3
Pineapple Banana Orange	5.5 oz	170	0	1
Strawberry Peach Banana	5.5 oz	150	0	1
Firefly				
Chill Out De-stress Drink	1 bottle (11.2 oz)	100	0	–
De-tox Morning After Drink	1 bottle (11.2 oz)	104	0	–
Five Alive				
Citrus	8 oz	120	0	–
Fresh Samantha				
Banana Strawberry	1 cup (8 oz)	130	0	6
Carrot Orange	1 cup (8 oz)	100	0	4
Desperately Seeking C	1 cup (8 oz)	110	0	7
The Big Bang	1 cup (8 oz)	100	0	8
Guzzler				
Citrus Punch	8 oz	140	0	–
Island Punch	8 oz	140	0	0
Hansen's				
Fruit Punch 100% Juice	1 box (4.23 oz)	60	0	–
Juice Slam Wild Berry	1 box	120	0	–
Hawaiian Punch				
Bodacious Berry	8 oz	110	0	–
Fruit Juicy Red	8 oz	80	0	–
Green Berry Rush	8 oz	120	0	–
Mazin Melon Mix	8 oz	110	0	–
Tropical Vibe	8 oz	110	0	–
Wild Purple Smash	8 oz	110	0	–
Hi-C				
Blast Berry Blue	1 bottle	170	0	–
Blast Fruit Pow	1 bottle	180	0	–
Blast Wild Berry	1 pkg	100	0	–
Flashin' Fruit Punch	1 box	90	0	–

FOOD	PORTION	CALS	CHOL	FIBER
Strive				
Crunchy Chocolate Smores	1 (2.1 oz)	200	0	0
Sweet Success				
Chewy Chocolate Brownie	1 (1.2 oz)	120	3	3
T.H.E. Bar				
Granola Raisin	1 (1.8 oz)	200	0	1
Think!				
Chocolate Almond Coconut Raisin	1 (2 oz)	243	9	2
Chocolate Fruit Harvest	1 (2 oz)	217	38	7
Zoe's				
Chocolate Delight	1 (1.7 oz)	190	0	5
Chocolate Peanut Butter Bliss	1 (1.7 oz)	200	0	5
Heavenly Apple	1	180	0	5
Peanut Butter Paradise	1 (1.7 oz)	190	0	5

ENERGY DRINKS
FOOD	PORTION	CALS	CHOL	FIBER
Accelerade				
All Flavors	8 oz	80	0	0
Amino Vital				
Amino Acid Supplement All Flavors	8 oz	35	0	–
Pro Fruit Punch	8 oz	35	0	–
Pro Tropic Fruit	8 oz	40	0	–
Puredge All Flavors	8 oz	50	0	–
AMP				
Energy Drink	1 can (8.4 oz)	120	0	0
Arizona				
Diet Green Tea Energy Drinks	8 oz	10	0	–
Extreme Energy Shot	1 bottle (8.3 oz)	130	0	–
Green Tea Energy Drink	8 oz	100	0	–
Pomegranate Lite	8 oz	70	0	–
Atkins				
Cafe Au Lait	1 can (11 oz)	170	15	3
Chocolate	1 can (11 oz)	170	15	3
Chocolate Royale	1 can (11 oz)	170	15	1
Strawberry	1 can (11 oz)	170	15	2
Vanilla	1 can (11 oz)	170	15	2

FOOD	PORTION	CALS	CHOL	FIBER
Shoutin' Orange Tangergreen	1 box	90	0	–
Strawberry Kiwi Kraze	1 box	100	0	–
Hog Wash				
All Flavors	1 bottle (10 oz)	37	0	0
Hood				
Fruit Punch	1 cup	120	0	0
Juici				
Sparkling All Flavors	1 bottle (12 oz)	105	0	–
Juicy Juice				
Apple Grape	1 box (8.45 oz)	140	0	0
Berry	1 box (8.45 oz)	130	0	0
Punch	1 box (4.23 oz)	70	0	0
Punch	1 box (8.45 oz)	140	0	0
Tropical	1 box (8.45 oz)	140	0	0
Kagome				
Burgundy Berry Blossom	8 oz	100	0	0
Golden Peach Garden	8 oz	100	0	1
Orange Carrot Blossom	8 oz	100	0	1
Purple Roots & Fruits	8 oz	130	0	1
Kool-Aid				
Jammers 10 All Flavors	1 pouch (6.75 oz)	10	0	0
L&A				
Pineapple Coconut	8 oz	140	0	1
Minute Maid				
Berry Kiwi	1 can (12 oz)	160	0	–
Cranberry Grape	8 oz	150	0	–
Light Guava Citrus	8 oz	5	0	–
Light Mango Tropical	8 oz	5	0	–
Light Orange Tangerine	8 oz	15	0	–
Orange Passion	8 oz	130	0	–
Orange Tangerine	8 oz	110	0	–
Tropical Punch Chilled	8 oz	110	0	–
Mott's				
Berry	1 box (8 oz)	100	0	–
Fruit Punch	1 box (8 oz)	110	0	–
Fruit Punch	8 oz	130	0	–
Naked Juice				
Berry Blast	8 oz	120	0	1

FOOD	PORTION	CALS	CHOL	FIBER
Blue Machine	8 oz	170	0	8
Green Machine	8 oz	130	0	1
Mango Acai	8 oz	190	0	3
Power C	8 oz	120	0	3
Protein Zone	8 oz	210	20	0
Red Machine	8 oz	160	0	4
Strawberry Banana C	8 oz	120	0	3
Very Berry	8 oz	130	0	1
Very Pro Berry	8 oz	190	15	1
Well Being	8 oz	140	0	0
Nantucket Nectars				
California Melonberry	8 oz	110	0	–
Cranberry Apple	8 oz	140	0	–
Fruit Punch	8 oz	130	0	–
Kiwi Berry	8 oz	120	0	–
Organic Blueberry Banana	8 oz	120	0	–
Organic Banana Mango Carrot	8 oz	120	0	–
Organic Cranberry Orange	8 oz	130	0	–
Peach Orange	8 oz	130	0	1
Pineapple Orange Guava	8 oz	120	0	–
Pomegranate Pear	8 oz	110	0	0
Watermelon Strawberry	8 oz	120	0	–
Newman's Own				
Orange Mango Tango	8 oz	150	0	–
Northland				
Cranberry Blueberry	1 cup (8 oz)	140	0	–
Oberweis				
Fruit Punch	8 oz	120	0	0
Ocean Spray				
Citrus Splash Spritzer	8 oz	160	0	–
Cran*Grape	8 oz	170	0	0
Cran*Raspberry	8 oz	140	0	0
Cran*Strawberry	8 oz	140	0	tr
Cranapple	8 oz	160	0	tr
Grape Cranberry	8 oz	170	0	–
Kiwi Strawberry	8 oz	120	0	0
Mandarin Magic	8 oz	120	0	0
Orange Citrus Spritzer	8 oz	160	0	–
Ruby Tangerine Spritzer	8 oz	160	0	–

FOOD	PORTION	CALS	CHOL	FIBER
White Cranberry Apple Juice	8 oz	120	0	–
Wildberry Spritzer	8 oz	160	0	–
Odwalla				
Carrot Orange Apple	8 oz	100	0	1
Rooty Fruity	8 oz	110	0	0
Strawberry Banana	8 oz	120	0	3
Phat Phruit				
Peach Mango	8 oz	40	0	0
Pineapple Orange	8 oz	40	0	0
Snapple				
Cranberry Raspberry	8 oz	120	0	–
Diet Carrot Apple	8 oz	10	0	–
Diet Plum-A-Granate	8 oz	0	0	–
Fruit Punch	8 oz	110	0	–
Go Bananas	8 oz	120	0	–
Kiwi Strawberry	8 oz	110	0	–
Snapricot Orange	8 oz	120	0	–
Soy20				
All Flavors	1 bottle (12 oz)	90	0	–
Squeezit				
Lemon Lime	1 bottle (7 oz)	110	0	0
Rockin' Red Puncher	1 bottle (7 oz)	110	0	0
TreeTop				
Apple Grape No Sugar Added	8 oz	130	0	–
Tropicana				
Fruit Punch	1 cup	130	0	0
Light Fruit Punch	8 oz	10	0	0
Orange Tangerine Juice	8 oz	110	0	0
Orchard Berry	8 oz	110	0	0
Twister Berry Blast	8 oz	120	0	0
Twister Citrus Spark	8 oz	120	0	0
Twister Fruit Fury	8 oz	120	0	0
Twister Light Strawberry Spiral	8 oz	40	0	0
V8				
Splash Fruit Medley	8 oz	80	0	–
Vruit				
Apple Carrot	1 box (8.45 oz)	120	0	–
Berry Veggie	1 box (8.45 oz)	110	0	–

FOOD	PORTION	CALS	CHOL	FIBER
Orange Veggie	1 box (8.45 oz)	110	0	–
Tropical Blend	1 box (8.45 oz)	110	0	–
Wadda Juice				
All Flavors	8 oz	50	0	–
Welch's				
White Grape Peach 100% Juice	8 oz	160	0	–

FRUIT MIXED (see also individual names)
CANNED

FOOD	PORTION	CALS	CHOL	FIBER
fruit cocktail in heavy syrup	½ cup	93	0	–
fruit cocktail juice pack	½ cup	56	0	–
fruit cocktail water pack	½ cup	40	0	–
fruit salad in heavy syrup	½ cup	94	0	–
fruit salad in light syrup	½ cup	73	0	–
fruit salad juice pack	½ cup	62	0	–
fruit salad water pack	½ cup	37	0	–
mixed fruit in heavy syrup	½ cup	92	0	–
tropical fruit salad in heavy syrup	½ cup	110	0	–
Del Monte				
Carb Clever Fruit Cocktail	½ cup	40	0	tr
Fruit Cocktail In 100% Juice	½ cup	60	0	1
Fruit Cocktail In Extra Light Syrup	½ cup	60	0	1
Fruit Cocktail In Heavy Syrup	½ cup	100	0	1
Fruit Cup Mixed In Extra Light Syrup	1 pkg (4 oz)	50	0	1
Fruit Naturals Tropical Medley	½ cup	70	0	tr
Orchard Select Premium Mixed	½ cup	80	0	tr
Snack Cups Strawberry Banana Peaches	1 pkg	70	0	tr
SunFresh Citrus Salad	½ cup	80	0	0
Dole				
FruitBowls Tropical Fruit	1 pkg (4 oz)	60	0	2
Tropical Fruit Salad	½ cup	80	0	1
Liberty Gold				
Fruit Cocktail In Heavy Syrup	½ cup	90	0	1

FOOD	PORTION	CALS	CHOL	FIBER
Mott's				
Fruitsations Banana	1 pkg (4 oz)	90	0	–
Fruitsations Cherry	1 pkg (4 oz)	70	0	–
Fruitsations Mango Peach	1 pkg (4 oz)	70	0	–
Fruitsations Mixed Berry	1 pkg (4 oz)	90	0	1
Fruitsations Pear	1 pkg (4 oz)	90	0	–
Fruitsations Strawberry	1 pkg (4 oz)	80	0	–
Fruitsations Tropical Fruit	1 pkg (4 oz)	70	0	–
Hearlthy Harvest Peach Medley	1 pkg (3.9 oz)	50	0	1
DRIED				
mixed	11 oz pkg	712	0	–
Goodniks				
Fruit Medley	¼ cup	110	0	2
Sun-Maid				
Mixed	¼ cup	100	0	3
Sunsweet				
Berry Blend	¼ cup (1.4 oz)	120	0	3
Orchard Mix	¼ cup (1.4 oz)	100	0	3
Tropical Mix	⅓ cup	150	0	2
FROZEN				
mixed fruit sweetened	1 cup	245	0	–
Tree of Life				
Organic Mixed Berries	¾ cup (5 oz)	60	0	3
FRUIT SNACKS				
fruit leather	1 (0.8 oz)	81	0	–
fruit leather pieces	1 oz	97	0	–
fruit leather pieces	1 pkg (0.9 oz)	92	0	–
fruit leather rolls	1 sm (0.5 oz)	49	0	–
fruit leather rolls	1 lg (0.7 oz)	73	0	–
CoolFruits				
Apple Grape	1 (0.5 oz)	51	0	1
Apple Strawberry	1 (0.5 oz)	51	0	1
Wild Blueberry	1 (0.5 oz)	51	0	1
Health Valley				
Fruit Bars Date	1	140	0	3
Stretch Island				
Fruit Leather Bountiful Blueberry	1 pkg (0.5 oz)	45	0	1

FOOD	PORTION	CALS	CHOL	FIBER
Fruit Leather Harvest Grape	1 pkg (0.5 oz)	45	0	1
Fruit Leather Truly Tropical	1 pkg (0.5 oz)	45	0	1
Fruit Leathers Mango Sunrise	1 pkg (0.5 oz)	45	0	1
Organic Smooshed Fruit Apple	1 piece (0.4 oz)	40	0	1
Organic Smooshed Fruit Strawberry	1 piece (0.4 oz)	40	0	tr
Tropicana				
Fruit Wise Bars All Flavors	1 (1.4 oz)	140	0	2
Fruit Wise Strips All Flavors	1 (0.7 oz)	70	0	1
Welch's				
White Grape Peach	20 pieces	110	0	–

GARLIC

clove	1	4	0	tr
fresh chopped	1 tbsp	18	0	tr
powder	1 tsp	9	0	tr
Dorot				
Crushed Cubes frzn	1 cube (4 g)	7	0	tr
Frieda's				
Elephant	1 tbsp	5	0	0
Vinegar Marinated	1 oz	30	0	0
McCormick				
Garlic Salt	¼ tsp	0	0	0

GEFILTE FISH

sweet	1 piece (1.5 oz)	35	12	–
Mrs. Adler's				
Pike'n Whitefish	1 piece (1.8 oz)	50	15	0

GELATIN
READY-TO-EAT
Del Monte

Mandarin Orange In Lite Orange Gel	1 pkg (4.5 oz)	60	0	0
Mixed Fruit In Cherry Gel	1 pkg (4.5 oz)	90	0	0
Peaches In Peach Gel	1 pkg (4.5 oz)	90	0	0
Peaches In Raspberry Gel	1 pkg (4.5 oz)	90	0	0
Peaches In Lite Strawberry Banana Gel	1 pkg (4.5 oz)	60	0	0

FOOD	PORTION	CALS	CHOL	FIBER
Hunt's				
Snack Pack Juicy Gels Raspberry Mixed Berry	1 serv (3.5 oz)	100	0	0
Snack Pack Juicy Gels Strawberry	1 serv (3.5 oz)	100	0	0
Snack Pack Juicy Gels Strawberry Orange	1 serv (3.5 oz)	100	0	0
Snack Pack Tropical Punch	1 serv (3.5 oz)	100	0	0
Jell-O				
Sugar Free Tropical Berry	1 serv (3.2 oz)	10	0	0
Kozy Shack				
Gel Treats Cherry	1 pkg (4 oz)	85	0	1
Gel Treats Lemon Lime	1 pkg (4 oz)	85	0	1
Gel Treats Orange	1 pkg (4 oz)	85	0	1
Gel Treats Strawberry	1 pkg (4 oz)	85	0	1
Gel Treats Sugar Free Orange	1 pkg (4 oz)	11	0	1
Gel Treats Sugar Free Strawberry	1 pkg (4 oz)	11	0	1
Swiss Miss				
Gels Berry Strawberry	1 pkg (3.5 oz)	79	0	0
Gels Berry Lemon	1 pkg (3.5 oz)	79	0	0
Gels Raspberry Orange	1 pkg (3.5 oz)	79	0	0
Gels Strawberry Raspberry	1 pkg (3.5 oz)	79	0	0
GIBLETS				
capon simmered	1 cup (5 oz)	238	629	0
chicken floured & fried	1 cup (5 oz)	402	647	–
chicken simmered	1 cup (5 oz)	228	570	–
turkey simmered	1 cup (5 oz)	243	606	–
GINGER				
ground	1 tsp	6	0	tr
pickled	0.5 oz	5	0	tr
root fresh	5 slices	9	0	tr
root fresh sliced	¼ cup	19	0	1
Eden				
Pickled w/ Shiso Leaves	1 tbsp	20	0	tr
Frieda's				
Crystallized	9 pieces (1.1 oz)	100	0	0
Galanga Thai Ginger	⅔ cup	60	0	2

FOOD	PORTION	CALS	CHOL	FIBER
McCormick				
Crystallized	¼ tsp	15	0	–
GINKGO NUTS				
canned	1 oz	32	0	–
dried	1 oz	99	0	–
raw	1 oz	52	0	–
GIZZARDS				
chicken simmered	1 cup (5 oz)	222	281	–
turkey simmered	1 cup (5 oz)	236	336	–
GNOCCHI				
Bellino				
W/ Potato	1 cup	240	0	2
GOAT				
roasted	3 oz	122	64	0
GOJI BERRIES				
dried	1 oz	106	0	2
GOOSE				
w/ skin roasted	½ goose (1.7 lbs)	2362	708	0
w/ skin roasted	6.6 oz	574	172	0
w/o skin roasted	5 oz	340	138	0
w/o skin roasted	½ goose (1.3 lbs)	1406	569	0
GOOSEBERRIES				
canned in light syrup	½ cup	93	0	–
fresh	1 cup	67	0	–
GRAPE JUICE				
bottled unsweetened	1 cup	154	0	tr
Ceres				
Hanepoot White Grape	8 oz	130	0	0
Daily				
Drink	8 oz	110	0	–
Hansen's				
White Grape 100% Juice	1 box (4.23 oz)	90	0	–
Juicy Juice				
Drink	1 box (4.23 oz)	70	0	–
Drink	1 box (8.45 oz)	140	0	0

FOOD	PORTION	CALS	CHOL	FIBER
Keto				
Kooler	½ tsp	0	0	0
Langers				
Plus 100% Juice	8 oz	160	0	–
White Grape Plus 100% Juice	8 oz	160	0	–
Mott's				
100% Juice	1 box (8 oz)	130	0	–
Grape Juice	8 oz	130	0	–
Nantucket Nectars				
Grapeade	8 oz	130	0	–
Organic Concord Grape	8 oz	130	0	–
Newman's Own				
Gorilla Grape	8 oz	140	0	–
Old Orchard				
Healthy Balance Brown	8 oz	35	0	–
Tang				
Drink Mix as prep	1 serv (8 oz)	110	0	0
Tropicana				
Grape	1 bottle (14 oz)	270	0	0
Welch's				
100% Juice	8 oz	170	0	–
100% White	8 oz	160	0	–
Light White Grape	8 oz	70	0	–
GRAPE LEAVES				
canned	1 (4 g)	3	0	–
fresh raw	1 (3 g)	3	0	tr
Sabra				
Stuffed Meatless	1	45	0	1
TAKE-OUT				
dolmas w/ beef & rice	1 (0.7 oz)	50	5	1
dolmas w/ lamb & rice	1 (0.7 oz)	56	5	1
dolmas w/ rice	1 (2 oz)	92	0	2
GRAPEFRUIT				
CANNED				
juice pack	½ cup	46	0	–
unsweetened	1 cup	93	0	–
water pack	½ cup	44	0	–
Del Monte				
Fruit Naturals Red	½ cup	60	0	tr

FOOD	PORTION	CALS	CHOL	FIBER
SunFresh Red	½ cup	80	0	2
SunFresh White In Real Fruit Juice	½ cup	45	0	2
FRESH				
pink	½	37	0	1
pink sections	1 cup	69	0	1
red	½	37	0	–
red sections	1 cup	69	0	–
white	½	39	0	1
white sections	1 cup	76	0	1
Ocean Spray				
Sweet Ruby	½ med	60	0	6
Sunkist				
Fresh	½ med	60	0	6
Oroblanco	½	100	0	4
GRAPEFRUIT JUICE				
fresh	1 cup	96	0	–
frzn as prep	1 cup	102	0	–
frzn not prep	6 oz	302	0	–
sweetened	1 cup	116	0	–
Crystal Light				
Sunrise Sunrise Ruby Red as prep	1 serv (8 oz)	5	0	0
Fresh Samantha				
Juice	1 cup (8 oz)	90	0	0
Izze				
Sparkling Grapefruit	8 oz	160	0	–
Minute Maid				
Frozen + Calcium	8 oz	100	0	–
Ruby Red	8 oz	130	0	–
Mott's				
100% Juice	8 oz	110	0	–
Nantucket Nectars				
100% Ruby Red	8 oz	100	0	–
Ocean Spray				
100% Juice Pink	8 oz	110	0	0
100% White Juice	8 oz	100	0	tr
Ruby Drink	8 oz	120	0	–
Ruby Red Drink	8 oz	130	0	0

FOOD	PORTION	CALS	CHOL	FIBER
Odwalla				
Juice	8 oz	90	0	0
Tao Tea				
Grapefruit Lemon Fusion	8 oz	72	0	–
Tropicana				
Sweet	8 oz	130	0	0
GRAPES				
seedless red or green	20	69	0	1
seedless red or green	1 cup	110	0	1
thompson seedless in heavy syrup	½ cup	93	0	1
thompson seedless water pack	½ cup	49	0	1
with seeds red or green	20	80	0	1
with seeds red or green	1 cup	106	0	1
Chiquita				
Grapes	1½ cups (4.8 oz)	90	0	1
Earthbound Farm				
Organic Black	½ cup	190	0	1
Frieda's				
Champagne	½ cup (3 oz)	50	0	1
GRAVY				
CANNED				
au jus	1 cup	38	1	–
beef	1 cup	124	7	–
beef	1 can (10 oz)	155	9	–
chicken	1 cup	189	5	–
mushroom	1 cup	120	0	–
turkey	1 cup	122	5	–
Boston Market				
Roasted Chicken	¼ cup	25	<5	–
Campbell's				
Beef	¼ cup	29	1	tr
Brown	¼ cup	46	tr	1
Chicken	¼ cup	42	3	1
Turkey	¼ cup	29	2	tr
Heinz				
Home Style Chicken	¼ cup	25	0	0
HomeStyle Roasted Turkey	¼ cup	25	<5	0

FOOD	PORTION	CALS	CHOL	FIBER
Pacific Foods				
Natural Beef	1 cup	20	0	0
Natural Chicken	¼ cup	25	0	–
Natural Mushroom	¼ cup	20	0	1
FROZEN				
Tofurky				
Giblet & Mushroom	2 tbsp	30	0	1
MIX				
au jus as prep w/ water	1 cup	32	1	–
brown as prep w/ water	1 cup	75	2	–
chicken as prep	1 cup	83	3	–
mushroom as prep	1 cup	70	1	–
onion as prep w/ water	1 cup	77	tr	–
pork as prep	1 cup	76	3	–
turkey as prep	1 cup	87	3	–
McCormick				
Beef & Herb as prep	¼ cup	30	<5	–
GREAT NORTHERN BEANS				
canned	1 cup	299	0	13
dried cooked	1 cup	209	0	12
Eden				
Organic	½ cup	110	0	8
GREEN BEANS				
CANNED				
drained	1 cup	27	0	3
Del Monte				
Cut	½ cup	20	0	2
Cut Italian	½ cup	30	0	3
Cut w/ Potatoes & Ham Flavor	½ cup	30	0	tr
French Style	½ cup	20	0	2
Whole	½ cup	20	0	2
S&W				
Blue Lake Cut	½ cup (4.2 oz)	20	0	2
French Style	½ cup (4.2 oz)	20	0	2
Whole Small	½ cup (4.2 oz)	20	0	2
Tillen Farms				
Crispy Dilly Beans Pickled	¼ cup	15	0	0

FOOD	PORTION	CALS	CHOL	FIBER
Veg-All				
French Style	½ cup	20	0	2
FRESH				
cooked w/o salt	1 cup	44	0	4
raw	1 cup	34	0	4
raw whole beans	10	17	0	2
GreenLine				
Fresh Trimmed	3 oz	25	0	2
FROZEN				
cooked	1 cup	38	0	4
Birds Eye				
Steamfresh Cut	½ cup	30	0	2
C&W				
French Cut	1 cup	30	0	2
Green Giant				
Green Bean Casserole	⅔ cup	110	0	1
Pictsweet				
Cut	⅔ cup	30	0	2
Tree Of Life				
Cut	⅔ cup (2.8 oz)	25	0	2
TAKE-OUT				
casserole w/ mushroom sauce	1 cup	108	2	3
pickled	½ cup	19	0	2
GREENS				
Ready Pac				
Microwave Leafy Greens as prep	½ cup	15	0	2
GROUNDCHERRIES				
fresh	½ cup	37	0	–
GROUPER				
cooked	1 fillet (7.1 oz)	238	95	0
cooked	3 oz	100	40	0
raw	3 oz	78	31	0
GUAR GUM				
Bob's Red Mill				
Guar Gum	1 tbsp	20	0	6

FOOD	PORTION	CALS	CHOL	FIBER
GUAVA				
fresh	1	45	0	–
guava sauce	½ cup	43	0	–
Frieda's				
Fresh	1 (3 oz)	45	0	5
GUAVA JUICE				
Ceres				
Guava	8 oz	120	0	0
Nantucket Nectars				
Guava	8 oz	130	0	0
GUINEA HEN				
w/o skin raw	½ hen (9.3 oz)	292	166	0
HADDOCK				
fresh broiled	4 oz	127	84	0
roe raw	1 oz	37	103	–
smoked	1 oz	33	22	0
TAKE-OUT				
breaded & fried	4 oz	229	88	1
HALIBUT				
atlantic & pacific cooked	½ fillet (5.6 oz)	223	65	0
atlantic & pacific cooked	3 oz	119	35	0
atlantic & pacific raw	3 oz	93	27	0
greenland baked	3 oz	203	50	0
greenland baked	5.6 oz	380	94	–
HAM				
boneless extra lean roasted	3 oz	123	45	0
boneless roasted	3 oz	151	50	0
canned extra lean roasted	3 oz	116	26	0
center slice lean & fat roasted	3 oz	173	46	0
deviled	¼ cup	188	35	0
ham salad spread	2 tbsp	65	11	0
patty grilled	1 patty (2 oz)	205	43	0
prosciutto	4 slices (1.3 oz)	72	26	0
sliced	3 slices (2.9 oz)	137	48	1
sliced extra lean	3 slices (2.2 oz)	69	30	0
whole roasted	3 oz	207	53	0

FOOD	PORTION	CALS	CHOL	FIBER
Alpine Lace				
Boneless Cooked 98% Fat Free	2 slices (2 oz)	60	25	0
Honey Ham 98% Fat Free	2 slices (2 oz)	60	25	0
Smoked Virginia 98% Fat Free	2 slices (2 oz)	60	25	0
Armour				
Lean Slices Brown Sugar	1 pkg (2.5 oz)	90	35	–
Boar's Head				
Black Forest Smoked	2 oz	60	30	0
Deluxe	2 oz	60	25	0
Deluxe 42% Lowered Sodium	2 oz	60	25	0
Fresh Seasoned	2 oz	90	35	0
Maple Glazed Honey	2 oz	60	20	0
Pepper	2 oz	60	20	0
Rosemary & Sundried Tomato	2 oz	70	10	0
Virginia Smoked	2 oz	60	25	0
Carl Buddig				
Ham Sliced w/ Natural Juices	1 pkg (2.5 oz)	120	40	–
Lean Slices Oven Roasted Honey Ham	1 pkg (2.5 oz)	90	35	–
Lean Slices Smoked	1 pkg (2.5 oz)	80	35	–
Hillshire				
Deli Select Honey Ham	6 slices (2 oz)	60	25	0
Oscar Mayer				
Brown Sugar	3 slices (1.8 oz)	60	25	0
Lunchables Ham Bagels	1 pkg	410	40	2
Lunchables Ham Wraps	1 pkg	430	35	2
Smoked	3 slices (2.2 oz)	60	25	0
Sara Lee				
Bavarian Oven Roasted Honey	2 oz	70	40	0
Brown Sugar	2 oz	70	20	0
Homestyle Baked	2 oz	60	25	0
Maple Honey	2 oz	70	20	0
Wampler				
Black Forest	2 oz	60	25	–

FOOD	PORTION	CALS	CHOL	FIBER
TAKE-OUT				
thick slice fried	1 (2.2 oz)	140	33	0
HAM DISHES				
TAKE-OUT				
croquette	1 (2.2 oz)	149	18	tr
salad	½ cup	287	237	tr
HAM SUBSTITUTES				
Yves				
Veggie Ham Deli Slices	1 serv (2.2 oz)	80	0	1
HAMBURGER				
Ian's				
Mini	2 (4.6 oz)	360	25	1
Mini Cheeseburger	2 (5 oz)	420	65	1
Kid Cuisine				
Cheeseburger Builder	1 meal	390	20	2
Lean Pockets				
Cheeseburger	1 (4.5 oz)	280	20	3
Oscar Meyer				
Lunchables All-Star Burgers	1 pkg	420	35	1
Wellshire				
Beef	1 (4 oz)	260	60	0
Turkey Burgers	1 (4 oz)	200	30	0
TAKE-OUT				
cheeseburger + condiments	1 reg (4.5 oz)	347	46	1
double hamburger + condiments	1 reg (5.8 oz)	384	66	2
single patty + condiments	1 reg (4 oz)	299	33	2
HAMBURGER SUBSTITUTES (*see also* MEAT SUBSTITUTES)				
Amy's				
All American Burger	1 (2.5 oz)	120	0	3
California Burger	1 (2.5 oz)	130	0	5
Chicago Burger	1 (2.5 oz)	160	5	3
Boca				
American Flame Grilled	1 (2.5 oz)	90	5	3
Cheeseburger	1 (2.5 oz)	100	5	3
Grilled Vegetable	1 (2.5 oz)	70	0	4
Ground Burger	1 serv (2 oz)	60	0	3

FOOD	PORTION	CALS	CHOL	FIBER
Original	1 (2.5 oz)	70	0	4
Original Vegan	1 patty (2.5 oz)	70	0	4
Dr. Praeger's				
California Burger	1 (2.7 oz)	100	0	4
Fantastic				
Natures Burger Mix not prep	¼ cup	170	0	5
Tofu Burger Mix not prep	3 tbsp	80	0	1
Franklin Farms				
Veggiburger Portabella	1 (3 oz)	120	0	4
Gardenburger				
Fire Roasted Vegetable	1 (2.5 oz)	120	10	2
Harmony Farms				
Soy Burger Onion	1 (2.5 oz)	90	0	3
Soy Burgers Garlic	1 (2.5 oz)	110	0	23
Soy Burgers Mushroom	1 (2.5 oz)	110	0	3
Soy Burgers Original	1 (2.5 oz)	110	0	4
Lightlife				
Light Burgers	1 (3 oz)	120	0	3
Smart Menu Burger	1	80	0	2
Morningstar Farms				
Classic Burger	1 (2.2 oz)	150	0	3
Garden Veggie Patties	1 patty (2.4 oz)	100	0	4
Harvest Burger	1	140	0	5
Okara Pattie	1 (2.2 oz)	120	0	3
Vegan Burger	1 (2.5 oz)	100	0	5
Superburgers				
Vegan Organic Original	1 (3 oz)	98	0	2
Vegan Organic Smoked	1 (3 oz)	98	0	2
Vegan Organic TexMex	1 (3 oz)	110	0	3
Tofurky				
SuperBurgers Original	1 (3.5 oz)	120	0	2
V'dora				
Vegetable BurgerLites	1 (3.3 oz)	58	0	0
VeggieLand				
Veggie Burger Original	1 (3.5 oz)	132	0	7
Veggie Burger Peppadew	1 (5 oz)	210	0	4
Yves				
Black Bean & Mushroom Burgers	1 (3 oz)	100	0	7

FOOD	PORTION	CALS	CHOL	FIBER
Garden Vegetable Patties	1 (3 oz)	90	0	7
Veggie Burger	1 (3 oz)	119	0	4

HAZELNUTS

dried blanched	1 oz	191	0	–
dried unblanched	1 oz	179	0	–
dry roasted unblanched	1 oz	188	0	–
oil roasted unblanched	1 oz	187	0	2
Kettle				
Butter Creamy Unsalted	2 tbsp	180	0	3
Love'n Bake				
Hazelnut Praline	2 tbsp	170	0	2
Low Carb Creations				
Soft Hazelnut Brittle	2 pieces (1 oz)	160	0	1
Torras				
Hazelnut Chocolate Spread	1 tsp	27	1	0
Twist				
Sugar Free Chocolate Hazelnut Spread	2 tbsp	180	0	0

HEART

beef simmered	3 oz	140	180	0
chicken cooked	1 (3 g)	5	6	0
chicken diced simmered	½ cup	134	175	0
lamb braised	3 oz	157	212	0
pork braised	1 (4.5 oz)	191	285	0
turkey simmered	½ cup	94	133	0
veal braised	3 oz	158	150	0

HEARTS OF PALM

canned	1 (1.2 oz)	9	0	1
canned	½ cup	20	0	2
Del Monte				
Hearts Of Palm	2-3 pieces	20	0	2

HEMP

HempNut				
Shelled Hempseed	1 oz	162	0	2
Nutiva				
Organic Protein Powder	2 scoops (1 oz)	120	0	14
Shelled Hempseed	2 tbsp	110	0	1

FOOD	PORTION	CALS	CHOL	FIBER
HERBAL TEA (see TEA/HERBAL TEA)				
HERBS/SPICES (see also individual names)				
garam masala	1 tsp	8	0	–
poultry seasoning	1 tsp	5	0	–
pumpkin pie spice	1 tsp	6	0	–
A Taste Of Thai				
Chicken & Rice Seasoning	¼ pkg (6 g)	15	0	0
Chef Paul Prudhomme's				
Magic Blackened Redfish	¼ tsp	0	0	0
Magic Fajita	¼ tsp	0	0	0
Magic Pork & Veal	¼ tsp	0	0	0
Magic Poultry	¼ tsp	0	0	0
Cut N Clean				
Greens Seasoning	1½ tsp	20	0	tr
Eden				
Shake Furikake	½ tsp	5	0	1
Emeril's				
Asian Essence	½ tsp	0	0	0
Bayou Blast!	½ tsp	0	0	0
Chicken Rub	½ tsp	0	0	0
Original Essence	½ tsp	0	0	0
Steak Rub	½ tsp	0	0	0
Gebhardt				
Menudo Mix	¼ tsp (0.4 g)	1	0	tr
Gringo Billy's				
Meat Rubs Chipotle	¼ tsp	0	0	0
Meat Rubs Montreau	¼ tsp	0	0	0
Tuna Seasoning	1 tsp	5	0	1
McCormick				
Blends Bon Appetit	¼ tsp	0	0	0
Cajun Seasoning	¼ tsp	0	0	0
Greek Seasoning	¼ tsp	0	0	0
Jamaican Jerk Seasoning	¼ tsp	0	0	0
Seafood Seasoning	¼ tsp	0	0	0
Mrs. Dash				
Grilling Blend Chicken	¼ tsp	0	0	0
Grilling Blend Steak	¼ tsp	0	0	0
Original Blend	¼ tsp	0	0	0

FOOD	PORTION	CALS	CHOL	FIBER
Nueva Cocina				
Picadillo	2 tsp	15	0	–
Taco Fresco	2 tsp	15	0	–
Ortega				
Burrito Seasoning	1½ tsp	20	0	tr
Fajita Seasoning	1½ tsp	20	0	–
Taco Seasoning	1 tbsp	20	0	–

HERRING

FOOD	PORTION	CALS	CHOL	FIBER
atlantic baked	4 oz	230	87	0
dried salted	1 fillet (1.4 oz)	161	61	0
pickled	1 oz	74	4	0
pickled in cream sauce	1 oz	72	5	0
roe	1 tbsp	39	105	0
smoked kippered	1 oz	620	23	0
Beach Cliff				
Kippered Snacks	1 can (4 oz)	220	135	0
TAKE-OUT				
breaded fried	1 serv (4 oz)	225	67	1

HIBISCUS

FOOD	PORTION	CALS	CHOL	FIBER
flowers dried sweetened	⅓ cup	100	0	2

HICKORY NUTS

FOOD	PORTION	CALS	CHOL	FIBER
dried	1 oz	187	0	–

HOMINY

FOOD	PORTION	CALS	CHOL	FIBER
CANNED				
white	1 cup (5.6 oz)	482	0	4
Van Camp's				
Golden	½ cup (4.3 oz)	80	0	1
White	½ cup (4.3 oz)	80	0	1

HONEY

FOOD	PORTION	CALS	CHOL	FIBER
honey	1 cup (11.9 oz)	1031	0	–
honey	1 tbsp (0.7 oz)	64	0	–
orange blossom	1 tbsp	60	0	0
wild honey	1 tbsp	60	0	–
Frieda's				
Honeycomb	½ cup (3 oz)	260	0	0
Steel's				
Sugar Free	1 tbsp	24	0	0

FOOD	PORTION	CALS	CHOL	FIBER
SueBee				
Clover	1 tbsp	60	0	–
HONEYDEW				
FRESH				
cubed	1 cup	60	0	–
wedge	1/10	46	0	–
Chiquita				
Wedge	1/10 melon (4.7 oz)	50	0	1
HORSE				
roasted	3 oz	149	58	–
HORSERADISH				
japanese wasabi	1/4 tsp	1	0	0
wasabi root raw	1 (5.9 oz)	184	0	12
wasabi root raw sliced	1 cup (4.6 oz)	142	0	10
Boar's Head				
Horseradish	1 tsp (5 g)	0	0	0
Horseradish & Beets	1 tsp	0	0	0
Eden				
Wasabi Powder	1 tsp	10	0	1
HOT CHOCOLATE				
Carnation				
Hot Cocoa 70 Calorie	1 pkg (0.7 oz)	70	0	tr
Hot Cocoa Double Chocolate Meltdown	1 pkg (1.2 oz)	150	0	1
Hot Cocoa Fat Free Raspberry	1 pkg (0.3 oz)	30	0	1
Hot Cocoa Fat Free w/ Marshmallows	1 pkg (0.4 oz)	45	0	tr
Hot Cocoa Lactose Free	1 pkg (1 oz)	120	0	1
Hot Cocoa Marshmallow Blizzard	1 pkg (1.5 oz)	180	<5	tr
Hot Cocoa Milk Chocolate	3 tbsp (1 oz)	110	<5	tr
Hot Cocoa Rich Chocolate as prep w/ 2% milk	1 pkg	200	21	tr
Hot Cocoa Rich Chocolate Fat Free	1 pkg (0.3 oz)	25	0	1
Hot Cocoa Rich Chocolate No Sugar Added	3 tbsp (0.5 oz)	50	<5	tr

FOOD	PORTION	CALS	CHOL	FIBER
Hot Cocoa Rich Chocolate w/ Marshmallows	3 tbsp (1 oz)	110	<5	tr
Country Choice Naturals				
Irish Chocolate Mint Cocoa	1 pkg	100	0	tr
Royal Chocolate Cocoa	1 pkg	100	0	tr
Soy Cocoa Irish Chocolate Mint	1 pkg	100	0	1
Soy Cocoa Royal Chocolate	1 pkg	100	0	1
Keto				
Hot Cocoa	1 tsp	12	0	1
Low Carb Creations				
Cocoa as prep	1 cup	30	0	0
White Hot Chocolate	1 cup	25	0	0
Nestle				
Hot Cocoa Rich Chocolate	1 pkg (1 oz)	110	0	tr
Hot Cocoa Rich w/ Marshmallows	1 pkg (1 oz)	110	0	tr
Sipper Sweets				
Sugar Free Low Carb Mix	1 serv	50	0	0
Swiss Miss				
Caramel Cream	1 serv	110	0	tr
Hot Cocoa And Cream	1 serv	153	6	1
Hot Cocoa Chocolate Sensation	1 serv	148	tr	1
Hot Cocoa Diet	1 serv	22	tr	1
Hot Cocoa Fat Free Marshmallow Lovers	1 serv	65	0	1
Hot Cocoa Lite	1 serv	76	0	2
Hot Cocoa Marshmallow Lovers	1 serv	142	2	1
Hot Cocoa Milk Chocolate Fat Free	1 pkg	50	0	tr
Hot Cocoa Milk Chocolate No Sugar Added	1 serv	55	1	1
Hot Cocoa Rich Chocolate	1 serv	110	1	1
Hot Cocoa w/ Marshmallows No Sugar Added	1 serv	56	1	1
Hot Cocoa White Chocolate	1 serv	109	1	tr
Milk Chocolate	1 pkg	120	0	1

FOOD	PORTION	CALS	CHOL	FIBER
Milk Chocolate w/ Marshmallows	1 pkg	120	tr	tr
Premiere Hot Cocoa Almond Mocha	1 serv	144	1	1
Premiere Hot Cocoa Raspberry Truffle	1 serv	144	1	1
Premiere Hot Cocoa Suisse Truffle	1 serv	142	1	1
Rich Hot Cocoa No Sugar Added	1 serv	54	1	1
Sidewalk Cafe Cappuccino	1 serv	119	1	1
Sidewalk Cafe Cinnamon	1 serv	126	1	1
Sidewalk Cafe French Vanilla	1 serv	121	1	tr
Sidewalk Cafe Mocha	1 serv	120	1	1
TAKE-OUT				
hot cocoa	1 cup	218	33	–
mexican hot chocolate	1 cup	173	18	1

HOT DOG

FOOD	PORTION	CALS	CHOL	FIBER
beef	1 (1.5 oz)	149	24	0
beef & pork	1 (1.5 oz)	137	23	1
beef low fat	1 (2 oz)	133	23	0
chicken	1 (1.5 oz)	116	45	0
fat free	1 (2 oz)	62	23	0
low fat	1 (2 oz)	88	25	0
low sodium	1 (2 oz)	180	35	0
pork and beef cheese smokie	1 (1.5 oz)	141	29	0
turkey	1 (1.5 oz)	102	48	0
Ball Park				
Franks	1 (2 oz)	180	40	0
Franks Beef	1 (2 oz)	180	35	0
Franks Bun Size	1 (2 oz)	180	40	0
Franks Smoked White Turkey	1 (1.8 oz)	45	10	0
Franks Fat Free	1 (1.8 oz)	40	10	0
Franks Lite	1 (1.8 oz)	100	25	0
Franks Singles Cheese	1 (1.6 oz)	150	30	0
Grillmaster Hearty Beef	1	250	50	0
Grillmaster Smokehouse	1	210	50	0

FOOD	PORTION	CALS	CHOL	FIBER
Boar's Head				
Beef	1 (2 oz)	160	30	0
Beef Lite	1 (1.6 oz)	90	25	0
Beef Cocktail	5 (2 oz)	170	30	0
Pork & Beef	1 (2 oz)	150	25	0
Health Is Wealth				
Uncured Beef	1 (1.5 oz)	80	20	–
Uncured Chicken	1 (1.5 oz)	100	30	–
Healthy Choice				
Beef Low Fat	1 (1.8 oz)	70	15	0
Low Fat Turkey Pork Beef	1 (1.4 oz)	60	10	–
Hebrew National				
97% Fat Free Beef	1 (1.7 oz)	45	15	0
Beef	1 (1.7 oz)	150	30	0
Cocktail Franks	5 (2 oz)	180	40	0
Dinner Frank	1 (4 oz)	350	70	0
Franks In A Blanket	5 (2.8 oz)	290	40	1
Reduced Fat Beef	1 (1.7 oz)	120	25	0
Ian's				
Popcorn Turkey Corn Dog	5 pieces (3 oz)	237	20	0
Organic Valley				
All-Natural Beef	1 (1.6 oz)	90	25	–
Oscar Mayer				
Corn Dogs	1 (3.2 oz)	260	35	1
Fat Free Turkey & Beef	1 (1.8 oz)	40	15	0
State Fair				
Corn Dogs	1 (2.67 oz)	180	15	1
Wampler				
Chicken	1 (2 oz)	120	60	1
Wellshire				
Beef Premium	1 (2 oz)	110	30	0
Cheese Franks	1 (2 oz)	110	30	0
Chicken Franks	1 (1.6 oz)	70	30	0
Turkey Franks	1 (1.6 oz)	110	30	0
TAKE-OUT				
corndog	1	460	79	–
w/ bun chili	1	297	51	–
w/ bun plain	1	242	44	–

FOOD	PORTION	CALS	CHOL	FIBER
HOT DOG SUBSTITUTES				
Lightlife				
Smart Dogs	1	45	0	1
Smart Franks	1 (2 oz)	110	0	0
Tofu Pups	1 (1.5 oz)	60	0	1
Loma Linda				
Big Franks	1 (1.8 oz)	110	0	2
Big Franks Low Fat Vegan	1 (1.8 oz)	80	0	2
Morningstar Farms				
Corn Dog Veggie	1 (2.5 oz)	170	0	3
Quorn				
Meat-Free Dogs	1 (1.5 oz)	70	5	2
Yves				
Good Dog	1 (1.8 oz)	70	0	1
Tofu Dogs	1 (1.3 oz)	45	0	0
Veggie Dogs	1 (1.6 oz)	60	0	1
Veggie Dogs Jumbo	1 (2.7 oz)	100	0	2
Veggie Dogs Jumbo Hot N' Spicy	1 (2.7 oz)	106	0	2
HUMMUS				
Athenos				
Black Olive	2 tbsp	50	0	1
Original	2 tbsp	50	0	1
Travelers Hummus & Pita	1 pkg	325	0	3
Guiltless Gourmet				
Roasted Garlic	2 tbsp	35	0	1
Sabra				
Homus	2 oz	110	0	3
Homus Spicy	½ cup	171	0	5
TAKE-OUT				
hummus	⅓ cup	140	0	–
HYACINTH BEANS				
dried cooked	1 cup	228	0	–

ICE CREAM AND FROZEN DESSERTS (*see also* ICES AND ICE POPS, SHERBET, YOGURT FROZEN)

FOOD	PORTION	CALS	CHOL	FIBER
chocolate	½ cup (4 oz)	143	22	–
dixie cup chocolate	1 (3.5 oz)	125	20	–
dixie cup strawberry	1 (3.5 oz)	112	17	–

FOOD	PORTION	CALS	CHOL	FIBER
dixie cup vanilla	1 (3.5 oz)	116	25	–
freeze dried ice cream chocolate strawberry & vanilla	1 pkg (0.75 oz)	158	1	1
strawberry	½ cup (4 oz)	127	19	–
vanilla	½ cup (4 oz)	132	29	–
vanilla soft serve	½ cup	111	10	–
Atkins				
Endulge Butter Pecan	½ cup	170	40	4
Endulge Chocolate	½ cup	140	45	5
Endulge Chocolate Peanut Butter Swirl	½ cup	170	40	5
Endulge Vanilla	½ cup	140	45	4
Endulge Vanilla Fudge	½ cup	140	40	4
Endulge Bars Chocolate Fudge	1	130	40	5
Endulge Bars Chocolate Fudge Swirl	1	180	30	4
Endulge Bars Peanut Butter Swirl	1	180	30	4
Endulge Bars Vanilla Fudge Swirl	1	180	30	4
Better Than Ice Creme				
Soy Vanilla as prep	½ cup	110	0	0
Blue Bunny				
Bar Candy Center Crunch	1 (3.2 oz)	370	20	1
Bar English Toffee	1 (1.4 oz)	130	15	0
Bar Homemade Vanilla	1 (2.3 oz)	190	20	0
Bar Orange Dream	1 (2.1 oz)	80	5	0
Bar Strawberry Sundae Crunch	1 (2.2 oz)	170	15	0
Blendz Peanut Butter Cup	1 (4.4 oz)	270	25	tr
Caramel Sundae Bite Size	4 bars (3.1 oz)	340	25	1
Chocolate	½ cup	130	25	0
Cone Bunny Tracks	1 (4.8 oz)	420	35	2
Cone The Champ Chocolate Lovers	1 (3.5 oz)	300	40	1
Cone Vanilla Nutty Sundae	1 (3 oz)	250	10	1
Cups Vanilla & Chocolate	1 (1.7 oz)	100	20	0
Mint Chip	½ cup	140	25	0

FOOD	PORTION	CALS	CHOL	FIBER
Neapolitan	½ cup	130	25	0
Orange Dream	½ cup	130	20	0
Premium All Natural Vanilla	½ cup	160	55	0
Premium Bunny Tracks	½ cup	190	25	tr
Premium Butter Pecan	½ cup	150	25	0
Premium Cookies & Cream	½ cup	150	25	0
Premium Double Strawberry	½ cup	140	25	0
Premium Exquisite Mint	½ cup	170	25	0
Premium Rocky Road	½ cup	150	20	0
Premium Toasted Almond Fudge	½ cup	160	25	tr
Sandwich Big Vanilla	1 (3.7 oz)	260	35	0
Sandwich Chips Galore	1 (3.4 oz)	310	35	1
Strawberry	½ cup	120	25	0
Bon Bons				
Dark Chocolate	5 pieces	190	15	0
Milk Chocolate	5 pieces	200	10	0
Breyers				
Almond Joy	½ cup	140	30	tr
Banana Fudge Chunk	½ cup	170	20	tr
Bar Light Creamy Vanilla Chocolate Coated	1	160	5	3
Butter Almond	½ cup	160	20	tr
Butter Pecan	½ cup	170	20	0
Butter Pecan Homemade	½ cup	170	50	0
Butter Pecan No Sugar Added	½ cup	120	10	tr
Caramel Praline Crunch	½ cup	180	20	0
Caramel Toffee Crunch	½ cup	180	50	0
CarbSmart Chocolate	½ cup	130	25	3
CarbSmart Strawberry	½ cup	130	25	3
CarbSmart Vanilla	½ cup	130	25	3
Cherry Chocolate Chip	½ cup	150	20	0
Cherry Vanilla	½ cup	140	20	0
Chocolate	½ cup	150	20	tr
Chocolate 98% Fat Free	½ cup	90	5	4
Chocolate Caramel No Sugar Added	½ cup	110	10	tr
Chocolate Chip	½ cup	160	20	0

FOOD	PORTION	CALS	CHOL	FIBER
Chocolate Chip Cookie Dough	½ cup	170	25	0
Chocolate Rainbow	½ cup	140	20	0
Coffee	½ cup	140	20	0
Cookies & Cream	½ cup	160	20	tr
Creamsicle	½ cup	130	15	0
Deep Chocolate Fudge	½ cup	200	30	1
Dulce De Leche	½ cup	150	20	0
French Vanilla	½ cup	150	50	0
French Vanilla Light	½ cup	120	35	0
French Vanilla No Sugar Added	½ cup	110	35	0
Fresh Banana	½ cup	140	15	0
Heath English Toffee	½ cup	190	20	0
Hershey w/ Almonds	½ cup	170	15	tr
Ice Cream Cake Oreo	1 slice	190	30	tr
Ice Cream Cake Vanilla	1 slice	190	40	0
Klondike Sandwich	½ cup	160	20	0
Mint Chocolate Chip	½ cup	160	20	0
Mint Chocolate Chip Light	½ cup	130	10	0
Mint Oreo	½ cup	170	15	0
Mocha Almond Fudge	½ cup	170	15	2
Oreo	½ cup	160	20	0
Peach	½ cup	130	15	0
Peanut Butter & Fudge	½ cup	170	20	tr
Reese's Peanut Butter Cups	½ cup	180	15	0
Rocky Road	½ cup	160	20	tr
SpongeBob Cookie Dough	½ cup	160	15	0
Strawberry	½ cup	120	15	0
Strawberry Shortcake	½ cup	160	15	0
Turtle Sundae	½ cup	190	30	tr
Vanilla	½ cup	140	20	0
Vanilla Calcium Rich	½ cup	130	20	0
Vanilla Caramel Brownie	½ cup	170	50	0
Vanilla Fudge Brownie	½ cup	180	25	tr
Vanilla Fudge Twirl	½ cup	140	20	tr
Vanilla Fudge Twirl No Sugar Added	½ cup	110	10	tr
Vanilla Homemade	½ cup	140	40	0
Vanilla Lactose Free	½ cup	130	20	0

FOOD	PORTION	CALS	CHOL	FIBER
Vanilla Light	½ cup	110	10	0
Vanilla Light 2% Milk	½ cup	130	30	0
Vanilla No Sugar Added	½ cup	100	15	0
Wild Berry Swirl	½ cup	140	20	0
Bubbies				
Mochi Mango	1 piece (1.3 oz)	110	15	0
Butterfinger				
Bar	1 (1.9 oz)	210	15	0
Carnation				
Cup Chocolate	1 (3 oz)	140	25	0
Cup Chocolate Malt	1 (12 oz)	270	20	1
Cup Strawberry	1 (3 oz)	100	20	0
Cup Vanilla	1 (5 oz)	170	35	0
Cup Vanilla	1 (3 oz)	100	20	0
Cup Vanilla Malt	1 (12 oz)	260	20	0
Sundae Cup Chocolate	1 (5 oz)	210	30	1
Sundae Cup Strawberry	1 (5 oz)	200	30	0
Celestial Seasonings				
Tea Dreams Bars Chocolate Caramel Chai	1 (2.7 oz)	240	0	2
Tea Dreams Cinnamon Apple Spice	½ cup	140	0	1
Tea Dreams Vanilla Ginger Spice Chai	½ cup	140	0	1
Cool Creations				
Cookies & Cream Sandwich	1 (3.5 oz)	240	15	1
Mickey Mouse Bar	1 (2.5 oz)	120	15	0
Mini Sandwich	1 (2.3 oz)	110	10	0
Dippin' Dots				
Chocolate	⅝ cup (3 oz)	190	40	0
Dove				
Beyond Vanilla	½ cup	240	50	0
Give In To Mint	½ cup	300	45	1
Irresistably Raspberry	½ cup	240	30	1
Milk Chocolate w/ Almonds	1 bar (3.3 oz)	340	35	1
Milk Chocolate w/ Vanilla Ice Cream	1 bar (3.3 oz)	330	40	1
Miniatures Milk Chocolate w/ Vanilla Ice Cream	5 pieces (3.1 oz)	300	30	1
Triple Chocolate	1 bar (2.8 oz)	200	25	3

FOOD	PORTION	CALS	CHOL	FIBER
Unconditional Chocolate	½ cup	290	40	2
Vanilla w/ A Chocolate Soul	½ cup	290	45	1
Drumstick				
Cone Chocolate	1 (4.6 oz)	320	25	2
Cone Chocolate Dipped	1 (4.6 oz)	320	25	1
Cone Vanilla	1 (4.6 oz)	340	20	2
Cone Vanilla Caramel	1 (4.6 oz)	360	25	2
Cone Vanilla Fudge	1 (4.6 oz)	360	20	2
Edy's				
Carb Benefit Butter Pecan	½ cup	170	30	6
Carb Benefit Chocolate	½ cup	150	30	7
Carb Benefit Chocolate Chip	½ cup	160	30	6
Carb Benefit Mint Chocolate Chip	½ cup	160	30	6
Carb Benefit Vanilla Bean	½ cup	140	30	6
Dips Chocolate	26 pieces	420	30	–
Dips Mint	26 pieces	420	25	–
Dips Vanilla	26 pieces	420	25	–
Grand Andes Cool Mint	½ cup	170	25	–
Grand Butter Pecan	½ cup	170	25	–
Grand Chocolate	½ cup	150	25	–
Grand Chocolate Caramel Swirl	½ cup	170	25	–
Grand Chocolate Chip	½ cup	160	20	–
Grand Chocolate Fudge Mousse	½ cup	160	25	–
Grand Chocolate Fudge Sundae	½ cup	170	20	–
Grand Coffee	½ cup	140	25	–
Grand Cookie Dough	½ cup	180	25	–
Grand Cookies 'N Cream	½ cup	160	25	–
Grand Double Fudge Brownie	½ cup	170	25	–
Grand Dulce De Leche	½ cup	150	25	–
Grand Espresso Chip	½ cup	150	25	–
Grand French Vanilla	½ cup	160	50	–
Grand Fudge Tracks	½ cup	180	25	–
Grand Ice Cream Sandwich	½ cup	150	25	–
Grand Mint Chocolate Chips	½ cup	170	25	–
Grand Peanut Butter Cup	½ cup	180	20	–

FOOD	PORTION	CALS	CHOL	FIBER
Grand Real Strawberry	½ cup	130	20	–
Grand Rocky Road	½ cup	170	30	–
Grand Spumoni	½ cup	150	25	–
Grand Toffee Bar Crunch	½ cup	170	25	–
Grand Toll House Cookie Swirl	½ cup	170	25	–
Grand Turtle Sundae	½ cup	160	25	–
Grand Utimate Caramel Cup	½ cup	170	20	–
Grand Vanilla	½ cup	140	25	–
Neapolitan	½ cup	140	25	–
Slow Churned Light Butter Pecan	½ cup	120	20	–
Slow Churned Light Caramel Delight	½ cup	120	20	–
Slow Churned Light Chocolate	½ cup	110	20	–
Slow Churned Light Chocolate Chip	½ cup	120	20	–
Slow Churned Light Chocolate Fudge Chunk	½ cup	120	20	–
Slow Churned Light Coffee	½ cup	105	20	–
Slow Churned Light Cookie Dough	½ cup	130	20	–
Slow Churned Light Cookies 'N Cream	½ cup	120	20	–
Slow Churned Light French Silk	½ cup	130	20	–
Slow Churned Light French Vanilla	½ cup	100	30	–
Slow Churned Light Fudge Tracks	½ cup	120	20	–
Slow Churned Light Mint Chocolate Chips	½ cup	120	20	–
Slow Churned Light Mocha Almond Fudge	½ cup	120	20	–
Slow Churned Light Neapolitan	½ cup	100	20	–
Slow Churned Light Rocky Road	½ cup	120	20	–

FOOD	PORTION	CALS	CHOL	FIBER
Slow Churned Light Strawberry	½ cup	110	15	–
Slow Churned Light Vanilla	½ cup	100	20	–
Slow Churned No Sugar Added Butter Pecan	½ cup	120	10	–
Slow Churned No Sugar Added Chocolate	½ cup	95	10	–
Slow Churned No Sugar Added Cookie Dough	½ cup	110	15	–
Slow Churned No Sugar Added Fat Free Chocolate Fudge	½ cup	100	0	–
Slow Churned No Sugar Added Fat Free Raspberry Vanilla Swirl	½ cup	90	0	–
Slow Churned No Sugar Added Fat Free Vanilla	½ cup	90	0	–
Slow Churned No Sugar Added Fat Free Vanilla Chocolate Swirl	½ cup	100	0	–
Slow Churned No Sugar Added Fudge Tracks	½ cup	110	10	–
Slow Churned No Sugar Added Mint Chocolate Chips	½ cup	110	10	–
Slow Churned No Sugar Added Neapolitan	½ cup	95	10	–
Slow Churned No Sugar Added Triple Chocolate	½ cup	110	10	–
Slow Churned No Sugar Added Vanilla	½ cup	90	10	–
Eskimo Pie				
Milk Chocolate	1 bar (1.8 oz)	160	20	0

FOOD	PORTION	CALS	CHOL	FIBER
Flintstones				
Cool Cream	1 (2.75 oz)	90	5	0
Push-Up Pebbles Treats	1 (2.75 oz)	120	20	0
Good Humor				
Bar Candy Center Crunch	1 (4 oz)	310	15	tr
Bar Oreo	1 (4 oz)	250	15	tr
Bar Reese's Peanut Butter	1 (4 oz)	310	20	tr
Bar Strawberry Shortcake	1 (4 oz)	230	10	tr
Bar Toasted Almond	1 (3 oz)	180	5	tr
Bar Vanilla Dark Chocolate	1 (3 oz)	190	10	tr
Bar Vanilla Milk Chocolate	1 (3 oz)	180	15	0
Chocolate Eclair Bar	1 (4 oz)	220	10	tr
Cone Premium Sundae	1 (4.3 oz)	270	15	tr
Cone Strawberry Shortcake	1 (4.3 oz)	230	5	tr
Giant Sandwich Neapolitan	1 (6 oz)	250	20	tr
Giant Sandwich Vanilla	1 (6 oz)	250	20	0
King Cone	1 (4.6 oz)	250	15	tr
Number 1 Bar	1 (4 oz)	200	10	tr
Sandwich Chocolate Chip Cookie	1 (4.5 oz)	290	20	1
Sandwich Vanilla	1 (3.5 oz)	160	10	0
Sundae Twist Cup	1 (6 oz)	160	10	0
GoodBody				
Chocolate Banana	1 (3.5 oz)	120	0	4
Chocolate Double Dutch	1 (3.5 oz)	130	0	4
Chocolate Peanut Butter	1 (3.5 oz)	180	0	5
Vanilla & Raspberry Sorbet	1 (3.5 oz)	120	0	4
Vanilla & Strawberry Sorbet	1 (3.5 oz)	120	0	4
Vanilla & Tropical Sorbet	1 (3.5 oz)	120	0	4
Haagen-Dazs				
Bars Chocolate & Almonds	1 (3.7 oz)	380	90	2
Bars Chocolate & Dark Chocolate	1 (3.6 oz)	350	65	2
Bars Chocolate Peanut Butter Swirl	1 (3 oz)	320	60	2
Bars Coffee & Almond Crunch	1 (3.7 oz)	370	90	tr
Bars Cookies & Cream Crunch	1 (3.6 oz)	370	85	tr

FOOD	PORTION	CALS	CHOL	FIBER
Bars Dulce De Leche Caramel	1 (3.7 oz)	370	75	0
Bars Tropical Coconut	1 (3.5 oz)	340	90	0
Bars Vanilla & Almonds	1 (3.7 oz)	380	90	1
Bars Vanilla & Dark Chocolate	1 (3.6 oz)	350	85	1
Bars Vanilla & Milk Chocolate	1 (3.5 oz)	340	90	tr
Butter Pecan	½ cup	310	110	tr
Cappuccino Commotion	½ cup	310	100	1
Cherry Vanilla	½ cup	240	100	0
Chocolate	½ cup	270	115	1
Chocolate Brownie w/ Walnuts	½ cup	290	100	1
Chocolate Chocolate Chip	½ cup	300	105	2
Chocolate Chocolate Fudge	½ cup	290	100	tr
Chocolate Swiss Almond	½ cup	300	100	2
Cinnamon	½ cup	250	110	0
Coffee	½ cup	270	120	0
Coffee Mocha Chip	½ cup	290	110	tr
Cookie Dough Chip	½ cup	310	95	0
Cookies & Cream	½ cup	270	105	0
Creme Caramel Pecan	½ cup	320	95	0
Dulce De Leche Caramel	½ cup	290	100	0
Low Fat Chocolate	½ cup	170	30	tr
Low Fat Coffee Fudge	½ cup	170	25	0
Low Fat Strawberry	½ cup	150	15	0
Low Fat Vanilla	½ cup	170	20	0
Macadamia Brittle	½ cup	300	110	0
Mango	½ cup	250	85	tr
Mint Chip	½ cup	300	105	tr
Pineapple Coconut	½ cup	230	90	0
Pistachio	½ cup	290	110	tr
Rum Raisin	½ cup	270	110	0
Strawberry	½ cup	250	95	tr
Vanilla	½ cup	270	120	0
Vanilla Chocolate Chip	½ cup	310	105	tr
Vanilla Fudge	½ cup	290	100	0
Vanilla Swiss Almond	½ cup	300	105	tr

FOOD	PORTION	CALS	CHOL	FIBER
Hawaiian Punch				
Cream Surfers	1	90	5	0
Healthy Choice				
Bar Sorbet & Cream	1	100	5	tr
Brownie Bliss	½ cup	130	10	1
Butter Pecan Crunch	½ cup	100	10	2
Cappuccino Chocolate Chunk	½ cup	120	10	tr
Caramel Fudge Brownie	½ cup	120	10	1
Cherry Chocolate Mambo	½ cup	130	10	1
Chocolate Chocolate Chunk	½ cup	120	5	1
Cookies 'N Cream	½ cup	120	5	tr
Crazy Caramel	½ cup	120	10	tr
Double Karma	½ cup	140	10	tr
French Silk	½ cup	120	5	2
Happy Together	½ cup	150	10	1
Jumpin' Java	½ cup	130	10	tr
Low Fat Bar Fudge	1	90	5	0
Low Fat Bar Mocha Fudge	1	90	5	2
Low Fat Bar Strawberry & Cream	1	90	5	tr
Mint Chocolate Chip	½ cup	120	10	tr
No Sugar Added Chocolate Fudge Brownie	½ cup	120	5	1
No Sugar Added Coffee Almond Fudge	½ cup	110	5	1
No Sugar Added Mint Chocolate Chip	½ cup	110	10	1
No Sugar Added Vanilla	½ cup	100	10	1
Peanut Butter Cup	½ cup	120	5	tr
Praline & Caramel	½ cup	120	10	tr
Rocky Road	½ cup	130	5	tr
Sandwich Caramel	1	140	5	tr
Sandwich Fudge Swirl	1	140	5	tr
Sandwich Vanilla	1	130	5	tr
Turtle Fudge Cake	½ cup	130	10	tr
Vanilla	½ cup	110	10	tr
Vanilla Bean	½ cup	120	10	tr
Vanilla Caramel Fudge	½ cup	140	10	tr
Hershey's				
Butter Pecan	½ cup	170	35	0

FOOD	PORTION	CALS	CHOL	FIBER
French Vanilla	½ cup	170	70	0
Neapolitan	½ cup	160	35	tr
Hood				
Butterscotch Blast	½ cup	160	25	0
Chocolate	½ cup	140	25	0
Chocolate Eclair	1 bar (2.2 oz)	150	5	0
Cookie Dough Delight	½ cup	160	25	0
Creamy Coffee	½ cup	140	30	0
Fat Free Chocolate Passion	½ cup	100	0	0
Fat Free Very Vanilla	½ cup	100	0	0
Fudge Twister	½ cup	150	25	0
Grasshopper Pie	½ cup	160	25	0
Hoodsie Cups	1 (1.7 oz)	100	20	0
Light Butter Pecan	½ cup	140	10	0
Light Creamy Vanilla	½ cup	110	10	0
Low Fat No Sugar Added Vanilla Dream	½ cup	90	5	3
Maple Walnut	½ cup	160	25	0
No Sugar Added Chocolate Chip	½ cup	100	5	3
Nutty Royale	1 cone (2.5 oz)	220	15	tr
Orange Cream	1 bar (2.2 oz)	90	5	0
Sandwich Vanilla	1	180	20	tr
Sandwich Vanilla Light	1 (2.2 oz)	160	10	tr
Sandwich Vanilla Lowfat	1 (2.8 oz)	80	<5	2
Spumoni	½ cup	140	25	0
Klondike				
Bar Almond	1	300	20	0
Bar Cappuccino	1	280	20	0
Bar Caramel & Peanut	1	290	15	tr
Bar Caramel Crunch	1	270	25	0
Bar Chocolate	1	280	20	tr
Bar Dark Chocolate	1	280	20	tr
Bar Heath	1	300	20	0
Bar Krunch	1	280	20	0
Bar Oreo	1	160	10	tr
Bar Original	1	280	20	0
Bar Peppermint Patty	1	280	20	tr
Bar Reese's	1	220	15	tr
Big Bear Cone Vanilla	1	330	15	1

FOOD	PORTION	CALS	CHOL	FIBER
Big Bear Cone Vanilla Caramel	1	360	15	1
Big Bear Cone Vanilla Fudge	1	380	15	1
Big Bear Sandwich Neapolitan	1	300	25	1
Big Bear Sandwich Vanilla	1	300	25	tr
CarbSmart Fudge Bar	1	60	20	1
CarbSmart Ice Cream Bar	1	130	15	2
Choco Taco	1	290	10	1
Cone Oreo	1	250	15	1
Cone Reese's	1	290	15	tr
Cookie Sandwich Chips	1	470	30	2
Cookie Sandwich Oreo	1	230	10	2
Minis	2 pieces	170	15	0
Sandwich Double Decker	1	370	30	1
Slim-A-Bear 98% Fat Free Sandwich Vanilla	1	130	5	3
Slim-A-Bear No Sugar Added Cone Vanilla	1	270	5	4
Slim-A-Bear No Sugar Added Fudge Bar	1	90	5	4
Slim-A-Bear No Sugar Added Reduced Fat Bar Vanilla	1	160	5	4
Slim-A-Bear No Sugar Added Sandwich Vanilla	1	120	5	2
Sundae Cup	1	280	35	tr
M&M's				
Cone	1 (2.8 oz)	250	20	1
Sandwich	1 (3 oz)	260	30	0
Vanilla Fudge	½ cup	180	15	0
Nestle Crunch				
Chocolate	1 bar (3 oz)	200	15	0
Crunch King	1 (4 oz)	270	20	0
Nuggets	8 pieces	310	20	0
Reduced Fat	1 (2.5 oz)	130	5	0
Vanilla	1 (3 oz)	200	15	0
No Pudge!				
Giant Chocolate Eclair Low Fat	1	110	<5	4

FOOD	PORTION	CALS	CHOL	FIBER
Giant Cone Chocolate No Sugar Added	1	110	<5	6
Giant Cone Cookies & Cream Low Fat	1	140	<5	3
Giant Cone Fudgy Brownie Low Fat	1	140	<5	4
Giant Cone Vanilla No Sugar Added	1	110	<5	5
Giant Cookie & Cream Low Fat No Sugar Added	1	100	<5	6
Giant Fudgy Fat Free No Sugar Added	1	60	0	6
Giant Sandwich Brownie Batter Low Fat	1	140	<5	3
Giant Sandwich Brownie Chunk Low Fat	1	140	<5	4
Giant Sandwich Vanilla & Chocolate No Sugar Added	1	130	<5	6
Giant Strawberry Shortcake 98% Fat Free	1	90	<5	4
Popsicle				
Bar Snoopy	1 (3.5 oz)	150	15	0
Bar Sprinklers	1 (2.1 oz)	130	10	0
Cone Crispy	1 (2.5 oz)	150	5	0
Creamsicle Pop	1 (1.75 oz)	70	5	0
Cup Cookies & Cream	1 (10 oz)	310	30	1
Fruit Juicee Cups	1 (4 oz)	80	0	–
Ice Cream Bar Vanilla	1 (3 oz)	160	15	1
Ice Cream Pops Minis	2 (2.8 oz)	190	15	0
Sandwich Cookie Rugrats	1 (2.5 oz)	140	10	tr
Sandwiches MInis	1 (2 oz)	100	5	0
Scribblers Ice Cream Pops	2 (2.4 oz)	130	15	0
Swirl Bar Bubble Gum	1 (2.6 oz)	60	0	–
WWE Bar	1 (3.6 oz)	180	10	tr
X-Men Wolverine Bar	1 (4 oz)	100	0	–
Rice Dream				
Bar Vanilla Nutty	1 (3.3 oz)	320	0	2
Bar Vanilla w/ Chocolate Coating	1 (3 oz)	230	0	tr

FOOD	PORTION	CALS	CHOL	FIBER
Carob Almond	½ cup	180	0	2
Frozen Pie Chocolate	1 (3.4 oz)	330	0	2
Mint Carob Chip	½ cup	170	0	0
Strawberry	½ cup	160	0	2
Silhouette				
The Skinny Cow Low Fat Ice Cream Sandwich Vanilla	1	130	0	2
Skinny Cow				
Sandwich Low Fat	1 (2.5 oz)	140	1	3
Slim-Fast				
Chocolate Fudge Bar	1	110	10	tr
Ice Cream Sandwich Chocolate	1	130	<5	tr
Ice Cream Sandwich Vanilla	1	130	<5	tr
Soy Dream				
Butter Pecan	½ cup	140	0	tr
Sandwich Lil' Dreamers Chocolate	1 (1.4 oz)	100	0	tr
Vanilla	½ cup	140	0	tr
Starbucks				
Caramel Cappuccino Swirl	½ cup	240	65	0
Classic Coffee	½ cup	230	65	0
Coffee Almond Fudge	½ cup	250	60	1
Frappuccino Bar Java Fudge	1	130	5	4
Frappuccino Bar Mocha	1	120	10	3
Java Chip	½ cup	250	60	0
Low Fat Latte	½ cup	170	10	0
Mud Pie	½ cup	240	55	1
White Chocolate Latte	½ cup	280	60	0
Tofutti				
Cuties Chocolate	1 (1.4 oz)	130	0	0
Cuties Vanilla	1 (1.4 oz)	120	0	0
Turkey Hill				
Black Cherry	½ cup	140	25	0
Black Raspberry	½ cup	140	30	–
Butter Pecan	½ cup	170	30	0
Carb IQ Vanilla Bean	½ cup	110	30	5
Chocolate Marshmallow	½ cup	160	30	–
Chocolate Mint Chip	½ cup	180	30	–
Chocolate Peanut Butter Cup	½ cup	180	30	–

FOOD	PORTION	CALS	CHOL	FIBER
Colombian Coffee	½ cup	140	30	–
Cookies 'N Cream	½ cup	160	30	0
Death By Chocolate	½ cup	160	30	–
Dutch Chocolate	½ cup	150	30	–
Egg Nog	½ cup	150	45	–
Fat Free No Sugar Added Caramel Fudge Decadence	½ cup	100	0	–
Fat Free No Sugar Added Cherry Vanilla Fudge	½ cup	90	0	–
Fat Free No Sugar Added Dutch Chocolate	½ cup	90	0	–
Fat Free No Sugar Added Vanilla Bean	½ cup	90	0	–
Fudge Ripple	½ cup	140	30	–
Light Butter Pecan	½ cup	130	15	0
Light Choco Mint Chip	½ cup	140	15	0
Light Tin Lizzie Sundae	½ cup	140	10	–
Light Vanilla & Chocolate	½ cup	110	15	0
Light Vanilla Bean	½ cup	110	15	0
Neapolitan	½ cup	150	30	0
Orange Swirl	½ cup	140	20	–
Original Vanilla	½ cup	140	30	–
Peanut Butter Ripple	½ cup	170	30	–
Philadelphia Style Butter Almond	½ cup	180	35	–
Philadelphia Style Chocolate	½ cup	170	35	–
Philadelphia Style Mint Chocolate Chip	½ cup	180	35	–
Philadelphia Style Sweet Cherry Vanilla	½ cup	160	30	–
Philadelphia Style Vanilla Bean	½ cup	170	35	–
Rocky Road	½ cup	170	30	0
Rum Raisin	½ cup	150	30	–
Sandwich Choco Mint Chip	1	200	25	–
Sandwich Vanilla	1	190	25	–
Strawberries 'N Cream	½ cup	140	25	–
Sundae Cones Rocky Road	1	340	25	–
Sundae Cones Tin Roof Sundae	1	290	25	–

FOOD	PORTION	CALS	CHOL	FIBER
Tin Roof Sundae	½ cup	160	30	0
Vanilla & Chocolate	½ cup	150	30	0
Vanilla Bean	½ cup	140	30	0
Twix				
Ice Cream	½ cup	160	20	0
Ice Cream Bar	1 (1.6 oz)	170	10	0
Weight Watchers				
English Toffee Crunch	1	110	<5	2
Smart Ones Giant Sundae	1 serv (8 oz)	150	5	7
TAKE-OUT				
cone vanilla light soft serve	1 (4.6 oz)	164	28	–
gelato chocolate hazelnut	½ cup (5.3 oz)	370	92	2
gelato vanilla	½ cup (3 oz)	211	151	0
sundae caramel	1 (5.4 oz)	303	25	–
sundae hot fudge	1 (5.4 oz)	284	21	–
sundae strawberry	1 (5.4 oz)	269	21	–

ICE CREAM CONES AND CUPS

wafer cone	1	17	0	tr
waffle cone	1 lg	121	0	1
Frookie				
Chocolate Crunch	1 (0.4 oz)	50	0	tr
Honey Crunch	1 (0.4 oz)	45	0	tr
Keebler				
Chocolatey Cone	1 (0.4 oz)	50	0	0
Ice Creme Cup	1 (0.2 oz)	15	0	0
Sugar Cone	1 (0.4 oz)	50	0	0
Waffle Cone	1 (0.4 oz)	50	0	0

ICE CREAM TOPPINGS

marshmallow cream	1 jar (7 oz)	615	0	–
marshmallow cream	1 oz	88	0	–
nuts in syrup	2 tbsp	184	0	1
pineapple	2 tbsp (1.5 oz)	106	0	–
pineapple	1 cup (11.5 oz)	861	0	–
strawberry	1 cup (11.5 oz)	863	0	–
strawberry	2 tbsp (1.5 oz)	107	0	–
Colac				
Passion Fruit	1 tbsp	31	0	0
Strawberry	1 tbsp	31	0	0

FOOD	PORTION	CALS	CHOL	FIBER
Hershey's				
Chocolate Shoppe Caramel	2 tbsp	100	0	–
Chocolate Shoppe Double Chocolate	1 tbsp	60	0	–
Chocolate Shoppe Hot Fudge	1 tbsp	70	<5	–
Chocolate Shoppe Hot Fudge Fat Free	2 tbsp	100	0	–
Sprinkles Candy Coated Milk Chocolate	1 tbsp	70	<5	–
Lollipop Tree				
Hot Fudge Sauce	1 tbsp	80	15	tr
Maple Walnut Cream	2 tbsp	190	30	0
Reese's				
Sprinkles Peanut Butter & Milk Chocolate	1 tbsp	70	0	–
Sanders				
Butterscotch Caramel	2 tbsp	90	10	0
Smucker's				
Butterscotch Caramel	2 tbsp	130	<5	tr
Dove Dark Chocolate	2 tbsp	140	0	1
Dove Milk Chocolate	2 tbsp	130	0	1
Dulce De Leche Milk Caramel Spread	2 tbsp	110	10	–
Hot Fudge	2 tbsp	140	0	tr
Hot Fudge Sugar Free Fat Free	2 tbsp	90	0	1
Magic Shell Caramel	2 tbsp	220	5	0
Magic Shell Chocolate	2 tbsp	210	0	1
Magic Shell Chocolate Fudge	2 tbsp	120	0	1
Magic Shell Turtle Delight	2 tbsp	210	0	1
Magic Shell Twix	2 tbsp	210	0	1
Steel's				
Sugar Free Butterscotch	2 tbsp	60	0	0
Sugar Free Chocolate Fudge	2 tbsp	45	10	2
Sugar Free Hot Fudge	2 tbsp	65	0	1
Sugar Free Peanut Butter Fudge	2 tbsp	75	7	2

FOOD	PORTION	CALS	CHOL	FIBER
ICED TEA				
MIX				
A La Source				
Organic as prep	8 oz	90	0	–
Organic Green Tea as prep	8 oz	90	0	–
Organic Herbal Tea Red Rooibos	8 oz	80	0	–
Atkins				
Sugar Free Lemon not prep	2 tbsp	0	0	0
Carb Options				
Lemon as prep	1 serv	0	0	0
Celestial Seasonings				
Blueberry Ice	1 cup	0	0	0
Crystal Light				
On The Go All Flavors as prep	1 serv	5	0	0
Sugar Free All Flavors as prep	1 serv	5	0	0
Lipton				
Chailatta Chocolate as prep	8 oz	120	<5	–
Chailatta Hazelnut as prep	8 oz	120	<5	–
Chailatta Original as prep	8 oz	120	<5	–
Chailatta Vanilla as prep	8 oz	120	<5	–
Decaffeinated Lemon Unsweetened as prep	1 serv	0	0	–
Decaffeinated Lemon as prep	1 serv	70	0	–
Diet Lemon as prep	1 serv	5	0	–
Diet Peach as prep	1 serv	5	0	–
Diet Raspberry as prep	1 serv	5	0	–
Green Tea as prep	1 serv	70	0	–
Lemon Sweetened as prep	1 serv	70	0	–
Sweetened All Fruit Flavors as prep	1 serv	80	0	–
To Go w/ Honey & Lemon	1 pkg	0	0	–
To Go w/ Lemon	1 pkg	0	0	–
To Go w/ Mandarin & Mango	1 pkg	0	0	–
Unsweetened as prep	1 serv	0	0	–
Nestea				
100% Tea	2 tsp (1 g)	0	0	0
100% Tea Decafe	2 tsp (1 g)	0	0	0

FOOD	PORTION	CALS	CHOL	FIBER
Ice Teasers Lemon	1 serv (0.5 oz)	5	0	0
Ice Teasers Orange	1 serv (0.5 oz)	5	0	0
Ice Teasers Wild Cherry	1 serv (0.5 oz)	5	0	0
Lemon	2 tsp (1 g)	5	0	0
Lemon & Sugar	2 tbsp (0.7 oz)	80	0	0
Lemonade Tea	2 tbsp (0.7 oz)	80	0	0
Sugar Free	2 tbsp (0.7 oz)	5	0	0
Sugar Free Decafe	1 tbsp (0.7 oz)	5	0	0
Sun Tea	1 tsp (1 g)	0	0	0
READY-TO-DRINK				
Anteadote				
All Flavors	8 oz	0	0	0
Apple & Eve				
Lemon Fruit	8 oz	100	0	–
Peach Fruit	8 oz	100	0	–
Raspberry Fruit	8 oz	100	0	–
Tangerine Fruit	8 oz	100	0	–
Arizona				
Green Tea w/ Ginseng & Honey	8 oz	70	0	0
Lemon	8 oz	90	0	0
Bolthouse Farms				
Perfectly Protein Vanilla Chai Tea	8 oz	160	0	0
Brazil Gourmet				
Nectar Tea All Flavors	8 oz	90	0	0
Nectar Tea Light Mango Passion	8 oz	60	0	0
C+Swiss				
Hemp Ice Tea	1 can (8.4 oz)	90	0	–
Crystal Light				
Sugar Free Lemon	8 oz	5	0	0
Delta Blues				
Spearmint Tea Punch	8 oz	90	0	0
Enviga				
All Flavors	1 can (12 oz)	5	0	0
Fuze				
LemonAID	8 oz	70	0	–
Slender Energy All Flavors	8 oz	20	0	–

FOOD	PORTION	CALS	CHOL	FIBER
Vitamin Tea Diet Peach	8 oz	5	0	0
Vitamin Tea Green Tea w/ Ginseng	8 oz	60	0	–
Vitamin Tea Lemon	8 oz	70	0	–
White Tea	8 oz	60	0	–
White Tea No Carb Diet Pomegranate	8 oz	0	0	0
Glaceau Vitamin Water				
Vital-T	8 oz	50	0	–
Hansen's				
Chai	8 oz	150	0	–
China Black	8 oz	90	0	–
Green	8 oz	70	0	–
Green Diet Lemon	8 oz	0	0	–
Green Diet Peach	8 oz	0	0	–
Green Lemon	8 oz	70	0	–
Green Peach	8 oz	70	0	–
Oolong	8 oz	70	0	–
Spice	8 oz	90	0	–
Hawaiian				
Iced Tea	1 can	120	0	0
Honest Tea				
Assam	8 oz	17	0	–
Black Forest Berry	8 oz	25	0	–
Gold Rush	8 oz	9	0	–
Green Dragon	8 oz	30	0	–
Kashmiri Chai	8 oz	17	0	–
Lori's Lemon	8 oz	30	0	–
Moroccan Mint	8 oz	17	0	–
Peach Oo-La-Long	8 oz	30	0	–
Hood				
Iced Tea	1 cup	100	0	0
Inko's				
White Tea All Flavors	1 bottle (16 oz)	56	0	–
White Tea Honeysuckle	1 bottle	0	0	–
Joe Tea				
All Flavors	8 oz	100	0	–
Kalahari				
Rooibos Red Tea All Flavors	8 oz	50	0	–

FOOD	PORTION	CALS	CHOL	FIBER
Kombucha				
Wonder Drink Asian Pear Ginger	1 bottle (8.5 oz)	60	0	–
Wonder Drink Rooibus Red Peach	1 bottle (8.5 oz)	60	0	–
Lipton				
Diet Green Tea w/ Citrus	8 oz	0	0	–
Diet Lemon	8 oz	0	0	–
Diet Sweet	8 oz	0	0	–
Extra Sweet	8 oz	100	0	–
Green Tea w/ Citrus	8 oz	80	0	–
Green Tea w/ Honey	8 oz	70	0	–
Lemon	8 oz	90	0	–
Original Unsweetened	8 oz	0	0	–
Orignal Sweetened	8 oz	70	0	–
Peach	8 oz	110	0	–
Raspberry	8 oz	110	0	–
Nantucket Nectars				
Diet	8 oz	5	0	–
Diet Green Tea	8 oz	5	0	–
Half & Half	8 oz	90	0	–
Iced Tea	8 oz	80	0	–
Matt Fee	8 oz	80	0	–
Raspberry	8 oz	90	0	–
Savannah	8 oz	80	0	–
New Leaf				
All Flavors	8 oz	75	0	–
Pacific Foods				
Organic Lemon	8 oz	70	0	0
Organic Peach	8 oz	70	0	0
Organic Raspberry	8 oz	70	0	0
Organic Sweetened Black Tea	8 oz	60	0	0
Organic Unsweetened Green Tea	8 oz	0	0	0
Republic Of Tea				
No Carb Unsweetened All Flavors	1 bottle (12 oz)	0	0	0
Snapple				
Diet Lemonade Ice Tea	8 oz	10	0	–

FOOD	PORTION	CALS	CHOL	FIBER
Diet Lime Green Tea	8 oz	0	0	–
Just Plain Tea	8 oz	0	0	–
Lemonade Ice Tea	8 oz	110	0	–
Lime Green Tea	8 oz	100	0	–
Mint	8 oz	110	0	–
Peach	8 oz	100	0	–
Raspberry	8 oz	100	0	–
Very Cherry	8 oz	100	0	–
SoBe				
Lean Diet Green Tea	8 oz	0	0	–
Lean Diet Peach Tea	8 oz	5	0	–
Lemon	8 oz	90	0	–
Solebury Home				
Organic All Flavors	8 oz	33	0	–
Soy20				
Lemon Green Tea	1 bottle (12 oz)	90	0	–
Sri Lankan				
Apple	8 oz	70	0	0
Lemon	8 oz	60	0	0
Sweet Leaf Tea				
Diet Sweet	8 oz	0	0	–
Hibiscus Herbal	8 oz	25	0	–
Lemon & Lime	8 oz	0	0	–
Mint & Honey Green	8 oz	60	0	–
Peach	8 oz	75	0	–
Raspberry & Tangerine	8 oz	75	0	–
Sweet Tea	8 oz	75	0	–
T42				
A Classic Earl Grey	8 oz	60	0	–
Herbal All Flavors	8 oz	70	0	–
Jamaican Ginger Green Tea	8 oz	70	0	–
Lemon And Honey Green Tea	8 oz	60	0	–
Wake-Up Blend English Breakfast	8 oz	45	0	–
With Lemon	8 oz	60	0	–
Tao Tea				
Grapefruit Green Tea	8 oz	71	0	–
Lemon Green Tea	8 oz	67	0	–

FOOD	PORTION	CALS	CHOL	FIBER
Tradewinds				
Diet Green Tea	8 oz	0	0	0
Diet Raspberry	8 oz	0	0	0
Mango Green Tea	8 oz	80	0	–
Turkey Hill				
Blueberry Oolong w/ Vitamins C & E	1 cup	100	0	–
Decaffeinated	1 cup	80	0	–
Decaffeinated Orange	1 cup	10	0	–
Diet	1 cup	0	0	–
Diet Decaffeinated	1 cup	0	0	–
Diet Green Tea w/ Ginseng & Honey	1 cup	5	0	–
Green Tea w/ Ginseng & Honey	1 cup	70	0	–
Lemon	1 cup	100	0	–
Mint Tea w/ Chamomile	1 cup	90	0	–
Oolong w/ Ginkgo Biloba & Ginseng	1 cup	100	0	–
Orange	1 cup	100	0	–
Peach	1 cup	110	0	–
Raspberry Tea	1 cup	110	0	–
Regular	1 cup	90	0	–
XS Energy				
Energy Tea Berry Typhoon	1 can (8.4 oz)	12	0	–

ICES AND ICE POPS
Blue Bunny

FOOD	PORTION	CALS	CHOL	FIBER
Bar Big Fudge	1 (2.7 oz)	110	5	0
Chill Cups Double Lemon	1 (4 oz)	100	0	0
FrozFruit Creamy Coconut	1 (3 oz)	150	25	tr
Frozfruit Strawberries & Cream	1 (4 oz)	190	20	tr
Pop Banana	1 (1.9 oz)	35	0	0
Pop Jolly Rancher	1 (4 oz)	120	0	0
Pop Root Beer	1 (1.9 oz)	40	0	0
The Original Bomb	1 (1.8 oz)	50	0	0
Breyers				
Fruit Bars No Sugar Added	1 (1.75 oz)	25	0	0
Juice Bar Strawberry	1 (3.75 oz)	120	0	tr

FOOD	PORTION	CALS	CHOL	FIBER
Soft Frozen Cup Lemonade	1 pkg (12 oz)	290	0	–
Soft Frozen Cup Strawberry	1 pkg (12 oz)	260	0	–
Carnation				
Cup Orange Sherbet	1 (5 oz)	150	5	0
Cup Orange Sherbet	1 (3 oz)	90	5	0
Cold Fusion				
Protein Juice Bar All Flavors	1 (3.8 oz)	130	0	0
Cool Creations				
Ice Pop	1 pop (2 oz)	50	0	0
Mickey Mouse Bar	1 (4 oz)	170	15	0
Surprise Pops	1 (2 oz)	60	0	0
CoolFruits				
Fruite Juice Freezer Pops Grape & Cherry	3 (3 oz)	70	0	0
Dole				
Fruit'n Juice Coconut	1 (4 oz)	210	10	0
Fruit'n Juice Lemonade	1 (4 oz)	120	0	0
Fruit'n Juice Lime	1 (4 oz)	110	0	0
Fruit'n Juice Peach Passion	1 (2.5 oz)	70	0	0
Fruit'n Juice Pineapple Coconut	1 (4 oz)	150	0	0
Fruit'n Juice Pineapple Orange Banana	1 (4 oz)	110	0	0
Fruit'n Juice Pineapple Orange Banana	1 (2.5 oz)	70	0	0
Fruit'n Juice Raspberry	1 (2.5 oz)	70	0	0
Fruit'n Juice Strawberry	1 (4 oz)	110	0	0
Fruit'n Juice Strawberry	1 (2.5 oz)	70	0	0
Grape No Sugar Added	1 (1.75 oz)	25	0	0
Raspberry	1 (1.75 oz)	45	0	0
Raspberry No Sugar Added	1 (1.75 oz)	25	0	0
Strawberry	1 (1.75 oz)	45	0	0
Strawberry No Sugar Added	1 (1.75 oz)	25	0	0
Edy's				
Sherbet Berry Rainbow	½ cup	130	5	–
Sherbet Key Lime	½ cup	130	0	–
Sherbet Orange Cream	½ cup	120	10	–
Sherbet Raspberry	½ cup	130	4	–
Sherbet Swiss Orange	½ cup	150	5	–
Sherbet Tropical Rainbow	½ cup	130	0	–

FOOD	PORTION	CALS	CHOL	FIBER
Whole Fruit Creamy Coconut	1	120	0	–
Whole Fruit Lemonade	1	80	0	–
Whole Fruit Lime	1	80	0	–
Whole Fruit Orange & Cream	1	80	5	–
Whole Fruit Peach	½ cup	90	0	–
Whole Fruit Strawberry	1	80	0	–
Whole Fruit Tangerine	1	80	0	–
Whole Fruit Tropical	1	100	0	–
Whole Fruit Wild Berry	1	80	0	–
Flintstones				
Push-Up Sherbet Treats	1 (2.75 oz)	100	5	0
Good Humor				
Great White	1 (3 oz)	70	0	–
Hyper Stripe	1 (2.7 oz)	80	0	–
Haagen-Dazs				
Sorbet Chocolate	½ cup	120	0	2
Sorbet Mango	½ cup	120	0	tr
Sorbet Orange	½ cup	120	0	tr
Sorbet Orchard Peach	½ cup	130	0	tr
Sorbet Raspberry	½ cup	120	0	2
Sorbet Strawberry	½ cup	120	0	1
Sorbet Zesty Lemon	½ cup	120	0	tr
Sorbet Bars Chocolate	1 (2.7 oz)	80	0	1
Sorbet Bars Orange	1 (2.5 oz)	120	35	0
Sorbet Bars Raspberry & Vanilla Yogurt	1 (2.5 oz)	90	0	tr
Sorbet Bars Strawberry & Vanilla Ice Cream	1 (2.5 oz)	110	35	0
Hawaiian Punch				
Artic Surfers	1	50	0	0
Hendrie's				
Citrus N' Berry Stix	1 (1.9 oz)	15	0	0
Fudge Stix Fat Free	1 (1.8 oz)	70	0	0
Hood				
Hoodsie Pop	1 (3.3 oz)	60	0	0
Minute Maid				
Fruit And Cream Swirl	1 tube (3 oz)	90	10	–
Fruit Bars	1	60	0	–

FOOD	PORTION	CALS	CHOL	FIBER
Natural Choice				
Organic Banana	½ cup (3.6 oz)	110	0	tr
Organic Blueberry	½ cup (3.6 oz)	100	0	tr
Organic Kiwi	½ cup (3.6 oz)	110	0	tr
Organic Lemon	½ cup (3.6 oz)	110	0	tr
Organic Mango	½ cup (3.6 oz)	110	0	tr
Organic Strawberry	½ cup (3.6 oz)	110	0	tr
Organic Strawberry Kiwi	½ cup (3.6 oz)	110	0	tr
Popsicle				
All Natural Ice Pops	1 (1.75 oz)	50	0	–
Bar Dora The Explorer	1 (4 oz)	100	0	–
Bar Fruti Holanda Lemon Lime	1 (3 oz)	90	0	–
Bar Fruti Holanda Strawberry	1 (3 oz)	90	0	–
Bar Incredible Hulk	1 (4 oz)	100	0	–
Bar Jimmy Neutron	1 (4 oz)	100	0	–
Bar Mega Warheads	1 (4 oz)	110	0	0
Bar Power Ranger	1 (4 oz)	100	0	–
Bar Spider Man	1 (4 oz)	100	0	–
Bar SpongeBob	1 (4 oz)	100	0	–
Big Stick Pops Big Reds	1 (3.5 oz)	70	0	–
Big Stick Pops Cherry Pineapple	1 (3.5 oz)	50	0	0
Bubble Play	1 (4 oz)	100	0	–
Creamsicle Bar	1 (2.5 oz)	100	5	0
Creamsicle Bar Sugar Free	2 (3.3 oz)	40	0	6
Creamsicle Pop No Sugar Added	1 (1.75 oz)	25	0	0
Cup Cherry	1 (12 oz)	240	0	–
Cup Frostee Fudge	1 (10 oz)	280	35	2
Cup Lemon	1 (12 oz)	230	0	–
Cup Screwball	1 (3.75 oz)	110	0	–
Firecracker	1 (1.6 oz)	35	0	–
Fudgsicle Bar	1 (2.5 oz)	90	5	tr
Fudgsicle Bar Fat Free	1 (1.75 oz)	60	0	tr
Fudgsicle Pop	1 (1.75 oz)	60	5	tr
Fudgsicle Pop No Sugar Added	2 (1.75 oz)	90	0	1
Minis Fudge Bar	2 (2.4 oz)	80	0	tr

FOOD	PORTION	CALS	CHOL	FIBER
Pop Great White	1 (1.75 oz)	45	0	–
Pop Lick-A-Color	1 (2 oz)	50	0	–
Pop Sherbet Cyclone	1 (1.8 oz)	50	0	0
Pop Towering Tornado	1 (3.5 oz)	90	0	–
Pop Ups Orange Burst	1 (2.75 oz)	80	<5	0
Pop Ups Reckless Rainbow	1 (2.75 oz)	90	<5	0
Pop Ups SpongeBob	1 (2.75 oz)	90	5	0
Pops Tropical Sugar Free	1 (1.75 oz)	15	0	–
Pops Wild Bunch	2 (2.2 oz)	60	0	–
Rainbow Floats	1 (1.75 oz)	60	5	0
Rainbow Pops	1 (1.75 oz)	45	0	–
Scribblers Juice Pops	2 (2.4 oz)	60	0	–
Snow Cone	1 (7 oz)	30	0	–
Sugar Free Pops Orange Cherry Grape	1 (1.75 oz)	15	0	–
Super Mario Bros Bar	1 (4 oz)	100	0	–
Swirl Bar Cotton Candy	1 (2.6 oz)	60	0	–
Tingle Twister Ice Pops	1 (1.75 oz)	45	0	–
Torpedo Pop Cherry	1 (1.75 oz)	35	0	–
Silhouette				
Fat Free Fudge Bars	1	90	0	–
Tropicana				
Fruit Juice Bar Orange	1	45	0	0
Fruit Juice Bar Raspberry	1	45	0	0
Strawberry	1	45	0	0
Wawona				
Peach	1	78	0	1
Strawberry	1	77	0	1

JACKFRUIT

fresh	3.5 oz	70	0	–

JALAPENO (see PEPPERS)

JAM/JELLY/PRESERVE

all flavors jam	1 tbsp (0.7 oz)	48	0	tr
all flavors jelly	1 tbsp (0.7 oz)	52	0	tr
all flavors preserve	1 pkg (0.5 oz)	34	0	tr
all flavors preserve	1 tbsp (0.7 oz)	48	0	tr
apple butter	1 tbsp (0.6 oz)	33	0	–
orange marmalade	1 pkg (0.5 oz)	34	0	–

FOOD	PORTION	CALS	CHOL	FIBER
orange marmalade	1 tbsp (0.7 oz)	49	0	–
strawberry jam	1 tbsp (0.7 oz)	48	0	tr
Colac				
Jelly All Flavors	1 tbsp	37	0	0
Eden				
Organic Apple Butter	1 tbsp	20	0	1
Organic Butter Apple Cherry	1 tbsp	25	0	tr
Organic Cherry Butter	1 tbsp	35	0	1
El Angel				
Strawberry Marmelade	1 tbsp	25	0	0
Jok'n'Al				
Low Carb Fruit Spreads All Flavors	1 tbsp	10	0	0
Lollipop Tree				
Butter Cranberry Pear	1 tbsp	25	0	–
Butter Pumpkin Maple Pecan	1 tbsp	30	0	tr
Jam Raspberry Peach	1 tbsp	50	0	–
Jam Triple Cherry	1 tbsp	50	0	–
Jelly Hot Pepper	1 tbsp	60	0	–
Jelly Wasabi Lime Pepper	1 tbsp	60	0	0
Matouk's				
Guava Jam	1 tbsp	50	0	–
Mango Jam	1 tbsp	50	0	–
Polaner				
All Fruit Apricot	1 tbsp	40	0	–
All Fruit Grape	1 tbsp	40	0	–
All Fruit Pineapple	1 tbsp	40	0	–
All Fruit Raspberry Seedless	1 tbsp	40	0	–
Sarabeth's				
Spreadable Fruit Orange Apricot	1 tbsp	30	0	–
Spreadable Fruit Peach Apricot	1 tbsp	40	0	1
Spreadable Fruit Strawberry Raspberry	1 tbsp	40	0	tr
Smucker's				
Cider Apple Butter	1 tbsp	45	0	–
Jam Concord Grape	1 tbsp	50	0	–
Jam Red Plum	1 tbsp	50	0	–
Jam Seedless Red Raspberry	1 tbsp	50	0	–

FOOD	PORTION	CALS	CHOL	FIBER
Jam Seedless Strawberry	1 tbsp	50	0	–
Jelly Apple	2 tbsp	50	0	–
Jelly Concord Grape	1 tbsp	50	0	–
Jelly Currant	1 tbsp	50	0	–
Jelly Guava	1 tbsp	50	0	–
Low Sugar All Flavors	1 tbsp	25	0	–
Preserves All Flavors	1 tbsp	50	0	–
Simply Fruit All Flavors	1 tbsp	40	0	–
Sugar Free All Flavors	1 tbsp	10	0	–
Welch's				
Grape Jam	1 tbsp	50	0	–
Wild Thyme Farms				
Fruit Spreads Blackberry Currant Ginger	1 tsp	8	0	–
Fruit Spreads Mango Apricot	1 tsp	7	0	–

JAPANESE FOOD (see ASIAN FOOD, SUSHI)

JELLY (see JAM/JELLY/PRESERVE)

JICAMA

fresh	1 sm (12.8 oz)	139	0	18
raw sliced	1 cup	46	0	6
Frieda's				
Jicama	¾ cup	35	0	1

JUJUBE

dried	1 oz	82	0	–

JUTE

cooked	1 cup	32	0	2

KALE

chopped cooked w/o salt	1 cup	36	0	3
fresh cooked w/ fat	1 cup	69	0	2
Glory				
Fresh Greens	1 serv (2.8 oz)	40	0	2
Seasoned canned	½ cup	35	0	1

KANGAROO

kangaroo	3 oz	120	56	–

KEFIR

kefir	8 oz	98	10	0

FOOD	PORTION	CALS	CHOL	FIBER
KETCHUP				
banana	1 tsp	10	0	0
ketchup	1 tbsp	15	0	0
ketchup	1 pkg (0.2 oz)	6	0	tr
low sodium	1 tbsp	15	0	0
Atkins				
Ketch-A-Tomato	1 tbsp	10	0	1
Del Monte				
Ketchup	1 tbsp	15	0	0
Estee				
No Sugar Added	1 tbsp	15	0	0
Healthy Choice				
Ketchup	1 tbsp (0.5 oz)	9	0	tr
Heinz				
Ketchup	1 tbsp	15	0	0
No Salt	1 tbsp	20	0	0
One Carb	1 tbsp	5	0	0
Organic	1 tbsp	20	0	0
Hunt's				
Ketchup	1 tbsp	15	0	0
No Salt Added	1 tbsp	20	0	0
Squeeze	1 tbsp	15	0	0
Keto				
Ketchup	1 tbsp	4	0	0
Muir Glen				
Organic	1 tbsp (0.6 oz)	15	0	0
Steel's				
Sugar Free	1 tbsp	10	0	0
Stokelys				
Tomato	1 tbsp	15	0	–
Tree of Life				
Ketchup	1 tbsp (0.5 oz)	10	0	–
Walden Farms				
Calorie Free	1 tbsp	0	0	0
KIDNEY				
beef simmered	3 oz	134	609	0
lamb braised	3 oz	116	480	0

FOOD	PORTION	CALS	CHOL	FIBER
pork braised	3 oz	128	408	0
veal braised	3 oz	139	672	0
KIDNEY BEANS				
canned	½ cup	108	0	6
dried cooked w/o salt	½ cup	112	0	6
Bush's				
Light Red	½ cup	110	0	7
Eden				
Chili Beans	½ cup	130	0	7
Organic	½ cup	100	0	10
Organic Cannellini	½ cup	100	0	5
Goya				
Dark	½ cup	90	0	7
Hunt's				
Kidney Beans	½ cup (4.5 oz)	94	0	5
Progresso				
Dark Red	½ cup (4.5 oz)	110	0	6
Red	½ cup	110	0	6
Rienzi				
Cannellini	½ cup	80	0	7
Red	½ cup	90	0	7
S&W				
Dark Red Premium	½ cup (4.6 oz)	100	0	6
Van Camp's				
Dark Red	½ cup (4.6 oz)	90	0	6
Light Red	½ cup (4.6 oz)	90	0	6
KIWI				
fresh	1 med (2.6 oz)	46	0	2
fresh	1 lg (3.2 oz)	56	0	3
Chiquita				
Fresh	2 med (5.2 oz)	100	0	4
Zespri				
Gold	2 med	80	0	2
Green	2 med	100	0	4
KIWI JUICE				
Auna				
Kiwifruit Juice	1 bottle (12 oz)	120	0	4

FOOD	PORTION	CALS	CHOL	FIBER
KNISH				
Gabila's				
Potato	1 (4.5 oz)	170	0	5
TAKE-OUT				
cheese	1 (2.1 oz)	205	56	1
meat	1 (1.8 oz)	174	53	1
potato	1 (2.1 oz)	212	59	1
potato	1 lg (7 oz)	332	72	1
KOHLRABI				
raw sliced	1 cup	36	0	4
sliced cooked w/o salt	1 cup	48	0	2
Frieda's				
Kohlrabi	⅔ cup	25	0	3
TAKE-OUT				
creamed	1 cup	150	6	1
KUMQUATS				
canned in syrup	1	13	0	1
fresh	1	13	0	1
KUZU				
Eden				
Root Starch	1 tbsp	30	0	–
LAMB				
cubed lean & fat braised	4 oz	253	122	0
cubed lean & fat broiled	4 oz	211	102	0
ground broiled	4 oz	321	110	0
leg roasted	4 oz	213	74	0
loin chop lean & fat broiled	1 chop (4 oz)	222	72	0
rib chop lean & fat broiled	1 chop (1.6 oz)	165	46	0
rib roast baked	4 oz	386	109	0
shank lean & fat braised	4 oz	360	157	0
shoulder chop lean & fat cooked	1 chop (5.5 oz)	274	91	0
shoulder w/ bone braised	4 oz	231	77	0
LAMB DISHES				
TAKE-OUT				
lamb curry	1 cup	257	90	1
moroccan pilaf w/ bulgur	1 serv	327	54	–

FOOD	PORTION	CALS	CHOL	FIBER
moussaka	4 in sq (16 oz)	659	96	8
stew w/ potatoes & vegetables	1 cup	260	58	4

LAMBSQUARTERS
chopped cooked w/ salt	1 cup	58	0	4

LEEKS
chopped cooked w/o salt	¼ cup	8	0	tr
cooked	1 (4.4 oz)	38	0	1
freeze dried	1 tbsp	1	0	0
Frieda's				
Fresh	1 cup	50	0	2

LEMON
fresh	1 med (4 oz)	22	0	5
peel	1 tsp	1	0	tr
peel	1 tbsp	3	0	1
wedge	1 (7 g)	2	0	tr
Sunkist				
Fresh	1 (2 oz)	15	0	tr
True Lemon				
Crystallized Lemon	1 pkg (1 g)	0	0	–

LEMON CURD
Lollipop Tree				
Lemon Curd	1 tbsp	50	20	–

LEMON EXTRACT
lemon extract	½ tsp	12	0	0
Virginia Dare				
Extract	1 tsp	22	0	–

LEMON JUICE
bottled	1 tbsp	3	0	tr
bottled	1 oz	6	0	tr
fresh	1 oz	8	0	tr
from 1 lemon	1.6 oz	12	0	tr
from wedge	6 g	1	0	0
Canarino				
Italian Hot Lemon Beverage	1 cup	0	0	0

FOOD	PORTION	CALS	CHOL	FIBER
Izze				
Sparkling Lemon	8 oz	150	0	–
LEMONADE				
FROZEN				
Tropicana				
Twister Light	8 oz	50	0	0
MIX				
A La Source				
Organic as prep	8 oz	110	0	–
Country Time				
Lemonade as prep	8 oz	60	0	–
Pink as prep	8 oz	60	0	–
Raspberry as prep	8 oz	80	0	–
Strawberry as prep	8 oz	80	0	–
Crystal Light				
Lemonade as prep	1 serv (8 oz)	5	0	0
On The Go as prep	1 pkg	5	0	0
Pink as prep	1 serv	5	0	0
Keto				
Kooler Pink	½ tsp	0	0	0
Low Carb Creations				
Lemonade as prep	1 serv	10	0	0
Raspberry as prep	1 serv	10	0	0
Sipper Sweets				
Sugar Free Low Carb	1 serv	8	0	0
READY-TO-DRINK				
Adina				
Hibiscus Lemon Bissap	8 oz	80	0	–
Bolthouse Farms				
Mango Lemonade	8 oz	120	0	tr
Crystal Light				
Sugar Free	8 oz	5	0	0
Hansen's				
Sparkling	8 oz	100	0	–
Sparkling Pink	8 oz	120	0	–
Hi-C				
Blast Pink	8 oz	120	0	–
Honest Ade				
Cranberry	8 oz	50	0	–

FOOD	PORTION	CALS	CHOL	FIBER
Hood				
Lemonade	1 cup	110	0	0
Minute Maid				
Chilled	8 oz	100	0	–
Coolers Pink	1 pouch (7 oz)	90	0	–
Light	8 oz	15	0	–
Naked Juice				
Just Made	8 oz	110	0	0
Nantucket Nectars				
Authentic	8 oz	120	0	–
Pink	8 oz	120	0	–
Nesbitt's				
Honey	1 bottle (12 oz)	180	0	–
Newman's Own				
Pink Virgin	8 oz	110	0	–
Roadside Virgin	8 oz	110	0	–
Virgin Lemon Aided	8 oz	110	0	–
Ocean Spray				
Spritzer	8 oz	160	0	–
Odwalla				
Pure Squeezed	8 oz	96	0	0
Santa Cruz				
Organic	1 can	160	0	–
Organic Raspberry	1 can	120	0	–
Snapple				
Lemonade	8 oz	110	0	–
Super Sour	8 oz	130	0	–
T42				
Lemonade	8 oz	90	0	–
Pink	8 oz	90	0	–
Three Drinks				
Sparkling	12 oz	12	0	–
Tropicana				
Light	1 cup	10	0	0
Orchard Style	8 oz	120	0	0
Twister Strawberry	8 oz	140	0	0
Turkey Hill				
Lemonade	1 cup	120	0	–
Raspberry	1 cup	120	0	–
Strawberry Kiwi	1 cup	120	0	–

FOOD	PORTION	CALS	CHOL	FIBER
Zeigler's				
Old Fashioned	8 oz	120	0	0
LEMONGRASS				
fresh	1 tbsp	5	0	–
LENTILS				
dried cooked	1 cup	230	0	16
Eden				
Organic Green w/ Onion & Bay Leaf	½ cup	90	0	4
Near East				
Lentil Pilaf as prep	1 cup	200	9	8
Sabra				
Dardara	2 oz	40	0	1
Shiloh Farms				
Organic Green not prep	¼ cup (1.6 oz)	150	0	7
TastyBite				
Bengal Lentils	½ pkg (5 oz)	190	0	1
Jodhpur Lentils	½ pkg (5 oz)	190	0	2
Madras Lentils	½ pkg (5 oz)	130	22	5
TAKE-OUT				
indian sambar	1 serv	236	10	9
lentil loaf	1 slice (1.6 oz)	83	0	3
middle eastern lentil salad	1 serv (4.5 oz)	158	0	–
yemiser selatta ethiopian lentil salad	1 serv (3 oz)	115	0	2
LETTUCE (see also SALAD)				
arugula	6 leaves (0.4 oz)	3	0	tr
arugula shredded	1 cup	5	0	tr
boston	1 head (5.7 oz)	21	0	2
boston chopped	6 leaves	7	0	1
cornsalad field salad	1 cup (1.9 oz)	7	0	1
iceberg	6 med leaves	7	0	1
iceberg	1 lg head (26.5 oz)	106	0	9
iceberg shredded	1 cup	10	0	1
looseleaf outer leaves	6 (5 oz)	22	0	2
looseleaf shredded	1 cup	5	0	1
red leaf	6 leaves (3.6 oz)	16	0	1
red leaf shredded	1 cup	4	0	tr

FOOD	PORTION	CALS	CHOL	FIBER
romaine	3 leaves (3 oz)	14	0	2
romaine heart	6 leaves (1.3 oz)	6	0	1
romaine shredded	1 cup	8	0	1
Andy Boy				
Romaine Hearts	6 leaves (3 oz)	20	0	1
Dole				
Classic Romaine	1½ cups (3 oz)	15	0	1
Shredded	1½ cups (3 oz)	15	0	1
Earthbound Farm				
Organic Baby Romaine Salad	2 cups	15	0	1
Frieda's				
Limestone	⅔ cup	10	0	1
Green Giant				
Hearts Of Romaine	6 leaves (3 oz)	14	0	2
Mann's				
Romaine Jumbo Hearts	3 oz	15	0	1
Ocean Mist				
Romaine Hearts	6 leaves	20	0	1
Ready Pac				
Baby Arugula	4 cups	20	0	2
Bella Romaine	1½ cups	15	0	1
River Ranch				
Hearts Of Romaine	1½ cups	12	0	1
Romaine Chopped	1½ cups	10	0	1
Romaine Hearts	1½ cups	10	0	1

LIMA BEANS
CANNED

FOOD	PORTION	CALS	CHOL	FIBER
lima beans	½ cup	95	0	6
Del Monte				
Green	½ cup	80	0	4
S&W				
Small Green	½ cup (4.4 oz)	80	0	4
Van Camp's				
Butter Beans	½ cup (4.6 oz)	110	0	7
Veg-All				
Baby Green	½ cup	90	0	3
DRIED				
cooked	½ cup	150	0	5

FOOD	PORTION	CALS	CHOL	FIBER
FROZEN				
C&W				
Baby	½ cup	110	0	5
LIME				
fresh	1 (2.4 oz)	20	0	1
wedge	1 (8 g)	2	0	tr
Sunkist				
Fresh	1 (2 oz)	20	0	2
LIME JUICE				
bottled	1 oz	6	0	tr
fresh	1 oz	8	0	tr
Adina				
Lime Mint Mojita	8 oz	70	0	–
Honest Ade				
Limeade	8 oz	50	0	–
Minute Maid				
Light Limeade	8 oz	15	0	–
Newman's Own				
Virgin Limeade	8 oz	140	0	–
Odwalla				
Summertime Lime	8 oz	90	0	0
LINGCOD				
baked	3 oz	93	57	0
fillet baked	5.3 oz	164	101	–
LIQUOR/LIQUEUR (see also BEER AND ALE, CHAMPAGNE, MALT, WINE)				
7&7	1 serv	178	0	0
alabama slammer	1 serv	103	0	tr
amaretto sour	1 serv	295	0	4
angel's kiss	1 serv	85	5	0
anisette	1 oz	111	0	0
antifreeze	1 serv	177	0	tr
apricot brandy	1 oz	96	0	0
apricot sour	1 serv	164	0	tr
b 52	1 serv	247	0	0
b&b	1 serv	75	0	0
bahama breeze	1 serv	70	0	tr
bahama mama	1 serv	153	0	tr

FOOD	PORTION	CALS	CHOL	FIBER
bailey's & amaretto	1 serv	184	0	0
banana colada	1 serv	376	0	3
bay breeze	1 serv	173	0	tr
bend me over	1 serv	242	0	tr
benedictine	1 oz	104	0	0
betsy ross	1 serv	206	0	0
black devil	1 serv	220	0	tr
black russian	1 serv	184	0	0
bloody mary	1 serv	150	0	1
blue whale	1 serv	222	0	0
bourbon & soda	1 serv (4 oz)	105	0	0
bourbon sour	1 serv	166	0	tr
brandy alexander	1 serv	266	20	0
brandy sour	1 serv	164	0	tr
bushwacker	1 serv	286	0	tr
coffee liqueur	1 serv (1.5 oz)	175	0	0
cognac	1 oz	67	0	0
cosmopolitan martini	1 serv	126	0	tr
creme de menthe	1 serv (1.5 oz)	186	0	0
curacao liqueur	1 oz	81	0	0
daiquiri	1 serv (2 oz)	112	0	tr
daiquiri banana	1 serv	277	0	1
dark & stormy	1 serv	64	0	0
doctor pepper	1 serv	95	0	0
frozen daiquiri pineapple	1 serv	186	0	2
frozen tequila screwdriver	1 serv	159	0	1
fuzzy navel	1 serv	247	0	tr
gimlet vodka	1 serv	150	0	1
gin	1 serv (1.5 oz)	110	0	0
gin & tonic	1 serv (7.5 oz)	171	0	–
gin ricky	1 serv	114	0	tr
grasshopper	1 serv	275	15	0
happy hawaiian	1 serv	434	0	tr
harvey wallbanger	1 serv	198	0	tr
head banger	1 serv	165	0	0
hot buttered rum	1 serv	219	10	4
hot toddy	1 serv	188	0	5
hurricane	1 serv	205	0	tr
kamikaze	1 serv	136	0	0
long island iced tea	1 serv	292	0	0

FOOD	PORTION	CALS	CHOL	FIBER
lynchburg lemonade	1 serv	465	0	1
mai tai	1 serv	165	0	tr
manhattan	1 serv	171	0	tr
margarita	1 serv	173	0	0
margarita strawberry	1 serv	106	0	1
martini	1 serv (3 oz)	206	0	0
martini apple	1 serv	147	0	tr
martini rum	1 serv	131	0	tr
mellow yellow	1 serv	95	0	0
mexican grasshopper	1 serv	638	66	0
mint julep	1 serv	136	0	tr
mississippi mud	1 serv	496	45	0
mudslide	1 serv	566	0	0
narragansett	1 serv	168	0	0
nutcracker	1 serv	730	0	0
old fashioned	1 serv	223	0	tr
orange crush	1 serv	461	0	tr
pain killer	1 serv	277	0	tr
peppermint pattie	1 serv	344	0	0
pina colada	1 serv (4.5 oz)	245	0	tr
planter's cocktail	1 serv	105	0	tr
planter's punch	1 serv	233	0	4
presbyterian	1 serv	170	0	tr
purple passion	1 serv	215	0	0
rob roy	1 serv	171	0	tr
rum	1 serv (1.5 oz)	97	0	0
rum boogie	1 serv	134	0	tr
rum cola	1 serv	209	0	tr
rum highball	1 serv	170	0	0
rum punch	1 serv	448	0	1
rusty nail	1 serv	159	0	0
sake	1 serv (1 oz)	39	0	0
salty dog	1 serv	210	0	tr
scotch & soda	1 serv	104	0	tr
screwdriver rum	1 serv	166	0	tr
sea breeze	1 serv	207	0	tr
sex on the beach	1 serv	190	0	tr
slippery nipple	1 serv	142	0	0
sloe gin fizz	1 serv (2.5 oz)	132	0	0
snake bite	1 serv	362	0	0

FOOD	PORTION	CALS	CHOL	FIBER
sour rum	1 serv	156	0	tr
swizzle rum	1 serv	187	0	0
tequila gimlet	1 serv	150	0	1
tequila sour	1 serv	156	0	tr
tequila stinger	1 serv	221	0	0
tequila sunrise	1 serv (6.8 oz)	232	0	0
tom collins	1 serv (7.5 oz)	121	0	–
vermouth cassis	1 serv	97	0	tr
vodka	1 serv (1.5 oz)	97	0	0
vodka sour	1 serv	138	0	tr
vodka stinger	1 serv	378	0	0
whiskey	1 serv (1.5 oz)	105	0	0
whiskey sour	1 serv (3.5 oz)	162	0	0
white russian	1 serv	290	31	0
zombie	1 serv	235	0	tr

LITCHI JUICE
Ceres
Litchi	8 oz	120	0	0

LIVER (see also PATE)
beef braised	1 slice (2.4 oz)	130	269	0
beef pan-fried	1 slice (2.8 oz)	142	309	0
chicken fried	3 oz	146	479	0
chicken simmered	3 oz	142	479	0
lamb braised	3 oz	187	426	0
lamb fried	3 oz	202	419	0
moose braised	3 oz	132	331	–
pork braised	3 oz	140	302	0
turkey simmered	1 liver (2.9 oz)	227	322	0
veal braised	1 slice (2.8 oz)	154	409	0
veal pan fried	1 slice (2.4 oz)	129	325	0

TAKE-OUT
calves liver w/ onions	1 serv (5 oz)	177	335	1

LLAMA
llama	3 oz	120	60	–

LOBSTER
northern cooked	1 cup	142	104	–
northern cooked	3 oz	83	61	–

FOOD	PORTION	CALS	CHOL	FIBER
spiny steamed	1 (5.7 oz)	233	146	–
spiny steamed	3 oz	122	76	–
Phillips Seafood				
Lobster Cake	1 (3 oz)	230	75	–
Progresso				
Lobster Sauce	½ cup (4.3 oz)	100	5	2
TAKE-OUT				
newburg	1 cup	485	455	–

LOGANBERRIES

frzn	1 cup	80	0	–

LONGANS

fresh	1	2	0	–

LOQUATS

fresh	1	5	0	–

LOTUS

root raw sliced	10 slices	45	0	–
root sliced cooked	10 slices	59	0	–
seeds dried	1 oz	94	0	–
Eden				
Dried Sliced	5 slices (0.3 oz)	35	0	2
Frieda's				
Lotus Root Fresh	1 cup	50	0	4

LOX (see SALMON)

LUPINES

dried cooked	1 cup	197	0	–

LYCHEES

fresh	1	6	0	–
Frieda's				
Fresh	6 to 8 (3.5 oz)	60	0	1

MACADAMIA NUTS

dry roasted w/ salt	10-12 (1 oz)	200	0	1
oil roasted	1 oz	204	0	–
Hawaiian Host				
White Choco	3 pieces (1.4 oz)	230	0	0

FOOD	PORTION	CALS	CHOL	FIBER
Mauna Loa				
Chocolate Trio	9 pieces	200	5	2
Dry Roasted Salted	¼ cup	200	0	2
Dry Roasted Unsalted	¼ cup	200	0	2
Honey Roasted	¼ cup	210	0	2
Kona Coffee Glazed	¼ cup	190	<5	1
Maui Onion & Garlic	¼ cup	200	0	3
Milk Chocolate Coated	3 pieces	230	5	1
Milk Chocolate Toffee	7 pieces	210	5	1
MACE				
ground	1 tsp	8	0	–
MACKEREL				
CANNED				
jack	1 can (12.7 oz)	563	285	0
jack	1 cup	296	150	0
Brunswick				
Jack In Water	2 oz	100	50	0
Chicken Of The Sea				
Jack In Tomato Sauce	¼ cup	70	45	0
Jack In Water	⅓ cup	90	55	0
Orleans				
Jack	¼ cup	90	55	0
DRIED				
Eden				
Bonito Flakes	2 tbsp	5	1	0
FRESH				
atlantic cooked	3 oz	223	64	0
atlantic raw	3 oz	174	60	0
jack baked	3 oz	171	51	–
jack fillet baked	6.2 oz	354	106	–
king baked	3 oz	114	58	0
king fillet baked	5.4 oz	207	105	0
pacific baked	3 oz	171	51	0
pacific fillet baked	6.2 oz	354	106	–
spanish cooked	1 fillet (5.1 oz)	230	107	0
spanish cooked	3 oz	134	62	0
spanish raw	3 oz	118	65	0
SMOKED				
atlantic	3.5 oz	296	93	0

FOOD	PORTION	CALS	CHOL	FIBER
MAHI MAHI				
fresh baked	4 oz	192	49	0
Phillips Seafood				
Coconut Mahi Mahi w/ Sauce	3 pieces	290	65	–
MALANGA				
dasheen mashed	1 cup	226	0	8
dasheen pieces boiled	1 cup	212	0	8
pieces fried	1 cup	304	0	8
root raw	1 (10.7 oz)	299	0	5
Frieda's				
Malanga	⅔ cup	90	0	2
MALT				
malt liquor	1 bottle (12 oz)	148	0	tr
nonalcoholic	1 bottle (12 oz)	133	0	0
MALTED MILK				
chocolate as prep w/ milk	1 cup	179	16	1
chocolate flavor powder	3 heaping tsp (0.7 oz)	79	0	1
natural flavor as prep w/ milk	1 cup	186	21	tr
natural flavor powder	3 heaping tsp (0.7 oz)	87	7	tr
MAMMY-APPLE				
fresh	1	431	0	–
MANGO				
fresh	1	135	0	–
C&W				
Chunks	¾ cup	90	0	3
Sunsweet				
Plillipine dried	6 pieces (1.5 oz)	130	0	2
Thailand dried	⅓ cup (1.4 oz)	140	0	1
Tomorrow's Tropicals				
Fresh	½ (3.6 oz)	70	0	1
MANGO JUICE				
Ceres				
Mango	8 oz	120	0	1
Fresh Samantha				
Mango Mama	1 cup (8 oz)	120	0	8

FOOD	PORTION	CALS	CHOL	FIBER
Guzzler				
Mango Passion	8 oz	140	0	–
Naked Juice				
Mighty Mango	8 oz	120	0	0
MANGOSTEEN				
canned in syrup	1 cup	143	0	4
MARGARINE				
squeeze	1 tsp	34	0	0
stick corn	1 stick (4 oz)	815	0	–
stick corn	1 tsp	34	0	0
tub corn	1 tsp	34	0	0
tub diet	1 tsp	17	0	0
Benecol				
Single Serve Light	1 pkg (0.3 oz)	30	0	–
Tub Light	1 tbsp (0.5 oz)	45	0	–
Tub Regular	1 tbsp (0.5 oz)	80	0	–
Blue Bonnet				
Light Stick	1 tbsp	50	0	0
Soft Spread	1 tbsp	60	0	0
Soft Spread Light	1 tbsp	40	0	0
Stick	1 tbsp	80	0	0
Brummel & Brown				
Made With Natural Yogurt	1 tbsp	45	0	0
Crystal Farms				
60/40 Margarine Butter	1 tbsp	100	5	0
Margarine	1 tbsp	100	0	0
Fleischmann's				
Soft Spread Light	1 tbsp	40	0	0
Soft Spread Original	1 tbsp	70	0	0
Soft Spread Unsalted	1 tbsp	70	0	0
Soft Spread w/ Olive Oil	1 tbsp	70	0	0
I Can't Believe It's Not Butter				
Regular Stick	1 tbsp	90	0	0
Soft Fat Free	1 tbsp	5	0	0
Soft Light	1 tbsp	50	0	0
Soft Regular	1 tbsp	80	0	0
Soft w/ Calcium	1 tbsp	50	0	0
Spray	5 sprays	0	0	0

FOOD	PORTION	CALS	CHOL	FIBER
Squeeze	1 tbsp	60	0	0
Stick Light	1 tbsp	50	0	0
Parkay				
Light Spread	1 tbsp	50	0	0
Original Spread	1 tbsp	60	0	0
Original Stick	1 tbsp	90	0	0
Spray	5 sprays	0	0	0
Spread + Calcium	1 tbsp	45	0	0
Squeeze	1 tbsp	70	0	0
Stick Light	1 tbsp	50	0	0
Promise				
Buttery Spread	1 tbsp	80	0	0
Stick	1 tbsp	90	0	0
Smart Balance				
37% Light	1 tbsp	45	0	0
67% Light	1 tbsp	25	0	0
Omega Plus w/ Flax Oil	1 tbsp	80	0	0
Spectrum				
Essential Omega	1 tbsp	80	0	0
Spread	1 tbsp	88	0	0
Take Control				
Light	1 tbsp	45	<5	–
Spread	1 tbsp (0.5 oz)	80	<5	0

MARINADE (see SAUCE)

MARJORAM

| dried | 1 tsp | 2 | 0 | – |

MARSHMALLOW

marshmallow	1 cup (1.6 oz)	146	0	–
marshmallow	1 reg (0.3 oz)	23	0	–
Gol D Lite				
Sugar Free	⅓ pkg (0.9 oz)	51	0	0

MATZO

brie	1 piece (0.5 oz)	54	21	tr
egg	1 (1 oz)	109	23	1
matzo ball	1 med (1.2 oz)	48	36	tr
plain	1 (1 oz)	111	0	1
whole wheat	1 (1 oz)	98	0	3

FOOD	PORTION	CALS	CHOL	FIBER
Eddyleon				
Dark Chocolate Coated Egg Matzo	1 oz	97	8	1
Milk Chocolate Coated Egg Matzo	1 oz	97	8	1
Horowitz Margareten				
Egg	1 (1.2 oz)	130	15	1
Manischewitz				
Dark Chocolate Coated Egg	½ (1.5 oz)	90	25	2
Egg	1 (1.2 oz)	120	15	1
Matzo Meal	¼ cup (1 oz)	130	0	1
Thin Unsalted	1 (0.8 oz)	90	0	0
Streit's				
Egg	1 (1.1 oz)	120	20	1
Egg & Onion	1 (1 oz)	100	5	1
Passover	1 (1 oz)	110	0	1

MAYONNAISE

FOOD	PORTION	CALS	CHOL	FIBER
mayonnaise	1 tbsp	99	8	–
mayonnaise	1 cup	1577	130	–
reduced calorie	1 tbsp	34	4	–
reduced calorie	1 cup	556	58	–
sandwich spread	1 tbsp	60	12	–
Blue Plate				
Squeeze	1 tbsp	100	10	0
Hellman's				
Mayonnaise	1 tbsp	90	5	0
Spectrum				
Canola Squeeze	1 tbsp	100	5	0
Canola Squeeze Light Eggless Vegan	1 tbsp	35	0	0
Organic Dijon	1 tbsp	90	0	0
Organic Olive Oil	1 tbsp	100	0	0
Organic Roasted Garlic	1 tbsp	100	0	0
Organic Squeeze	1 tbsp	100	10	0
Organic Wasabi	1 tbsp	100	0	0

MAYONNAISE TYPE SALAD DRESSING

FOOD	PORTION	CALS	CHOL	FIBER
mayonnaise type salad dressing	1 cup	916	60	–

FOOD	PORTION	CALS	CHOL	FIBER
mayonnaise type salad dressing	1 tbsp	57	4	–
reduced calorie w/o cholesterol	1 cup	1084	0	–
reduced calorie w/o cholesterol	1 tbsp	68	0	–
Carb Options				
Whipped Dressing	1 tbsp	50	5	0
Nasoya				
Fat Free Nayonaise	1 tbsp	10	0	0
Nayonaise	1 tbsp	35	0	0
MEAT STICKS				
jerky beef	1 piece (0.7 oz)	82	10	tr
pork jerky	1 strip (0.5 oz)	62	7	tr
venison jerky	1 strip (0.5 oz)	55	18	0
Jack Link's				
Beef Jerky Teriyaki	1 oz	80	20	0
Pemmican				
Homestyle Tender All Flavors	1 oz	80	35	1
Kippered Beef Original	1 pkg (1 oz)	60	25	0
Kippered Beef Peppered	1 pkg (1 oz)	60	25	0
Kippered Beef Sweet & Hot	1 pkg (1 oz)	70	15	0
Kippered Beef Teriyaki	1 pkg (1 oz)	60	20	0
Long Lasting Hot & Spicy	1 oz	60	10	0
Long Lasting Original	1 oz	60	10	0
Long Lasting Peppered	1 oz	60	10	0
Long Lasting Teriyaki	1 oz	70	10	0
Premium Cut Beef Jerky	1 oz	80	35	1
Premium Cut Turkey Peppered	1 oz	70	25	0
Premium Cut Turkey Sweet Smoked	1 oz	70	25	0
Shredded Beef Jerky All Flavors	¼ cup	80	35	1
Steak Tips All Flavors	1 oz	70	20	0
Rustlers Roundup				
Beef Jerky	1 serv (5 g)	20	5	tr
Flamin' Hot	1 serv (8 g)	40	10	tr
Smoky Steak	1 serv (0.8 oz)	60	20	0
Spicy	1 serv (0.5 oz)	70	20	tr

FOOD	PORTION	CALS	CHOL	FIBER
Wellshire				
Matt's Select Pepperoni	1 stick (0.9 oz)	90	20	0
Tom Tom Snack Hot n' Spicy Turkey	1 stick (0.8 oz)	50	20	0

MEAT SUBSTITUTES (*see also* BACON SUBSTITUTES, CANADIAN BACON SUBSTITUTES, CHICKEN SUBSTITUTES, HAMBURGER SUBSTITUTES, MEATBALL SUBSTITUTES, SAUSAGE SUBSTITUTES, TURKEY SUBSTITUTES)

FOOD	PORTION	CALS	CHOL	FIBER
Fantastic				
Sloppy Joe Mix not prep	¼ cup	70	0	3
Taco Filling not prep	¼ cup	80	0	4
Ken & Robert's				
Veggie Pockets Bar B Que	1 (4.5 oz)	290	0	5
Veggie Pockets Greek	1 (4.5 oz)	250	0	4
Veggie Pockets Pizza	1 (4.5 oz)	270	0	4
Veggie Pockets Pot Pie	1 (4.5 oz)	250	0	2
Veggie Pockets Potato & Cheddar	1 (4.5 oz)	260	0	2
Veggie Pockets Santa Fe	1 (4.5 oz)	250	0	5
Veggie Pockets Tex Mex	1 (4.5 oz)	260	0	6
Lightlife				
Balogna	4 slices (2 oz)	60	0	2
Gimme Lean Ground Beef	1 serv (2 oz)	50	0	2
Smart BBQ	¼ cup	70	0	1
Smart Cutlet Salisbury Steak	1 (4.5 oz)	130	0	6
Smart Deli Country Ham	4 slices (2 oz)	90	0	1
Smart Deli Pastrami Style	4 slices (2 oz)	60	0	0
Smart Deli Pepperoni Style	13 slices (1 oz)	45	0	1
Smart Ground Original	⅓ cup (1.9 oz)	80	0	3
Smart Ground Taco Burrito	⅓ cup (2 oz)	70	0	4
Smart Menu Crumbles	⅓ cup	80	0	3
Smart Menu Meatless Meatballs	5	160	0	2
Smart Menu Steak Strips	1 serv (3 oz)	80	0	5
Smart Tex Mex	¼ cup	50	0	2
Loma Linda				
Dinner Cuts	2 slices (3.2 oz)	90	0	2
Swiss Stake	1 piece (3.2 oz)	130	0	3
Tender Bits	6 pieces (3 oz)	110	0	3
Vita Burger Chunks not prep	¼ cup (0.7 oz)	70	0	3

FOOD	PORTION	CALS	CHOL	FIBER
Morningstar Farms				
Meal Starters Steak Strips	12 pieces (3 oz)	140	0	1
Quorn				
Grounds	⅔ cup (3 oz)	80	0	4
Soy7				
Burger Bits as prep	½ cup	60	0	2
Burger Mix as prep	1 serv (3.2 oz)	120	0	3
Recipe Strips as prep	¾ cup	70	0	3
Taco Mix as prep	¼ cup	70	0	3
VeggieLand				
Crumbles Beef	½ cup	70	0	–
Veg-T-Balls	3 (3 oz)	113	0	5
Viana				
Cowgirl Veggie Steaks	1 (3.7 oz)	260	0	4
Veggie Cevapcici	4 pieces (2.8 oz)	240	0	3
Veggie Gyros	24 strips (3 oz)	220	0	2
Veggie Kebab	½ cup	210	0	2
Worthington				
Bolono	3 slices (2 oz)	80	0	2
Choplets	2 slices (3.2 oz)	90	0	2
Corned Beef Vegetarian	3 slices (2 oz)	140	0	0
Dinner Roast	1 slice (3 oz)	180	0	3
Multigrain Cutlets	2 slices (3.2 oz)	100	0	3
Prime Stakes	1 piece (3.2 oz)	120	0	1
Vegetable Skallops	½ cup (3 oz)	90	0	3
Wham	2 slices (2 oz)	110	0	0
Yves				
Veggie Bologna	4 slices (2.2 oz)	70	0	0
Veggie Ground Italian	⅓ cup (2 oz)	60	0	3
Veggie Ground Round Italian	⅓ cup (1.9 oz)	60	0	3
Veggie Ground Round Original	2 oz	60	0	3
Veggie Pizza Pepperoni Slices	1 serv (1.7 oz)	70	0	3
Veggie Salami Deli Slices	1 serv (2.2 oz)	90	0	1
MEATBALL SUBSTITUTES				
meatless	2 (1.3 oz)	71	0	2
Loma Linda				
Tender Rounds	6 (2.8 oz)	120	0	1

FOOD	PORTION	CALS	CHOL	FIBER
Quorn				
Meatballs	4 (2.4 oz)	110	5	1
MEATBALLS				
beef	1 med (1 oz)	74	25	0
beef	1 lg (1.5 oz)	111	37	0
beef cocktail	1 (0.2 oz)	18	6	0
Shady Brook				
Italian Beef	3 oz	260	55	1
Turkey Meatballs Appetizer Size	3 oz	190	65	1
Turkey Meatballs Italian Style	3 (3 oz)	190	65	tr
TastyBite				
Meatballs Vindaloo	1 pkg (9.5 oz)	270	25	4
TAKE-OUT				
albondigas w/ sauce	3 + sauce (5.3 oz)	372	102	1
porcupine + tomato sauce	3 + sauce	160	34	1
swedish w/ cream sauce	3 + sauce (4.7 oz)	215	86	tr
sweet & sour	3 + sauce (4.5 oz)	188	67	1
MELON				
Frieda's				
Camouflage	1 cup (5 oz)	50	0	1
SpriteMelon	1 (10.5 oz)	115	0	2
Temptation	1/10 melon (4.7 oz)	55	0	1
MEXICAN FOOD (see SALSA, SPANISH FOOD, TORTILLA)				
MILK				
CANNED				
condensed sweetened	1 cup	982	104	–
evaporated	1/2 cup	169	37	–
evaporated skim	1/2 cup	99	5	–
Carnation				
Evaporated	2 tbsp	40	10	–
Evaporated Fat Free	2 tbsp	25	0	–
Evaporated Lowfat 2%	2 tbsp	25	5	–
Meyenberg				
Evaporated Goat Milk	8 oz	145	27	–
Pet				
Evaporated	2 tbsp	40	10	–

FOOD	PORTION	CALS	CHOL	FIBER
DRIED				
buttermilk	1 tbsp	25	5	–
nonfat instantized	1 pkg (3.2 oz)	244	12	–
Carnation				
Instant Nonfat as prep	1 cup	80	<5	0
Meyerberg				
Instant Goat Milk as prep	1 cup	142	25	–
Sanalac				
Powder	¼ cup (0.8 oz)	85	6	0
REFRIGERATED				
1%	1 cup	102	10	–
1% protein fortified	1 qt	477	39	–
1% protein fortified	1 cup	119	10	–
2%	1 cup	121	18	–
2%	1 qt	485	73	–
buttermilk	1 cup	99	9	–
buttermilk	1 qt	396	34	–
goat	1 cup	168	28	–
goat	1 qt	672	111	–
human	1 cup	171	34	–
indian buffalo	1 cup	236	46	–
low sodium	1 cup	149	33	–
nonfat	1 cup	86	4	–
whole	1 cup	150	33	–
Active Lifestyle				
Fat Free w/ Plant Sterols	8 oz	90	<5	0
Borden				
Fat Free Skim	1 cup	80	5	0
Farmland				
Buttermilk	8 oz	160	20	0
Far Free	8 oz	80	5	0
Special Request 1% Plus Omega-3	8 oz	130	10	0
Special Request Skim Plus	8 oz	110	5	0
Special Request Skim Plus 100% Lactose Free	8 oz	110	5	0
Whole	8 oz	160	20	0
Hood				
1%	1 cup	110	15	0
2%	1 cup	130	20	0

FOOD	PORTION	CALS	CHOL	FIBER
Buttermilk Fat Free	1 cup	90	<5	0
Calorie Countdown 2 %	8 oz	90	20	0
Calorie Countdown Fat Free	8 oz	45	0	0
Fat Free	1 cup	80	<5	0
Simply Smart 0% Fat	1 cup	90	<5	0
Simply Smart 1% Fat	1 cup	120	15	0
Whole	1 cup	150	35	0
Horizon Organic				
Fat Free	8 oz	90	<5	0
Lactaid				
1% Lowfat	1 cup	110	10	0
2% Reduced Fat	1 cup	130	20	0
Calcium Fortified	1 cup	80	<5	0
Fat Free	1 cup	90	<5	0
Whole	1 cup	150	35	0
Land O Lakes				
1% Lowfat	1 carton (10 oz)	120	15	–
Fat Free	1 carton (10 oz)	100	5	–
Whole	1 carton (10 oz)	180	45	–
Meyenberg				
Goat Milk	8 oz	142	25	–
Goat Milk Low Fat	8 oz	89	8	–
Organic Valley				
Reduced Fat	1 cup	130	20	0
Whole	1 cup	150	30	0
Skinny Cow				
Fat Free	8 oz	110	0	0
Stonyfield Farm				
Organic Whole Milk	1 cup (8 oz)	180	40	0
Organic Whole Milk Vanilla	1 cup (8 oz)	230	30	0
Turkey Hill				
Cool Moos 2% Reduced Fat	1 cup	130	20	–
Cool Moos Whole Milk	1 cup	160	35	–
Tuscan				
Whole	8 oz	150	35	0
Welsh Farms				
Fat Free	8 oz	80	5	0
SHELF-STABLE				
Parmalat				
2% Reduced Fat	8 oz	130	20	0

FOOD	PORTION	CALS	CHOL	FIBER
Fat Free	8 oz	80	5	0
Lactose Free 2% Reduced Fat	8 oz	130	20	0

MILK DRINKS

FOOD	PORTION	CALS	CHOL	FIBER
chocolate milk	1 cup	208	30	–
chocolate milk	1 qt	833	122	–
chocolate milk 1%	1 cup	158	7	–
chocolate milk 2%	1 cup	179	17	–
Bravo!				
Blenders Creamy Double Chocolate	1 bottle (11 oz)	180	20	2
Blenders Creamy French Vanilla	1 bottle (11 oz)	160	20	2
Cal-C				
Orange Tangerine	8 oz	70	0	–
Peach Mango	8 oz	70	0	–
Strawberry Citrus	8 oz	70	0	–
Cocio				
Chocolate Milk	1 bottle	225	25	tr
Farmland				
Really Really Good! Chocolate Milk	8 oz	160	10	0
Garelick				
Colossal Coffee	1 cup	145	15	0
Ultimate Chocolate	1 cup	150	15	1
Hershey's				
Chocolate Milk Fat Free	1 bottle	160	5	tr
Chocolate Milk Reduced Fat	1 bottle	200	20	1
Hood				
Calorie Countdown Chocolate 2%	8 oz	90	15	1
Chocolate Lowfat	1 cup	170	15	tr
Chocolate Milk	1 cup	230	35	tr
Coffee Lowfat Milk	1 cup	170	15	0
Horizon Organic				
Lowfat Chocolate Milk	8 oz	170	15	tr
Strawberry	8 oz	200	20	0
Land O Lakes				
Chocolate	1 cup (8.4 oz)	200	30	0

FOOD	PORTION	CALS	CHOL	FIBER
Nesquik				
Chocolate as prep w/ lowfat milk	1 cup	210	18	1
Chocolate No Sugar as prep w/ lowfat milk	1 cup	130	3	1
Double Chocolate as prep w/ lowfat milk	1 cup	210	18	1
Ready-To-Drink Banana	1 cup	200	20	0
Ready-To-Drink Chocolate	1 cup	200	15	tr
Ready-To-Drink Double Chocolate	1 cup	200	15	tr
Ready-To-Drink Fat Free Chocolate	1 cup	160	0	tr
Ready-To-Drink Strawberry	1 cup	200	15	tr
Ready-To-Drink Very Vanilla	1 cup	200	15	tr
Strawberry as prep w/ lowfat milk	1 cup	210	18	0
Vanilla as prep w/ lowfat milk	1 cup	210	18	0
Organic Valley				
Chocolate Milk Reduced Fat	1 cup	180	10	0
Parmalat				
Chocolate Milk 2% Reduced Fat	1 cup	190	20	1
Quaker				
Chocolate	8 oz	140	16	3
Strawberry	8 oz	130	17	tr
Vanilla	8 oz	130	17	tr
Quik				
Banana Lowfat	1 cup (8.4 oz)	200	20	0
Banana Powder	2 tbsp (0.8 oz)	90	0	0
Chocolate	1 cup (8.4 oz)	230	30	1
Chocolate Lowfat	1 carton (8.4 oz)	200	20	0
Cookies n Cream Powder	2 tbsp (0.8 oz)	100	0	1
Strawberry	1 cup (8.4 oz)	230	30	0
Strawberry Lowfat	1 carton (8.4 oz)	210	20	0
Strawberry Powder	2 tbsp (0.8 oz)	90	0	0
Rosa's Original				
Horchata All Flavors	8 oz	160	5	0

FOOD	PORTION	CALS	CHOL	FIBER
Turkey Hill				
Cool Moos Chocolate 1% Lowfat	1 cup	180	10	–
Cool Moos Orange Cream 1% Lowfat	1 cup	190	10	–
Cool Moos Strawberry 1% Lowfat	1 cup	160	10	–
Cool Moos Vanilla 1% Lowfat	1 cup	160	10	–
MILK SUBSTITUTES				
imitation milk	1 cup	150	tr	–
imitation milk	1 qt	600	2	–
8th Continent				
Soymilk Chocolate	8 oz	140	0	1
Soymilk Original	8 oz	80	0	0
Soymilk Vanilla	8 oz	100	0	0
Soymilk Fat Free Original	8 oz	60	0	0
Soymilk Fat Free Vanilla	8 oz	70	0	0
Soymilk Light Chocolate	8 oz	90	0	tr
Soymilk Light Original	8 oz	50	0	0
Soymilk Light Vanilla	8 oz	60	0	0
Almond Breeze				
Chocolate	8 oz	115	0	1
Original	8 oz	57	0	1
Original Unsweetened	8 oz	40	0	1
Vanilla	8 oz	91	0	1
Better Than Milk				
Rice Original	2 tbsp (0.66 oz)	78	0	1
Rice Original Light	2 tbsp (0.66 oz)	66	0	1
Rice Vanilla	2 tbsp (0.66 oz)	78	0	1
Rice Vanilla Light	2 tbsp (0.66 oz)	66	0	1
Soy Carob	2 tbsp (1 oz)	90	0	2
Soy Chocolate	2 tbsp (1.1 oz)	112	0	1
Soy Light	2 tbsp (0.66 oz)	73	0	1
Soy Original	2 tbsp (0.8 oz)	100	0	0
Soy Vanilla	2 tbsp (0.7 oz)	77	0	1
DariFree				
Fat Free as prep	8 oz	70	0	0
Fat Free Chocolate as prep	8 oz	110	5	tr

FOOD	PORTION	CALS	CHOL	FIBER
EdenBlend				
Organic	8 oz	120	0	tr
Edensoy				
Organic Carob	8 oz	170	0	tr
Organic Chocolate	8 oz	180	0	tr
Organic Light Vanilla	8 oz	110	0	0
Organic Original	8 oz	140	0	tr
Organic Original Light	8 oz	100	0	0
Organic Original Unsweetened	8 oz	120	0	tr
Organic Vanilla	8 oz	150	0	tr
Hansen's				
Soy Smoothie Lemon Chiffon	8 oz	150	0	tr
Soy Smoothie Orange Dream	8 oz	150	0	tr
Harmony Farms				
Original Rice Beverage	1 cup (8 oz)	90	0	0
Harmony House				
Enriched Rice Beverage	1 cup (8 oz)	90	0	0
Enriched Soy Beverage	1 cup (8 oz)	90	0	0
Original Soy Beverage	1 cup (8 oz)	90	0	0
Keto				
Low Carb Mix	1 scoop	54	30	–
Pacific Foods				
Almond Low Fat Original	1 cup	70	0	1
Almond Low Fat Vanilla	1 cup	100	0	1
Multi Grain Low Fat Original	1 cup	160	0	1
Oat Organic Low Fat Original	1 cup	130	0	2
Oat Organic Low Fat Vanilla	1 cup	130	0	2
Rice Low Fat Plain	1 cup	130	0	0
Rice Low Fat Vanilla	1 cup	130	0	0
Soy Organic Unsweetened Original	1 cup	90	0	2
Soy Select Low Fat Plain	1 cup	70	0	tr
Soy Select Low Fat Vanilla	1 cup	80	0	tr
Soy Ultra	1 cup	130	0	1
Soy Ultra Plain	1 cup	120	0	1

FOOD	PORTION	CALS	CHOL	FIBER
Rice Dream				
Carob	8 oz	150	0	tr
Heartwise Vanilla	8 oz	140	0	3
Horchata	8 oz	130	0	2
Original	8 oz	120	0	0
Original Enriched	8 oz	120	0	0
Vanilla Enriched	8 oz	130	0	0
Silk				
Chocolate	1 cup	140	0	0
Organic Plain	1 cup	100	0	0
Vanilla	1 bottle (11 oz)	140	0	0
Sno*e				
Tofu as prep	8 oz	80	0	0
Tofu Low Fat as prep	8 oz	70	0	0
Soy Dream				
Classic Vanilla	8 oz	140	0	2
Original Enriched	8 oz	100	0	2
Tree Of Life				
Original Rice Beverage	1 cup	90	0	0
Vitamite				
Non-Dairy	1 cup (8 oz)	110	0	0
Vitasoy				
Classic Original	8 oz	120	0	1
Complete Original	8 oz	70	0	4
Complete Vanilla	8 oz	50	0	4
Creamy Original	8 oz	110	0	1
Green Tea Soymilk	8 oz	120	0	1
Light Chocolate	8 oz	100	0	0
Light Original	8 oz	60	0	0
Lite Vanilla	8 oz	70	0	0
Original Unsweetened	8 oz	80	0	tr
Rich Chocolate	8 oz	160	0	1
Smooth Vanilla	8 oz	120	0	1
Vanilla Delight	8 oz	120	0	1
White Wave				
Mocha	1 cup	140	0	1
MILKFISH (AWA)				
baked	3 oz	162	57	0

FOOD	PORTION	CALS	CHOL	FIBER
MILKSHAKE				
chocolate	1 serv (10 oz)	393	42	2
malted milk shake	1 serv (10 oz)	402	51	1
vanilla	10 serv (10 oz)	379	48	1
Ben & Jerry's				
Cherry Garcia	1 bottle (8 oz)	320	40	–
Chocolate Fudge Brownie	1 bottle (8 oz)	340	40	–
Chunky Monkey	1 bottle (8 oz)	330	35	–
Breyers				
Quick Vanilla	1 serv (10 oz)	320	45	0
Carb Options				
Chocolate Delite	1 can (11 oz)	190	15	4
Creamy Vanilla	1 can (11 oz)	190	15	4
Hershey's				
Chocolate	1 bottle	270	20	tr
Cookies 'N' Cream	1 bottle	280	20	0
Strawberry	1 bottle	280	20	10
Vanilla Cream	1 bottle	320	20	0
Nesquik				
Ready-To-Drink Chocolate	1 cup	170	15	tr
MILLET				
cooked	1 cup (6.1 oz)	207	0	2
MISO				
miso	½ cup	284	0	7
Eden				
Hacho	1 tbsp	40	0	tr
Organic Genmai	1 tbsp	25	0	2
Organic Mugi	1 tbsp	25	0	tr
Organic Shiro	1 tbsp	30	0	tr
Tekka	1 tsp	5	0	0
MOLASSES				
blackstrap	1 cup (11.5 oz)	771	0	–
blackstrap	1 tbsp (0.7 oz)	47	0	–
molasses	1 cup (11.5 oz)	873	0	–
molasses	1 tbsp (0.7 oz)	53	0	–
Brer Rabbit				
Dark	1 tbsp	60	0	–

FOOD	PORTION	CALS	CHOL	FIBER
Grandma's				
Robust	1 tbsp	60	0	–
Mott's				
Sulphured	1 tbsp	50	0	–
Unsulphured	1 tbsp	50	0	–
MONKFISH				
baked	3 oz	82	27	0
MOOSE				
roasted	3 oz	114	66	0
MOTH BEANS				
dried cooked	1 cup	207	0	–
MOUSSE				
TAKE-OUT				
chocolate	½ cup (7.1 oz)	447	299	–
orange	½ cup	87	1	–
MUFFIN				
MIX				
blueberry	1 (1.75 oz)	149	23	–
corn	1 (1.75 oz)	160	31	–
wheat bran as prep	1 (1.75 oz)	138	34	–
Betty Crocker				
Apple Cinnamon as prep	1	170	36	–
Apple Streusel as prep	1	210	18	–
Banana Nut as prep	1	170	18	1
Cranberry Orange as prep	1	150	18	–
Double Chocolate as prep	1	220	27	–
Golden Corn as prep	1	160	36	–
Lemon Poppyseed as prep	1	180	36	–
Sunkist Lemon Poppyseed as prep	1	190	18	–
Twice The Blueberries as prep	1	140	18	1
Wild Blueberry as prep	1	170	18	tr
Carbsense				
Honey Bran not prep	1 serv (1.3 oz)	120	0	12
Glory				
Golden Sweet Corn as prep	1	170	36	1

FOOD	PORTION	CALS	CHOL	FIBER
Gold Medal				
Corn	1	160	35	0
Jiffy				
Apple Cinnamon as prep	1	190	33	1
Banana Nut as prep	1	180	27	2
Blueberry as prep	1	190	36	1
Bran w/ Dates as prep	1	170	36	3
Corn as prep	1	180	30	1
Raspberry as prep	1	180	42	1
Ketogenics				
Apple Cinnamon Bran as prep	1	190	54	7
Chocolate Chip as prep	1	215	36	5
Wild Blueberry as prep	1	190	36	4
King Arthur				
Cranberry Orange Whole Grain not prep	¼ cup	180	0	3
MiniCarb				
Apple Cinnamon as prep	1	225	35	4
Sweet Corn as prep	1	225	35	6
Miracle Maize				
Country Style as prep	1	155	15	1
Sweet as prep	1	180	15	1
Robin Hood				
Apple Cinnamon	1	170	35	0
Banana Nut	1	170	35	0
Blueberry	1	160	35	0
Caramel Nut	1	170	35	0
Sweet Rewards				
Low Fat Apple Cinnamon as prep	1	140	16	–
READY-TO-EAT				
blueberry	1 (2 oz)	158	17	2
oat bran wheat free	1 (2 oz)	154	0	4
Atkins				
Blueberry	1 (3.5 oz)	210	0	6
Fred's Incredible Muffins				
All Flavors	1 (2.5 oz)	100	55	–
Natural Ovens				
Blueberry	1 (2.5 oz)	180	0	2

FOOD	PORTION	CALS	CHOL	FIBER
Carrot Nut	1 (2.5 oz)	170	0	2
Raisin Bran	1 (2.5 oz)	170	0	5
Otis Spunkmeyer				
Apple Cinnamon	1 (4 oz)	420	70	tr
Cheese Streusel	½ muffin (2 oz)	220	25	tr
Low Fat Wild Blueberry	1 (2.25 oz)	200	35	tr
Mayport Almond Poppy Seed	½ muffin (2 oz)	210	40	tr
Mayport Banana Nut	1 (2.25 oz)	270	30	tr
Mayport Chocolate Chip	½ muffin (2 oz)	240	35	tr
Mayport Chocolate Chocolate Chip	1 (2.25 oz)	260	40	1
Mayport Cinnamon Spice	½ muffin (2 oz)	230	40	1
Mayport Corn	½ muffin (2 oz)	230	50	0
Mayport Harvest Bran	1 (2.25 oz)	240	35	3
Mayport Lemon	½ muffin (2 oz)	230	40	1
Mayport Low Fat Apple Cinnamon	1 (4 oz)	380	65	1
Mayport Low Fat Banana Nut	1 (4 oz)	350	65	1
Mayport Orange	½ muffin (2 oz)	230	40	tr
Mayport Pineapple	½ muffin (2 oz)	210	40	1
Mayport Wild Blueberry	1 (2.25 oz)	230	45	1
Uncle Wally's				
Chocolate Passion	1 (2 oz)	130	0	1
Cranberry Orange Supreme	1 (2 oz)	130	0	1
Fat Free Apple Cinnamon Delight	1 (2 oz)	110	0	1
Fat Free Wild Blueberry Bliss	1 (2 oz)	120	0	1
Golden Waves Of Corn	1 (2 oz)	120	0	1
Honey Raisin Bran	1 (2 oz)	130	0	1
No Nut Banana	1 (2 oz)	130	0	1
VitaMuffin				
Apple Berry Bran	1 (2 oz)	100	0	5
Blue Bran	1 (2 oz)	100	0	4
Cran Bran	1 (2 oz)	100	0	4
Deep Chocolate	1 (4 oz)	200	0	12
Multi Bran	1 (2 oz)	100	0	4
VitaTops Apple Berry Bran	1 (2 oz)	100	0	5
VitaTops Blue Bran	1 (2 oz)	100	0	4
VitaTops Cran Bran	1 (2 oz)	100	0	4

FOOD	PORTION	CALS	CHOL	FIBER
VitaTops Deep Chocolate	1 (2 oz)	100	0	6
VitaTops MultiBran	1 (2 oz)	100	0	4
Weight Watchers				
Low Fat Chocolate Chip	1 (2.5 oz)	180	0	2
TAKE-OUT				
corn	1 lg (2.5 oz)	214	31	2
raisin bran lowfat	1 (4 oz)	270	0	5

MULBERRIES
fresh	1 cup	61	0	–

MULLET
striped cooked	3 oz	127	54	0
striped raw	3 oz	99	42	0

MUNG BEANS
dried cooked	1 cup	213	0	–

MUNGO BEANS
dried cooked	1 cup	190	1	–

MUSHROOMS
FOOD	PORTION	CALS	CHOL	FIBER
CANNED				
caps	8 (1.6 oz)	12	0	1
caps pickled	6 (0.8 oz)	5	0	tr
chanterelle	3.5 oz	12	0	6
pickled	1 cup	33	0	1
pieces	½ cup	20	0	1
straw	1 cup	58	0	5
Green Giant				
Pieces & Stems	½ cup	30	0	2
Sunny Dell				
Portabella Sliced	½ cup	20	0	2
DRIED				
chanterelle	1 oz	25	0	17
shiitake	1 (3.6 g)	11	0	tr
tree ear	½ cup (0.4 oz)	36	0	–
Eden				
Maitake Sliced	10 pieces (0.3 oz)	35	0	4
Shitake	3 (0.4 oz)	35	0	5
Shitake Sliced	3 pieces (0.3 oz)	35	0	5

FOOD	PORTION	CALS	CHOL	FIBER
Frieda's				
Chanterelle	2 pieces (4 g)	15	0	1
Wood Ear	3 pieces (4 g)	15	0	1
FRESH				
brown italian or crimini sliced	1 cup	19	0	tr
brown italian or crimini whole	1 (0.7 oz)	5	0	tr
chanterelle	3.5 oz	11	0	6
enoki raw	1 lg (5 g)	2	0	tr
enoki sliced	1 cup	29	0	2
enoki whole	1 cup	28	0	2
maitake diced	1 cup	26	0	2
maitake whole	1 (6.6 g)	2	0	tr
morel	3.5 oz	9	0	7
oyster	1 sm (0.5 oz)	5	0	tr
oyster sliced	1 cup	30	0	2
portabella raw	1 cap (3 oz)	22	0	1
portabella sliced grilled	1 cup (4.2 oz)	42	0	3
raw sliced	½ cup	8	0	tr
shiitake pieces cooked	1 cup	81	0	3
shitake cooked	4 (2.5 oz)	40	0	2
white	1 (0.6 oz)	4	0	tr
white sliced cooked	1 cup	28	0	2
Frieda's				
Enoki	¼ pkg (1 oz)	10	0	1
FROZEN				
Alexia				
Mushroom Bites	1 serv (2 oz)	110	0	1
TAKE-OUT				
battered fried	1 lg (0.6 oz)	39	1	tr
creamed	1 cup	171	7	3
stuffed	1 (0.8 oz)	67	3	1
MUSSELS				
blue raw	3 oz	73	24	–
blue raw	1 cup	129	42	–
fresh blue cooked	3 oz	147	48	–
MUSTARD				
dry mustard	1 tsp	15	0	–

FOOD	PORTION	CALS	CHOL	FIBER
organic yellow	1 tsp	5	0	0
yellow ready-to-use	1 tsp	5	0	–
Annie's Naturals				
Organic Horseradish Mustard	1 tsp	5	0	–
Boar's Head				
Delicatessen Style	1 tsp (5 g)	0	0	0
Honey	1 tsp (5 g)	10	0	0
Country Cupboard				
Smokey Garlic or Horseradish	1 tsp	10	0	0
Eden				
Organic Brown	1 tsp	0	0	0
Yellow	1 tsp	0	0	0
Emeril's				
Horseradish	1 tbsp	5	0	0
Smooth Honey	1 tbsp	10	0	–
French's				
Classic Yellow	1 tsp	0	0	0
Honey	1 tsp	10	0	–
Honey Dijon	1 tsp	10	0	–
Horseradish	1 tsp	5	0	0
Spicy Brown	1 tsp	5	0	0
Gulden's				
Spicy Brown	1 tsp	5	0	0
Hebrew National				
Deli	1 tsp	4	0	0
Hunt's				
Mustard	1 tsp (5 g)	3	0	tr
Kosciusko				
Spicy Brown	1 tsp	0	0	0
Luzianne				
Creole Mustard	1 tbsp	10	0	0
Sara Lee				
Country Honey	1 tbsp	10	0	0
Cranberry Honey	1 tbsp	10	0	0
Tree Of Life				
Dijon	1 tsp (5 g)	0	0	–
Dijon Imported	1 tsp (5 g)	5	0	–
Stone Ground	1 tsp (5 g)	0	0	–
Yellow	1 tsp (5 g)	0	0	–

FOOD	PORTION	CALS	CHOL	FIBER
Wild Thyme Farms				
Chili Pepper Garlic	1 tsp	5	0	–
Dill Horseradish	1 tsp	5	0	–
MUSTARD GREENS				
fresh chopped cooked	½ cup	11	0	–
fresh raw chopped	½ cup	7	0	–
frozen chopped cooked	½ cup	14	0	–
Allen's				
Seasoned Southern Style	½ cup	30	0	2
Glory				
Seasoned canned	½ cup	35	0	1
NATTO				
natto	½ cup	187	0	–
NAVY BEANS				
CANNED				
navy	1 cup	296	0	–
Eden				
Organic	½ cup	110	0	7
DRIED				
cooked	1 cup	259	0	–
NECTARINE				
fresh	1	67	0	2
Chiquita				
Fresh	1 med (4.9 oz)	70	0	2
Sunsweet				
Dried	3 pieces (1.4 oz)	100	0	3
NEUFCHATEL				
neufchatel	1 oz	74	22	–
neufchatel	1 pkg (3 oz)	221	65	–
Back To Nature				
Organic	⅛ pkg (1 oz)	70	20	0
Organic Valley				
Neufchatel	1 oz	70	20	0
NOODLE DISHES (*see also* PASTA DINNERS)				
TAKE-OUT				
bami goreng indonesian noodle dish	1 cup	170	0	4

FOOD	PORTION	CALS	CHOL	FIBER
NOODLES				
cellophane	1 cup	492	0	–
chow mein	1 cup (1.6 oz)	237	0	2
egg	1 cup (38 g)	145	36	–
egg cooked	1 cup (5.6 oz)	213	53	2
japanese soba cooked	1 cup (4 oz)	113	0	–
japanese somen cooked	1 cup (6.2 oz)	231	0	–
rice cooked	1 cup (6.2 oz)	192	0	2
spinach/egg cooked	1 cup (5.6 oz)	211	53	4
A Taste Of Thai				
Rice Wide	2 oz	200	0	2
Annie Chun's				
Chow Mein	2 oz	200	0	3
Noodle Bowl Teriyaki	1 pkg	310	0	2
Noodle Express Chinese Chow Mein	½ pkg	160	0	1
Noodle Express Singapore Curry	½ pkg	160	0	2
Noodle Express Spicy Szechuan	½ pkg	170	0	1
Noodle Express Teriyaki	½ pkg	160	0	1
Noodle Express Thai Peanut	½ pkg	200	0	1
Rice	2 oz	210	0	0
Rice Pad Thai	2 oz	210	0	0
Azumaya				
Asian Style Thin Cut	1 cup	210	0	2
Chun King				
Chow Mein	½ cup (1 oz)	137	0	1
Hodgson Mill				
Egg Whole Wheat not prep	2 oz	190	30	4
La Choy				
Chow Mein	½ cup (1 oz)	137	0	1
Chow Mein Crispy Wide	½ cup (1 oz)	148	0	1
Rice	½ cup (1 oz)	121	0	tr
Manischewitz				
Egg Medium	1¼ cups	220	65	2
Fine Yolk Free	1½ cups	210	0	2
Fine Egg	1½ cups	220	65	2
Wide Yolk Free	1¾ cups	210	0	2

FOOD	PORTION	CALS	CHOL	FIBER
Nasoya				
Chinese	1 cup	210	0	2
Japanese	1 cup	210	0	2
No Yolks				
Extra Broad	2 oz	210	0	3
Pennsylvania Dutch				
Yolk Free Ribbons as prep	1½ cups	210	0	2

NUTMEG

ground	1 tsp	12	0	–

NUTRITION SUPPLEMENTS (see also CEREAL BARS, ENERGY BARS, ENERGY DRINKS)

FOOD	PORTION	CALS	CHOL	FIBER
Amino Vital				
Jel All Flavors	1 pkg (4.9 oz)	70	0	1
Boost				
Breeze	8 oz	160	0	–
Clif				
Shot Energy Gel All Flavors	1 pkg (1.1 oz)	100	0	0
DiabetiTrim				
Shake French Vanilla	1 pkg	90	5	4
Enlive!				
Drink All Flavors	1 box (8.1 oz)	300	<5	0
Ensure				
Creamy Milk Chocolate Shake	1 can (8 oz)	350	<5	tr
Plus Vanilla Shake	1 bottle (8 oz)	350	<5	0
GeniSoy				
Soy Natural Protein Powder	1 scoop (1 oz)	100	0	0
Glucerna				
Shakes All Flavors	1 can (8 oz)	220	<5	3
Jelly Belly				
Sport Beans Berry Blue	1 pkg (1 oz)	100	0	0
Joint Juice				
Tropical Fruit	1 can (8 oz)	30	0	–
Kindercal				
Vanilla	1 can (8 oz)	250	5	0
Met-Rx				
Lite	1 pkg (1.6 oz)	170	30	1
Original	1 pkg (2.5 oz)	250	15	tr

FOOD	PORTION	CALS	CHOL	FIBER
Protein Shake	1 can	200	10	2
Ultra	1 pkg (2.6 oz)	250	50	2
Nestle				
Additions	2⅓ tsp (0.7 oz)	100	0	0
PermaLean				
Protein Powder Bodacious Berry	1 scoop (1 oz)	104	0	–
Protein Powder Chocoholic Chocolate	1 scoop (1 oz)	104	0	–
Pounds Off				
All Flavors	1 bar (2.1 oz)	210	0	2
PowerBar				
Powergel All Flavors	1 pkg (1.4 oz)	120	0	–
Pria				
Complete Shake Creamy Milk Chocolate	1 pkg (11.6 oz)	170	10	7
Complete Shake French Vanilla	1 pkg (11.6 oz)	170	10	7
Resource				
Beneprotein Protein Powder	1 scoop	25	0	0
Optisource High Protein Drink	1 box (4 oz)	100	<5	0
Slim-Fast				
Optima Ready-To-Drink Creamy Milk Chocolate	1 can (11 oz)	190	5	5
Optima Shake Mix Chocolate Royale as prep with fat free milk	1 serv	190	5	4
Optima Shake Mix French Vanilla as prep w/ fat free milk	1 serv	200	5	4
Vitasoy				
Weight Management Meal All Flavors	1 bottle (10 oz)	200	0	8
NUTS MIXED (see also individual names)				
dry roasted w/ peanuts salted	¼ cup	203	0	3
dry roasted w/ peanuts w/o salt	¼ cup	203	0	3

FOOD	PORTION	CALS	CHOL	FIBER
mixed nuts chocolate covered	¼ cup (1.5 oz)	240	5	2
oil roasted w/o peanuts salted	¼ cup	221	0	2
oil roasted w/o peanuts w/o salt	¼ cup	221	0	2
Estee				
Chocolate Covered Fruit & Nut Mix Fructose Sweetened	¼ cup	210	<5	2
Good Sense				
Deluxe Mix	¼ cup	180	0	2
Here's Howe				
Royal Mixed Nuts	1 oz	180	0	2
Judy's				
Sugar Free Mixed Nut Brittle	¼ piece (1 oz)	120	<5	tr
Kind				
Nut Delight	1 bar (1.4 oz)	203	0	3
Maranatha				
Cashew Macadamia Butter	2 tbsp	210	0	2
Tamari Organic	¼ cup	160	0	2
Tamari Roasted	¼ cup	160	0	2
Mauna Loa				
Macadamia Mixed	¼ cup	190	0	2
Macadamias & Cashews	¼ cup	180	0	1
Organic Trails				
Tamari Roasted Nuts & Seeds	¼ cup	190	0	5
Peanut Better				
Mixed Nut Butter Creamy & Crunchy	2 tbsp	190	0	3
Planters				
Nut-rition Energy Mix	¼ cup	180	0	3
Nut-rition Heart Healthy Mix	1 (0.9 oz)	170	0	3
OCA				
Frieda's				
Oca	½ cup	70	0	1
OCTOPUS				
fresh steamed	3 oz	140	82	–

FOOD	PORTION	CALS	CHOL	FIBER
OHELOBERRIES				
fresh	1 cup	39	0	–
OIL				
almond	1 tbsp	120	0	0
almond	1 cup	1927	0	0
apricot kernel	1 tbsp	120	0	0
apricot kernel	1 cup	1927	0	0
avocado	1 cup	1927	0	0
avocado	1 tbsp	124	0	0
babassu palm	1 tbsp	120	0	0
butter oil	1 cup	1795	524	0
butter oil	1 tbsp	112	33	0
canola	1 cup	1927	0	0
canola	1 tbsp	124	0	0
coconut	1 tbsp	117	0	0
corn	1 tbsp	120	0	0
corn	1 cup	1927	0	0
cottonseed	1 cup	1927	0	0
cottonseed	1 tbsp	120	0	0
cupu assu	1 tbsp	120	0	0
garlic oil	1 tbsp	150	0	0
grapeseed	1 tbsp	120	0	0
hazelnut	1 cup	1927	0	0
hazelnut	1 tbsp	120	0	0
mustard	1 tbsp	124	0	0
mustard	1 cup	1927	0	0
oat	1 tbsp	120	0	0
olive	1 cup	1909	0	0
olive	1 tbsp	119	0	0
palm	1 cup	1927	0	0
palm	1 tbsp	120	0	0
palm kernel	1 tbsp	117	0	0
palm kernel	1 cup	1879	0	0
peanut	1 cup	1909	0	0
peanut	1 tbsp	119	0	0
peppermint	1 tsp	42	0	0
poppyseed	1 tbsp	120	0	0
rice bran	1 tbsp	120	0	0
safflower	1 cup	1927	0	0

FOOD	PORTION	CALS	CHOL	FIBER
safflower	1 tbsp	120	0	0
sesame	1 tbsp	120	0	0
sheanut	1 tbsp	120	0	0
soybean	1 cup	1927	0	0
soybean	1 tbsp	120	0	0
soybean organic	1 tbsp	120	0	0
sunflower	1 tbsp	120	0	0
sunflower	1 cup	1927	0	0
teaseed	1 tbsp	120	0	0
tomatoseed	1 tbsp	120	0	0
vegetable	1 cup	1927	0	0
vegetable	1 tbsp	120	0	0
walnut	1 tbsp	120	0	0
walnut	1 cup	1927	0	0
wheat germ	1 tbsp	120	0	0
Alpha				
Hazelnut	1 oz	257	0	0
Asoyia				
Soybean Ultra Low Lin	1 tbsp	129	0	0
Botticelli				
Olive	1 tbsp	120	0	0
Carapelli				
Grapeseed	1 tbsp	120	0	0
Olive Extra Virgin	1 tbsp	120	0	0
Consorzio				
Dipping Oil	1 tbsp	120	0	–
Olive Basil	1 tbsp	120	0	0
Olive Roasted Pepper	1 tbsp	120	0	0
Organic Extra Virgin Olive Meyer Lemon	1 tbsp	120	0	0
Eden				
Olive Extra Virgin	1 tbsp	120	0	0
Organic Safflower	1 tbsp	120	0	0
Organic Soybean	1 tbsp	120	0	0
Toasted Sesame	1 tbsp	120	0	0
Enova				
Oil	1 tbsp	120	0	0
Hollywood				
Safflower	1 tbsp	120	0	0

FOOD	PORTION	CALS	CHOL	FIBER
House Of Tsang				
Mongolian Fire	1 tsp	45	0	0
Wok Oil	1 tbsp	130	0	0
Iowa Natural				
Soybean 1% Linolenic	1 tbsp	129	0	0
Loriva				
5 Pepper Hot	1 tbsp	120	0	–
Avocado	1 tbsp	120	0	–
Basil Flavored	1 tbsp	120	0	–
Canola	1 tbsp	120	0	–
Canolive	1 tbsp	120	0	–
Garlic Flavored	1 tbsp	120	0	–
Grapeseed	1 tbsp	120	0	–
Olive	1 tbsp	120	0	–
Olive Organic Extra Virgin	1 tbsp	120	0	–
Peanut	1 tbsp	120	0	–
Rice Bran	1 tbsp	120	0	–
Safflower	1 tbsp	120	0	–
Sesame	1 tbsp	120	0	–
Sunflower	1 tbsp	120	0	–
Toasted Sesame	1 tbsp	120	0	–
Walnut	1 tbsp	120	0	–
Mazola				
Corn	1 tbsp	120	0	0
No Stick Spray	⅓ sec spray	0	0	0
Pure Cooking Spray Canola All Flavors	¼ sec spray	0	0	0
Right Blend	1 tbsp	120	0	0
Vegetable	1 tbsp	120	0	0
Monini				
Olive Extra Virgin	1 tbsp	118	0	0
Nutiva				
Organic Coconut Extra Virgin	1 tbsp	120	0	0
Organic Hemp Cold Pressed	1 tbsp	120	0	0
Nutrium				
Soybean Low Linolenic	1 tbsp	129	0	0
Olivo				
Spray Olive Oil 100% Extra Virgin	⅓ sec spray	0	0	0

FOOD	PORTION	CALS	CHOL	FIBER
Orville Redenbacher's				
Popping & Topping	1 tbsp	120	0	0
Pacifica Culinaria				
Avocado	1 tbsp	120	0	−
Avocado Blood Orange	1 tbsp	120	0	−
Pam				
Cooking Spray All Types	⅓ sec spray	0	0	0
Pompeian				
Olive	1 tbsp	130	0	−
Progresso				
Olive Extra Mild	1 tbsp (0.5 oz)	120	0	0
Olive Extra Virgin	1 tbsp (0.5 oz)	120	0	0
Olive Riviera Blend	1 tbsp (0.5 oz)	120	0	0
Smart Balance				
Omega Oil	1 tbsp	120	0	0
Spectrum				
Almond	1 tbsp	120	0	0
Apricot Kernel	1 tbsp	120	0	0
Avocado	1 tbsp	120	0	0
Canola Organic	1 tbsp	120	0	0
Coconut Organic	1 tbsp	120	0	0
Corn	1 tbsp	120	2	0
Grapeseed	1 tbsp	120	1	0
Grapeseed Oil Spray	⅓ sec spray	0	0	0
Hazelnut Toasted Organic	1 tbsp	120	0	0
Mediterranean Olive Organic	1 tbsp	120	0	0
Organic Extra Virgin Oil Spray	⅓ sec spray	0	0	0
Peanut	1 tbsp	120	0	0
Pumpkin Seed Organic	1 tbsp	120	0	0
Sesame Organic	1 tbsp	120	0	0
Sesame Toasted Organic	1 tbsp	120	0	0
Soy Organic	1 tbsp	120	0	0
Sunflower Organic	1 tbsp	120	0	0
Walnut	1 tbsp	120	0	0
Walnut Organic	1 tbsp	120	0	0
Tree Of Life				
Olive Extra Virgin Organic	1 tbsp (0.5 g)	130	0	−

FOOD	PORTION	CALS	CHOL	FIBER
Vistive				
Soybean Low Linolenic	1 tbsp	129	0	0
Wesson				
Canola	1 tbsp	120	1	0
OKRA				
CANNED				
pickled	6 pods (2.3 oz)	18	0	2
Glory				
Cut	½ cup	25	0	2
FRESH				
cooked w/ salt	8 pods	19	0	2
luffa chinese okra cooked	1 cup	39	0	4
sliced cooked w/ salt	½ cup	18	0	2
FROZEN				
McKenzie's				
Breaded Okra	1 serv (2.8 oz)	90	0	–
Cut	1 serv (3 oz)	25	0	3
TAKE-OUT				
batter dipped fried	10 pieces (2.6 oz)	142	2	2
OLIVES				
green	3 extra lg	15	0	tr
green	4 med	15	0	tr
green olive tapenade	1 tbsp	25	0	0
ripe	1 sm	4	0	tr
ripe	1 lg	5	0	tr
ripe	1 jumbo	7	0	–
ripe	1 colossal	12	0	–
spanish stuffed	5 (0.5 oz)	15	0	0
Peloponnese				
Amfissa	3	45	0	0
Ionian Green	3	25	0	0
Kalamata Pitted	5	45	0	0
Kalamata Spread	1 tsp	15	0	0
Progresso				
Olive Salad (drained)	2 tbsp (0.8 oz)	25	0	tr
Vlasic				
Ripe Colossal Pitted	2 (0.6 oz)	20	0	0
Ripe Jumbo Pitted	3 (0.6 oz)	25	0	0
Ripe Large Pitted	4 (0.5 oz)	25	0	0

FOOD	PORTION	CALS	CHOL	FIBER
Ripe Medium Pitted	5 (0.5 oz)	25	0	0
Ripe Sliced	¼ cup (0.5 oz)	25	0	0
Ripe Small Pitted	6 (0.5 oz)	25	0	0

ONION
CANNED
cocktail	½ cup	41	0	2

Boar's Head
Sweet Vidalia In Sauce	1 tbsp	10	0	0

French's
Original French Fried	2 tbsp	45	0	0

DRIED
flakes	1 tbsp	17	0	1
powder	1 tsp	7	0	tr
shallots	1 tbsp	3	0	–

FRESH
cooked w/o salt	1 sm (2 oz)	26	0	1
cooked w/o salt	1 med (3.3 oz)	41	0	1
cooked w/o salt	1 lg (4.5 oz)	56	0	2
cooked w/o salt chopped	1 tbsp	7	0	tr
raw chopped	1 tbsp	4	0	tr
raw chopped	½ cup	32	0	1
raw slice	1 (0.5 oz)	6	0	tr
raw sliced	½ cup	23	0	1
scallions raw	1 med (0.5 oz)	5	0	tr
scallions raw chopped	¼ cup	8	0	1
shallots raw chopped	¼ cup	29	0	–
sweet whole raw	1 (11.6 oz)	106	0	3
whole raw	1 sm (2.5 oz)	28	0	1
whole raw	1 med (4 oz)	44	0	2
whole raw	1 lg (5.3 oz)	60	0	3

Antioch Farms
Vidalia	1 med	60	0	3

Arrowfarms
Cipoline	2 (1.1 oz)	20	0	5

Earthbound Farm
Organic Green Onions	¼ cup	10	0	1
Organic Red	1 med (5.2 oz)	60	0	3

Frieda's
Cipolline	3 (3 oz)	30	0	2

FOOD	PORTION	CALS	CHOL	FIBER
Maui	⅓ cup (1.1 oz)	10	0	1
Pearl	⅔ cup (3 oz)	30	0	2
Nature's Harvest				
Onion	1 med (5.2 oz)	60	0	3
OsoSweet				
Onion	1 med (5 oz)	60	0	3
FROZEN				
Alexia				
Onion Rings	6 (3 oz)	230	0	4
C&W				
Petite Whole	⅔ cup (3 oz)	30	0	tr
Ian's				
Rings & Strings	5-9 pieces (2.5 oz)	152	0	1
McKenzie's				
Onion Rounds	1 serv (3.2 oz)	220	0	6
TAKE-OUT				
creamed	1 cup	187	7	2
fried	½ cup	57	0	1
rings breaded & fried	8 to 9 (3 oz)	276	14	–

ORANGE
CANNED
Del Monte

FOOD	PORTION	CALS	CHOL	FIBER
SunFresh Mandarin	½ cup	80	0	tr
Dole				
Fruit Bowls Mandarin Oranges	1 pkg	70	0	0
FRESH				
california navel	1	65	0	3
california valencia	1	59	0	3
florida	1	69	0	4
peel	1 tbsp	6	0	–
sections	1 cup	85	0	4
Frieda's				
Cara Cara	1 med (5 oz)	70	0	3
Mandarin Delite	1 cup (5 oz)	60	0	3
Mandarin Page	1 cup (5 oz)	60	0	3
Mandarin Pixie	1 cup (5 oz)	60	0	3
Mandarin Satsuma	1 (5 oz)	60	0	3
Melogold	½ (6 oz)	50	0	2
Seville	1 (3 oz)	40	0	2

FOOD	PORTION	CALS	CHOL	FIBER
Sunkist				
Cara Cara Navel	1 med	80	0	7
Minneola Tangelo	1 (3.8 oz)	70	0	2
Moro	1 (5.4 oz)	70	0	3
Orange	1 med	80	0	7
Satsuma Mandarin	1 (3.8 oz)	50	0	2
ORANGE EXTRACT				
Virginia Dare				
Extract	1 tsp	22	0	–
ORANGE JUICE				
canned	1 cup	104	0	–
chilled	1 cup	110	0	–
fresh	1 cup	111	0	–
frzn as prep	1 cup	112	0	1
frzn not prep	6 oz	339	0	2
orange drink	6 oz	94	0	–
After The Fall				
24 Karrot Orange	8 oz	120	0	–
Big Juicy				
Drink	8 oz	110	0	–
Bright & Early				
Orange Drink	8 oz	110	0	–
Crystal Light				
Sunrise Sunrise Sugar Free Mix as prep	1 serv	5	0	0
Dole				
100% Juice	8 oz	110	0	–
Florida's Natural				
Calcium & Vitamin D	8 oz	110	0	0
Fresh Samantha				
Juice	1 cup (8 oz)	100	0	0
Hi-C				
Blast Orange Drink	8 oz	120	0	–
Orange Lavaburst	1 box	90	0	–
Hood				
100% Juice	1 cup	120	0	0
Italian Volcano				
Blood Orange Organic	1 serv (6.75 oz)	84	0	1

FOOD	PORTION	CALS	CHOL	FIBER
Juicy Juice				
Punch	1 box (4.23 oz)	60	0	0
Punch	1 box (8.45 oz)	130	0	0
Minute Maid				
Country Style	8 oz	110	0	–
Heart Wise	8 oz	110	0	–
Kids+	8 oz	110	0	–
Light	8 oz	50	0	–
Original	8 oz	110	0	–
Plus Calcium	8 oz	110	0	–
W/ Extra Vitamin C & E Plus Zinc	8 oz	110	0	–
Mott's				
100% Juice	8 oz	130	0	–
100% Juice	1 box (8 oz)	130	0	–
Naked Juice				
Just OJ	8 oz	110	0	0
Ocean Spray				
100% Juice	8 oz	120	0	0
Odwalla				
Organic	8 oz	110	0	–
Simply Orange				
Calcium Pulp Free	8 oz	110	0	–
Snapple				
Orangeade	8 oz	120	0	–
Tang				
Orange Drink as prep	1 serv	90	0	0
Sugar Free Orange as prep	1 serv (8 oz)	5	0	0
Tropicana				
Antioxidant Advantage	8 oz	110	0	0
Calcium + Vitamin D	8 oz	110	0	0
Fiber	8 oz	120	0	3
Healthy Heart	8 oz	120	0	0
Healthy Kids	8 oz	110	0	0
Light 'n Healthy w/ Calcium	8 oz	50	0	0
Light'N Healthy w/ Pulp	8 oz	50	0	0
No Pulp	8 oz	110	0	0
Orangeade	8 oz	111	0	0
Turkey Hill				
Orangeade	1 cup	120	0	–

FOOD	PORTION	CALS	CHOL	FIBER
Welsh Farms				
Juice	8 oz	110	0	–
TAKE-OUT				
orange julius	1 serv (24 oz)	443	0	1

OREGANO
ground	1 tsp	5	0	–

ORGAN MEATS (*see* BRAINS, GIBLETS, GIZZARD, HEART, KIDNEY, LIVER, SWEETBREAD)

OSTRICH
cooked	3 oz	120	74	–

OYSTERS
canned eastern	1 cup	112	89	0
eastern baked	6 med	47	22	0
eastern raw	6 med	50	21	0
eastern sauteed	6 med	76	36	0
smoked	6	33	26	0
Brunswick				
Smoked	1 can (3 oz)	140	23	1
Bumble Bee				
Smoked	¼ cup	120	35	0
Whole	¼ cup	70	45	0
Chicken Of The Sea				
Smoked In Oil	1 can (3.75 oz)	140	45	–
Smoked In Water	1 can (3.75 oz)	120	55	0
Smoked Teriyaki	1 can (3.75 oz)	120	55	1
Whole	½ can (2 oz)	80	35	0
TAKE-OUT				
breaded & fried	6	368	108	–
fritter	1 (1.4 oz)	121	36	tr
oysters rockefeller	1 cup	302	90	4
stew	1 cup	208	78	0

PANCAKE/WAFFLE SYRUP
lite	¼ cup	98	0	0
pancake syrup	¼ cup	209	0	0
Atkins				
Sugar Free	¼ cup	0	0	0
Aunt Jemima				
Original	¼ cup	210	0	–

FOOD	PORTION	CALS	CHOL	FIBER
Country Cupboard				
Boysenberry	¼ cup	0	0	0
Maple Butter	¼ cup	0	0	0
Strawberry	¼ cup	0	0	0
Eggo				
Lite	¼ cup	110	0	–
Original	¼ cup	240	0	–
Estee				
Maple	¼ cup	30	0	–
Hungry Jack				
Lite	¼ cup	100	0	0
Original	¼ cup	210	0	0
Karo				
Pancake Syrup	¼ cup	240	0	–
Keto				
Maple Butter	¼ cup	0	0	0
Ketogenics				
Zero Carb	¼ cup	0	0	0
Log Cabin				
Lite	¼ cup	100	0	–
Original	¼ cup	210	0	0
Mrs. Butterworth's				
Lite	¼ cup	100	0	–
Original	¼ cup (2 oz)	230	0	–
Smucker's				
Breakfast Syrup Sugar Free	¼ cup	30	0	–
Stonewall Kitchen				
Maine Maple	¼ cup	210	0	0

PANCAKES
FROZEN

FOOD	PORTION	CALS	CHOL	FIBER
Eggo				
Buttermilk	3	280	15	1
Minis	11	260	10	1
Golden				
Potato	1 (1.3 oz)	70	5	1
Ian's				
Blueberry	1 (1.3 oz)	100	<5	1
Pancake	1 (1.3 oz)	100	<5	1

FOOD	PORTION	CALS	CHOL	FIBER
Inland Valley				
Potato	1 (2 oz)	120	20	2
McCain				
Homestyle BabyCakes	4 pieces (2.6 oz)	150	0	2
MIX				
Atkins				
Quick Quisine Buttermilk not prep	⅓ cup	100	0	5
Quick Quisine Original not prep	¼ cup	80	5	3
Aunt Jemima				
Buttermilk Pancake & Waffle Mix not prep	⅓ cup	160	10	1
Pancake & Waffle Mix Whole Wheat as prep	3 pancakes	200	57	3
Aunt Paula's				
Pancake & Waffle Mix as prep	2	132	0	4
Betty Crocker				
Buttermilk as prep	3	200	10	1
Original as prep	3	200	10	2
Big Train				
Low Carb Pancake & Waffle Mix as prep	3	190	108	5
Bisquick				
Shake 'N Pour Blueberry as prep	3	210	0	1
Bruce				
Sweet Potato Pancakes	2	210	0	2
Carbsense				
Buckwheat not prep	½ cup	140	0	7
Buttermilk not prep	½ cup	140	0	7
Don's Chuck Wagon				
Buckwheat Mix	⅓ cup	160	0	1
Hodgson Mill				
Buckwheat not prep	⅓ cup	140	0	3
Whole Wheat Buttermilk not prep	⅓ cup	120	0	4
Ketogenics				
Low Carb not prep	⅔ cup	185	94	6

FOOD	PORTION	CALS	CHOL	FIBER
King Arthur				
Multi-Grain Buttermilk not prep	6 tbsp	160	5	5
MiniCarb				
Apple Cinnamon as prep	2	150	10	13
TAKE-OUT				
buckwheat	1 (7 in)	142	45	2
plain	1 (7 in)	183	7	1
potato	1 (1.3 oz)	70	26	1
w/ butter & syrup	2 (8.1 oz)	520	58	–
whole wheat	1 (7 in)	183	47	3

PANCREAS (see SWEETBREAD)

PAPAYA

fresh	1	117	0	–
Del Monte				
In Extra Light Syrup w/ Passion Fruit Puree	½ cup	70	0	1
Frieda's				
Mexican	1 cup (5 oz)	50	0	3

PAPAYA JUICE

nectar	1 cup	142	0	–
Ceres				
Papaya	8 oz	120	0	0
Langers				
Papaya Delight 100% Juice	8 oz	130	0	1
Nantucket Nectars				
Cocktail	8 oz	120	0	–

PAPRIKA

paprika	1 tsp	6	0	–

PARSLEY

dry	1 tbsp	1	0	–
fresh chopped	½ cup	11	0	–
Dorot				
Chopped Cubes frzn	1 cube (4 g)	5	0	tr
Frieda's				
Parsley Root	⅔ cup	10	0	1

FOOD	PORTION	CALS	CHOL	FIBER
PARSNIPS				
fresh cooked	1 (5.6 oz)	130	0	–
fresh sliced cooked	½ cup	63	0	–
raw sliced	½ cup	50	0	–
Frieda's				
Sliced	1 cup	100	0	7
PASSION FRUIT				
purple fresh	1	18	0	–
PASSION FRUIT JUICE				
purple	1 cup	126	0	–
yellow	1 cup	149	0	–
Ceres				
Passion Fruit	8 oz	120	0	0
PASTA (*see also* NOODLES, PASTA DINNERS, PASTA SALAD)				
DRY				
corn cooked	1 cup (4.9 oz)	176	0	7
corn spaghetti	2 oz	180	0	3
elbows	1 cup	389	0	–
elbows cooked	1 cup (4.9 oz)	197	0	2
shells small cooked	1 cup (4 oz)	162	0	2
spaghetti cooked	1 cup (4.9 oz)	197	0	2
spinach spaghetti cooked	1 cup (4.9 oz)	182	0	–
spirals cooked	1 cup (4.7 oz)	189	0	2
vegetable cooked	1 cup (4.7 oz)	172	0	6
whole wheat all shapes cooked	1 cup	174	0	4
Annie Chun's				
Soba Noodles	2 oz	200	0	3
Atkins				
All Shapes not prep	2 oz	230	0	9
Quick Quisine All Shapes as prep	¾ cup	210	0	8
Barilla				
Pastina	2 oz	210	65	2
Penne	1 cup (2 oz)	200	0	2
Plus Penne	2 oz	200	0	4
Tortelloni Porcini Mushroom	¾ cup	240	50	5

FOOD	PORTION	CALS	CHOL	FIBER
Tortelloni Ricotta & Asparagus	¾ cup	240	60	5
Tortelloni Ricotta & Spinach	¾ cup	240	50	4
Bella Vita				
Low Carb Penne Rigate	2 oz	190	0	8
Catelli				
Bistro Cracked Black Pepper Fettucine	¼ pkg	320	0	2
Bistro Italian Herb Fettuccine	¼ pkg	310	0	3
Bistro Lemon Pepper Linguine	¼ pkg	320	0	3
Bistro Rainbows	3 oz	320	0	2
Bistro Spinach Lasagne	3 oz	320	0	3
Bistro Sun Dried Tomato & Basil Spaghettini	¼ pkg	320	0	3
Bistro Vegetable Fusilli	3 oz	320	0	2
Healthy Harvest Flax Omega-3	3 oz	290	0	6
Healthy Harvest Multigrain	3 oz	310	0	6
Healthy Harvest Organic Whole Wheat	3 oz	320	0	3
Healthy Harvest Whole Wheat All Shapes	3 oz	310	0	5
Darielle				
All Shapes not prep	2 oz	160	0	8
DaVinci				
Rotini	1 cup	210	0	2
Spaghetti	2 oz	210	0	2
DeCecco				
Spaghetti w/ Spinach	⅛ pkg (2 oz)	200	0	2
Dreamfields				
Lasagna not prep	2 pieces (2 oz)	190	0	5
Rotini not prep	⅔ cup (2 oz)	190	0	5
Due Amici				
Pasta Lite Low Carb Fusilli	2 oz	160	0	7
Eden				
Bifun Pasta not prep	2 oz	200	5	0
Harusame Pasta not prep	2 oz	190	0	0
Kudzu	2 oz	200	0	2

FOOD	PORTION	CALS	CHOL	FIBER
Organic Gemelli Spelt & Buckwheat not prep	½ cup (2 oz)	210	0	4
Organic Ribbons Artichoke not prep	½ cup (2 oz)	210	0	2
Organic Rigatoni Kamut & Buckwheat not prep	½ cup (2 oz)	200	0	5
Organic Spaghetti 100% Whole Wheat not prep	2 oz	210	0	6
Organic Spirals Flax Rice not prep	½ cup (2 oz)	200	0	4
Organic Spirals Kamut Vegetable not prep	½ cup (2 oz)	210	0	6
Organic Spirals Rye not prep	½ cup (2 oz)	200	0	8
Organic Spirals Spinach not prep	½ cup (2 oz)	210	0	5
Organic Udon not prep	¼ pkg	200	0	3
Organic Udon Spelt not prep	¼ pkg	200	0	2
Organic Vegetable Alphabets not prep	½ cup (2 oz)	210	0	4
Organic Vegetable Shells not prep	½ cup (2 oz)	210	0	4
Organic Ziti Rigati Spelt not prep	½ cup (2 oz)	210	0	5
Soba Japanese 100% Buckwheat not prep	2 oz	200	0	3
Soba Japanese Lotus Root not prep	2 oz	190	0	4
Soba Japanese Mugwort not prep	2 oz	190	0	2
Soba Japanese Wild Yam not prep	2 oz	190	0	2
Udon Japanese Brown Rice not prep	2 oz	190	0	2
Udon Japanese not prep	2 oz	190	0	3
Food For Life				
Ezekiel 4:9 Sprouted Grain	2 oz	210	0	7
Goya				
Coditos not prep	½ cup	230	0	3

FOOD	PORTION	CALS	CHOL	FIBER
Hodgson Mill				
Lasagne Whole Wheat not prep	2 oz	190	0	6
Organic Fettuccine Whole Wheat w/ Milled Flax Seed not prep	2 oz	200	0	6
Pasta Ribbons Whole Wheat not prep	2 oz	190	0	5
Spaghetti Whole Wheat not prep	2 oz	190	0	6
Veggie Bows not prep	2 oz	200	0	1
Wagon Wheels Veggie not prep	2 oz	200	0	1
Keto				
Elbows not prep	1.6 oz	108	0	1
Spaghetti not prep	1.3 oz	130	0	2
LifeStream				
Organic All Shapes	2 oz	208	0	8
Lundberg				
Spaghetti Organic Brown Rice	2 oz	210	0	3
Mueller's				
Elbow Macaroni not prep	½ cup	210	0	2
Multi Grain Rotini not prep	1 cup (2 oz)	190	0	5
Notta Pasta				
Rice Pasta All Shapes	2 oz	200	0	2
Real Torino				
Tirali not prep	1 cup (2 oz)	210	0	2
Revival				
Soy Penne	⅙ box	200	0	1
Soy Thin Spaghetti	⅙ box	200	0	1
Rice Select				
Orzo Original not prep	⅓ cup	210	0	–
Ronzoni				
Elbows not prep	½ cup (2 oz)	210	0	2
Healthy Harvest Multigrain Spaghetti	½ pkg (2 oz)	190	0	5
Healthy Harvest Whole Wheat Blend Spaghetti	½ pkg (2 oz)	180	0	6

FOOD	PORTION	CALS	CHOL	FIBER
Healthy Harvest Whole Wheat Rotini not prep	¾ cup (2 oz)	180	0	6
Lasagne	2½ pieces (2 oz)	210	0	2
San Giorgio				
Elbows not prep	½ cup	210	0	2
Soy7				
Pasta All Shapes	2 oz	200	0	2
Whey Cool				
High Protein Xtreme Rotini	1 serv (2 oz)	210	5	1
FRESH				
cooked	2 oz	75	33	–
spinach cooked	2 oz	74	19	–
REFRIGERATED				
Buitoni				
Angel Hair	1¼ cup	230	50	2
Fettuccine	1¼ cup	240	55	2
Fettuccine Spinach	1¼ cup	260	75	2
Linguine	1¼ cup	240	55	2
Ravioletti Three Cheese	1 cup	270	35	2
Ravioli Doublestuffed Mozzarella & Herb	1.5 cup	340	55	3
Ravioli Four Cheese	1¼ cups	330	60	3
Ravioli Chicken & Roasted Garlic	1¼ cup	340	50	2
Ravioli Chicken Parmesan	1¼ cup	310	55	2
Ravioli Classic Beef	1¼ cup	340	60	2
Ravioli Garden Vegetable	1 cup	250	40	2
Ravioli Light Four Cheese	1¼ cup	230	35	2
Tortellini Herb Chicken	1 cup	340	40	2
Tortellini Mixed Cheese	1 cup	320	60	3
Tortellini Spinach Cheese	1 cup	320	55	3
Tortellini Three Cheese	1 cup	320	40	3
Tortelloni Cheese & Roasted Garlic	1 cup	270	35	2
Tortelloni Chicken & Prosciutto	1 cup	320	40	2
Tortelloni Mozzarella & Herb	1 cup	330	40	2
Tortelloni Portabello Mushroom & Cheese	1 cup	290	25	3
Tortelloni Sun Dried Tomato	1 cup	310	25	3

FOOD	PORTION	CALS	CHOL	FIBER
Tortelloni Sweet Italian Sausage	1 cup	330	35	3

PASTA DINNERS (see also PASTA SALAD)
CANNED
Annie's Homegrown

FOOD	PORTION	CALS	CHOL	FIBER
Organic All Stars	1 cup	150	0	tr
Organic BernieOs	1 cup	150	0	tr
Organic Cheesy Ravioli	1 cup	180	5	3
Organic P'sghetti Loops	1 cup	190	0	2
Campbell's				
SpaghettiOs Sliced Franks	1 cup	230	20	5
Chef Boyardee				
99% Fat Free Beef Ravioli	1 cup	170	10	2
99% Fat Free Cheese Ravioli	1 cup (8.8 oz)	210	<5	4
Beef Ravioli	1 cup	240	15	3
Beefaroni	1 cup	260	25	3
Macaroni & Cheese	½ can (7.5 oz)	180	20	2
Mini Ravioli	1 cup	250	15	3
Spaghetti & Meat Balls	1 cup	270	20	2
Tortellini Cheese	½ can (7 oz)	230	15	5
Tortellini Meat	½ can (7 oz)	260	30	4
Franco-American				
Beef Raviolios	1 can (7.7 oz)	250	12	4
Beefy Mac	1 can (7.5 oz)	228	10	3
Elbow Macaroni & Cheese	1 can (7.5 oz)	187	7	2
Spaghetti 'N Beef	1 can (7.5 oz)	226	14	3
Spaghetti w/ Meatballs	1 can (7.2 oz)	249	14	4
Hunt's				
Noodles & Chicken	1 cup (8.7 oz)	176	37	2
Noodles & Beef	1 cup (8.7 oz)	151	17	5
Lunch Bucket				
Beef Ravioli In Tomato Sauce	1 pkg (7.5 oz)	180	5	3
Italian Pasta w/ Chicken	1 pkg (7.5 oz)	130	10	2
Lasagna 'n Meatsauce	1 pkg (7.5 oz)	160	5	2
Macaroni 'n Beef in Meatsauce	1 pkg (7.5 oz)	180	10	8
Macaroni'n Cheese	1 pkg (7.5 oz)	190	20	2
Pasta'n Chicken	1 pkg (7.5 oz)	150	20	2
Spaghetti'n Meatsauce	1 pkg (7.5 oz)	160	5	2

FOOD	PORTION	CALS	CHOL	FIBER
Progresso				
Beef Ravioli	1 cup (9.1 oz)	260	5	4
Cheese Ravioli	1 cup (9.1 oz)	220	<5	4
FROZEN				
Amy's				
Bowl Stuffed Pasta Shells	1 pkg (10 oz)	300	30	5
Cannelloni w/ Vegetables	1 pkg (9 oz)	330	15	6
Lasagna Cheese	1 pkg (10.25 oz)	330	35	5
Lasagna Garden Vegetable	1 pkg (10.25 oz)	290	20	5
Macaroni & Cheese	1 pkg (9 oz)	410	50	3
Macaroni & Soy Cheese	1 pkg (9 oz)	370	0	4
Pasta & Vegetable Alfredo	1 cup	220	20	4
Pasta Primavera	1 pkg (9 oz)	300	45	3
Ravioli w/ Sauce	1 pkg (8 oz)	340	25	3
Rice Mac & Cheese	1 pkg (9 oz)	140	50	3
Skillet Meals	1 cup	250	5	3
Tofu Vegetable Lasagna	1 pkg (9.5 oz)	300	0	6
Vegetable Lasagna	1 pkg (9.5 oz)	280	20	3
Banquet				
Chicken Pasta Primavera	1 meal (9.5 oz)	320	25	6
Family Size Egg Noodles w/ Beef & Brown Gravy	1 serv	150	35	2
Family Size Lasagna w/ Meat Sauce	1 cup	270	45	2
Family Size Macaroni & Cheese	1 cup	230	10	3
Fettuccine Alfredo	1 meal (9.5 oz)	350	25	4
Homestyle Noodles & Chicken	1 meal (12 oz)	390	50	7
Lasagna w/ Meat Sauce	1 meal (9.5 oz)	260	15	3
Macaroni & Cheese	1 meal (12 oz)	420	20	5
Bertolli				
Meatballs Pomodoro & Penne	1 serv (12 oz)	600	50	6
Boca				
Lasagna Meatless	1 pkg (9.4 oz)	290	15	5
Celentano				
Cheese Ravioli	4 (4.3 oz)	230	30	2
Contessa				
Ravioli Portobello	6 (6.7 oz)	360	65	2

FOOD	PORTION	CALS	CHOL	FIBER
Glory				
Macaroni & Cheese	1 pkg	480	90	1
Golden Cuisine				
Cheese Manicotti	1 pkg	360	50	6
Spaghetti & Meatballs	1 pkg	490	33	12
Tuna Casserole	1 pkg	386	41	8
Healthy Choice				
Beef Macaroni	1 meal (8.5 oz)	220	20	5
Breaded Chicken Breast Strips w/ Macaroni & Cheese	1 meal (8 oz)	270	40	1
Breaded Chicken Breast w/ Mac & Cheese	1 pkg	290	40	3
Cheese Ravioli Parmigiana	1 meal (9 oz)	260	20	6
Fettuccine Alfredo	1 pkg	280	15	3
Fettuccini Alfredo Chicken	1 pkg	290	45	3
Lasagna Bake	1 pkg (9 oz)	270	20	4
Macaroni & Cheese	1 meal (9 oz)	240	20	3
Macaroni & Cheese	1 pkg	290	15	5
Manicotti	1 pkg	280	45	4
Manicotti w/ Three Cheeses	1 meal (11 oz)	300	35	5
Rigatoni w/ Broccoli & Chicken	1 pkg	270	40	5
Spaghetti & Sauce w/ Seasoned Beef	1 meal (10 oz)	260	30	5
Spaghetti w/ Meat Sauce	1 pkg	310	25	7
Stuffed Pasta Shells	1 pkg	290	20	5
Joseph's Pasta				
Grilled Chicken Ravioli w/ Roasted Red Pepper Sauce	1 pkg (14 oz)	540	150	6
Kashi				
Chicken Pasta Promodoro	1 pkg (10 oz)	280	25	6
Kid Cuisine				
Cheese Blaster Mac & Cheese	1 meal	380	16	5
Twist & Twirl Spaghetti w/ Mini Meatballs	1 meal	460	19	6
Lean Cuisine				
Cafe Classics Bow Tie Pasta & Chicken	1 pkg (9.5 oz)	240	45	3

FOOD	PORTION	CALS	CHOL	FIBER
Cafe Classics Bowl Three Cheese Stuffed Ragatoni	1 pkg (10 oz)	260	20	4
Cafe Classics Cheese Lasagna w/ Chicken Breast Scallopini	1 pkg (10 oz)	290	30	3
Cafe Classics Four Cheese Cannelloni	1 pkg (9.1 oz)	260	20	3
Cafe Classics Grilled Chicken & Penne Pasta	1 pkg (12 oz)	320	40	4
Cafe Classics Jumbo Rigatoni w/ Meatballs	1 pkg (15.4 oz)	400	40	6
Cafe Classics Lasagna w/ Meat Sauce	1 pkg (10.5 oz)	310	30	4
Cafe Classics Macaroni & Beef	1 pkg (9.5 oz)	270	20	3
Cafe Classics Macaroni & Cheese	1 pkg (10 oz)	300	20	1
Cafe Classics Penne Pasta w/ Tomato Basil Sauce	1 pkg (10 oz)	270	0	5
Cafe Classics Roasted Chicken w/ Lemon Pepper Fettuccini	1 pkg (8.1 oz)	250	30	2
Cafe Classics Shrimp & Angel Hair Pasta	1 pkg (10 oz)	240	50	2
Cafe Classics Spaghetti w/ Meat Sauce	1 pkg (11.5 oz)	280	15	3
Cafe Classics Spaghetti w/ Meatballs	1 pkg (9.5 oz)	270	25	3
Dinnertime Selects Chicken Fettuccini	1 pkg (12 oz)	360	45	4
One Dish Favorites Alfredo Pasta w/ Chicken & Broccoli	1 pkg (10 oz)	270	40	3
One Dish Favorites Angel Hair Pasta Marinara	1 pkg (10 oz)	260	5	4
One Dish Favorites Cheese Ravioli	1 pkg (8.5 oz)	250	35	3
One Dish Favorites Chicken Fettuccini	1 pkg (9.25 oz)	280	35	2
One Dish Favorites Lasagna Cheese Florentine Bake	1 pkg (10 oz)	270	25	3

FOOD	PORTION	CALS	CHOL	FIBER
One Dish Favorites Lasagna Chicken Florentine	1 pkg (10 oz)	270	25	3
One Dish Favorites Lasagna Classic Five Cheese	1 pkg (11.5 oz)	330	25	4
Skillet Chicken Alfredo	1 serv	180	25	3
Marie Callender's				
Cheese Ravioli In Marinara Sauce w/ Spirals & Garlic Bread	1 meal (16 oz)	750	30	11
Extra Cheese Lasagna	1 meal (15 oz)	590	50	7
Fettuccine Alfredo & Garlic Bread	1 meal (14 oz)	920	90	3
Fettuccine Alfredo Supreme	1 meal (13 oz)	450	80	4
Fettuccine Primavera w/ Tortellini	1 meal (14 oz)	750	65	6
Fettuccine w/ Broccoli & Chicken	1 meal (13 oz)	710	85	6
Macaroni & Cheese	1 meal (12 oz)	540	50	5
Meat Lasagna	1 cup	240	45	2
Skillet Meal Chicken Alfredo	½ pkg	490	75	7
Skillet Meal Penne Pasta & Meatballs	½ pkg	600	45	4
Skillet Meal Rigatoni Vegetables In Cheese Sauce	1 cup	290	30	4
Spaghetti w/ Meat Sauce & & Garlic Bread	1 meal (17 oz)	670	35	9
Stuffed Pasta Trio	1 meal (10.5 oz)	380	50	5
Michelina's				
Lasagna w/ Meat Sauce	1 pkg (9 oz)	340	35	3
Morton				
Macaroni & Cheese	1 serv (8 oz)	240	20	3
Spaghetti w/ Meat Sauce	1 meal (8.5 oz)	200	5	4
Savvy Faire				
Lasagna Florentine	1 pkg (9.2 oz)	300	5	5
Seeds Of Change				
Chicken Fettuccine Alfredo	1 pkg (10 oz)	340	50	3
Lasagna Creamy Spinach	1 pkg (11 oz)	370	35	7
Lasagne Vegetable	1 pkg (11 oz)	310	20	5
Penne Marinara	1 pkg (11 oz)	290	10	5

FOOD	PORTION	CALS	CHOL	FIBER
Slim-Fast				
Fettuccine Alfredo	1 pkg	240	20	5
Rotini w/ Tomato & Italian Herb	1 pkg	240	<5	4
Shells & Creamy Cheese Sauce	1 pkg	240	20	5
South Beach Diet				
Penne & Chicken In Roasted Red Pepper Sauce w/ Broccoli	1 pkg	290	50	8
Stouffer's				
Lasagna w/ Meat Sauce	1 cup	260	30	3
Yves				
Veggie Lasagna	1 pkg (10.5 oz)	300	0	4
Veggie Macaroni	1 pkg (10.5 oz)	230	0	3
Veggie Penne	1 pkg (10.5 oz)	220	0	4
MIX				
A Taste Of Thai				
Coconut Ginger	1 cup	280	0	1
Pad Thai For Two	½ pkg	345	0	4
Peanut Noodles as prep	1 cup	330	0	1
Red Curry Noodles as prep	1 cup	280	5	2
Annie's Homegrown				
Gluten Free Rice Pasta & Cheddar as prep	1 cup	330	10	0
Organic Skillet Meals Beef Stroganoff as prep	1 cup	320	51	1
Organic Skillet Meals Cheddar & Herb Chicken as prep	1 cup	310	75	1
Organic Skillet Meals Cheese Lasagna as prep	1 cup	280	36	1
Organic Skillet Meals Cheeseburger Macaroni as prep	1 cup	350	51	1
Organic Skillet Meals Chicken Fettuccine as prep	1 cup	330	84	1
Organic Skillet Meals Creamy Tuna Spirals as prep	1 cup	260	30	1
Organic Shells & Real Aged Wisconsin Cheddar as prep	1 cup	370	39	2

FOOD	PORTION	CALS	CHOL	FIBER
Organic Whole Wheat Shells & Cheddar as prep	1 cup	360	42	5
Shells & Real Aged Wisconsin Cheddar as prep	1 cup	290	10	1
Shells & White Cheddar as prep	1 cup	290	10	1
Aramana				
Cheddar Cheeseburger as prep	1 cup	260	55	4
Creamy Chicken Alfredo as prep	1 cup	260	55	5
Mild Mexican as prep	1 cup	260	55	5
Atkins				
Quick Quisine Elbows & Cheese as prep	1 cup	250	10	9
Quick Quisine Fettuccine Alfredo as prep	1 cup	210	10	9
Quick Quisine Pesto Cream as prep	1 cup	240	5	10
Back To Nature				
Alfredo & Gemelli as prep	1 cup	340	30	1
Macaroni & Cheese as prep	1 cup	320	24	1
White Cheddar & Spirals as prep	1 cup	330	30	1
Carapelli				
Penne Alfredo as prep	1 cup	240	5	4
Spirals Creamy Tomato as prep	1 cup	240	0	4
Hamburger Helper				
Ravioli as prep	1 cup	280	50	1
Ravioli w/ White Cheese Topping as prep	1 cup	310	50	1
Near East				
Angel Hair w/ Spicy Tomato as prep	1 cup	240	0	3
Radiatore Basil & Herb as prep	1 cup	240	3	3
Vermicelli Garlic & Oil as prep	1 cup	310	3	3

FOOD	PORTION	CALS	CHOL	FIBER
Whey Cool				
High Protein Macaroni & Cheese as prep	1 serv	260	15	1
REFRIGERATED				
Country Crock				
Elbow Macaroni & Cheese	1 cup	380	0	1
SHELF-STABLE				
It's Pasta Anytime				
Penne With Tomato Italian Sausage Sauce	1 pkg (15.25 oz)	540	<5	12
TAKE-OUT				
lasagna meatless	1 piece (9 oz)	356	38	3
lasagna w/ meat	1 piece (8 oz)	362	56	3
lasagna w/ vegetables	1 serv (9 oz)	315	33	4
macaroni & cheese w/ ham	1 cup	542	61	3
manicotti cheese filled marinara sauce	1 (5 oz)	229	83	1
manicotti cheese filled w/ meat sauce	1 (5 oz)	239	86	3
pasta w/ pesto sauce	1 cup	370	10	2
ravioli cheese & spinach filled w/ cream sauce	1 cup	362	160	2
ravioli meat filled w/ marinara sauce	1 cup	372	168	3
ravioli cheese w/ tomato sauce	1 cup	335	158	2
rigatoni w/ sausage sauce	¾ cup	260	59	3
spaghetti w/ red clam sauce	1 cup	285	17	3
spaghetti w/ sauce & meatballs	2 cups	670	114	12
spaghetti w/ white clam sauce	1 cup	456	50	3
tortellini cheese w/ tomato sauce	1 cup	332	158	2
tortellini meat filled w/ marinara sauce	1 cup	281	90	2
tortellini spinach filled w/ marinara sauce	1 cup	238	72	2

FOOD	PORTION	CALS	CHOL	FIBER
PASTA SALAD				
MIX				
Dole				
Veggie Pasta Salads Broccoli Ranch	1½ cups	230	5	2
Veggie Pasta Salads Cheddar Bacon Ranch	1½ cups	370	25	3
Veggie Pasta Salads Garden Vegetable	1½ cups	240	0	2
Veggie Pasta Salads Italian Herb	1½ cups	270	5	2
Suddenly Salad				
Classic Pasta	¾ cup	250	0	2
Classic Pasta Reduced Fat Recipe	¾ cup	210	0	2
Garden Italian 98% Fat Free	¾ cup	140	0	2
TAKE-OUT				
pasta salad w/ crab vegetables mayonnaise	1 cup	317	32	2
tortellini salad cheese filled w/ vinaigrette dressing	1 cup	333	144	1
PATE				
chicken liver canned	1 tbsp	26	51	0
liver w/ truffle	1 serv (2 oz)	183	59	–
mushroom anchovy pate	1 can (2.25 oz)	130	5	1
pate de foie gras smoked canned	1 tbsp	60	20	0
pork pate	1 oz	107	51	0
pork pate en croute	1 oz	91	32	tr
rabbit pate	1 oz	66	21	–
shrimp	1 can (2.25 oz)	140	25	0
PEACH				
CANNED				
halves in heavy syrup	1 half	60	0	–
halves in light syrup	1 half	44	0	–
halves juice pack	1 half	34	0	–
halves water pack	1 half	18	0	–
peachsauce	½ cup	120	0	1

FOOD	PORTION	CALS	CHOL	FIBER
spiced in heavy syrup	1 cup	180	0	–
spiced in heavy syrup	1 fruit	66	0	–
Del Monte				
Carb Clever Sliced	½ cup	30	0	1
Freestone Lite Slices	½ cup	60	0	1
Freestone Sliced	½ cup	100	0	1
Fruit Cup Diced Extra Light Syrup	1 pkg (4 oz)	50	0	1
Fruit Cup Diced In Heavy Syrup	1 serv (4 oz)	80	0	1
Fruit Naturals Chunks	½ cup	70	0	tr
Fruit To Go Banana Berry Peaches	1 pkg (4 oz)	70	0	1
Halves In Heavy Syrup	½ cup	100	0	1
Orchard Select Sliced Cling	½ cup	80	0	tr
Sliced In 100% Juice	½ cup	60	0	1
Sliced Light Syrup Raspberry Flavor	½ cup	80	0	tr
Dole				
All Natural Yellow Cling Sliced	½ cup	80	0	tr
Liberty Gold				
Sliced Cling In Heavy Syrup	½ cup	100	0	1
S&W				
Slices Lightly Sweetened Juice	½ cup	80	0	1
Yellow Cling In Heavy Syrup	½ cup	100	0	1
DRIED				
halves	10	311	0	11
halves	1 cup	383	0	13
halves cooked w/ sugar	½ cup	139	0	–
halves cooked w/o sugar	½ cup	99	0	–
Crispy Green				
Crispy Peaches	1 pkg (0.36 oz)	38	0	tr
FRESH				
peach	1	37	0	1
sliced	1 cup	73	0	–
Chiquita				
Peach	1 med (3.4 oz)	40	0	2

FOOD	PORTION	CALS	CHOL	FIBER
FROZEN				
slices sweetened	1 cup	235	0	–
C&W				
Ulimate Sliced	¾ cup	50	0	2
PEACH JUICE				
nectar	1 cup	134	0	–
After The Fall				
Georgia Peach	8 oz	130	0	–
Ceres				
Peach	8 oz	120	0	0
Nantucket Nectars				
The Original	8 oz	120	0	–
PEANUT BUTTER				
chunky	1 cup	1520	0	17
chunky	2 tbsp	188	0	2
chunky w/o salt	2 tbsp	188	0	2
chunky w/o salt	1 cup	1520	0	17
smooth	2 tbsp	188	0	2
smooth	1 cup	1517	0	15
smooth w/o salt	2 tbsp	188	0	2
smooth w/o salt	1 cup	1517	0	15
Carb Options				
Creamy	2 tbsp	190	0	2
Cream-Nut				
Natural	2 tbsp	190	0	2
Estee				
Creamy Low Sodium	2 tbsp	180	0	2
Jif				
Creamy	2 tbsp	190	0	2
Creamy To Go	1 pkg (2.25 oz)	270	0	4
Extra Crunchy	2 tbsp	190	0	2
Peanut Butter & Honey	2 tbsp	190	0	2
Reduced Fat Creamy	2 tbsp	190	0	2
Reduced Fat Crunchy	2 tbsp	190	0	2
Simply	2 tbsp	190	0	2
Kettle				
Organic Unsalted	2 tbsp	170	0	2
Maranatha				
Salted	2 tbsp	190	0	2

FOOD	PORTION	CALS	CHOL	FIBER
P.B.				
Slices	1 slice (1 oz)	170	0	1
Peanut Better				
Cinnamon Currant	2 tbsp	180	0	3
Deep Chocolate	2 tbsp	170	0	2
Hickory Smoked	2 tbsp	190	0	3
Onion Parsley	2 tbsp	180	0	3
Peanut Praline	2 tbsp	180	0	3
Rosemary Garlic	2 tbsp	180	0	3
Spicy Southwestern	2 tbsp	190	0	3
Sweet Molasses	2 tbsp	180	0	2
Thai Ginger & Red Pepper	2 tbsp	180	0	3
Vanilla Cranberry	2 tbsp	170	0	2
Peanut Butter & Co.				
Cinnamon Raisin Swirl	2 tbsp	143	0	2
Crunch Time	2 tbsp	200	0	2
Dark Chocolate Dreams	2 tbsp	175	0	2
Smooth Operator	2 tbsp	200	0	2
The Heat Is On	2 tbsp	164	0	2
White Chocolate Wonderful	1 tbsp	165	0	2
Peanut Wonder				
Low Sodium	2 tbsp	100	0	0
Regular	2 tbsp	100	0	0
Reese's				
Creamy	2 tbsp	200	0	2
Peanut Butter Chips	1 tbsp	80	0	–
Skippy				
Creamy	2 tbsp	190	0	2
Creamy w/ 2 slices white bread	1 sandwich	340	0	–
Reduced Fat Creamy	2 tbsp	190	0	2
Roasted Honey Nut	2 tbsp	190	0	2
Roasted Honey Nut Super Chunk	2 tbsp	190	0	2
Squeeze Stix	1 pkg	140	0	2
Squeeze Stix Chocolate	1 pkg	140	0	2
Squeez'lt	2 tbsp	190	0	2
Super Chunk	2 tbsp	190	0	2
Super Chunk Reduced Fat	2 tbsp	190	0	2

FOOD	PORTION	CALS	CHOL	FIBER
Smucker's				
Goober All Flavors	3 tbsp	240	0	2
Natural Chunky	2 tbsp	210	0	2
Natural Creamy	2 tbsp	210	0	2
Natural Honey	2 tbsp	200	0	2
Natural No Salt Added Creamy	2 tbsp	210	0	2
Natural Reduced Fat Creamy	2 tbsp	200	0	2
Teddies				
Old Fashioned	2 tbsp	190	0	3
Tropical Source				
Chips Dairy Free	13 pieces (1.5 oz)	80	0	0
PEANUTS				
chocolate coated	¼ cup	193	3	2
cooked w/ salt	½ cup	286	0	8
dry roasted w/ salt	28 nuts (1 oz)	164	0	1
dry roasted w/ salt	1 oz	166	0	2
dry roasted w/o salt	28 (1 oz)	164	0	2
dry roasted w/o salt	¼ cup	214	0	3
honey roasted	¼ cup	191	0	3
milk chocolate coated	1	21	0	tr
sugar coated	¼ cup	203	0	2
yogurt coated	¼ cup	230	0	2
A Taste Of Thai				
Spicy Peanut Bake	¼ pkg	45	0	1
At Last!				
Chocolate Covered	1 pkg (0.9 oz)	150	0	5
Brach's				
Double Dippers Chocolate Covered	15 pieces	210	10	2
Estee				
Chocolate Coated Fructose Sweetened	¼ cup	170	<5	1
Frito Lay				
Salted	1 oz	160	0	2
Salted w/ Shells	½ cup	160	0	2
Judy's				
Sugar Free Coconut Peanut Brittle	¼ piece (1 oz)	90	0	1

FOOD	PORTION	CALS	CHOL	FIBER
Low Carb Creations				
Soft Peanut Brittle	2 pieces (1 oz)	140	0	2
Planters				
Cocktail	1 oz	170	0	2
Dry Roasted	1 oz	170	0	2
Sweet Delight				
Peanut Roasters	⅓ pkg (1 oz)	160	0	3
Tom's				
Double Coated	1 pkg (1.35 oz)	220	0	1
PEAR				
CANNED				
halves in heavy syrup	1 half	68	0	–
halves in heavy syrup	1 cup	188	0	–
halves in light syrup	1 half	45	0	–
halves juice pack	1 cup	123	0	–
halves water pack	1 half	22	0	–
Del Monte				
Carb Clever Sliced	½ cup	40	0	1
Fruit Cup Diced In Heavy Syrup	1 pkg (4 oz)	80	0	1
Fruit Cup Diced Extra Light Syrup	1 pkg (4 oz)	50	0	1
Fruit To Go Peachy Peaches	1 pkg (4 oz)	70	0	1
Halves In 100% Juice	½ cup	60	0	1
Halves In Light Syrup	½ cup	60	0	1
Orchard Select Sliced Bartlett	½ cup	80	0	2
S&W				
Halves In Lightly Sweetened Juice	½ cup	80	0	2
DRIED				
halves	10	459	0	–
halves	1 cup	472	0	–
halves cooked w/ sugar	½ cup	196	0	–
halves cooked w/o sugar	½ cup	163	0	–
FRESH				
asian	1 (4.3 oz)	51	0	–
pear	1	98	0	4
sliced w/ skin	1 cup	97	0	4

FOOD	PORTION	CALS	CHOL	FIBER
Chiquita				
Pear	1 med (5.8 oz)	100	0	4
PEAR JUICE				
nectar	1 cup	149	0	–
Ceres				
Pear	8 oz	120	0	0
Izze				
Sparkling Pear	8 oz	130	0	–
Langers				
Kid's 100% Juice	4 oz	60	0	–
PEAS				
CANNED				
green	½ cup	59	0	–
green low sodium	½ cup	59	0	–
Del Monte				
Sweet	½ cup	60	0	4
Sweet Very Young Small	½ cup	60	0	4
Green Giant				
Sweet	½ cup	60	0	3
Libby's				
No Salt No Sugar Added	½ cup	70	0	3
S&W				
Petite	½ cup (4.4 oz)	70	0	4
Small	½ cup (4.4 oz)	70	0	4
Tillen Farms				
Crispy Snapper Pickled	¼ cup	15	0	1
Veg-All				
Tender Sweet	½ cup	60	0	3
DRIED				
split cooked	1 cup	231	0	–
FRESH				
green cooked	½ cup	67	0	–
green raw	½ cup	58	0	–
snap peas cooked	½ cup	34	0	2
snap peas raw	½ cup	30	0	2
Frieda's				
Snow Peas	1 cup	35	0	2
Sugar Snap	⅔ cups (3 oz)	35	0	2

FOOD	PORTION	CALS	CHOL	FIBER
River Ranch				
Sugar Snap	1½ cups	35	0	2
FROZEN				
green cooked	½ cup	63	0	–
snap peas cooked	½ cup	42	0	–
Birds Eye				
Steamfresh Garlic Baby Peas & Mushrooms	¾ cup	80	0	3
Steamfresh Sweet Peas	⅓ cup	70	0	4
C&W				
Alfredo	½ cup	110	15	4
Early Harvest Petite No Salt Added	⅔ cup	70	0	4
Sugar Snap	⅔ cup	40	0	2
Green Giant				
Sweet	⅔ cup	70	0	4
La Choy				
Snow Pea Pods	½ pkg (3 oz)	35	0	2
Pictsweet				
Green Peas	⅔ cup	70	0	4
Tree Of Life				
Peas	⅔ cup (3.1 oz)	70	0	4
SHELF-STABLE				
TastyBite				
Agra Peas & Greens	½ pkg (5 oz)	260	0	1
PECANS				
candied	1 oz	190	0	5
dry roasted	1 oz	187	0	–
dry roasted salted	1 oz	187	0	–
halves dry roasted w/ salt	20 (1 oz)	200	0	3
halves dried	1 cup	721	0	7
oil roasted	1 oz	195	0	–
oil roasted salted	1 oz	195	0	–
Emerald				
Glazed Pecan Pie	¼ cup	150	0	1
Sweet Delights				
Pecan Roasters	⅓ pkg (1 oz)	210	0	2

FOOD	PORTION	CALS	CHOL	FIBER
PECTIN				
liquid	1 oz	3	0	1
powder	1 pkg (1.75 oz)	162	0	4
Slim Set				
Packet	1 pkg	208	0	14
Powder	1 tbsp	3	0	tr
Sure Jell				
For Lower Sugar Recipes	1 tsp (2.8 g)	20	0	0
Fruit Pectin	1 tsp (3.6 g)	20	0	0
PEPEAO				
dried	¼ cup	18	0	–
raw sliced	1 cup	25	0	–
PEPPER				
black	1 tsp	5	0	–
cayenne	1 tsp	6	0	–
red	1 tsp	6	0	–
white	1 tsp	7	0	–
Emeril's				
Kicked Up Red Sauce	1 tsp	0	0	0
McCormick				
Lemon & Pepper Seasoning Salt	¼ tsp	0	0	0
PEPPERS				
CANNED				
chili green	1 cup (5.5 oz)	29	0	2
chili green hot chopped	½ cup	17	0	–
chili red hot	1 (2.6 oz)	18	0	–
chili red hot chopped	½ cup	17	0	–
green halves	½ cup	13	0	–
jalapeno chopped	½ cup	17	0	–
red halves	½ cup	13	0	–
B&G				
Cherry Hot	1 (1 oz)	10	0	–
Cherry Sweet	1 (1 oz)	10	0	–
Hot Pepper Rings	7 pieces (1 oz)	0	0	–
Pepperoncini	3 pieces (1 oz)	10	0	–
Roasted w/ Balsamic Vinegar	½ piece (1 oz)	10	0	–

FOOD	PORTION	CALS	CHOL	FIBER
Las Palmas				
Diced Green Chiles	2 tbsp	5	0	1
Jalapenos Sliced	3 tbsp	10	0	0
Old El Paso				
Green Chiles Chopped	2 tbsp (1 oz)	5	0	1
Progresso				
Cherry Sliced & So Hot	2 tbsp (1 oz)	25	0	1
Hot Cherry	1 (1 oz)	10	0	tr
Pepper Salad (drained)	2 tbsp (1 oz)	15	0	tr
Roasted	1 piece (1 oz)	10	0	0
Sweet Fried w/ Onions	2 tbsp (0.9 oz)	20	0	1
Tuscan	3 (1 oz)	10	0	1
Rosarita				
Chilies Diced Green	2 tbsp (1 oz)	6	0	1
Chilies Green Strips	¼ cup (1.2 oz)	5	0	1
Chilies Whole Green	2 tbsp (1.2 oz)	5	0	1
Jalapenos Diced	2 tbsp (1 oz)	5	0	1
Jalapenos Nacho Sliced	2 tbsp (1 oz)	2	0	tr
Jalapenos Whole w/ Escabeche	¼ cup (1.2 oz)	8	0	1
Tillen Farms				
Bell Peppers Pickled Sweet	¼ cup	25	0	0
Vlasic				
Hot Sliced Cherry	1 oz	5	0	–
Jalapeno Sliced	1 oz	10	0	–
Mild Cherry	1 oz	5	0	–
Pepper Rings Hot	1 oz	5	0	–
Pepper Rings Mild	1 oz	5	0	–
DRIED				
ancho	1 tsp	3	0	tr
ancho	1 (0.6 oz)	48	0	4
casabel	1 tsp	3	0	tr
chipotle smoked	1 tsp	3	0	tr
green	1 tbsp	1	0	–
guajillo	1 tsp	3	0	tr
mulato	1 tsp	3	0	tr
pasilla	1 tsp	3	0	tr
pasilla	1 (7 g)	24	0	2
red	1 tbsp	1	0	–

FOOD	PORTION	CALS	CHOL	FIBER
Frieda's				
California Chili	2 tbsp	15	0	0
FRESH				
banana	1 (4 in) (1.2 oz)	9	0	1
banana	1 cup (4.4 oz)	33	0	4
chili green hot	1	18	0	–
chili green hot chopped	½ cup	30	0	–
chili red chopped	½ cup	30	0	–
chili red hot	1 (1.6 oz)	18	0	–
green	1 (2.6 oz)	20	0	1
green chopped	½ cup	13	0	1
green chopped cooked	½ cup	19	0	–
green cooked	1 (2.6 oz)	20	0	–
habanero chile	1 tsp	9	0	1
hungarian	1 (0.9 oz)	8	0	0
jalapeno	1 (0.5 oz)	4	0	tr
jalapeno sliced	1 cup (3.2 oz)	27	0	3
red	1 (2.6 oz)	20	0	1
red chopped	½ cup	13	0	1
red chopped cooked	½ cup	19	0	–
red cooked	1 (2.6 oz)	20	0	–
serrano	1 (6 g)	2	0	tr
serrano chopped	1 cup (3.7 oz)	34	0	4
yellow	1 (6.5 oz)	50	0	–
yellow	10 strips	14	0	–
Chiquita				
Pepper	1 med (5.2 oz)	30	0	2
Frieda's				
Peppadew	⅓ cup	40	0	3
FROZEN				
green chopped	1 oz	6	0	–
red chopped	1 oz	6	0	–
C&W				
Strips	¾ cup	25	0	1
Roast Works				
Flame Roasted Red	1 serv (3 oz)	45	0	3
PERCH				
FRESH				
cooked	3 oz	99	98	0

FOOD	PORTION	CALS	CHOL	FIBER
cooked	1 fillet (1.6 oz)	54	53	0
ocean perch atlantic cooked	1 fillet (1.8 oz)	60	27	0
ocean perch atlantic cooked	3 oz	103	46	0

PERSIMMONS
dried japanese	1 (1.2 oz)	93	0	5
fresh	1 (6 oz)	118	0	6
Frieda's				
Dried Fuyu	⅓ cup (1.4 oz)	140	0	3

PHEASANT
breast cooked	½ breast (4.5 oz)	312	113	0
leg cooked	1 (2.6 oz)	184	67	0

PHYLLO
sheet	1 (0.7 oz)	57	0	tr
Ekizian				
Sheets	¼ lb	433	62	–
Fillo Factory				
Fillo Dough Spelt Vegan	3 sheets (2 oz)	180	0	4
Fillo Dough Vegan	3 sheets (2 oz)	170	0	1
Fillo Dough Whole Wheat Vegan	3 sheets (2 oz)	190	0	3
Pastry Shells Vegan	3 (0.4 oz)	45	0	0

PICANTE (see SALSA)

PICKLES
bread & butter	6 slices	39	0	1
dill	1 lg (4.7 oz)	24	0	2
dill low sodium	1 med (2.3 oz)	12	0	1
dill sliced	6 slices	7	0	1
gherkins	1 oz	6	0	–
sweet gherkin	1 (1.2 oz)	41	0	tr
B&G				
Bread & Butter	3 slices (1 oz)	25	0	–
Kosher Dill	⅓ pickle (1 oz)	0	0	0
Kosher Dill No Salt	½ pickle (1 oz)	10	0	–
Sour	½ pickle (1 oz)	0	0	0
Sweet Gerkins	1 (1 oz)	35	0	–
Claussen				
Bread 'N Butter Chips	4 slices (1 oz)	20	0	0

FOOD	PORTION	CALS	CHOL	FIBER
Deli Style Hearty Garlic Whole	½ (1 oz)	5	0	0
Kosher Dill Spears	1 spear (1.2 oz)	5	0	0
Kosher Dills Halves	1 half (1 oz)	5	0	0
Kosher Dills Mini	1 (0.8 oz)	5	0	0
Kosher Dills Whole	½ (1 oz)	5	0	0
New York Deli Style Half Sours Whole	½ (1 oz)	5	0	0
Sandwich Slices Bread 'N Butter	2 (1.2 oz)	25	0	0
Sandwich Slices Deli Style Hearty Garlic	2 (1.2 oz)	5	0	0
Sandwich Slices Kosher Dills	2 (1.2 oz)	5	0	0
Super Slices For Burgers	1 (0.8 oz)	5	0	0
Del Monte				
Dill Halves	1 piece (1 oz)	5	0	1
Hamburger Dill Chips	1 serv (1 oz)	0	0	0
Sweet	1 serv (1 oz)	40	0	tr
Sweet Gerkins	1 serv (1 oz)	40	0	tr
Tiny Kosher Dill	1 serv (1 oz)	5	0	tr
Hebrew National				
Dill	1	23	0	–
Mt Olive				
Bread & Butter No Sugar Added	1 oz	0	0	0
Vlasic				
Hamburger Dill Chips	1 oz	5	0	–
Kosher Cross Cuts	1 oz	5	0	–
Kosher Spears	1 oz	5	0	–
Kosher Whole	1 oz	5	0	–
Sweet Butter Chips	1 oz	30	0	–
Sweet Gerkins	1 oz	35	0	–
Whole Dills	1 oz	5	0	–

PIE (see also PIE CRUST, PIE FILLING)
FROZEN
Amy's

Apple	1 serv (4 oz)	240	25	2
Edwards				
Pie Slices Chocolate Creme	1 slice (2.7 oz)	290	10	tr

FOOD	PORTION	CALS	CHOL	FIBER
Pie Slices Key Lime	1 slice (3.2 oz)	330	35	0
Pie Slices Oreo Cream	1 slice (2.6 oz)	290	10	1
Mrs. Smith's				
Apple	1 slice (4.3 oz)	350	0	3
Blueberry	1 slice (4.6 oz)	330	0	3
Cappuccino	1 slice (4.2 oz)	300	0	2
Cherry	1 slice (4.3 oz)	320	0	2
Cherry Crumb	1 slice (4.2 oz)	320	0	1
Chocolate Cream	1 slice (4.6 oz)	340	15	2
Chocolate Mint Cream	1 slice (4.3 oz)	360	0	2
Coconut Custard	1 slice (4.4 oz)	260	70	tr
Cookies 'N Cream	1 slice (4.3 oz)	360	0	2
Dutch Apple	1 slice (3.3 oz)	260	0	1
French Silk	1 slice (4.4 oz)	560	55	1
Key West Lime	1 slice (4.3 oz)	430	15	1
Lemon Cream	1 slice (5 oz)	440	0	tr
Lemonade	1 slice (4.3 oz)	340	0	1
Mince	1 slice (4.6 oz)	380	0	2
Mixed Berry	1 slice (4.2 oz)	300	0	2
Peach	1 slice (4.6 oz)	320	0	2
Peach Lattice	1 slice (4.2 oz)	290	0	2
Peanut Butter Silk	1 slice (4.6 oz)	600	55	2
Pecan	1 slice (4.8 oz)	560	65	2
Pumpkin Custard	1 slice (4.6 oz)	270	40	2
Raspberry	1 slice (4.6 oz)	330	0	1
S'Mores Cream	1 slice (4.3 oz)	360	0	2
Strawberry Banana	1 slice (4.3 oz)	330	0	1
Sweet Potato Custard	1 slice (4.6 oz)	340	40	2
Sara Lee				
Apple	1 slice (4.6 oz)	340	0	1
Cherry	1 slice (4.6 oz)	320	0	0
Coconut Cream	1 slice (4.8 oz)	330	5	2
French Silk	1 slice (4.8 oz)	340	10	2
Key West Lime	1 slice (4.2 oz)	400	5	2
Lemon Meringue	1 slice (5 oz)	220	0	1
Mince	1 slice (4.6 oz)	370	0	2
Pumpkin	1 slice (4.6 oz)	260	30	2
Southern Pecan	1 slice (4.2 oz)	520	45	3
Southern Sweet Potato	1 slice (4.6 oz)	280	35	2
Sulce de Leche Caramel Swirl	1 slice (4.4 oz)	400	5	2

FOOD	PORTION	CALS	CHOL	FIBER
READY-TO-EAT				
Entenmann's				
Peach Raspberry Melba	⅛ pie (2.6 oz)	250	10	tr
SNACK				
Tom's				
Apple	1 pkg (3 oz)	330	5	1
Banana Marshmallow	1 pkg (2.75 oz)	320	0	0
Cherry	1 pkg (3 oz)	320	5	1
Chocolate Marshmallow	1 pkg (2.75 oz)	320	0	tr
TAKE-OUT				
apple	⅛ of 9 in pie (5.4 oz)	411	0	3
banana cream	⅛ of 9 in pie (5.2 oz)	398	75	–
blueberry	⅛ of 9 in pie (5.2 oz)	360	0	–
butterscotch	⅛ of 9 in pie (4.5 oz)	355	78	–
cherry	⅛ of 9 in pie (6.3 oz)	486	0	–
chocolate creme	1 slice (4 oz)	344	6	–
coconut creme	⅛ of 9 in pie (4.7 oz)	396	77	–
coconut custard	⅙ of 8 in pie (3.6 oz)	271	36	–
custard	⅛ of 9 in pie (4.5 oz)	262	87	2
key lime	1 slice (5 oz)	420	25	tr
lemon meringue	1 slice (4.5 oz)	303	51	1
mince	⅛ of 9 in pie (5.8 oz)	477	0	–
pecan	1 slice (4 oz)	452	36	4
pumpkin	1 slice (3.8 oz)	229	22	3
vanilla cream	⅛ of 9 in pie (4.4 oz)	350	78	–
PIE CRUST				
FROZEN				
baked	9 in crust	884	0	2
baked	⅛ of 9 in pie	113	0	tr
puff pastry shell	1 (1.4 oz)	223	0	1
tart shell	1 (1 oz)	149	0	tr
Pet-Ritz				
Deep Dish	⅛ pie (0.7 oz)	90	<5	0
MIX				
Betty Crocker				
Pie Crust as prep	⅛ crust	110	0	–
Jiffy				
Pie Crust Mix	½ crust	180	<5	tr

FOOD	PORTION	CALS	CHOL	FIBER
MiniCarb				
Pie Crust Mix	1 slice	105	40	0
READY-TO-EAT				
chocolate crumb	⅛ of 9 in pie	132	0	tr
chocolate crumb	1 (9 in crust)	1063	2	3
graham cracker	1 (9 in crust)	1037	0	3
graham cracker	⅛ of 9 in pie	109	0	tr
graham cracker dessert shell	1 (1.1 oz)	148	0	tr
Keebler				
Graham Single Serve	1 (0.8 oz)	120	0	tr
Reduced Fat Graham	⅛ pie (0.7 oz)	90	0	0
REFRIGERATED				
All Ready				
Crust	⅛ pie (0.9 oz)	120	5	0
PIE FILLING				
apple	1 can (21 oz)	599	0	6
apple	⅛ can (2.6 oz)	74	0	1
cherry	1 can (21 oz)	683	0	–
cherry	⅛ can (2.6 oz)	85	0	–
pumpkin pie mix	1 cup	282	0	–
Colac				
All Flavors	1 tbsp	19	0	0
Comstock				
Blueberry	⅓ cup	100	0	1
Country Cherry	⅓ cup	90	0	1
Light Cherry	⅓ cup	60	0	1
Framer's Market				
Organic Pumpkin Pie Mix	½ cup	120	0	2
Libby's				
Pumpkin Pie Mix	⅓ cup	90	0	2
PIEROGI				
pierogi	¾ cup (4.4 oz)	307	49	–
Health Is Wealth				
Potato & Cheddar	2 (2.8 oz)	140	0	3
Potato & Onion	2 (2.8 oz)	140	0	3
Mrs. T's				
Broccoli & Cheddar	3 (4.2 oz)	200	10	2
Jalapeno & Cheddar	3 (4.2 oz)	190	10	2
Potato & American Cheese	3 (4.2 oz)	220	15	2

FOOD	PORTION	CALS	CHOL	FIBER
Potato & Roasted Garlic	3 (4.2 oz)	190	5	2
Potato & 4 Cheese Blend	3 (4.2 oz)	230	10	1
Potato & Onion	3 (4.2 oz)	180	0	2
Rogies Cheddar & Bacon	7 (3 oz)	140	5	1
Rogies Jalapeno & Cheddar	7 (3 oz)	120	5	1
Rogies Potato & Cheddar	7 (3 oz)	130	5	1

PIGEON PEAS

dried cooked	1 cup	204	0	–
dried cooked	½ cup	102	0	–

PIG'S FEET

feet cooked	1	201	93	0
pickled	1	177	70	0

PIKE

northern cooked	3 oz	96	43	0
northern cooked	½ fillet (5.4 oz)	176	78	0
northern raw	3 oz	75	33	0
roe raw	1 oz	37	103	–
walleye baked	3 oz	101	94	0
walleye fillet baked	4.4 oz	147	137	0

PILLNUTS

canarytree dried	1 oz	204	0	–

PIMIENTOS

canned	1 slice	0	0	–
canned	1 tbsp	3	0	–

PINE NUTS

pignolia dried	1 oz	146	0	–
pignolia dried	1 tbsp	51	0	–
pinyon dried	1 oz	161	0	–
Frieda's				
Pine Nuts	¼ cup	150	0	1
Good Sense				
Pignolias	¼ cup	190	0	4
Progresso				
Pignoli	1 jar (1 oz)	170	0	0

FOOD	PORTION	CALS	CHOL	FIBER
PINEAPPLE				
CANNED				
chunks in heavy syrup	1 cup	199	0	–
chunks juice pack	1 cup	150	0	–
crushed in heavy syrup	1 cup	199	0	–
slices in heavy syrup	1 slice	45	0	–
slices in light syrup	1 slice	30	0	–
slices juice pack	1 slice	35	0	–
slices water pack	1 slice	19	0	–
tidbits in heavy syrup	1 cup	199	0	–
tidbits in juice	1 cup	150	0	–
tidbits in water	1 cup	79	0	–
Del Monte				
Chunks In Heavy Syrup	½ cup	90	0	1
Chunks In Its Own Juice	½ cup	70	0	1
Crushed In Heavy Syrup	½ cup	90	0	1
Crushed In Its Own Juice	½ cup	70	0	1
Fruit Cup Tidbits	1 pkg (4 oz)	50	0	1
Fruit Naturals Chunks	½ cup	70	0	tr
Dole				
All Natural Chunks	½ cup	60	0	tr
Chunks Juice Pack	½ cup	60	0	1
Liberty Gold				
Crushed No Sugar Added	½ cup	80	0	2
Slices Natural Juice	½ cup	80	0	2
DRIED				
Sunsweet				
Pineapples	⅓ cup (1.4 oz)	130	0	1
FRESH				
diced	1 cup	77	0	2
slice	1 slice	42	0	1
Bonita Hill				
Golden Extra Sweet	2 slices (3.9 oz)	60	0	1
Cala Fruit				
Golden Sliced	1 serv (3.5 oz)	50	0	1
Frieda's				
Zululand Queen	1 cup (5 oz)	70	0	2
Frosty Fresh				
Peeled & Cored	½ cup	60	0	1

FOOD	PORTION	CALS	CHOL	FIBER
FROZEN				
chunks sweetened	½ cup	104	0	–
Europe's Best				
Aloha Gold	1 cup	70	0	2
Roast Works				
Flame Roasted	1 serv (3 oz)	80	0	1
PINEAPPLE JUICE				
canned	1 cup	139	0	–
frzn as prep	1 cup	129	0	–
frzn not prep	6 oz	387	0	–
Adina				
Pineapple Ginger Gin-Jah	8 oz	80	0	–
Ceres				
Pineapple	8 oz	120	0	2
Del Monte				
Juice	6 oz	80	0	0
Langers				
100% Juice	8 oz	130	0	–
PINK BEANS				
dried cooked	1 cup	252	0	–
PINTO BEANS				
CANNED				
pinto	1 cup	186	0	–
Progresso				
Pinto Beans	½ cup (4.6 oz)	110	0	7
DRIED				
cooked	1 cup	235	0	–
FROZEN				
cooked	3 oz	152	0	–
PISTACHIOS				
dry roasted w/ salt	49 nuts (1 oz)	161	0	3
dry roasted w/o salt	49 nuts (1 oz)	162	0	3
in shells	½ cup	165	0	3
Love'n Bake				
Pistachio Paste	2 tbsp	160	0	2
Sweet Delights				
Pistachio Roasters	⅓ pkg (1 oz)	190	0	3

FOOD	PORTION	CALS	CHOL	FIBER
PITANGA				
fresh	1 cup	57	0	–
fresh	1	2	0	–
PIZZA (see also PIZZA CRUST, PIZZA SAUCE)				
Alexia				
Pizza Snack Sweet Italian Sausage Roasted Peppers & Parmesan	6 pieces (3 oz)	210	10	1
Pizza Snacks Pesto Chicken w/ Fresh Mozzarella	6 pieces (3 oz)	220	10	1
Amy's				
Cheese	⅓ pie	300	15	2
Mushroom & Olive	¼ pie	250	10	2
Pesto	⅓ pie	310	10	2
Pocket Sandwich Cheese Pizza	1 (4.5 oz)	300	15	4
Pocket Sandwich Vegetarian Pizza	1 (4.5 oz)	250	10	4
Roasted Vegetable	⅓ pie	260	0	2
Snacks Cheese	5-6 pieces	180	10	2
Soy Cheese	⅓ pie	290	0	2
Spinach	⅓ pie	300	15	2
Veggie Combo	⅓ pie	280	10	2
Banquet				
Pepperoni	1 pie (6.75 oz)	490	35	5
Pizza Snack Cheese	6 pieces (7.5 oz)	200	20	2
Pizza Snack Pepperoni	6 pieces (7.5 oz)	230	20	2
Pizza Snack Pepperoni & Sausage	6 pieces (7.5 oz)	210	20	2
Boca				
Supreme w/ Rising Crust Sausage & Pepperoni	⅓ pkg (4.3 oz)	280	10	3
Celeste				
4 Cheese	1 (5.7 oz)	360	30	2
Ellio's				
All Cheesy	1 slice	160	10	1
Cheese	1 slice	150	10	1
Microwave Single Slice	1 slice	360	15	4
Pepperoni	1 slice	160	10	1

FOOD	PORTION	CALS	CHOL	FIBER
Freschetta				
Pepperoni	½ pie (5.8 oz)	470	45	2
Health Is Wealth				
Pizza Munchees	6 (3 oz)	190	0	1
Healthy Choice				
French Bread Cheese	1 piece (6 oz)	340	15	5
French Bread Cheese	1 pie	340	10	5
French Bread Pepperoni	1 piece (6 oz)	340	20	6
French Bread Pepperoni	1 pie	340	20	5
French Bread Sausage	1 piece (6 oz)	320	25	5
French Bread Supreme	1 piece (6.35 oz)	330	20	6
French Bread Supreme	1 pie	340	20	5
French Bread Vegetable	1 pie	320	10	6
Ian's				
Cheese	1 slice (1.5 oz)	100	10	1
Jeno's				
Crisp 'N Tasty Cheese	1 pie (6.8 oz)	460	20	2
Jiffy				
Crust Mix as prep	⅕ crust	180	0	2
Kid Cuisine				
Cheese Pizza Painter	1 meal	320	10	5
Dip & Dunk Cheese Pizza Strips	1 meal	510	20	9
Primo Pepperoni Pizza	1 meal	400	10	6
Lean Cuisine				
Casual Eating Deluxe	1 pkg (6 oz)	370	25	3
Casual Eating Four Cheese	1 pkg (6 oz)	400	15	3
Casual Eating French Bread Cheese	1 serv (6 oz)	320	20	3
Casual Eating French Bread Deluxe	1 pkg (6.1 oz)	310	20	3
Casual Eating French Bread Pepperoni	1 pkg (5.25 oz)	300	15	2
Casual Eating Margherita	1 pkg (6 oz)	320	5	4
Casual Eating Pepperoni	1 pkg (6 oz)	380	25	3
Casual Eating Roasted Vegetable	1 pkg (6 oz)	330	10	3
Casual Eating Spinach & Mushroom	1 pkg (6.1 oz)	310	15	4
Casual Eating Three Meat	1 pkg (6.4 oz)	350	25	4

FOOD	PORTION	CALS	CHOL	FIBER
Lean Pockets				
Pepperoni	1 (4.5 oz)	280	25	3
Sausage & Pepperoni	1 (4.5 oz)	280	45	3
Marie Callender's				
French Bread Cheese	1 (7.2 oz)	530	60	4
French Bread Pepperoni	1 (7.5 oz)	570	65	4
French Bread Supreme	1 (7.5 oz)	510	50	4
Mr. P's				
Cheese	1 pie (6.5 oz)	410	25	5
Red Baron				
Deep Dish Single Pepperoni	1 pizza	460	35	2
French Bread Supreme	1 pie (5.8 oz)	370	30	2
South Beach Diet				
Deluxe w/ Wheat Crust	1 pie	340	25	10
Four Cheese w/ Wheat Crust	1 pie	340	20	10
Grilled Chicken & Vegetable w/ Wheat Crust	1 pie	330	25	10
Pepperoni w/ Wheat Crust	1 pie	350	25	9
Tony's				
Pizza For One Cheese	1 (6.5 oz)	500	20	3
Totino's				
Crisp Crust Cheese	½ pie	320	20	2
TAKE-OUT				
cheese	16 in pie	3384	294	23
cheese	⅛ of 16 in pie	423	37	3
cheese deep dish individual	1 (5.5 oz)	460	20	2
cheese & vegetables	⅛ of 16 in pie	428	19	3
ground beef	16 in pie	3753	299	20
ham & pineapple	⅛ of 16 in pie	439	29	3
no cheese	⅛ of 16 in pie	262	0	2
pepperoni	⅛ of 16 in pie	469	37	3
white pizza	⅛ of 16 in pie	484	38	2

PIZZA CRUST

crust	1 slice (1.7 oz)	130	0	1
whole wheat	⅛ crust	140	0	1
Alvarado Street Bakery				
Sprouted Wheat California Style	⅛ pie	190	0	1

FOOD	PORTION	CALS	CHOL	FIBER
Betty Crocker				
Italian Herb Crust Mix	¼ crust (1.6 oz)	180	0	1
Boboli				
Thin Crust	⅕ crust (2 oz)	160	0	1
Carbsense				
Garlic & Herb as prep	1 slice	100	0	4
MiniCarb				
Parmesan Herb Mix as prep	1 slice	130	0	3
Robin Hood				
Crust	¼ crust	160	0	1
PIZZA SAUCE				
Hunt's				
Family Favorites	¼ cup	25	0	1
Muir Glen				
Organic	¼ cup (2.2 oz)	40	0	2
Progresso				
Pizza Sauce	¼ cup (2.1 oz)	20	0	1
PLANTAINS				
cooked mashed	1 cup	232	0	5
sliced cooked	1 cup	179	0	4
Chester's				
Chips	1 oz	150	0	2
TAKE-OUT				
mofongo	1 serv	320	7	5
sweet baked w/ ice cream	1 serv	285	0	3
PLUMS				
canned in heavy syrup	1 cup	163	0	3
canned purple juice pack	1 cup	146	0	2
canned purple water pack	1 cup	102	0	2
dried japanese	1	9	0	tr
fresh	1	30	0	1
pickled	1	34	0	tr
Eden				
Umeboshi Plum Paste	1 tsp	5	0	0
Umeboshi Plums	1 (8 g)	5	0	0
FRESH				
Chiquita				
Purple	2 med (4.6 oz)	80	0	2

FOOD	PORTION	CALS	CHOL	FIBER
POI				
poi	½ cup	134	0	–
POKEBERRY SHOOTS				
cooked	½ cup	16	0	–
fresh	½ cup	18	0	–
POLENTA				
Frieda's				
Organic	2 slices (3.5 oz)	70	0	1
Original	4 oz	80	0	2
Melissa's				
Original	4 oz	80	0	2
POLLACK				
altantic fillet baked	5.3 oz	178	137	0
atlantic baked	3 oz	100	77	0
POMEGRANATE				
fresh	1 (5.4 oz)	105	0	1
POMEGRANATE JUICE				
Izze				
Sparkling Pomegranate	8 oz	80	0	–
Langers				
All Pomegranate	8 oz	140	0	–
Naked Juice				
Pomegranate Passion	8 oz	150	0	0
Odwalla				
PomaGrand Berry	8 oz	140	0	0
PomaGrand Mango	8 oz	160	0	0
POM				
100% Juice	8 oz	140	0	0
Pomegranate Blueberry	8 oz	140	0	0
Pomegranate Cherry	8 oz	140	0	0
Pomegranate Mango	8 oz	140	0	0
Pomegranate Tangerine	8 oz	150	0	0
POMPANO				
broiled	4 oz	192	49	0
smoked	2 oz	109	33	0
steamed	4 oz	232	71	0

FOOD	PORTION	CALS	CHOL	FIBER
TAKE-OUT				
battered & fried	4 oz	304	67	tr
breaded & fried	4 oz	361	94	1
POPCORN (see also POPCORN CAKES)				
air-popped	1 cup (0.3 oz)	31	0	2
caramel coated w/ peanuts	⅔ cup (1 oz)	114	0	1
cheese	1 cup (0.4 oz)	58	1	1
oil popped	1 cup (0.4 oz)	55	0	1
Cape Cod				
White Cheddar	2⅓ cups	170	8	2
Chester's				
Microwave Butter	3 cups	170	0	3
Microwave Cheddar Cheese	3 cups	200	<5	2
Cracker Jack				
Butter Toffee	¾ cup	140	0	1
Original	½ cup	120	0	1
Dale & Thomas				
Caramel	½ cup	75	0	0
Hall Of Fame Kettlecorn	½ cup	34	0	1
North Country Cheddar	½ cup	73	1	1
Peanut Butter & White Chocolate Drizzlecorn	½ cup	115	0	1
Purepopped Natural	½ cup	26	0	1
Sweet Georgia Pecan	½ cup	96	3	1
Toffee Crunch Drizzlecorn	½ cup	107	1	1
Husman's				
Cheese Corn	2¼ cups (1 oz)	160	<5	1
Jolly Time				
American's Best 94% Fat Free	5 cups	100	0	5
American's Best White	5 cups	100	0	6
American's Best Yellow	5 cups	90	0	9
Blast O Butter Light	4 cups	120	0	4
Butter Licious Light	5 cups	130	0	4
Crispy'n White Light	5 cups	125	0	7
Healthy Pop 94% Fat Free	5 cups	100	0	5
Healthy Pop Caramel Apple	5 cups	110	0	6
Healthy Pop Kettle	4 cups	100	0	4
Healthy Pop Minis	4 cups	90	0	8

FOOD	PORTION	CALS	CHOL	FIBER
Mallow Magic	2.5 cups	180	0	3
The Big Cheez	3.5 cups	140	0	6
White	5 cups	100	0	6
Yellow	5 cups	100	0	6
Judy's				
Sugar Free Popcorn Nut Brittle	¼ piece (1 oz)	100	0	tr
LesserEvil				
Black&White	1 cup	120	0	1
KettleCorn	1 cup	120	5	2
MaplePecan	1 cup	120	0	3
PeanutButter & Choco	1 cup	120	0	1
SinNamon	1 cup	120	5	2
Mauna Loa				
Macadamia Nut Butter Corn Crunch	1 oz	150	1	1
Newman's Own				
Microwave 94% Fat Free	3½ cups	110	0	4
Microwave Butter	3½ cups	130	0	3
Microwave Butter Boom	3½ cups	130	0	3
Microwave Light Butter	3½ cups	120	0	4
Microwave Low Sodium Butter	3½ cups	130	0	3
Microwave Natural	3½ cups	130	0	3
Organic Pop's Corn Butter	3½ cups	160	0	1
Organic Pop's Corn No Butter No Salt 94% Fat Free	3½ cups	120	0	1
Oogie's				
Romano & Pesto	1 oz	138	0	3
Smoked Gouda	1 oz	132	0	3
Spicy Chipotle & Lime	1 oz	143	0	3
White Cheddar	1 oz	142	0	3
Orville Redenbacher's				
Gourmet Original	3 cups	92	0	5
Hot Air	1 cup	15	0	1
Kernel Original	1 cup	15	0	1
Microwave Butter Light	1 cup	20	0	1
Microwave Kettle Korn Sweet	1 cup	35	tr	1
Microwave Movie Theater Butter Light	1 cup	20	0	1

FOOD	PORTION	CALS	CHOL	FIBER
Microwave Movie Theater Extra Butter	1 cup	35	0	1
Microwave Natural Light	1 cup	20	0	1
Microwave Pour Over Butter	1 cup	40	0	1
Microwave Pour Over Cheddar	1 cup	50	0	1
Microwave Regular Butter	1 cup	35	0	1
Microwave Regular Corn On The Cob	1 cup	35	0	1
Microwave Regular Natural	1 cup	15	0	1
Microwave Regular Old Fashioned Butter	1 cup	35	0	1
Microwave Regular Tender White	1 cup	40	0	1
Microwave Smart Pop Butter	1 cup	15	0	1
Microwave Smart Pop Kettle Korn	1 cup	20	0	1
Microwave Smart Pop Movie Theater Butter	1 cup	20	0	1
Microwave Sweet Caramel	1 cup	90	0	4
Microwave Sweet Cinnabon	1 cup	50	0	tr
Microwave Sweet Honey Butter	1 cup	35	0	1
Microwave Sweet 'N Buttery	1 cup	40	tr	1
Microwave Ultimate Butter	1 cup	30	0	1
White	1 cup	15	0	1
Pop Secret				
94% Fat Free Butter	1 cup (5 g)	20	0	tr
94% Fat Free Natural	1 cup (5 g)	20	0	tr
Butter	1 cup (7 g)	35	0	tr
Cheddar Cheese	1 cup (6 g)	30	0	tr
Jumbo Pop Butter	1 cup (7 g)	40	0	tr
Jumbo Pop Movie Theater Butter	1 cup (7 g)	40	0	tr
Light Movie Theater Butter	1 cup (5 g)	25	0	tr
Light Natural	1 cup (5 g)	25	0	tr
Movie Theater Butter	1 cup (7 g)	40	0	tr
Nacho Cheese	1 cup (6 g)	30	0	tr
Natural	1 cup (7 g)	35	0	tr
Real Butter	1 cup (7 g)	35	0	tr

FOOD	PORTION	CALS	CHOL	FIBER
Poppycock				
The Original	½ cup	160	10	1
Smart Balance				
Light as prep	4 cups	120	0	4
Low Fat as prep	5 cups	120	0	5
Movie Style as prep	3.5 cups	170	0	3
Smartfood				
Reduced Fat White Cheddar	3 cups	140	<5	3
White Cheddar	1 pkg	160	5	2
Snyder's Of Hanover				
Butter	⅝ oz	110	0	0
Utz				
Hulless Puff'N Corn	2 cups (1 oz)	180	0	0
Hulless Puff'N Corn Cheese	2 cups (1 oz)	170	<5	0
Hulless Puff'N Corn Hot Cheese	1 pkg (1.75 oz)	290	0	0
Wise				
Butter	1 pkg (0.5 oz)	80	0	1
Hot Cheese	1 oz	150	<5	2
POPCORN CAKES				
Orville Redenbacher's				
Butter	2	60	0	2
Caramel	1	40	0	tr
Chocolate	1	45	0	tr
Mini Butter	8	60	0	1
Mini Caramel	7	50	0	1
Mini Peanut Caramel Crunch	6	60	0	1
Mini Peanut Crunch	6	60	0	2
Mini Sour Cream & Onion	8	60	0	2
White Cheddar	2	60	0	2
POPOVER				
home recipe as prep w/ 2% milk	1 (1.4 oz)	87	46	–
home recipe as prep w/ whole milk	1 (1.4 oz)	90	47	–
POPPY SEEDS				
poppy seeds	1 tsp	15	0	–

FOOD	PORTION	CALS	CHOL	FIBER
Love'n Bake				
Poppy Seed Filling	2 tbsp	120	0	tr
PORK (*see also* HAM, PORK DISHES)				
FRESH				
boneless loin lean & fat roasted	3.5 oz	195	80	0
center loin chop bone in broiled	1 (3 oz)	178	71	0
center rib chop lean & fat bone in broiled	1 (3 oz)	189	57	0
country style ribs bone in lean & fat braised	3.5 oz	288	110	0
dehydrated oriental style	1 cup (0.8 oz)	135	15	0
fresh ham rump half lean & fat roasted	4 oz	278	106	0
fresh ham shank half lean & fat roasted	4 oz	319	102	0
fresh ham whole lean & fat roasted	4 oz	302	104	0
ground cooked	4 oz	328	104	0
ham hock cooked	1	167	56	0
shoulder chop bone in braised	1 (3 oz)	229	84	0
sirloin roast lean & fat bone in roasted	4 oz	231	89	0
spareribs bone in roasted	3 oz	304	89	0
tail simmered	3 oz	336	110	0
tenderloin roast boneless lean & fat roasted	4 oz	145	73	0
top loin chop boneless lean & fat broiled	1 (3.5 oz)	195	73	0
Boar's Head				
Smoked Shoulder Butt Roast	3 oz	170	55	–
Freirich				
Porkette	4 oz	220	70	0
Smithfield				
Smoked Pork Chop	3 oz	100	30	0

FOOD	PORTION	CALS	CHOL	FIBER
READY-TO-EAT				
Sara Lee				
Oven Roasted	2 oz	70	40	0
TAKE-OUT				
chicharrones pork cracklings fried	1 cup	492	100	0
chop breaded & fried	1 lg (5 oz)	441	126	1
chop breaded & fried	1 med (3.4 oz)	304	87	1
chop stewed	1 lg (4.6 oz)	315	106	0
PORK DISHES				
Hormel				
Extra Lean Apple Burbon	1 serv (4 oz)	140	50	0
Extra Lean Teriyaki	4 oz	140	50	0
Pork Roast Au Jus	1 serv (5 oz)	180	85	0
Morton's Of Omaha				
Tender Pork Roast w/ Gravy & Vegetables	1 serv (5 oz)	210	70	1
Smithfield				
Pulled Pork w/ Barbecue Sauce	2 oz	90	20	–
Tenderloin Garlic & Herb	3 oz	100	60	tr
Tenderloin Hickory Sweet	4 oz	110	60	0
Tyson				
Lemon Pepper Pork Roast	1 serv (3 oz)	110	30	0
Wellshire				
Baby Back Ribs w/ Sauce	2 ribs (5 oz)	260	81	0
TAKE-OUT				
spareribs barbecued w/ sauce	2 med (2.8 oz)	248	70	tr
PORK RINDS (see SNACKS)				
POT PIE				
Amy's				
Broccoli	1 (7.5 oz)	430	45	4
Country Vegetable	1 (7.5 oz)	370	40	4
Shepard's	1 (8 oz)	160	0	5
Vegetable	1 (7.5 oz)	420	50	4
Vegetable Non-Dairy	1 (7.5 oz)	320	0	4

FOOD	PORTION	CALS	CHOL	FIBER
Banquet				
Beef	1 (7 oz)	400	30	1
Cheesy Potato & Broccoli w/ Ham	1 (7 oz)	410	25	2
Chicken	1 (7 oz)	380	40	1
Family Size Hearty Chicken	1 cup	460	35	2
Macaroni & Cheese	1 pkg (6.5 oz)	210	10	1
Turkey	1 (7 oz)	370	45	3
Vegetable Cheese	1 (7 oz)	340	10	1
Hot Pockets				
Pot Pie Express Chicken	1 piece (4.5 oz)	350	15	3
Ian's				
Chicken	1 pkg (9.4 oz)	510	65	2
Marie Callender's				
Beef	1 (9.5 oz)	680	20	1
Chicken	1 (9.5 oz)	680	20	3
Chicken & Broccoli	1 (9.5 oz)	670	25	4
Chicken Au Gratin	1 (9.5 oz)	690	30	4
Turkey	1 (9.5 oz)	680	15	5
Morton				
Macaroni & Cheese	1 (6.5 oz)	210	10	1
Vegetable w/ Beef	1 (7 oz)	340	20	2
Vegetable w/ Chicken	1 (7 oz)	320	25	2
Vegetable w/ Turkey	1 (7 oz)	310	25	2
Swanson				
Beef	1 (7 oz)	376	22	5
Chicken	1 (7 oz)	416	19	2
Turkey	1 (7 oz)	440	18	2
TAKE-OUT				
beef	1 (8 in pie) 14.6 oz	938	67	5
chicken	1 (8 in pie) 14.6 oz	897	113	6
ham	1 serv (11 oz)	752	38	4
oyster	1 serv (11.5 oz)	817	89	3

POTATO (*see also* CHIPS, KNISH, PANCAKES)

FOOD	PORTION	CALS	CHOL	FIBER
CANNED				
potatoes	½ cup	54	0	–
Del Monte				
New Whole	2 med (5.5 oz)	60	0	2
Savory Sides Au Gratin	½ cup	80	0	1

FOOD	PORTION	CALS	CHOL	FIBER
Lunch Bucket				
Scalloped w/ Ham Chunks	1 pkg (7.5 oz)	170	10	3
S&W				
Whole Small	2 (5.5 oz)	60	0	2
FRESH				
baked skin only	1 skin (2 oz)	115	0	2
baked w/ skin	1 (6.5 oz)	220	0	–
baked w/o skin	1 (5 oz)	145	0	2
baked w/o skin	½ cup	57	0	1
boiled	½ cup	68	0	1
microwaved	1 (7 oz)	212	0	–
microwaved w/o skin	½ cup	78	0	–
raw w/o skin	1 (3.9 oz)	88	0	–
Arrowfarms				
Yukon Gold	1 med (5 oz)	100	0	3
Dole				
Idaho	1 (5.3 oz)	100	0	3
Frieda's				
Fingerling	4 (5 oz)	100	0	3
Green Giant				
Red Potatoes	1 med (5 oz)	100	0	3
Lucinda's				
Red "C"	1 med (5.2 oz)	100	0	3
SunLite				
SunLite	1 (5 oz)	87	0	4
FROZEN				
french fries	10 strips	111	0	2
french fries thick cut	10 strips	109	0	–
potato puffs	½ cup	138	0	–
potato puffs as prep	1	16	0	–
Alexia				
Hashed Brown	1 serv (3 oz)	80	0	2
Mashed Red w/ Garlic & Parmesan	½ cup	150	0	2
Mashed Yukon Gold & Sea Salt	½ cup	150	20	2
Oven Crinkles Classic	1 serv (3 oz)	120	0	3
Oven Crinkles Salt & Pepper	1 serv (3 oz)	120	0	3
Oven Fries Garlic	12 pieces	140	0	2
Oven Reds	1 serv (3 oz)	120	0	2

FOOD	PORTION	CALS	CHOL	FIBER
Waffle Fries	8 pieces	150	0	3
Yukon Gold Fries w/ Sea Salt	1 serv (3 oz)	130	0	2
Fillo Factory				
Petite Fillo Puffs Potato & Herb	7 (4.6 oz)	280	15	1
Healthy Choice				
Cheddar Broccoli Potatoes	1 pkg	270	20	7
Ian's				
Alphatots	1 serv (3.5 oz)	156	0	1
Fries Sweet Potato	7 pieces (2.5 oz)	70	0	1
Inland Valley				
Crinkle Cuts	15 pieces (3 oz)	150	0	2
Crisscut Fries	13 pieces (3 oz)	160	0	2
Curly QQQ's	1⅓ cups (3 oz)	180	0	2
Fajita Fries	17 pieces (3 oz)	170	0	2
French Fries	15 pieces (3 oz)	130	0	2
Hash Browns	⅔ cup	70	0	2
Home Browns	1 patty (2.2 oz)	130	0	2
Mashed Homestyle	⅔ cup	160	5	3
Simply Shreds	1 cup	70	0	2
Stix	5 pieces (3 oz)	170	0	2
Stuffed Spudz w/ Cheese	5 pieces	210	20	2
Tater Babies	8 pieces (3 oz)	130	0	2
Tater Puffs	10 pieces	160	0	2
Twice Baked	1 (5.2 oz)	230	30	2
Twice Baked Sour Cream Bacon & Chives	1 (5.2 oz)	240	10	3
Twice Baked Triple Cheese	1 (5.2 oz)	250	20	3
Larry's				
Mashed Broccoli & Cheddar Cheese	1 serv (5 oz)	180	0	2
Mashed Cheddar Cheese	1 serv (5 oz)	190	5	2
Mashed Old Fashioned Butter	1 serv (5 oz)	190	10	2
Mashed Sour Cream & Chives	1 serv (5 oz)	180	5	2
Mashed Sweet Potatoes	1 serv (4 oz)	140	10	2
Lean Cuisine				
One Dish Favorites Deluxe Cheddar	1 pkg (10.4 oz)	260	25	5

FOOD	PORTION	CALS	CHOL	FIBER
McCain				
French Fries Crinkle Cut	18 pieces (3 oz)	130	0	2
Mash-Bites	1 serv (3 oz)	50	0	1
Roasters All American	1 serv (3 oz)	120	0	tr
Roasters Grilled Garlic & Onion	1 serv (3 oz)	120	0	2
Seasoned Wedges Skin On	1 serv (3 oz)	120	0	2
Shoestring French Fries	45 pieces (3 oz)	140	0	2
Smiles	6 pieces (3 oz)	160	0	2
Steak Fries	8 pieces (3 oz)	120	0	2
Tasti Tater	1 serv (3 oz)	160	0	3
Oh Boy!				
Stuffed w/ Onion Sour Cream & Chives	1 (5 oz)	110	<5	2
Roast Works				
Roasted Seasoned Wedge	1 serv (3 oz)	100	0	1
Roasted Wedges Rosemary Redskin	1 serv (3 oz)	110	0	2
Roasted Wedges Yukon Gold	1 serv (3 oz)	110	0	1
Tree of Life				
Organic French Fries	20 pieces (3 oz)	110	0	1
MIX				
au gratin as prep	½ cup	160	29	–
instant mashed flakes as prep w/ whole milk & butter	½ cup	118	15	–
instant mashed flakes not prep	½ cup	78	0	–
instant mashed granules as prep w/ whole milk & butter	½ cup	114	15	–
instant mashed granules not prep	½ cup	372	0	–
scalloped	½ cup	105	14	–
Betty Crocker				
Au Gratin as prep	½ cup	150	5	1
Au Gratin Low Fat Recipe	½ cup	110	<5	1
Cheddar & Bacon	½ cup	150	<5	1
Cheddar & Bacon Low Fat Recipe	½ cup	120	0	1
Cheddar & Sour Cream	½ cup	130	5	1

FOOD	PORTION	CALS	CHOL	FIBER
Chicken & Vegetable	⅔ cup	140	<5	2
Chicken & Vegetable Low Fat Recipe	⅔ cup	120	<5	2
Hash Browns	½ cup	190	0	3
Homestyle Broccoli Au Gratin	½ cup	140	<5	2
Homestyle Broccoli Au Gratin Low Fat Recipe	½ cup	110	0	2
Homestyle Cheddar Cheese	½ cup	120	<5	1
Homestyle Cheddar Cheese Stove Top Recipe	½ cup	140	5	1
Homestyle Cheesy Scalloped	½ cup	140	<5	2
Homestyle Cheesy Scalloped Low Fat Recipe	½ cup	110	<5	3
Julienne	½ cup	150	<5	1
Mashed Butter & Herb	½ cup	160	3	1
Mashed Butter & Herb Reduced Fat Recipe	½ cup	130	<5	1
Mashed Chicken & Herb	½ cup	150	<5	1
Mashed Chicken & Herb Reduced Fat Recipe	½ cup	120	0	1
Mashed Four Cheese	½ cup	150	<5	2
Mashed Four Cheese Reduced Fat Recipe	½ cup	120	0	2
Mashed Potato Buds	⅔ cup	160	<5	1
Mashed Potato Buds Reduced Fat Recipe	⅔ cup	120	0	1
Mashed Roasted Garlic	½ cup	150	<5	2
Mashed Roasted Garlic Reduced Fat Recipe	½ cup	130	0	2
Mashed Sour Cream & Chives	½ cup	150	5	1
Mashed Sour Cream & Chives Reduced Fat Recipe	½ cup	120	<5	1
Potato Shakers Original	⅔ cup	140	<5	2
Potato Shakers Original Low Fat Recipe	⅔ cup	120	<5	2

FOOD	PORTION	CALS	CHOL	FIBER
Ranch	½ cup	160	<5	2
Scalloped	½ cup	150	<5	1
Scalloped Low Fat Recipe	⅔ cup	110	0	1
Sour Cream'n Chives	½ cup	160	5	2
Three Cheese	½ cup	150	<5	1
Twice Baked Cheddar & Bacon as prep	⅔ cup	210	85	1
Twice Baked Cheddar & Bacon Low Fat Recipe	⅔ cup	130	<5	1
Idahoan				
AuGratin as prep	½ cup	150	3	2
Hash Browns as prep	½ cup	160	0	1
Hash Browns Cheesy not prep	½ cup	120	0	2
Mashed Baked as prep	½ cup	110	0	2
Mashed Butter & Herb as prep	½ cup	110	0	1
Mashed Buttery Homestyle as prep	½ cup	110	0	1
Mashed Four Cheese as prep	½ cup	100	0	1
Mashed Southwest as prep	½ cup	110	0	2
Roasted Garlic as prep	½ cup	600	0	1
Scalloped as prep	½ cup	150	3	1
REFRIGERATED				
Country Crock				
Garlic Mashed	⅔ cup	170	0	3
Homestyle Mashed	⅔ cup	190	20	3
PurelyIdaho				
Cheddar Crusted	¾ cup	120	3	2
Oven Roasts	1 serv (3 oz)	70	0	2
Simply Potatoes				
Diced w/ Onion	⅔ cup	60	0	1
Homestyle Slices	⅔ cup	70	0	1
Mashed	⅔ cup	170	20	1
Mashed Sweet Potatoes	⅔ cup	160	0	2
Red Potato Wedges	½ cup	50	0	2
Shredded Hash Browns	½ cup	50	0	tr

FOOD	PORTION	CALS	CHOL	FIBER
SHELF-STABLE				
TastyBite				
Bombay Potatoes	½ pkg (5 oz)	190	0	6
Mumbai Pav Bhaji	½ pkg (5 oz)	229	0	7
Simla Potatoes	½ pkg (5 oz)	180	0	1
TAKE-OUT				
au gratin w/ cheese	½ cup	178	18	–
baked topped w/ cheese sauce	1	475	19	–
baked topped w/ cheese sauce & bacon	1	451	30	–
baked topped w/ cheese sauce & broccoli	1	402	20	–
baked topped w/ cheese sauce & chili	1	481	31	–
baked topped w/ sour cream & chives	1	394	23	–
french fries	1 reg	235	0	–
hash brown	½ cup (2.5 oz)	151	9	–
indian yogurt potatoes	1 serv	315	18	0
mashed	½ cup	111	2	–
o'brien	1 cup	157	7	–
potato pancakes	1 (1.3 oz)	101	35	–
potato salad	½ cup	179	85	2
red new boiled	5 sm (5 oz)	120	0	2
scalloped	½ cup	127	7	–
twice baked w/ cheese	1 half (10 oz)	392	54	4
POTATO STARCH				
potato starch	1 oz	96	0	–
POUT				
ocean baked	3 oz	86	57	0
ocean fillet baked	4.8 oz	139	91	0
PRETZELS				
chocolate covered	1 (0.4 oz)	47	1	tr
soft	1 lg (5 oz)	483	4	2
twists salted	10 (2.1 oz)	229	0	2
twists w/o salt	10 (2.1 oz)	229	0	2
whole wheat	2 sm (1 oz)	103	0	2

FOOD	PORTION	CALS	CHOL	FIBER
yogurt covered	1 (4 g)	19	0	tr
yogurt covered	1 cup (3 oz)	391	1	1
Aramana				
Soy Pretzels	15 (1 oz)	100	5	4
Bachman				
Thin'n Right	12 (1 oz)	120	0	1
Cape Cod				
Pretzels	25	130	0	tr
Combos				
Cheddar Cheese Cracker	1 pkg (1.7 oz)	240	0	1
Nacho Cheese	1 pkg (1.7 oz)	230	0	1
Pizzeria Pretzel	1 pkg (1.7 oz)	230	0	1
Gardetto's				
Mustard	1 pkg (0.5 oz)	50	0	tr
Glenny's				
Organic Original Salted	8 (1 oz)	110	0	1
Organic Sourdough	6 (1 oz)	110	0	1
Goodniks				
Yogurt Pretzels	15	180	0	0
Handi-Snack				
Mister Salty Pretzels 'N Cheese	1 pkg	90	5	0
Healthy Handfuls				
Python Pretzels	1 box (1.5 oz)	170	0	1
Landies Candies				
Sugar Free Chocolate	4 (1.5 oz)	220	<5	tr
Newman's Own				
Organic Bavarian Sour Dough	1	90	0	1
Organic Hi Protein	22	120	0	4
Organic Salt & Pepper Rounds	8	100	0	1
Organic Salt & Pepper Thins	10	120	0	tr
Organic Salted Nuggets	20	120	0	2
Organic Salted Rods	4	120	0	2
Organic Salted Rounds	8	110	0	tr
Organic Salted Sticks	13	110	0	1
Organic Salted Thins	10	110	0	1
Organic Spelt	20	120	0	4
Organic Unsalted Rounds	8	110	0	tr

FOOD	PORTION	CALS	CHOL	FIBER
Quinlan				
Low Fat Mini	1 oz	110	0	tr
Rold Gold				
Braided Twists	8	110	0	1
Braided Twists Honey Wheat	8	110	0	1
Checkers	20	110	<5	1
Rods	3	110	0	1
Sourdough Hard	1	100	0	1
Sourdough Specials	5	110	0	1
Sticks	48	100	0	1
Thins	9 pieces	110	0	1
Tiny Twists	18 pieces	110	0	1
Tiny Twists Cheddar	20	110	0	1
Tiny Twists Honey Mustard	13	110	0	1
Snyder's Of Hanover				
100 Calorie Pack Snaps	1 pkg (0.9 oz)	100	0	tr
100 Calorie Pack Stick	1 pkg (0.9 oz)	100	0	tr
Dips White Fudge	1 oz	130	0	0
Hard Sourdough	1 oz	100	0	1
Hard Sourdough Unsalted	1 oz	100	0	1
Logs	1 oz	110	0	tr
Mini	1 pkg (0.9 oz)	100	0	tr
Mini Unsalted	1 oz	110	0	tr
Nibblers	1 oz	120	0	tr
Nibblers Oat Bran	1 oz	130	0	3
Nibblers Unsalted	1 oz	120	0	tr
Oat Bran	1 oz	100	0	2
Old Fashioned Dipping Stix	1 oz	100	0	1
Olde Tyme	1 oz	120	0	1
Olde Tyme Stix	1 oz	120	0	1
Old Tyme Unsalted	1 oz	120	0	1
Pieces Buttermilk Ranch	1 oz	130	0	tr
Pieces Cheddar Cheese	1 oz	190	0	tr
Pieces Honey Mustard & Onions	1 oz	140	0	tr
Pieces Peppered Pizza	1 oz	150	0	tr
Rods	1 oz	120	0	tr
Thin	1 oz	130	0	tr
Whole Wheat Honey	1 oz	120	0	2

FOOD	PORTION	CALS	CHOL	FIBER
Spinzels				
Braided	1 pkg (0.5 oz)	55	0	tr
Utz				
Rods	3 (1 oz)	120	0	1
Wege				
Honey Wheat	1 (0.8 oz)	120	0	1
Wise				
Fat Free Sticks	1 oz	100	0	tr
Low Fat Honey Wheat Braided Twists	1 oz	110	0	1
PRUNE JUICE				
jarred	1 cup	182	0	3
L&A				
100% Juice	8 oz	180	0	3
Langers				
Plus 100% Juice	8 oz	180	0	1
Ocean Spray				
100% Juice	8 oz	180	0	0
Sunsweet				
100% Juice	8 oz	180	0	3
PlumSmart	8 oz	160	0	3
PRUNES				
cooked w/o sugar	½ cup	133	0	4
dried	1	20	0	1
Love'n Bake				
Prune Lekvar	2 tbsp	90	0	1
Newman's Own				
Organic	½ cup	110	0	2
St Dalfour				
French Prunes	3	100	0	3
Sunsweet				
Pitted Dried	5	100	0	3
PUDDING				
MIX				
Betty Crocker				
Rice as prep	1 serv	200	9	–
Jell-O				
Vanilla as prep w/ 2% milk	½ cup (5.1 oz)	150	9	0

FOOD	PORTION	CALS	CHOL	FIBER
Keto				
Banana not prep	½ scoop	62	10	2
Chocolate not prep	½ scoop	66	10	3
French Vanilla not prep	½ scoop	62	10	2
Louisiana Purchase				
Bread	1 serv (1.3 oz)	150	0	2
Lundberg				
Elegant Rice Cinnamon Raisin	½ cup (3.9 oz)	70	0	1
Elegant Rice Coconut	½ cup (3.9 oz)	70	0	1
Elegant Rice Honey Almond	½ cup (3.9 oz)	70	0	1
Uncle Ben's				
Rice Pudding Cinnamon & Raisins as prep	½ cup	160	0	1
Rice Pudding French Vanilla as prep	½ cup	120	0	1
READY-TO-EAT				
Boost				
Vanilla	1 pkg (5 oz)	240	<5	0
Healthy Choice				
Low Fat Chocolate Almond	½ cup (3.5 oz)	109	0	0
Low Fat Chocolate Raspberry	½ cup (3.5 oz)	102	0	0
Low Fat Double Chocolate Fudge	½ cup (3.5 oz)	101	0	0
Low Fat French Vanilla	½ cup (3.5 oz)	98	0	0
Low Fat Tapioca	½ cup (3.5 oz)	101	1	0
Hunt's				
Dessert Favorites Banana Cream Pie	1 serv (3.5 oz)	140	0	0
Dessert Favorites Chocolate Brownie	1 serv (3.5 oz)	190	0	0
Dessert Favorites Chocolate Mud Pie	1 serv (3.5 oz)	170	0	0
Dessert Favorites Chocolate Peanut Butter Pie	1 serv (3.5 oz)	190	0	0
Dessert Favorites Dulce De Leche Caramel Cream	1 serv (3.5 oz)	140	0	0
Dessert Favorites Lemon Merinque Pie	1 serv (3.5 oz)	130	0	0
Snack Pack Butterscotch	1 serv (3.5 oz)	130	0	0

FOOD	PORTION	CALS	CHOL	FIBER
Snack Pack Chocolate	1 serv (3.5 oz)	104	1	0
Snack Pack Chocolate Fudge	1 serv (3.5 oz)	150	1	0
Snack Pack Chocolate Marshmallow	1 serv (3.5 oz)	130	1	0
Snack Pack Fat Free Chocolate	1 serv (3.5 oz)	90	0	0
Snack Pack Fat Free Tapioca	1 serv (3.5 oz)	80	0	0
Snack Pack Fat Free Vanilla	1 serv (3.5 oz)	80	0	0
Snack Pack Lemon	1 serv (3.5 oz)	120	0	0
Snack Pack Swirl Chocolate Caramel	1 serv (3.5 oz)	140	0	0
Snack Pack Swirl S'mores	1 serv (3.5 oz)	140	0	0
Snack Pack Tapioca	1 serv (3.5 oz)	130	0	0
Snack Pack Vanilla	1 serv (3.5 oz)	130	1	0
Jell-O				
100 Calorie Pack Fat Free Chocolate Vanilla Swirl	1 serv (4 oz)	100	0	tr
100 Calorie Pack Fat Free Tapioca	1 serv (4 oz)	100	0	0
Fat Free Chocolate Fudge & Caramel	1 serv (4 oz)	100	0	0
Fat Free Vanilla Caramel	1 serv (4 oz)	100	0	0
Tapioca	1 serv (4 oz)	110	0	0
Kozy Shack				
Banana	1 pkg (4 oz)	132	17	0
Chocolate	1 pkg (4 oz)	139	13	1
Chocolate No Sugar Added	1 pkg (4 oz)	93	9	1
Rice	1 pkg (4 oz)	135	20	0
Tapioca	1 pkg (4 oz)	130	15	0
Tapioca No Sugar Added	1 pkg	90	15	4
Vanilla	1 pkg (4 oz)	130	17	0
Vanilla No Sugar Added	1 pkg (4 oz)	90	9	0
Swiss Miss				
Butterscotch	1 pkg (4 oz)	156	1	0
Chocolate	1 pkg (4 oz)	166	1	0
Chocolate Fudge	1 pkg (4 oz)	175	1	0
Fat Free Chocolate	1 pkg (4 oz)	98	0	0
Fat Free Chocolate Fudge	1 pkg (4 oz)	101	0	0
Fat Free Vanilla	1 pkg (4 oz)	93	0	0

FOOD	PORTION	CALS	CHOL	FIBER
Fat Free Parfait Vanilla Chocolate	1 pkg (4 oz)	96	0	0
Lemon Meringue Pie	1 pkg (4 oz)	150	0	–
Low Fat Tapioca	1 pkg (4 oz)	130	0	0
Low Fat Vanilla	1 serv (4 oz)	120	0	–
Milk Chocolate	1 pkg (4 oz)	166	1	0
Parfait Vanilla Chocolate	1 pkg (4 oz)	164	1	0
Swirl Chocolate Caramel	1 pkg (4 oz)	169	1	1
Swirl Chocolate Vanilla	1 pkg (4 oz)	169	1	0
Tapioca	1 pkg (4 oz)	138	1	0
Vanilla	1 pkg (4 oz)	156	1	0
TAKE-OUT				
bread w/ raisins	1 cup	306	124	2
coconut	1 cup	291	15	2
corn	1 cup	328	185	4
indian pudding	½ cup	156	40	1
noodle pudding kugel	1 cup	297	144	2
plum pudding	1 slice (1.5 oz)	125	22	1
rice pudding	1 cup	302	14	1
sweet potato	1 cup	215	2	5
tapioca	1 cup	236	156	0
yorkshire	1 serv (3 oz)	177	57	tr
PUMMELO				
fresh	1	228	0	–
sections	1 cup	71	0	–
Sunkist				
Fresh	¼	90	0	4
PUMPKIN				
butter	1 tbsp	32	0	–
canned	½ cup	41	0	–
cooked mashed	½ cup	24	0	–
flowers cooked	½ cup	10	0	–
flowers raw	1	0	0	–
leaves cooked	½ cup	7	0	–
leaves raw	½ cup	4	0	–
raw cubed	½ cup	15	0	–
Farmer's Market				
Organic Puree	½ cup	50	0	4
Libby's				
Puree	½ cup	40	0	5

FOOD	PORTION	CALS	CHOL	FIBER
PUMPKIN SEEDS				
dried	1 oz	154	0	–
roasted	¼ cup	296	0	–
salted & roasted	¼ cup	296	0	–
whole roasted	1 oz	127	0	–
whole roasted	¼ cup	71	0	–
whole salted roasted	¼ cup	71	0	–
David				
All Natural	¼ cup	160	0	1
Eden				
Dry Roasted & Salted	¼ cup	200	0	5
Good Sense				
Roasted & Salted	½ cup	160	0	1
PURSLANE				
cooked	1 cup	21	0	–
fresh	1 cup	7	0	–
QUAIL				
cooked bone removed	1 (2.7 oz)	177	65	0
QUICHE				
Atkins				
Crustless Bacon & Onion	1 serv	320	175	0
Crustless Four Cheese	1 serv	290	45	0
Crustless Smoked Ham & Cheese	1 serv	290	170	0
TAKE-OUT				
cheese pie	⅛ of 9 in pie	566	240	1
lorraine pie	⅛ of 9 in pie	568	242	1
spinach pie	⅛ of 9 in pie	342	157	1
QUINCE				
fresh	1	53	0	–
QUINOA				
quinoa not prep	1 cup (6 oz)	636	0	10
Eden				
Quinoa not prep	¼ cup	180	0	11
Seeds Of Change				
French Herb Quinoa Blend as prep	1 cup	290	0	3

FOOD	PORTION	CALS	CHOL	FIBER
RABBIT				
domestic w/o bone roasted	3 oz	167	70	–
wild w/o bone stewed	3 oz	147	104	–
RADICCHIO				
raw shredded	½ cup	5	0	–
RADISHES				
chinese dried	½ cup	157	0	–
chinese raw	1 (12 oz)	62	0	–
chinese raw sliced	½ cup	8	0	–
chinese sliced cooked	½ cup	13	0	–
daikon dried	½ cup	157	0	–
daikon raw	1 (12 oz)	62	0	–
daikon raw sliced	½ cup	8	0	–
daikon sliced cooked	½ cup	13	0	–
red raw	10	7	0	–
red sliced	½ cup	10	0	–
white icicle raw	1 (0.5 oz)	2	0	–
white icicle raw sliced	½ cup	7	0	–
Eden				
Daikon Dried Shredded	2 tbsp	45	0	3
Daikon Pickled	2 slices (0.5 oz)	5	0	–
Frieda's				
Black	¾ cup	15	0	1
Chinese Lo Bok	⅔ cup	25	0	2
Daikon	½ cup	15	0	0
Korean Moo	⅔ cup	15	0	1
TAKE-OUT				
moo namul saengche korean salad	1 serv (3.7 oz)	34	0	2
RAISINS				
cinnamon coated	¼ cup	108	0	1
cooked	¼ cup	162	0	1
golden seedless	¼ cup	109	0	1
jumbo golden	¼ cup	130	0	2
milk chocolate coated	¼ cup	176	1	2
milk chocolate coated	28 (1 oz)	109	1	1
seedless	55 (1 oz)	86	0	1

FOOD	PORTION	CALS	CHOL	FIBER
Brach's				
California Chocolate Covered	35 pieces	170	10	1
Dole				
CinnaRaisins	1 pkg (1 oz)	95	0	2
Earthbound Farm				
Organic Jumbo Flame Seedless	¼ cup	120	0	2
Estee				
Chocolate Covered Fructose Sweetened	¼ cup	180	<5	1
Goodniks				
Yogurt Raisins	3 tbsp	145	0	1
Mariana				
Fruitn Yogurt Milk Chocolate Covered Raisins	32 pieces (1 oz)	130	0	2
Nestle				
Chocolate Covered	1⅓ tbsp	70	0	tr
Newman's Own				
Organic	¼ cup	130	0	2
Sun-Maid				
California Golden	¼ cup	130	0	2
California Seedless	¼ cup	130	0	2
Sunsweet				
Red Flame	¼ cup	130	0	2
Tree Of Life				
Organic	¼ cup (1.4 oz)	130	0	2
RASPBERRIES				
canned in heavy syrup	½ cup	117	0	–
fresh	1 cup	61	0	–
fresh	1 pint	154	0	–
frozen sweetened	1 cup	256	0	–
frozen sweetened	1 pkg (10 oz)	291	0	–
frzn unsweetened	¾ cup	130	0	2
C&W				
Ultimate Red	¾ cup	70	0	7
Europe's Best				
Raspberries frzn	¾ cup	60	0	2

FOOD	PORTION	CALS	CHOL	FIBER
Frieda's				
Dried	⅓ cup (1.4 oz)	145	0	6
RASPBERRY JUICE				
Crystal Light				
Raspberry Ice Sugar Free	8 oz	5	0	0
Naked Juice				
Raspberry Ade	8 oz	90	0	0
Nantucket Nectars				
Organic Very Raspberry	8 oz	120	0	–
Newman's Own				
Razz-Ma-Tazz Raspberry	8 oz	120	0	–
RED BEANS				
CANNED				
Hunt's				
Small	½ cup (4.5 oz)	89	0	6
Van Camp's				
Red Beans	½ cup (4.6 oz)	90	0	5
MIX				
Bean Cuisine				
Pasta & Beans Barcelona Red With Radiatore	1 serv	210	0	4
RELISH				
cranberry orange	½ cup	246	0	–
hamburger	1 tbsp	19	0	–
hamburger	½ cup	158	0	–
hot dog	1 tbsp	14	0	–
hot dog	½ cup	111	0	–
sweet	1 tbsp	19	0	–
sweet	½ cup	159	0	–
B&G				
India	1 tbsp	15	0	–
Piccalilli	1 tbsp	20	0	–
Sweet	1 tbsp	15	0	–
Claussen				
Sweet Pickle	1 tbsp (0.5 oz)	15	0	0
Del Monte				
Hamburger	1 tbsp	20	0	tr
Hot Dog	1 tbsp	15	0	tr
Sweet Pickle	1 tbsp	20	0	0

FOOD	PORTION	CALS	CHOL	FIBER
Frieda's				
Kim Chee	¼ cup	15	0	1
Matouk's				
Hot Chow	2 tbsp	20	0	0
Kuchela	1 tsp	9	0	0
Patak's				
Brinjal Eggplant Sweet Spicy	1 tbsp	70	0	1
Garlic	1 tbsp	45	0	0
Lime Mild	1 tbsp	30	0	0
Mango Mild	1 tbsp	40	0	0
Poloponnese				
Sun Dried Tomato	1 tbsp	25	0	0
Vlasic				
Fancy Sweet	1 tbsp	15	0	–
RHUBARB				
fresh	½ cup	13	0	–
frozen	½ cup	60	0	–
frzn as prep w/ sugar	½ cup	139	0	–
RICE (see also RICE CAKES, WILD RICE)				
arborio	½ cup	100	0	–
brown long grain cooked	1 cup (6.8 oz)	216	0	4
brown medium grain cooked	1 cup (6.8 oz)	218	0	4
glutinous cooked	1 cup (6.1 oz)	169	0	2
starch	1 oz	98	0	–
white long grain cooked	1 cup (5.5 oz)	205	0	1
white long grain instant cooked	1 cup (5.8 oz)	162	0	1
white medium grain cooked	1 cup (6.5 oz)	242	0	1
white short grain cooked	1 cup (6.5 oz)	242	0	–
A Taste Of Thai				
Coconut Garlic Basil as prep	¾ cup	160	0	0
Coconut Ginger as prep	¾ cup	190	0	2
Jasmine not prep	¼ cup	160	0	0
Yellow Curry as prep	¾ cup	180	0	0
Amy's				
Bowls Brown Rice & Vegetables	1 pkg (10 oz)	240	0	5

FOOD	PORTION	CALS	CHOL	FIBER
Buitoni				
Risotto Garden Vegetable	1 serv	210	0	0
Risotto Portobello Mushrooms	1 serv	210	0	0
Risotto Rosemary & Potatoes	1 serv	210	10	2
Risotto Tomato Basil	1 serv	210	0	0
Carolina				
Black Beans & Rice Mix as prep	1 serv	200	0	5
Gold as prep	1 cup	160	0	tr
Spanish Rice Mix as prep	1 serv	180	0	2
Chun King				
Fried Rice Mix	½ cup (1.4 oz)	126	0	1
Country Crock				
Chicken Rice w/ Herbs	1 cup	210	<5	1
Fantastic				
Arborio not prep	¼ cup	160	0	tr
Basmati not prep	¼ cup	160	0	tr
Jasmine not prep	¼ cup	160	0	tr
Gourmet House				
Brown & White not prep	¼ cup	160	0	1
La Choy				
Fried Rice	1 cup (4.9 oz)	236	0	2
Lundberg				
One-Step Curry	1 cup (7.4 oz)	160	0	5
Risotto Tomato Basil	1 serv	140	0	1
Mahatma				
Jambalaya as prep	1 cup	190	0	1
Nacho Cheese Mix as prep	1 serv	250	5	tr
Thai Jasmine as prep	¾ cup	160	0	2
Marrakesh Express				
Pilaf Tomato & Basil as prep	1 cup	190	0	0
Risotto Parmesan as prep	1 cup	200	0	1
Minute				
Instant Brown as prep	⅔ cup	170	0	2
Near East				
Creative Grains Chicken & Herb as prep	1 cup	270	0	6
Creative Grains Creamy Parmesan as prep	1 cup	280	18	3

FOOD	PORTION	CALS	CHOL	FIBER
Creative Grains Roasted Garlic as prep	1 cup	220	0	5
Creative Grains Roasted Pecan as prep	1 cup	240	0	4
Long Grain & Wild Rice Garlic & Herb as prep	1 cup	220	9	2
Long Grain & Wild Rice Roasted Vegetable & Chicken as prep	1 cup	220	9	2
Pilaf Brown Rice as prep	1 cup	210	9	3
Pilaf Chicken as prep	1 cup	220	9	2
Pilaf Mix Curry as prep	1 cup	220	9	2
Pilaf Mix Garlic & Herb as prep	1 cup	220	0	1
Pilaf Mix Long Grain & Wild as prep	1 cup	220	9	2
Pilaf Mix Rice as prep	1 cup	220	9	1
Pilaf Mix Roasted Chicken & Garlic as prep	1 cup	220	6	2
Pilaf Mix Spanish Rice as prep	1 cup	310	21	2
Pilaf Mix Toasted Almond as prep	1 cup	230	9	2
Pilaf Mix Wild Mushroom & Herb as prep	1 cup	220	9	2
Nueva Cocina				
Arroz Con Pollo	1 cup	150	0	1
Gallo Pinto	1/3 pkg	220	0	3
Moros Y Cristianos	1/3 pkg	220	0	3
Paella	1/3 pkg	160	0	1
Pacific Foods				
Ready-To-Serve Lemon & Herb	1/2 pkg	240	0	1
Ready-To-Serve Roasted Chicken	1/2 pkg	240	0	1
Ready-To-Serve Spanish Style	1/2 pkg	230	0	1
Ready-To-Serve Wild Rice & Mushroom	1/2 pkg	230	0	1
Patak's				
Basmati	1 pkg	430	0	2

FOOD	PORTION	CALS	CHOL	FIBER
Coconut	1 pkg	500	0	4
Yellow	1 pkg	440	0	2
Rice Expressions				
Indian Basmati	1 cup	180	0	tr
Organic Brown	1 cup	160	0	3
Organic Long Grain	1 cup	180	0	tr
Organic Rice Pilaf	1 cup	170	0	2
Organic Tex Mex	1 cup	190	0	tr
Rice Select				
Jasmati	1 serv	150	0	–
Risotto	1 serv	150	0	–
Royal Blend w/ Lentils	1 serv	130	0	1
Royal Blend w/ Red Beans	1 serv	130	0	2
Sushi Rice not prep	¼ cup	190	0	–
Texmati Royal Blend Brown & Wild	1 serv	160	0	–
River Rice				
Brown Long Grain not prep	¼ cup	150	0	tr
S&W				
Arborio as prep	¾ cup	150	0	tr
Basmati Mix as prep	¾ cup	160	0	0
Brown Long Grain not prep	¼ cup	150	0	1
Long Grain Organic not prep	¼ cup	150	0	0
Seeds Of Change				
Moroccan Lentil Rice Pilaf as prep	1 cup	180	0	3
Tuscan Rice & Beans as prep	1 cup	180	0	2
Success				
Boil-In-Bag Brown as prep	1 cup	150	0	2
Boil-In-Bag Jasmine as prep	¾ cup	150	0	0
Boil-In-Bag White as prep	1 cup	190	0	1
Ready To Serve Brown	1 cup	170	0	2
Ready To Serve White	1 pkg	190	0	0
Ready To Serve Yellow Rice Mix	1 pkg	190	0	1
Whole Grain Herb Roasted Chicken as prep	1 cup	230	5	3
Whole Grain Multigrain Pilaf as prep	1 cup	230	10	3

FOOD	PORTION	CALS	CHOL	FIBER
Whole Grain Portobello Mushroom as prep	1 cup	220	0	3
TastyBite				
Pilaf Curried Vegetable	½ pkg (4.5 oz)	180	0	9
Pilaf Green Peas	½ pkg (4.5 oz)	208	0	4
Pilaf Vegetable Kofta	½ pkg (4.5 oz)	229	0	7
Uncle Ben's				
Boil-In-Bag	1 cup	190	0	1
Brown Natural as prep	1 cup	170	0	–
Country Inn Chicken & Broccoli as prep	1 cup	190	0	1
Country Inn Chicken & Vegetables as prep	1 cup	200	0	1
Country Inn Mexican Fiesta as prep	1 cup	200	0	1
Country Inn Oriental Fried as prep	1 cup	200	0	1
Country Inn Three Cheese as prep	1 cup	200	5	1
Country Inn Wheat	1 cup	200	0	1
Fast & Natural	1 cup	190	0	2
Flavorful Four Cheese as prep	1 cup	190	5	1
Flavorful Garlic & Butter as prep	1 cup	200	0	tr
Flavorful Lemon & Herb as prep	1 cup	200	0	tr
Flavorful Spanish as prep	1 cup	200	0	tr
Instant	1 cup	190	0	1
Long Grain & Wild Butter Herb as prep	1 cup	190	0	1
Long Grain & Wild Fast Cook as prep	1 cup	200	0	1
Long Grain & Wild Original as prep	1 cup	200	0	1
Long Grain & Wild Roasted Garlic as prep	1 cup	200	0	1
Ready Rice Long Grain & Wild as prep	1 cup	240	0	1
Ready Rice Original as prep	1 cup	230	0	1

FOOD	PORTION	CALS	CHOL	FIBER
Ready Rice Roasted Chicken as prep	1 cup	230	0	1
Ready Rice Teriyaki as prep	1 cup	190	0	1
Ready Rice Whole Grain Brown	1 cup	220	0	1
White Original as prep	1 cup	170	0	0
Van Camp's				
Spanish	½ cup (4.5 oz)	90	0	2
Water Maid				
White Medium Grain not prep	¼ cup	160	0	tr
Zatarain's				
Dirty Rice Mix as prep w/o meat and oil	½ cup	130	0	0
Red Beans & Rice as prep w/o oil	½ cup	100	0	4
TAKE-OUT				
nasi goreng indonesian rice & vegetables	1 cup (4.9 oz)	130	0	1
paella	1 serv (7 oz)	308	92	3
pilaf	½ cup	84	22	3
spanish	¾ cup	363	35	–

RICE CAKES (see also POPCORN CAKES)

FOOD	PORTION	CALS	CHOL	FIBER
Lundberg				
Nutra Farmed Brown Rice	1 (0.7 oz)	70	0	–
Nutra Farmed Sesame Tamari	1 (0.7 oz)	70	0	2
Organic Koku Semsame	1 (0.7 oz)	80	0	2
Mr. Krispers				
Baked Rice Krisps Barbecue	37	110	0	1
Baked Rice Krisps Nacho	37	120	0	1
Baked Rice Krisps Sea Salt & Pepper	37	110	0	1
Baked Rice Krisps Sour Cream & Onion	37	110	0	1
Tastemorr				
Rice Crisps Caramel	7	55	0	0

ROCKFISH

FOOD	PORTION	CALS	CHOL	FIBER
pacific cooked	3 oz	103	38	0

FOOD	PORTION	CALS	CHOL	FIBER
pacific cooked	1 fillet (5.2 oz)	180	66	0
pacific raw	3 oz	80	29	0

ROE (see also individual fish names)

fresh baked	1 oz	58	136	0

ROLL
FROZEN
Alexia

Ciabatta	1 (1.5 oz)	100	0	1
French	1 (1.5 oz)	100	0	1
Three Cheese Focaccia	1 (1.5 oz)	110	0	tr
Whole Grain	1 (1.5 oz)	90	0	3

Eggo

Toaster Swirlz Cinnamon Roll Minis	4 (1.6 oz)	120	5	tr

Pepperidge Farm

Hearth Fired Hearty Wheat Dinner Roll	1	120	0	2

Pillsbury

Dinner Rolls Crusty French	1	110	0	0

Sara Lee

Deluxe Cinnamon Rolls w/ Icing	1 (2.7 oz)	320	40	1

READY-TO-EAT

bialy	1 (2.2 oz)	138	0	1
brioche sweet roll	1 (3.5 oz)	410	190	3
brown & serve	1 (1 oz)	85	0	–
cinnamon raisin	1 (2¾ in)	223	40	1
dinner	1 (1 oz)	85	0	–
french	1 (1.3 oz)	105	0	–
hamburger multi-grain	1 (1.5 oz)	113	0	2
hamburger reduced calorie	1 (1.5 oz)	84	0	3
hard	1 (3½ in)	167	0	–
hotdog reduced calorie	1 (1.5 oz)	84	0	3
hotdog whole wheat	1 (1.5 oz)	110	0	2
kaiser	1 (3½ in)	167	0	–
oat bran	1 (1.2 oz)	78	0	1
rye	1 (1 oz)	81	0	–
submarine	1 (4.7 oz)	155	tr	–

FOOD	PORTION	CALS	CHOL	FIBER
wheat	1 (1 oz)	77	0	–
whole wheat	1 (1 oz)	75	0	–
Alvarado Street Bakery				
Sprouted Wheat Burger Bun	1 (2.2 oz)	140	0	3
Bread Du Jour				
Cracked Wheat	1 (1.2 oz)	100	0	1
Italian	1 (1.2 oz)	90	0	0
Sourdough	1 (1.2 oz)	90	0	0
Country Kitchen				
Wheat Light	1	80	0	4
Natural Ovens				
Best Burger Bun	1	178	0	3
Better Wheat Buns	1	140	0	5
Gourmet Dinner	1	70	0	4
Pepperidge Farm				
Dinner Rolls Finger Poppy	1 (0.9 oz)	80	<5	tr
Kaiser Soft 100% Whole Wheat	1	200	1	3
Sara Lee				
Hamburger Bun Classic	1 (2.6 oz)	200	0	1
Hamburger Bun Classic Wheat	1 (2.6 oz)	200	0	3
Heart Healthy Hamburger Bun Wheat	1 (2.6 oz)	190	0	3
Hot Dog Gourmet	1 (1.5 oz)	120	0	tr
Super Bakery				
Daily Donut Reduced Fat	1 (2.2 oz)	200	15	1
Organic Sandwich Bun	1 (3.6 oz)	250	0	10
Sub Roll	1 (3.6 oz)	250	0	10
Wonder				
Brown & Serve	1 (1 oz)	80	0	0
Brown & Serve Wheat	1 (1 oz)	80	0	0
Club French	1 (1.6 oz)	120	0	0
Club Grain	1 (1.6 oz)	120	0	1
Club Sourdough	1 (1.6 oz)	120	0	0
Dinner	2 (1.6 oz)	130	0	1
Hamburger Wheat	1 (1.5 oz)	120	0	1
Hoagie French	1 (3 oz)	220	0	1
Hoagie Grain	1 (3 oz)	220	0	2
Hoagie Sourdough	1 (3 oz)	220	0	1

FOOD	PORTION	CALS	CHOL	FIBER
Kaiser	1 (2.2 oz)	180	0	1
Kaiser Hoagie	1 (3 oz)	220	0	1
REFRIGERATED				
crescent	1 (1 oz)	98	0	–
Pillsbury				
Crecents Reduced Fat	1 (1 oz)	100	0	0
Crescent	1 (1.7 oz)	170	0	tr
ROSE APPLE				
fresh	3.5 oz	32	0	–
ROSE HIP				
fresh	1 oz	26	0	–
ROSELLE				
fresh	1 cup	28	0	–
ROSEMARY				
dried	1 tsp	4	0	–
ROUGHY				
orange baked	3 oz	75	22	0
RUBS (see HERBS/SPICES)				
RUTABAGA				
cooked mashed	½ cup	41	0	–
raw cubed	½ cup	25	0	–
Glory				
Cut Fresh	1 cup	50	0	4
SABLEFISH				
baked	3 oz	213	53	0
smoked	1 oz	72	18	0
SAFFLOWER				
seeds dried	1 oz	147	0	–
SAFFRON				
saffron	1 tsp	2	0	–
SAGE				
ground	1 tsp	2	0	–

FOOD	PORTION	CALS	CHOL	FIBER
SALAD (see also SALAD TOPPINGS)				
Dole				
American Blend	1½ cups	15	0	1
Baby Spinach Salad	1½ cup (3 oz)	20	0	2
Butter & Red Leaf	1½ cups (3 oz)	10	0	1
Classic Iceberg	1½ cups (3 oz)	15	0	1
Classic Romaine	1½ cups (3 oz)	15	0	1
European Blend	1½ cups (3 oz)	15	0	1
Field Greens	1½ cups (3 oz)	15	0	2
French Blend	1½ cups (3 oz)	15	0	2
Greener Selection	1½ cups (3 oz)	15	0	1
Hearts Delight	1½ cups (3 oz)	15	0	1
Italian Blend	1½ cups (3 oz)	15	0	1
Kits Asian Crunch	1½ cups (3.5 oz)	120	0	2
Kits Bacon Lettuce Toss	1½ cups (3.5 oz)	130	10	1
Kits Caesar	1½ cups (3 oz)	170	10	2
Kits Caesar Light	1½ cups (3 oz)	100	0	1
Kits Fall Harvest	1½ cups (3.5 oz)	150	0	–
Kits Romano	1½ cups (3 oz)	150	0	2
Kits Spring Garden	1½ cups (3.5 oz)	140	0	2
Kits Sunflower Ranch	1½ cups (3 oz)	160	5	2
Mediterranean Blend	1½ cups	15	0	2
Very Veggie Blend	1½ cups (3 oz)	20	0	1
Earthbound Farm				
Organic Baby Arugula Salad	2 cups	20	0	1
Organic Baby Lettuce Salad	2 cups	15	0	1
Organic Baby Spinach Salad	2 cups	10	0	7
Organic Fresh Herb Salad	2 cups	15	0	2
Organic Mixed Baby Greens	2 cups	15	0	2
Fresh Express				
Baby Spinach Trio	4 cups (3 oz)	20	0	1
Krakus				
Bordeaux	1 pkg (5 oz)	35	0	2
Mann's				
Rainbow	3 oz	25	0	2
Ready Pac				
All American	2½ cups	15	0	1
Bowl Salad Chef	1 pkg	350	70	2
Bowl Salad Chicken Caesar	1 pkg	380	75	2
Bowl Salad Greek	1 pkg	400	20	3

FOOD	PORTION	CALS	CHOL	FIBER
Bowl Salad Spinach Bacon	1 pkg	300	155	1
Bowl Salad Spring Mix Veggie	1 pkg	330	15	3
Caesar Romaine	1½ cups	15	0	1
Classic Crisp Salad	2¼ cups	10	0	tr
Continental	3 cups	20	0	2
Costa Brava	3 cups	15	0	2
Hearty Green Salad	2½ cups	10	0	tr
Lafayette	3 cups	10	0	1
Milano	3 cups	15	0	2
Organic Caesar Romaine	2¼ cups	15	0	tr
Organic Mesclun Blend	1 pkg (4.5 oz)	35	0	3
Organic Monterey	3 cups	15	0	2
Parisian	2 cups	20	0	1
Portofino	1 pkg (5 oz)	25	0	2
Santa Barbara	3½ cups	15	0	tr
Spring Mix	1 pkg (5 oz)	35	0	3
River Ranch				
American Bland	1½ cups	15	0	1
Caesar Kit	1½ cups	110	6	2
European Blend	1¾ cups	10	0	1
Garden	1½ cups	15	0	1
Garden Supreme	1½ cups	15	0	1
Italian Blend	1¾ cups	15	0	1
Raspberry Vinaigrette Kit	1¾ cups	130	0	2
Riviera Blend	1½ cups	10	0	tr
Suddenly Salad				
Caesar	¾ cup	220	0	1
Caesar Low Fat Recipe	¾ cup	170	0	1
Italian Pepperoni	1 cup	190	0	2
Italian Pepperoni Low Fat Recipe	1 cup	180	0	2
Ranch & Bacon	¾ cup	330	15	1
Ranch & Bacon Low Fat Recipe	¾ cup	180	<5	1
TAKE-OUT				
7-layer salad	2 cups	557	119	3
caesar	4 cups	734	173	7
chef w/o dressing	3 cups	535	280	–
chef w/o dressing	1½ cups	386	244	–

FOOD	PORTION	CALS	CHOL	FIBER
cobb w/ dressing	4 cups	645	294	11
greek w/ dressing	4 cups	424	475	4
mixed salad greens shredded	1 cup	9	0	1
somen w/ lettuce egg fish pork	2 cups	550	429	4
spinach no dressing	4 cups	429	308	6
tossed w/ avocado w/o dressing	2 cups	90	0	5
tossed w/ chicken w/o dressing	3 cups	194	86	2
tossed w/ egg w/o dressing	2 cups	93	183	2
tossed w/ seafood w/o dressing	3 cups	120	145	3
tossed w/ shrimp & egg w/o dressing	3 cups	185	430	2
tossed w/o dressing	2 cups	22	0	2
waldorf	1 cup	242	7	3
wilted lettuce w/ bacon dressing	1 cup	99	11	1

SALAD DRESSING
MIX
A Taste Of Thai

FOOD	PORTION	CALS	CHOL	FIBER
Peanut Dressing as prep	2 tbsp	40	0	1

Et Tu

Caesar Salad Kit	1 serv	140	5	0

Good Seasons

Italian as prep	2 tbsp	130	0	–
Italian not prep	⅛ pkg (3 g)	5	0	–

READY-TO-EAT

french reduced calorie	1 tbsp	22	1	–
italian reduced calorie	1 tbsp	16	1	–
russian reduced calorie	1 tbsp	23	1	–
sesame seed	1 tbsp	68	0	–
thousand island reduced calorie	1 tbsp	24	2	–

Annie's Naturals

Organic Buttermilk	2 tbsp	70	10	–

FOOD	PORTION	CALS	CHOL	FIBER
Organic No Fat Yogurt w/ Dill	2 tbsp	20	0	–
Bernstein's				
Chunky Blue Cheese	2 tbsp	120	5	0
Creamy Caesar	2 tbsp	120	15	0
Italian Restaurant Recipe	2 tbsp	120	5	0
Light Fantastic Roasted Garlic Balsamic	2 tbsp	45	0	0
Red Wine & Garlic Italian	2 tbsp	110	0	0
Carb Options				
Italian	2 tbsp	70	0	0
Ranch	2 tbsp	150	10	0
Consorzio				
Balsamic Vinaigrette	2 tbsp	60	0	0
Caesar Parmesan & Romano	2 tbsp	120	20	–
Honey Mustard	2 tbsp	100	0	0
Italian	2 tbsp	60	0	0
Mango	1 tbsp	15	0	0
Raspberry & Balsamic	1 tbsp	15	0	0
Strawberry & Balsamic	1 tbsp	10	0	0
David Burke				
Flavor Spray Ranch	2 sprays	0	0	0
Drew's				
Low Carb Garlic Italian	1 tbsp	80	0	0
Low Carb Lemon Tahini Goddess	1 tbsp	80	0	0
Low Carb Sesame Orange	1 tbsp	80	0	0
Girard's				
White Balsamic Vinaigrette	2 tbsp	140	0	–
Ken's				
Bacon Ranch	2 tbsp	140	0	0
Caesar	2 tbsp	170	0	0
Country French w/ Vermont Honey	2 tbsp	150	0	0
Fat Free Italian	2 tbsp	25	0	0
Fat Free Raspberry Pecan	2 tbsp	50	0	0
Honey Mustard	2 tbsp	130	15	0
Italian w/ Aged Romano	2 tbsp	110	0	0
Lite Italian	2 tbsp	50	0	0
Lite Ranch	2 tbsp	80	10	0

FOOD	PORTION	CALS	CHOL	FIBER
Lite Red Wine Vinegar & Olive Oil	2 tbsp	50	0	0
Lite Vinaigrette Balsamic & Basil	2 tbsp	50	0	0
Lite Chunky Blue Cheese	2 tbsp	80	0	0
Red Wine Vinegar & Olive Oil	2 tbsp	120	0	0
Russian	2 tbsp	140	15	0
Thousand Island	2 tbsp	140	15	0
Kraft				
Free French	2 tbsp	50	0	0
Free Ranch	2 tbsp	50	0	1
Free Thousand Island	2 tbsp	45	0	0
LaMartinique				
Blue Cheese Vinaigrette	2 tbsp	160	5	0
Poppy Seed	2 tbsp	170	0	0
Nasoya				
Creamy Dill	1 tbsp	30	0	0
Creamy Italian	2 tbsp	70	0	0
Garden Herb	2 tbsp	60	0	0
Sesame Garlic	2 tbsp	60	0	0
Newman's Own				
Balsamic Vinaigrette	2 tbsp	90	0	0
Caesar	2 tbsp	150	0	0
Creamy Caesar	2 tbsp	150	<5	0
Family Recipe Italian	2 tbsp	120	0	0
Lighten Up Balsamic Vinaigrette	2 tbsp	45	0	0
Lighten Up Caesar	2 tbsp	70	5	0
Lighten Up Honey Mustard	2 tbsp	70	0	0
Lighten Up Italian	2 tbsp	60	0	0
Lighten Up Low Fat Sesame Ginger	2 tbsp	35	0	0
Lighten Up Raspberry & Walnut	2 tbsp	70	0	0
Lighten Up Red Wine Vinegar & Olive Oil	2 tbsp	110	0	–
Olive Oil & Vinegar	2 tbsp	150	0	0
Parmesan & Roasted Garlic	2 tbsp	110	0	0
Ranch	2 tbsp	140	10	0
Two Thousand Island	2 tbsp	140	10	0

FOOD	PORTION	CALS	CHOL	FIBER
Old Dutch				
Sweet & Sour	2 tbsp	50	0	0
Paul's				
No-Fat Raspberry & Balsamic	2 tbsp	20	0	–
No-Oil Orange & Basil	2 tbsp	15	0	0
San-J				
Tamari Mustard	2 tbsp	25	0	–
Seeds Of Change				
Vinaigrette Balsamic	2 tbsp	60	0	0
Vinaigrette Greek Feta	2 tbsp	60	0	0
Vinaigrette Roasted Garlic	2 tbsp	60	0	0
Vinaigrette Sweet Basil	2 tbsp	60	0	0
Sonoma				
Creamy Tomato Bacon	2 tbsp	150	5	0
South Beach Diet				
Balsamic Vinaigrette	2 tbsp	50	0	0
Italian	2 tbsp	60	0	0
Ranch	2 tbsp	70	0	0
Spectrum				
Honey Dijon	2 tbsp	35	0	0
Organic Creamy Dill	2 tbsp	25	0	0
Organic Creamy Garlic	2 tbsp	20	0	0
Organic Greek Goddess	2 tbsp	110	0	0
Organic Omega 3 Balsamic Vinaigrette	2 tbsp	80	0	0
Organic Omega 3 Ginger Garlic Vinaigrette	2 tbsp	80	0	0
Organic Omega 3 Raspberry Vinaigrette	2 tbsp	80	0	0
Organic Porcini Mushroom Vinaigrette	2 tbsp	70	0	0
Organic Rocky Mountain Ranch	2 tbsp	130	20	0
Organic Sweet Onion & Garlic	2 tbsp	15	0	0
Organic Toasted Sesame	2 tbsp	15	0	0
Provencal Garlic Lover's	2 tbsp	50	0	0
Zesty Italian	2 tbsp	30	0	0

FOOD	PORTION	CALS	CHOL	FIBER
Steel's				
Honey Mustard	1 tbsp	90	0	0
Sweet Ginger Lime	1 tbsp	68	0	1
Wishbone				
Blue Cheese w/ Gorgonzola	2 tbsp	140	<5	0
Caesar w/ Aged Romano	2 tbsp	80	0	0
Classic Ranch Extra Thick	2 tbsp	140	10	0
Creamy Caesar	2 tbsp	170	10	0
Creamy Italian	2 tbsp	110	0	0
Deluxe French	2 tbsp	50	0	tr
Fat Free Chunky Blue Cheese	2 tbsp	35	0	tr
Fat Free Italian	2 tbsp	20	0	0
Fat Free Ranch	2 tbsp	30	0	tr
Fat Free Western	2 tbsp	45	0	–
Five Cheese Italian	2 tbsp	120	0	0
Italian	2 tbsp	90	0	0
Just 2 Good Blue Cheese	2 tbsp	45	0	0
Just 2 Good Creamy Caesar	2 tbsp	50	10	0
Just 2 Good Deluxe French	2 tbsp	50	0	tr
Just 2 Good Italian	2 tbsp	35	0	0
Just 2 Good Ranch	2 tbsp	40	0	0
Just 2 Good Thousand Island	2 tbsp	50	5	0
Just 2 Good Western	2 tbsp	70	0	0
Light Ranch Extra Thick	2 tbsp	70	10	0
Light Vinaigrette Asian Sesame	2 tbsp	70	0	0
Light Vinaigrette Raspberry Walnut	2 tbsp	80	0	0
Ranch	2 tbsp	160	10	0
Russian	2 tbsp	110	0	0
Salad Spritzers Balsamic Breeze	10 sprays	10	0	0
Salad Spritzers Italian	10 sprays	10	0	0
Salad Spritzers Red Wine Mist	10 sprays	10	0	0
Thousand Island	2 tbsp	130	10	0
Vinaigrette Berry	2 tbsp	50	0	0
Vinaigrette Lemon Garlic & Herb	2 tbsp	70	0	0

FOOD	PORTION	CALS	CHOL	FIBER
Vinaigrette Olive Oil	2 tbsp	60	0	0
Western	2 tbsp	160	0	0
TAKE-OUT				
vinegar & oil	1 tbsp	72	0	–

SALAD TOPPINGS
Salad Pizazz!

FOOD	PORTION	CALS	CHOL	FIBER
Asian Medley	1 tbsp	40	0	tr
Cherry Cranberry Pecano	1 tbsp	35	0	tr
Honey Toasted Delites	1 tbsp	40	0	1
Orange Cranberry Almondine	1 tbsp	35	0	tr
Raspberry Cranberry Walnut Frisco	1 tbsp	30	0	0
Tomato 'N Bacon Parmesano	1 tbsp	30	0	tr
Tomato Pinenut Tuscano	1 tbsp	130	0	tr

SALMON
CANNED

FOOD	PORTION	CALS	CHOL	FIBER
w/ bone	½ cup	106	39	0
Bumble Bee				
Blueback	¼ cup	110	40	0
Keta	¼ cup	90	40	0
Pink	¼ cup	90	40	0
Red	¼ cup	110	40	0
Skinless & Boneless	¼ cup	50	20	0
Smoked Fillets In Oil	⅓ cup	150	55	0
Chicken Of The Sea				
Pink	1 pkg (3 oz)	90	30	0
Pink Skinless Boneless	¼ cup	60	20	0
Red	¼ cup	110	40	0
Smoked Pacific	1 pkg (3 oz)	120	45	0
Libby's				
Alaskan Sockeye Red	¼ cup	110	40	0
Pink Skinless Boneless	¼ cup	50	20	0
Red	¼ cup	110	40	0
FRESH				
atlantic farmed baked	4 oz	233	71	0
coho wild poached	4 oz	209	65	0
pink baked	4 oz	169	76	0
sockeye baked	4 oz	245	99	0

FOOD	PORTION	CALS	CHOL	FIBER
FROZEN				
Phillips Seafood				
Salmon Cakes	1 (3 oz)	180	40	–
SMOKED				
lox	1 oz	33	7	0
Lascco				
Nova Sliced	2 oz	60	20	0
TAKE-OUT				
guisado stew salmon	1 serv (7.4 oz)	320	66	3
roulette w/ spinach stuffing	1 serv (4 oz)	160	45	tr
salmon cake	1 (4.2 oz)	264	56	1
salmon loaf	1 slice (3.7 oz)	206	120	tr
SALSA				
black bean & corn	2 tbsp	15	0	tr
cirtus	2 tbsp (1 oz)	10	0	0
peach	2 tbsp	15	0	0
tomato-less corn & chile	2 tbsp	45	0	tr
Cape Cod				
Medium & Mild	2 tbsp	15	0	1
Del Salsa				
Fire Roasted All Flavors	2 tbsp	8	0	0
Emeril's				
Original Recipe	2 tbsp	10	0	0
Gringo Billy's				
Salsa Mix	1 tsp	5	0	1
Hunt's				
Alfresco All Varieties	2 tbsp (1.1 oz)	10	0	tr
Hot	2 tbsp (1.1 oz)	27	0	1
Medium	2 tbsp (1.1 oz)	27	0	1
Mild	2 tbsp (1.1 oz)	27	0	1
Picante All Varieties	2 tbsp (1.1 oz)	11	0	tr
Squeeze Mild & Medium	2 tbsp (1.1 oz)	27	0	1
Muir Glen				
Black Bean & Corn Medium	2 tbsp (1.1 oz)	15	0	tr
Chipotle Medium	2 tbsp (1.1 oz)	10	0	0
Fire Roasted Tomato Medium	2 tbsp (1.1 oz)	10	0	0
Garlic Cilantro Medium	2 tbsp (1.1 oz)	10	0	0
Habanero Hot	2 tbsp (1.1 oz)	10	0	0

FOOD	PORTION	CALS	CHOL	FIBER
Organic Medium	2 tbsp (1.1 oz)	10	0	0
Organic Mild	2 tbsp (1.1 oz)	10	0	0
Roasted Garlic Medium	2 tbsp (1.1 oz)	10	0	0
Newman's Own				
Bandito Mild	2 tbsp	10	0	1
Bandito Peach	2 tbsp	25	0	tr
Bandito Pineapple	2 tbsp	15	0	1
Bandito Roasted Garlic	2 tbsp	10	0	1
Bandito Tequila Lime	2 tbsp	15	0	–
Ortega				
Garden Style Mild	2 tbsp	10	0	tr
Picante Mild	2 tbsp	10	0	–
Pace				
Picante Mild or Medium	2 tbsp	10	0	0
Thick & Chunky Mild or Medium	2 tbsp	10	0	0
Rosarita				
Extra Chunky Medium	2 tbsp (1 oz)	7	0	tr
Green Tomatillo Medium	2 tbsp (1 oz)	8	0	1
Picante Zesty Jalapeno Hot	2 tbsp (1 oz)	8	0	1
Picante Zesty Jalapeno Medium	2 tbsp (1 oz)	9	0	1
Picante Zesty Jalapeno Mild	2 tbsp (1 oz)	8	0	tr
Roasted Mild	2 tbsp (1 oz)	10	0	1
Traditional Medium	2 tbsp (1 oz)	7	0	1
Traditional Mild	2 tbsp (1 oz)	7	0	1
Seeds Of Change				
Black Bean & Tomato Mild	2 tbsp	15	0	tr
Garlic & Cilantro Mild	2 tbsp	15	0	tr
Snyder's Of Hanover				
Mild	2 tbsp	10	0	0
Tostitos				
All Natural	2 tbsp	15	0	1
Con Queso	2 tbsp	40	<5	tr
Monterey Jack Queso	2 tbsp	40	<5	0
Restaurant Style	2 tbsp	15	0	tr
Tree Of Life				
Medium	2 tbsp (1 oz)	10	0	–
Mild	2 tbsp (1 oz)	10	0	–

FOOD	PORTION	CALS	CHOL	FIBER
Utz				
Chunky	2 tbsp (1 oz)	60	0	4
SALSIFY				
fresh sliced cooked	½ cup	46	0	–
Frieda's				
Salsify	¾ cup	70	0	3
SALT SUBSTITUTES				
AlsoSalt				
Butter Flavored	¼ tsp	1	0	0
Garlic Flavored	¼ tsp	1	0	0
Salt Substitute	¼ tsp	tr	0	0
Chef Paul Prudhomme's				
Magic Salt Free Seasoning	¼ tsp	0	0	0
Eden				
Organic Seaweed Gomasio Sesame Salt	1 tsp	15	0	0
Organic Gomasio Sesame Salt	1 tsp	15	0	0
French's				
No Salt	¼ cup	0	0	0
Halsosalt				
All Flavors	¼ tsp (7 g)	1	0	–
Molly McButter				
Lite Sodium	1 tsp	5	0	–
SALT/SEASONED SALT				
salt	1 tsp (6 g)	0	0	0
salt	1 tbsp (18 g)	0	0	0
sea salt coarse	¼ tsp	0	0	0
sea salt fine	¼ tsp	0	0	0
Eden				
French Celtic Salt	¼ tsp	0	0	0
Portuguese Coast Salt	¼ tsp	0	0	0
McCormick				
Celery Salt	¼ tsp	0	0	0
Morton				
Iodized	¼ tsp	0	0	0
Kosher	1 tsp	0	0	–
Non-Iodized	1 tsp	0	0	–

FOOD	PORTION	CALS	CHOL	FIBER

SANDWICHES
Amy's

FOOD	PORTION	CALS	CHOL	FIBER
Pocket Sandwich Broccoli & Cheese	1 (4.5 oz)	270	15	3
Pocket Sandwich Roasted Vegetables	1 (4.5 oz)	220	0	4
Pocket Sandwich Spinach Feta	1 (4.5 oz)	250	20	3
Pocket Sandwich Tofu Scramble	1 (4 oz)	160	0	tr
Pocket Sandwich Vegetable Pie	1 (5 oz)	300	0	3
Toaster Pops Grilled Cheese	1	180	20	0
Guiltless Gourmet				
Wrap California Veggie	1 (5.7 oz)	270	0	4
Wrap Mediterranean Spinach	1 (5.7 oz)	270	<5	4
Ian's				
Mini Chicken Patty	2 (5.3 oz)	368	34	1
Lean Pockets				
Bacon Egg & Cheese	1 (4.5 oz)	150	40	2
Barbecue Sauce w/ Beef	1 (4.5 oz)	290	20	3
Chicken Cheddar & Broccoli	1 (4.5 oz)	260	20	3
Chicken Fajita	1 (4.5 oz)	260	25	3
Chicken Parmesan	1 (4.5 oz)	280	30	3
Ham & Cheese	1 (4.5 oz)	280	25	3
Meatballs & Mozzarella	1 (4.5 oz)	290	20	3
Philly Steak & Cheese	1 (4.5 oz)	280	25	3
Sausage Egg & Cheese	1 (4.5 oz)	140	45	2
Steak Fajita	1 (4.5 oz)	260	25	3
Three Cheese & Chicken Quesadilla	1 (4.5 oz)	280	25	3
Turkey & Ham w/ Cheddar	1 (4.5 oz)	280	30	3
Turkey Broccoli & Cheese	1 (4.5 oz)	270	25	3
Madalena's Masterpiece				
Calzone Artichoke Parmesan	1 (10 oz)	570	45	2
Calzone Grilled Chicken	1 (10 oz)	520	75	1
Calzone Sausage Pepperoni	1 (10 oz)	640	90	tr
Panini Garlic Chicken	1 (8 oz)	450	85	2
Panini Honey Ham	1 (8 oz)	520	50	tr

FOOD	PORTION	CALS	CHOL	FIBER
Panini Turkey Pesto	1 (8 oz)	500	55	0
Panini Veggie	1 (8 oz)	480	40	1
Quesabake Mexican Sausage	1 (7 oz)	510	45	2
Quesabake Roasted Veggie	1 (7 oz)	460	35	1
Smucker's				
Uncrustables Grilled Cheese	1 (1.8 oz)	150	15	tr
Uncrustables Peanut Butter & Grape Jelly	1 (2 oz)	210	0	2
Uncrustables Peanut Butter & Strawberry Jam	1 (2 oz)	210	0	2
South Beach Diet				
Breakfast Wraps All American	1 serv (4.6 oz)	200	15	15
Breakfast Wraps Denver	1 serv (4.6 oz)	180	15	15
Breakfast Wraps Southwestern	1 serv (4.6 oz)	160	10	15
Breakfast Wraps Vegetable Medley	1 serv (4.6 oz)	160	5	15
Wrap Kit Deli Ham & Turkey	1 pkg	220	40	15
Wrap Kit Grilled Chicken Caesar	1 pkg	230	50	14
Wrap Kit Sesame Chicken	1 pkg (6.4 oz)	220	40	15
Wrap Kit Southwestern Style Chicken	1 pkg	250	55	15
Wrap Kits Turkey & Bacon Club	1 pkg	250	40	15
TAKE-OUT				
bacon & egg	1 (6.2 oz)	388	421	1
bacon lettuce & tomato w/ mayo	1 (5.8 oz)	344	21	3
beef barbecue w/ bun	1 (6.7 oz)	417	69	2
calzone beef & cheese	1 (14 oz)	1476	187	6
calzone cheese	1 (15 oz)	1632	254	5
chicken salad	1 (5 oz)	333	49	2
crab cake w/ bun	1	308	97	2
croque monsieur	1 (12.4 oz)	765	152	2
egg salad	1 (5.6 oz)	485	329	1
french dip w/ roll	1 (6.8 oz)	357	54	1
fried egg	1 (3.4 oz)	226	206	1

FOOD	PORTION	CALS	CHOL	FIBER
grilled cheese	1 (2.9 oz)	290	22	1
gyro	1 (13.7 oz)	593	82	4
ham & egg	1 (4.4 oz)	272	222	2
ham w/ cheese w/ lettuce & mayo	1 (5.4 oz)	369	57	2
peanut butter & jelly	1 (3.3 oz)	327	0	3
reuben w/ sauerkraut & cheese	1 (6.4 oz)	463	81	4
roast beef w/ gravy	1 (7.8 oz)	386	69	2
sloppy joe pork on bun	1 (6.5 oz)	318	50	2
tuna melt	1 (5.3 oz)	350	34	1
tuna salad w/ lettuce	1 (5.9 oz)	289	22	2
turkey w/ mayo	1 (5 oz)	329	67	1

SAPODILLA

FOOD	PORTION	CALS	CHOL	FIBER
fresh	1	140	0	–
fresh cut up	1 cup	199	0	–

SAPOTES

FOOD	PORTION	CALS	CHOL	FIBER
fresh	1	301	0	–

SARDINES
CANNED

FOOD	PORTION	CALS	CHOL	FIBER
atlantic in oil w/ bone	1 can (3.2 oz)	192	131	0
atlantic in oil w/ bone	2	50	34	0
pacific in tomato sauce w/ bone	1 can (13 oz)	658	225	0
pacific in tomato sauce w/ bone	1	68	23	0
Beach Cliff				
In Louisiana Hot Sauce	1 can (3.7 oz)	150	110	0
In Mustard Sauce	1 can (3.7 oz)	150	110	0
In Olive Oil	1 can (3.7 oz)	200	105	0
In Tomato Sauce	1 can (3.7 oz)	140	90	0
In Water	1 can (3.7 oz)	150	115	0
Small In Soybean Oil	1 can (3.7 oz)	200	115	0
With Hot Green Chilies	1 can (3.7 oz)	180	100	0
Brunswick				
In Louisiana Hot Sauce	1 can (3.7 oz)	150	110	0
In Mustard Sauce	1 can (3.7 oz)	150	110	0
In Soybean Oil	1 can (3.7 oz)	110	115	0

FOOD	PORTION	CALS	CHOL	FIBER
In Spring Water	1 can (3.7 oz)	150	115	0
In Tomato Sauce	1 can (3.7 oz)	150	100	0
With Hot Tabasco Peppers	1 can (3.7 oz)	110	110	0
Bumble Bee				
In Hot Sauce	¼ cup	90	30	0
In Mustard	¼ cup	70	20	1
In Oil	1 can (3.7 oz)	130	35	0
In Water	1 can (3.7 oz)	120	35	0
Chicken Of The Sea				
In Hot Sauce	1 can (3.75 oz)	130	60	2
In Mustard Sauce	1 can (3.75 oz)	150	60	2
In Oil	1 can (3.75 oz)	190	45	0
In Tomato Sauce	1 can (3.75 oz)	130	60	2
In Water	1 can (3.75 oz)	100	45	0
Goya				
In Tomato Sauce	2 pieces (2.2 oz)	50	45	2
King Oscar				
In Olive Oil	1 can (3.75 oz)	150	120	0
Skinless Boneless In Soya Oil	3 pieces (1.9 oz)	120	20	0
Season				
Brisling In Water	1 can (3.75 oz)	145	120	0

SAUCE (*see also* BARBECUE SAUCE, GRAVY, PIZZA SAUCE, SPAGHETTI SAUCE)
JARRED

FOOD	PORTION	CALS	CHOL	FIBER
fish sauce vietnamese nuoc mam	1 tbsp	6	0	0
hoisin	1 tbsp	35	0	tr
morroccan tagine	½ cup (4 oz)	70	0	1
oyster	1 tbsp	8	0	0
teriyaki	1 tbsp	15	0	–
A Taste Of Thai				
Chili Sauce Sweet Red	1 tsp	10	0	0
Fish Sauce	1 tbsp	15	0	–
Peanut Satay	2 tbsp	80	0	1
A1				
Bold Steak Sauce	1 tbsp	20	0	–
Annie Chun's				
Marinade & Dressing Lemongrass Herb	1 tbsp	25	0	0

FOOD	PORTION	CALS	CHOL	FIBER
Noodle Sauce & Dressing Sesame Cilantro	1 tbsp	60	0	0
Shiitake Mushroom	1 tbsp	15	0	0
Annie's Naturals				
Organic Worcestershire	1 tbsp	20	0	–
Asian Gourmet				
Duck Sauce Peking Style	2 tbsp	40	0	–
Atkins				
Steak Sauce	1 tbsp	5	0	0
Teriyaki	1 tbsp	10	0	0
Boar's Head				
Ham Glaze Sugar & Spice	2 tbsp	120	0	0
Horseradish Sauce Pub Style	1 tsp	15	5	0
Carb Options				
Alfredo	¼ cup	110	30	0
Cheese	¼ cup	90	25	0
Garden Style	½ cup	80	0	2
Steak Sauce	1 tbsp	5	0	0
Chun King				
Sweet And Sour	2 tbsp (1.2 oz)	58	0	0
Teriyaki	1 tbsp (0.6 oz)	17	0	0
Teriyaki Hot	1 tbsp (0.6 oz)	17	0	0
Consorzio				
Marinade Dijon Peppercorn	1 tbsp	15	0	–
Marinade Jamaican Jerb	1 tbsp	10	0	–
Marinade Roasted Garlic	1 tbsp	35	0	0
Marinade Southwestern Chipotle	1 tbsp	30	0	0
Marinade Tropical Grill	1 tbsp	40	0	0
Del Monte				
Seafood Cocktail	¼ cup	100	0	0
Sloppy Joe Hickory Flavor	¼ cup	60	0	0
Sloppy Joe Original	¼ cup	50	0	0
Eden				
Ponzu Sauce	1 tbsp	5	0	–
Emeril's				
Steak Sauce	1 tbsp	20	0	–
Fage				
Tzatziki	2 tbsp	30	5	0

FOOD	PORTION	CALS	CHOL	FIBER
Frank's				
Buffalo Wing Sauce	1 tbsp	5	0	0
RedHot Chile & Lime Sauce	1 tsp	0	0	0
RedHot Original Cayenne Pepper Sauce	1 tsp	0	0	0
RedHot X-tra Hot	1 tsp	0	0	0
French's				
Worchestershire	1 tsp	0	0	0
Gebhardt				
Enchilada Sauce	¼ cup (2.2 oz)	35	0	1
Hot Dog Chili Sauce	¼ cup (2.2 oz)	60	1	2
Hot Sauce	1 tsp (5 g)	1	0	0
Gringo Billy's				
Chipotle Dipping & Grilling Sauce	1 tsp	5	0	0
House Of Tsang				
General Tsao	1 tsp	45	0	0
Hoisin	1 tsp	15	0	0
Kobe Steak Grill	1 tbsp	50	0	0
Korean Teriyaki Stir Fry	1 tbsp	35	0	0
Peanut Sauce Bangkok Padang	1 tbsp	45	0	0
Spicy Brown Bean	1 tbsp	15	0	0
Sweet & Sour	1 tbsp	35	0	0
Sweet Ginger Sesame	1 tbsp	40	0	0
Thai Peanut	1 tbsp	50	0	0
Jok'n'Al				
Cocktail	¼ cup	29	0	–
Plum	1 tbsp	10	0	–
Just Rite				
Hot Dog	¼ cup (2.2 oz)	50	2	2
Ken's				
Marinade Herb & Garlic	1 tbsp	20	0	0
Marinade Lemon & Pepper	1 tbsp	10	0	0
Marinade Teriyaki	1 tbsp	20	0	0
Kikkoman				
Teriyaki	1 tbsp	15	0	0
La Choy				
Duck Sauce Sweet & Sour	2 tbsp (1.3 oz)	61	0	0

FOOD	PORTION	CALS	CHOL	FIBER
Sweet & Sour	2 tbsp (1.2 oz)	58	0	0
Teriyaki	1 tbsp (0.6 oz)	17	0	0
Las Palmas				
Enchilada Green	¼ cup	25	0	0
Enchilada Mild	¼ cup	20	0	1
Red Chili	¼ cup	20	0	1
Lea & Perrins				
Worcestershire	1 tsp	5	0	–
Lee Kum Kee				
Plum Sauce	2 tbsp	100	0	–
Lollipop Tree				
Grilling & Glazing Chipotle	1 tbsp	50	0	0
Grilling & Glazing Mango Garlic	2 tbsp	60	0	0
Manwich				
Bold	¼ cup (2.2 oz)	62	0	1
Mexican	¼ cup (2.2 oz)	27	0	1
Original	¼ cup (2.2 oz)	32	0	1
Taco Season	¼ cup (2.2 oz)	27	0	1
Thick & Chunky	¼ cup (2.3 oz)	44	0	1
Matouk's				
Calypso	1 tsp	0	0	0
Flambeau Sauce	1 tsp	0	0	0
Nando's				
Curry Coconut	¼ cup	71	4	1
Fresh Lemon	¼ cup	61	3	0
Marinade Lime & Cilantro	1 tbsp	27	0	0
Marinade Sundried Tomato	1 tbsp	15	0	0
Peri-Peri Pepper Extra Hot	1 oz	17	0	–
Peri-Peri Pepper Garlic	1 oz	12	0	–
Peri-Peri Pepper Hot	1 oz	16	0	–
Peri-Peri Pepper Wild Herb	1 oz	14	0	–
Roasted Red	¼ cup	70	0	1
Sweet Apricot	¼ cup	51	0	0
Newman's Own				
Fra Diavolo	½ cup	70	0	3
Steak Sauce	1 tbsp	20	0	0
Old El Paso				
Enchilada Mild	¼ cup	25	0	0

FOOD	PORTION	CALS	CHOL	FIBER
Open Range				
Hot Dog Chili	¼ cup (2.2 oz)	61	3	2
Ortega				
Enchilada	¼ cup	15	0	tr
Taco	1 tbsp	10	0	–
Pace				
Enchilada Sauce	¼ cup	36	0	0
Taco Sauce	¼ cup	32	0	0
Patak's				
Dopiaza	½ cup	90	0	0
Jalfrezi Sweet Peppers & Coconut	½ cup	140	0	1
Korma Rich Creamy Coconut	½ cup	240	15	1
Rogan Josh Spicy Tomato & Cardamon	½ cup	90	0	2
Tikka Masala Tangy Lemon & Cilantro	½ cup	120	0	1
Progresso				
Alfredo	½ cup (4.4 oz)	200	50	1
San-J				
Japanese Steak	1 tbsp	13	0	–
Sweet & Tangy	1 tbsp	50	0	–
Szechuan	1 tsp	5	0	–
Teriyaki	1 tbsp	10	0	–
Sara Lee				
Horseradish	1 tbsp	20	0	0
Sauce Arturo				
Original	¼ cup (2.2 oz)	50	0	0
South Beach Diet				
Steak Sauce	1 tbsp	5	0	0
Steel's				
Sugar Free Cocktail w/ Dill & Lemon	¼ cup	36	0	1
Sugar Free Hoisin	2 tbsp	15	0	1
Sugar Free Mango Curry	1 tbsp	13	0	tr
Sugar Free Sweet & Sour	2 tbsp	10	0	0
Tostitos				
Beef Fiesta Nacho	2.4 oz	120	10	tr
Chicken Quesadilla Topping	2.5 oz	90	10	tr

FOOD	PORTION	CALS	CHOL	FIBER
Ty Ling				
Duck	2 tbsp	70	0	1
Walden Farms				
Calorie Free Seafood Sauce	1 tbsp	0	0	0
Scampi Sauce Calorie Free	2 tbsp	0	0	0
Wild Thyme Farms				
Chili Ginger Honey	1 tbsp	30	0	–
MIX				
cheese as prep w/ milk	1 cup	307	53	–
curry as prep	1 cup	120	0	–
curry as prep w/ milk	1 cup	270	35	–
mushroom as prep w/ milk	1 cup	228	34	–
sour cream as prep w/ milk	1 cup	509	91	–
stroganoff as prep	1 cup	271	38	–
sweet & sour as prep	1 cup	294	0	–
teriyaki as prep	1 cup	131	0	–
white as prep w/ milk	1 cup	241	34	–
A Taste Of Thai				
Pad Thai Sauce	2 tbsp	90	0	1
Peanut Sauce	¼ pkg	45	0	1
Durkee				
A La King as prep	1 cup	60	0	0
Cheese as prep	¼ cup	25	2	0
Hollandaise as prep	2 tbsp	10	0	0
White as prep	¼ cup	20	0	0
Manwich				
Mix	¼ oz	22	0	tr
McCormick				
Chicken Dijon Blend	1⅔ tbsp (10 g)	40	<5	–
Hollandaise Blend	2 tsp (4 g)	15	15	–
TAKE-OUT				
adobo fresco	2 tbsp	81	0	1
bearnaise	1 oz	177	21	tr
cucumber yogurt sauce	1.5 tbsp	20	2	0
enchilada sauce green	¼ cup	46	11	1
enchilada sauce red	¼ cup	79	22	1

SAUERKRAUT

FOOD	PORTION	CALS	CHOL	FIBER
canned	½ cup	22	0	–

FOOD	PORTION	CALS	CHOL	FIBER
B&G				
Sauerkraut	2 tbsp (1 oz)	6	0	1
Boar's Head				
Sauerkraut	2 tbsp (1 oz)	5	0	tr
Claussen				
Sauerkraut	¼ cup (1.1 oz)	5	0	1
Del Monte				
Bavarian Style	2 tbsp	15	0	0
Sauerkraut	2 tbsp	0	0	tr
Eden				
Organic	½ cup	25	0	3
Hebrew National				
Sauerkraut	2 tbsp	5	0	1
S&W				
Canned	2 tbsp (1 oz)	5	0	0
Red Cabbage	2 tbsp (1 oz)	15	0	0
Silver Floss				
Sauerkraut	½ cup	20	0	4
SAUSAGE				
beef & pork	1 link (2.3 oz)	196	51	0
beef & pork w/ cheddar cheese	1 link (2.7 oz)	228	49	0
bratwurst pork cooked	1 link (2.5 oz)	226	44	0
brotwurst pork & beef	1 link (2.5 oz)	226	44	0
chipolata	3.5 oz	342	66	0
chorizo	1 link (2.1 oz)	273	53	0
free range chicken breakfast	2 links (2.7 oz)	110	45	0
italian pork cooked	1 (2.4 oz)	230	38	1
knockwurst pork & beef	1 (2.5 oz)	221	43	0
polish kielbasa	2 oz	127	39	0
pork cooked	2 links (1.7 oz)	163	40	0
vienna canned	1 link (0.5 oz)	37	14	0
vienna canned	1 can (4 oz)	260	98	0
Al Fresco				
Apple Maple	1 (1.2 oz)	70	25	–
Buffalo Style	1 (3 oz)	160	50	–
Country Style	1 (1.2 oz)	60	35	–
Italian Sweet	1 (3 oz)	170	65	–
Roasted Garlic	1 (3 oz)	170	70	–

FOOD	PORTION	CALS	CHOL	FIBER
Spicy Jalapeno	1 (3 oz)	120	65	–
Sundried Tomato & Basil	1 (3 oz)	180	70	–
Sweet Apple	1 (3 oz)	160	65	–
Teriyaki Ginger	1 (3 oz)	180	70	–
Wild Blueberry	1 (1.2 oz)	90	25	–
Armour				
Brown'N Serve Lite Original	3	120	45	0
Brown'N Serve Turkey	3 links	120	35	0
Vienna Sausage 25% Less Fat	3 (1.9 oz)	130	50	0
Vienna Sausage Hot'n Spicy	3 (2.1 oz)	150	50	0
Vienna Sausage In BBQ Sauce	3 (2.1 oz)	150	50	0
Vienna Sausage In Beef Stock	3 (1.9 oz)	150	50	0
Bilinski's				
Chicken Bratworst w/ Wild Rice	1 (2 oz)	70	25	0
Chicken Cajun-Style Andouille	2 oz	80	60	0
Chicken Italian w/ Peppers	1 (2 oz)	70	60	0
Chicken w/ Apples & Chardonnay	2 oz	70	60	0
Chicken w/ Cilantro	2 oz	70	40	1
Chicken w/ Jalapenos	2 oz	70	55	0
Chicken w/ Pesto	2 oz	90	40	0
Chicken w/ Spinach	2 oz	70	40	1
Chicken w/ Sun-Dried Tomato	2 oz	70	40	0
Boar's Head				
Bratwurst	1 (4 oz)	300	75	0
Hot Smoked	1 (3.2 oz)	250	55	0
Kielbasa	2 oz	120	50	0
Knockwurst Beef	1 (4 oz)	310	70	0
Hebrew National				
Knockwurst Beef	1 (3 oz)	260	55	0
Jennie-O				
Italian Hot	1 (3.9 oz)	160	60	–
Turkey Italian Sweet	1 link (3.9 oz)	160	60	0

FOOD	PORTION	CALS	CHOL	FIBER
Jones				
Light 50% Less Fat	2 (1.6 oz)	110	25	–
Little Pork	3	190	45	–
Murray's				
Chicken Hot Italian	3 oz	130	85	–
Chicken Spinach & Garlic	3 oz	100	50	–
Chicken Sun Dried Tomato	3 oz	110	55	–
Chicken Sweet Italian	3 oz	130	85	–
Perdue				
Hot Italian Turkey Cooked	1 link (2.4 oz)	150	60	–
Sweet Italian Turkey Cooked	1 link (2.4 oz)	150	60	–
Shady Brook				
Turkey Breakfast	1 (2.3 oz)	80	35	0
Turkey Sweet Italian	1 (2.5 oz)	110	50	–
Turkey Bratwurt	3 oz	160	75	–
Soy Lean				
Pork Breakfast Patty	1 (2 oz)	75	15	–
Turkey Store				
Breakfast	2 links (2 oz)	140	45	–
Wampler				
Breakfast Turkey	2 (2.4 oz)	110	45	–
Italian Turkey	1 (2.7 oz)	120	50	–
Wellshire				
Andouille	1 link (3 oz)	197	84	0
Andouille Turkey	2 oz	59	14	0
Chorizo	1 piece (2 oz)	130	50	0
Chorizo Dried	1 oz	100	30	0
Italian Turkey Mild	1 link (2 oz)	70	25	0
Kielbasa Polska	1 piece (2 oz)	130	50	0
Kielbasa Turkey	1 piece (2 oz)	59	14	0
Turkey Maple Breakfast	1 link (2 oz)	70	25	0

SAUSAGE DISHES
TAKE-OUT

italian sausage w/ peppers & onions	1 cup	210	70	–

SAUSAGE SUBSTITUTES

meatless	1 link (0.9 oz)	64	0	1
meatless	1 patty (1.3 oz)	98	0	1

FOOD	PORTION	CALS	CHOL	FIBER
Boca				
Bratwurst	1 (2.5 oz)	140	0	1
Breakfast Patties	1 (1.3 oz)	60	0	2
Breakfast Links	2 (1.6 oz)	70	0	2
Italian	1 (2.5 oz)	130	0	1
Lightlife				
Gimme Lean	2 oz	50	0	2
Smart Brats	1 (2 oz)	120	0	1
Smart Links Breakfast	2 (2 oz)	100	0	4
Smart Links Italian	1 (2 oz)	120	0	3
Smart Menu Breakfast Patty	1	45	0	1
Morningstar Farms				
Breakfast Links	2	60	0	2
Breakfast Patties	1 (1.3 oz)	80	0	1
Quron				
Links	2 (1.6 oz)	70	0	1
Tofurky				
Turkey Beerbrats	1 (3.5 oz)	280	0	5
Turkey Breakfast Links	1 (1.6 oz)	130	0	4
Turkey Italian Sweet	1 (3.5 oz)	280	0	8
Turkey Kielbasa	1 (3.5 oz)	240	0	8
Worthington				
Saucettes Breakfast Links	1 (1.3 oz)	90	0	1
Yves				
Veggie Breakfast Links	1 (1.6 oz)	60	0	2
Veggie Breakfast Patties	1 (2 oz)	70	0	2
SAVORY				
ground	1 tsp	4	0	–
SCALLOP				
raw	3 oz	75	28	–
TAKE-OUT				
breaded & fried	2 lg	67	19	–
SCONE				
Finnegan's				
Irish Raisin	1 (2 oz)	170	0	1
Health Valley				
Cinnamon Raisin	1	180	0	5

FOOD	PORTION	CALS	CHOL	FIBER
King Arthur				
Cranberry Orange as prep	1	248	47	0
English Cream Tea Scone not prep	⅓ cup	180	0	tr
TAKE-OUT				
blueberry	1 (3 oz)	270	10	2
orange poppy	1 (3 oz)	260	30	2
raisin	1 (3 oz)	270	10	2

SEA CUCUMBER

FOOD	PORTION	CALS	CHOL	FIBER
dried	1 oz	74	17	0
fresh	1 oz	20	14	0

SEAWEED

FOOD	PORTION	CALS	CHOL	FIBER
agar dried	1 oz	87	0	–
agar fresh	1 oz	tr	0	–
hijiki dried	1 tbsp	9	0	1
irishmoss fresh	1 oz	14	0	–
kelp fresh	1 oz	12	0	–
kombu fresh	1 oz	12	0	–
laver fresh	1 oz	10	0	–
nori fresh	1 oz	10	0	–
nori sheet dried	1 (8 x 8 in)	5	0	1
seahair dried	1 tbsp	13	0	tr
spirulina dried	1 oz	83	0	–
spirulina fresh	1 oz	7	0	–
tangle fresh	1 oz	12	0	–
wakame fresh	1 oz	13	0	–
Eden				
Agar Agar Bars	1 (7 g)	25	0	5
Agar Agar Flakes	1 tbsp	0	0	1
Arame Wild	½ cup	30	0	7
Hiziki Wild	½ cup	30	0	6
Kombu Wild	½ piece (3.3 g)	5	0	1
Organic Dulse Flakes	1 tsp	3	0	0

SEITAN (*see* WHEAT)

SEMOLINA

FOOD	PORTION	CALS	CHOL	FIBER
dry	1 cup (5.9 oz)	601	0	7

FOOD	PORTION	CALS	CHOL	FIBER
SESAME				
seeds	1 tsp	16	0	–
sesame butter	1 tbsp	95	0	1
sesame crunch candy	1 oz	146	0	–
tahini from roasted & toasted kernels	1 tbsp	89	0	–
tahini from stone ground kernels	1 tbsp	86	0	–
tahini from unroasted kernels	1 tbsp	85	0	–
Maranatha				
Raw Tahini	2 tbsp	190	0	3
Roasted Tahini	2 tbsp	210	0	2
Peloponnese				
Tahini	1 tbsp	100	0	1
Sabra				
Tahini Sauce Taratore	1 oz	80	0	0
SESBANIA				
flower	1	1	0	–
flowers cooked	1 cup	23	0	–
SHAD				
cooked	1 oz	55	121	0
SHALLOTS				
Christopher Ranch				
Fresh	1 (1 oz)	20	0	1
Frieda's				
Fresh	1 tbsp (1 oz)	20	0	0
SHARK				
raw	3 oz	111	43	0
TAKE-OUT				
batter-dipped & fried	3 oz	194	50	–
SHELLFISH (see individual names, SHELLFISH SUBSTITUTES)				
SHELLFISH SUBSTITUTES				
crab imitation	1 cup (4.4 oz)	144	60	tr
scallop imitation	3 oz	84	18	–
shrimp imitation	3 oz	86	31	–

FOOD	PORTION	CALS	CHOL	FIBER
surimi	1 oz	28	8	–
surimi	3 oz	84	25	–
Chicken Of The Sea				
Imitation Crab	1 pkg (2.5 oz)	40	9	1
Louis Kemp				
Crab Delights	½ cup (3 oz)	80	10	0
Crab Delights Chunk Style	½ cup (3 oz)	80	10	0
Crab Delights Easy Shred	½ cup (3 oz)	80	10	0
Crab Delights Leg Style	½ cup (3 oz)	80	10	0
Lobster Delights Chunk or Salad Style	½ cup (3 oz)	80	10	0
Scallop Delights Bay Style	½ cup (3 oz)	80	10	0
TAKE-OUT				
crab salad	1 cup	395	77	1
SHELLIE BEANS				
canned	½ cup	37	0	–
SHERBET				
orange	1 bar (2.75 oz)	91	3	–
orange	½ cup (4 oz)	132	5	–
orange	½ gal	2158	113	–
Blue Bunny				
Cool Tubes Orange Sherbet	1 (3 oz)	110	5	0
Lime	½ cup	110	0	0
Rainbow	½ cup	110	0	0
Raspberry	½ cup	110	0	0
Breyers				
Orange	½ cup	120	5	0
Rainbow	½ cup	120	5	0
Hood				
Orange Burst	½ cup	120	<5	0
Turkey Hill				
Fruit Rainbow	½ cup	120	5	–
Orange Grove	½ cup	120	5	–
SHRIMP				
CANNED				
canned	1 can (6 oz)	136	195	0
chinese shrimp paste	1 tbsp	15	45	–

FOOD	PORTION	CALS	CHOL	FIBER
Bumble Bee				
Broken Shrimp	¼ cup	40	115	0
Medium Or Large Or Jumbo	¼ cup	40	115	0
Small	¼ cup	40	115	0
Tiny	¼ cup	40	115	0
Chicken Of The Sea				
Tiny Small or Medium	½ can (2 oz)	45	145	0
DRIED				
dried	10	15	22	0
FRESH				
broiled	6 med	46	55	0
steamed	6 med	41	59	0
FROZEN				
Chicken Of The Sea				
Cooked Large Peeled Deveined Tail On	3 oz	80	165	0
Large Raw Cleaned Tail Off	4 oz	120	170	0
Contessa				
Orange Shrimp	11 to 13 (6 oz)	250	95	5
Ragin' Cajun	8 to 10 (4 oz)	170	100	3
Shrimp Scampi	8 to 10 (4 oz)	290	85	2
Gorton's				
Popcorn Garlic & Herb	22 pieces (3.6 oz)	270	90	–
Popcorn Original	20 pieces (3.2 oz)	240	65	–
Margaritaville				
Calypso Coconut + Sauce	5 pieces	350	70	0
Island Lime	6 pieces	130	155	0
Jammin' Jerk	7 pieces	140	145	0
Paradise Cocktail + Sauce	5 pieces	85	130	tr
Sunset Scampi	1 serv (½ pkg)	270	130	0
Surfside Skewers + Sauce	2 skewers	105	185	0
Phillips Seafood				
Breaded Shrimp	5 pieces	230	50	–
Buffalo Shrimp	5 pieces	260	50	–
Coconut Shrimp	5 pieces	330	100	–
Crab Stuffed Shrimp	3 pieces	160	125	–
TAKE-OUT				
breaded & fried	6 med (2.3 oz)	162	121	tr
cocktail w/ sauce	4 shrimp	87	78	2
curried	1 cup	295	175	tr

FOOD	PORTION	CALS	CHOL	FIBER
gingered	4	80	140	–
jambalaya	1 cup	309	180	1
scampi	1 cup	310	246	0
shrimp newburg	1 serv (6.4 oz)	456	313	tr
shrimp salad	¾ cup	212	152	1
shrimp w/ crab stuffing	5	158	126	tr

SMELT
rainbow cooked	3 oz	106	76	0
rainbow raw	3 oz	83	60	0

SMOOTHIES (see also FRUIT DRINKS, YOGURT DRINKS)
8th Continent
Refresher Orange Pineapple Banana	8 oz	150	0	0
Refresher Strawberry Banana	8 oz	150	0	0

Bolthouse Farms
Strawberry Banana Fruit	8 oz	124	0	tr

C&W
Berry Blend	½ cup	90	10	2
Peach	½ cup	80	10	1

E4B
100% Fruit Puree Blueberry Raspberry	4 oz	70	0	3
100% Fruit Puree Kiwi	4 oz	70	0	1
100% Fruit Puree Mango	4 oz	70	0	1
100% Fruit Puree Pear Caramel	4 oz	70	0	1
100% Fruit Puree Strawberry Banana	4 oz	70	0	1

Hansen's
Apricot Nectar	1 can	170	0	–
Cranberry Twist	1 can	180	0	–
Energy Island Blast	1 can	170	0	–
Guava Strawberry	1 can	170	0	–
Lite Cranberry Raspberry	1 can	50	0	–
Mango Pineapple	1 can	170	0	–
Peach Berry	1 can	170	0	–
Pineapple Coconut	1 can	180	0	–
Strawberry Banana	1 can	180	0	–

FOOD	PORTION	CALS	CHOL	FIBER
Tropical Passion	1 can	170	0	–
Whipped Orange	1 can	180	0	–
Horizon Organic				
Tropical Punch	1 bottle (6.2 oz)	120	0	1
Jammin' Juice				
Mambo Mango	6 oz	92	0	1
Jammin' Nectars				
C-Beta Carrot	6 oz	96	0	1
Ginger Party	6 oz	6	0	1
Guanabana Limbo	6 oz	78	0	2
Pure Passion	6 oz	78	0	1
Razz-Ade	6 oz	89	0	1
Kidz Dream				
Orange Cream	1 box	120	0	tr
LightFull				
Satiety Smoothie Cafe Latte	1 (11 oz)	90	0	5
Satiety Smoothie Chocolate Fudge	1 (11 oz)	90	0	6
Satiety Smoothie Peaches & Cream	1 (11 oz)	100	0	6
Satiety Smoothie Strawberries & Cream	1 (11 oz)	90	0	6
Naked Juice				
Chocolate Karma	8 oz	190	0	3
Vanilla Chai	8 oz	170	0	2
Nutiva				
Organic HempShake Amazon Acai not prep	4 tbsp	100	0	8
Organic HempShake Chocolate not prep	4 tbsp	80	0	12
Odwalla				
Blackberry Fruit Shake	8 oz	140	0	1
Orange Pina	8 oz	140	0	1
Sambazon				
Acai Energy Mango Banana	8 oz	190	0	3
Acai Soy Energy	8 oz	210	0	4
Amazon Cherry	8 oz	156	0	1
Mango Uprising	8 oz	190	0	3
Protein Warrior Chocolate	8 oz	215	0	3
Protein Warrior Vanilla	8 oz	215	0	3

FOOD	PORTION	CALS	CHOL	FIBER
Purple Power	1 bottle (1.05 oz)	155	0	2
Shaman's Immunity	8 oz	90	0	1
Strawberry Sensation	8 oz	210	0	2
Supergreens Revolution	8 oz	200	0	3
Smooze				
Mango + Coconut	1 box (8.5 oz)	250	0	0
Passion Fruit + Coconut	1 box (8.5 oz)	225	0	3
Pineapple + Coconut	1 box (8.5 oz)	200	0	0
Soy Blendz				
Mango Orange Dream	1 bottle (10 oz)	220	0	3
Mixed Berry Medley	1 bottle (10 oz)	210	0	3
Orange Citrus Splash	1 bottle (10 oz)	220	0	3
Strawberry Banana Blast	1 bottle (10 oz)	230	0	3
Tree Of Life				
Organic Smoothie Banana Raspberry Strawbery	⅔ cup (5 oz)	90	0	3
Organic Smoothie Mango Strawberry Raspberry	⅔ cup (5 oz)	70	0	4
Organic Smoothie Strawberry Banana	⅔ cup (5 oz)	90	0	3
Organic Smoothie Strawberry Blueberry Banana	⅔ cup (5 oz)	90	0	3
Tropicana				
Fruit Smoothie Mixed Berry	1 bottle (11 oz)	220	0	2
Fruit Smoothie Tropical Fruit	1 bottle (11 oz)	220	0	1
WholeSoy & Co.				
Organic Soy Peach	8 oz	210	0	0
Organic Soy Raspberry	8 oz	210	0	0
Organic Soy Strawberry	8 oz	210	0	0
Yoplait				
Go-Gurt All Fruit Flavors	1 bottle (5 oz)	120	5	0
Light All Flavors	1 bottle (8.3 oz)	90	5	3
Smoothie All Flavors	1 bottle (8.3 oz)	220	15	3

SNACKS

FOOD	PORTION	CALS	CHOL	FIBER
cheese puffs	1 oz	157	1	tr
corn puffs cheese	1 bag (8 oz)	1256	9	2
corn twists cheese	1 bag (8 oz)	1256	9	2
corn twists cheese	1 oz	157	1	tr
oriental mix	1 oz	155	0	–

FOOD	PORTION	CALS	CHOL	FIBER
pork skins	1 oz	154	27	0
pork skins barbecue	1 oz	152	33	–
trail mix	1 cup (5.3 oz)	693	0	–
trail mix	1 oz	131	0	–
trail mix tropical	1 oz	115	0	–
Baken-ets				
Fried Pork Skins	9 pieces	80	20	0
Fried Pork Skins Hot'n Spicy	9 pieces	80	20	tr
Fried Pork Skins Sweet & Tangy BBQ	9 pieces	80	20	0
Pork Cracklins	8 pieces	90	15	tr
Pork Cracklins Hot'n Spicy	8 pieces	80	20	tr
Barbara's Bakery				
Cheese Puffs Bakes	1½ cups (1 oz)	160	0	0
Cheese Puffs Jalapeno	¾ cup (1 oz)	150	0	0
Cheese Puffs Original	¾ cup (1 oz)	150	0	0
Bowlby's				
Bits Almond	½ cup	100	0	1
Bits Pecan	½ cup	200	0	1
Bits Ranch	½ cup	170	0	0
Bits Salsa	½ cup	170	0	0
Bits Sour Cream Onion & Dill	½ cup	170	0	0
Bits'N'Pops	¾ cup	130	13	1
Mix-Ups Country Mix	½ cup	170	0	1
Mix-Ups Nuttyest-Of-All	½ cup	160	0	1
Mix-Ups Trail Mix	½ cup	165	0	1
Bugles				
Baked Original	1⅓ cup	130	0	–
Chile Con Queso	1⅓ cups	160	0	–
Nacho	1½ cups	160	0	–
Original	1½ cups	160	0	tr
Smokin'BBQ	1⅓ cups	150	0	–
Cheetos				
Asteriods Go Snack	¾ cup (1 oz)	160	0	1
Baked Crunchy	34 pieces (1 oz)	130	0	0
Crunchy	21 pieces (1 oz)	160	0	tr
Natural White Cheddar	32 pieces (1 oz)	150	<5	tr
Puffs	13 pieces (1 oz)	160	0	0
Twisted	7 pieces (1 oz)	160	0	0

FOOD	PORTION	CALS	CHOL	FIBER
Chester's				
Puffcorn Butter	3 cups	160	0	tr
Puffcorn Cheese	3 cups	160	0	0
Chex Mix				
Cheddar	⅔ cup	140	0	2
Hot'N Spicy	⅔ cup	130	0	2
Nacho Fiesta	⅔ cup	120	0	1
Party Blend Bold	⅔ cup	140	0	2
Peanut Lovers	⅔ cup	140	0	1
Traditional	⅔ cup	130	0	1
Funyuns				
Mini Onion Rings Go Snacks	1 pkg	260	0	1
Onion Rings	13 pieces	140	0	tr
Garden Of Eatin'				
Organic Baked Cheese Puffs	32 pieces	150	<5	1
Organic Baked Chunchitos	35 pieces	140	<5	1
Good Sense				
Organic Trail Mix Tropical	⅓ cup	160	0	2
Snack Mix Cajun Corn 'N Sesame	¼ cup	150	0	2
Trail Mix Dietary Snack Mix	¼ cup	130	0	2
J&J				
Microwave Pork Rinds All Flavors	1 oz	130	0	0
Kangaroo				
Pita Snackers Crispy Cinnamon	10 pieces (1 oz)	90	0	1
Pita Snackers Sea Salt	10 pieces (1 oz)	90	0	1
Maranatha				
High Energy Mix	¼ cup	120	0	2
Organic Harvest Mix	¼ cup	150	0	2
Organic Nature Mix	¼ cup	150	0	2
Snack Attack Mix	¼ cup	140	0	2
Trail Mix Deluxe	¼ cup	150	0	2
Trail Mix Navajo	¼ cup	140	0	4
Trail Mix Olympic w/ Chocolate	¼ cup	140	0	2
Trail Mix Organic Delight	¼ cup	150	0	2
Trail Mix Organic Raw	¼ cup	140	0	2

FOOD	PORTION	CALS	CHOL	FIBER
Mauna Loa				
Tropical Nut & Fruit	¼ cup	180	0	2
Munchies				
Snack Mix Flamin' Hot	1 oz	140	0	tr
Snack Mix Kids	1 oz	130	0	1
Old Dutch Foods				
Baked Cheese Curls	2 cups (1.1 oz)	180	0	tr
Cheese Puffcorn Curls	2 cups (1.1 oz)	170	0	0
Organic Trails				
Trail Mix Summit Blend	¼ cup	150	0	2
Planters				
Trail Mix Berry Nut & Chocolate	3 tbsp (1 oz)	120	0	1
Pumpkorn				
Caramel	⅓ cup	150	0	2
Chili	⅓ cup	150	0	2
Curry	⅓ cup	150	0	2
Maple Vanilla	⅓ cup	150	0	2
Mesquite	⅓ cup	150	0	2
Original	⅓ cup	150	0	2
Sabritones				
Chile & Lime	23 pieces	150	0	1
Snyder's Of Hanover				
Cheese Twists	1 oz	230	0	0
Fried Pork Skins	1 oz	80	30	0
Fried Pork Skins Barbecue	1 oz	80	20	0
Kruncheez	1.25 oz	200	0	tr
Onion Toasters	1 oz	188	0	tr
SunRise				
Trail Mix Honey Coated	3 tbsp (1 oz)	137	1	4
Trail Mix w/ Fruit	3 tbsp (1 oz)	130	0	2
Tumaro's				
Organic Krispy Crunchy Puffs Cheddar	22	120	0	1
Organic Krispy Crunchy Puffs Natural Corn	22	120	0	1
Organic Krispy Crunchy Puffs Ranch & Herb	22	130	0	tr
Organic Krispy Crunchy Puffs Tangy BBQ	22	120	0	tr

FOOD	PORTION	CALS	CHOL	FIBER
Utz				
Caramel Corn Clusters	1⅛ cups (1 oz)	120	0	tr
Pork Cracklins	0.5 oz	90	15	–
Pork Cracklins Hot & Spicy	0.5 oz	80	15	–
Pork Rinds	0.5 oz	80	15	0
Pork Rinds BBQ	0.5 oz	80	15	–
Wise				
Cheez Doodles Crunchy	1 pkg (1 oz)	150	0	0
Cheez Doodles Crunchy Reduced Fat	1 oz	130	<5	tr
Cheez Doodles Puffed	1 pkg (0.7 oz)	110	0	0
Doodle O's	1 oz	160	<5	0
Onion Rings	1 oz	140	0	0
Pork Rinds Original	1 oz	90	25	0
SNAIL				
cooked	3 oz	233	110	–
raw	3 oz	117	55	–
TAKE-OUT				
escargot cooked	5	25	15	0
SNAP BEANS				
FRESH				
Frieda's				
Purple Wax	⅔ cup	25	0	3
SNAPPER				
cooked	1 fillet (6 oz)	217	80	0
cooked	3 oz	109	40	0
raw	3 oz	85	31	0
SODA				
club	12 oz	0	0	0
cola	12 oz	151	0	–
cream	12 oz	191	0	–
diet cola	12 oz	2	0	–
diet cola w/ equal	12 oz	2	0	–
diet cola w/ saccharin	12 oz	2	0	–
ginger ale	12 oz can	124	0	–
grape	12 oz	161	0	–
lemon lime	12 oz	149	0	–
orange	12 oz	177	0	–

FOOD	PORTION	CALS	CHOL	FIBER
pepper type	12 oz	151	0	–
quinine	12 oz	125	0	–
root beer	12 oz	152	0	–
shirley temple	1 serv	159	0	0
tonic water	12 oz	125	0	–
7 Up				
Diet	8 oz	0	0	–
Original	8 oz	100	0	–
Plus	1 can (12 oz)	10	0	–
A & W				
Root Beer	1 can (12 oz)	170	0	–
AJ Stephans				
Birch Beer	1 bottle	170	0	–
Black Cherry	1 bottle	180	0	–
Cream	1 bottle	170	0	–
Jamaican Style Ginger Beer	1 bottle	170	0	–
Lemon & Lime	1 bottle	190	0	–
Olde Style Root Beer	1 bottle	170	0	–
Barq's				
Diet French Vanilla Creme	8 oz	1	0	–
Diet Red Creme	8 oz	4	0	–
Diet Root Beer	8 oz	1	0	–
Floatz	8 oz	127	0	–
French Vanilla Creme	8 oz	112	0	–
Red Creme	8 oz	113	0	–
Root Beer	8 oz	111	0	–
Barritts				
Ginger Beer	1 bottle (12 oz)	200	0	–
Big Red				
Vanilla Float	1 can	180	0	–
Blumers				
Black Cherry	1 bottle (12 oz)	138	0	–
Blueberry Cream	1 bottle (12 oz)	190	0	–
Cream	1 bottle (12 oz)	181	0	–
Orange Cream	1 bottle (12 oz)	187	0	–
Root Beer	1 bottle (12 oz)	190	0	–
Bong Water				
Chronic Tonic	12 oz	144	0	–
Cottonmouth Quencher	12 oz	165	0	–

FOOD	PORTION	CALS	CHOL	FIBER
Green Dreams	12 oz	165	0	–
Purple Haze	12 oz	165	0	–
Briar's				
Black Cherry	1 bottle (12 oz)	180	0	–
Cream	1 bottle (12 oz)	180	0	–
Diet Root Beer	8 oz	4	0	–
Orange Cream	8 oz	120	0	–
Red Birch	8 oz	104	0	–
Root Beer	1 bottle (12 oz)	168	0	–
Bubble Yum				
All Flavors	8 oz	110	0	–
Canada Dry				
Ginger Ale	1 can (12 oz)	140	0	0
Tonic Water	8 oz	90	0	0
Capt'n Eli's				
Root Beer	8 oz	165	0	–
Carver's				
Ginger Ale	8 oz	94	0	–
Chronic 187				
Orange	1 bottle (12 oz)	300	0	–
Coca-Cola				
Blak	1 bottle (8 oz)	45	0	–
C2	8 oz	45	0	–
Classic	1 can (12 oz)	140	0	–
W/ Lime	8 oz	98	0	–
Zero	8 oz	0	0	–
Coke				
Cherry	8 oz	104	0	–
Diet	8 oz	1	0	–
Diet Cherry	8 oz	1	0	–
Diet Vanilla	8 oz	1	0	–
Diet w/ Lime	8 oz	2	0	–
Vanilla	8 oz	100	0	–
Dr Pepper				
Diet	1 oz	tr	0	–
Original	1 can (12 oz)	150	0	0
DRY				
Kumquat	1 bottle (12 oz)	50	0	–
Lavender	1 bottle (12 oz)	70	0	–
Lemongrass	1 bottle (12 oz)	50	0	–
Rhubarb	1 bottle (12 oz)	60	0	–

FOOD	PORTION	CALS	CHOL	FIBER
Fanta				
Apple	8 oz	121	0	–
Black Cherry	8 oz	110	0	–
Cherry	8 oz	117	0	–
Citrus	8 oz	91	0	–
Grape	8 oz	122	0	–
Lemon	8 oz	112	0	–
Orange	8 oz	111	0	–
Peach	8 oz	29	0	–
Pineapple	8 oz	120	0	–
Pink Grapefruit	8 oz	113	0	–
Strawberry	8 oz	120	0	–
Firefighter				
Backdraft Root Beer	8 oz	90	0	–
Courageous Cola	8 oz	90	0	–
Flashover Orange	8 oz	20	0	–
Incendiary Citrus	8 oz	90	0	–
Rolling Code Black Cherry	8 oz	90	0	–
Fresca				
Soda	8 oz	3	0	–
Frostie				
Diet Cherry Limeade	1 bottle (12 oz)	0	0	–
Diet Root Beer	1 bottle (12 oz)	0	0	0
Vanilla Root Beer	1 bottle (12 oz)	180	0	–
Hansen's				
Black Cherry	8 oz	110	0	–
Diet All Flavors	1 can	0	0	–
Ginger Beer	8 oz	100	0	–
Natural Black Cherry	1 can	160	0	–
Natural Cherry Vanilla	1 can	140	0	–
Natural Creamy Root Beer	1 can (12 oz)	160	0	–
Natural Ginger Ale	1 can	140	0	–
Natural Grapefruit	1 can	130	0	–
Natural Key Lime	1 can	130	0	–
Natural Kiwi Strawberry	1 can	130	0	–
Natural Mandarin Lime	1 can	130	0	–
Natural Orange Mango	1 can	170	0	–
Natural Raspberry	1 can	130	0	–
Natural Tangerine	1 can	160	0	–
Natural Tropical Passion	1 can	160	0	–

FOOD	PORTION	CALS	CHOL	FIBER
Natural Vanilla Cola	1 can	140	0	–
Orange Creme	8 oz	110	0	–
Sangria	8 oz	110	0	–
Sarsaparilla	8 oz	110	0	–
Sparkling Orangeade	8 oz	100	0	–
Vanilla Creme	8 oz	110	0	–
Hiball				
Club	1 bottle (10 oz)	5	0	0
Tonic Water	1 bottle (10 oz)	120	0	–
IBC				
Cream	1 bottle (12 oz)	180	0	–
Root Beer	1 can	160	0	–
Inca Kola				
Diet	8 oz	1	0	–
Soda	8 oz	96	0	–
Jolt				
Blue	8 oz	120	0	–
Cherry Bomb	8 oz	90	0	–
Cola	8 oz	100	0	–
Red	8 oz	120	0	–
Ultra	8 oz	0	0	0
Jones Soda				
Sugar Free All Flavors	1 bottle (12 oz)	0	0	–
Kutztown				
Birch Beer	1 bottle (12 oz)	160	0	–
Red Cream	1 bottle (12 oz)	150	0	–
Sarsaparilla	1 bottle (12 oz)	150	0	–
Like				
Cola	1 oz	13	0	–
Lucozade				
Soda	7 oz	136	0	0
Maine Root				
All Flavors	1 bottle (12 oz)	165	0	–
Manzana Mia				
Soda	8 oz	99	0	–
Mello Yellow				
Cherry	8 oz	118	0	–
Diet	8 oz	3	0	–
Melon	8 oz	119	0	–
Soda	8 oz	118	0	–

FOOD	PORTION	CALS	CHOL	FIBER
Mountain Dew				
Pitch Black	8 oz	110	0	–
Mr. Pibb				
Diet	8 oz	1	0	–
Nesbitt's				
Orange	1 bottle (12 oz)	190	0	–
Northern Neck				
Diet Ginger Ale	8 oz	4	0	–
Ginger Ale	8 oz	94	0	–
Nuky				
Rose Soda	8 oz	120	0	–
Olde Brooklyn				
Coney Island Cream	8 oz	130	0	–
Flatbush Orange	8 oz	130	0	–
Williamsburg Root Beer	8 oz	120	0	–
Olde Philadelphia				
Black Cherry	1 bottle (12 oz)	180	0	–
Cream	1 bottle (12 oz)	190	0	–
Cream Diet	1 bottle (12 oz)	0	0	–
Grape	1 bottle (12 oz)	180	0	–
Orange Cream	1 bottle (12 oz)	190	0	–
Pineapple	1 bottle	190	0	–
Root Beer	1 bottle (12 oz)	180	0	–
Orangina				
Sparkling Citrus	8 oz	90	0	–
Pennsylvania Dutch				
Birch Beer	8 oz	110	0	–
Pepsi				
Blue Berry Cola Fusion	8 oz	100	0	–
Diet	1 can (12 oz)	0	0	–
Edge	1 can (12 oz)	70	0	–
Regular	1 can (12 oz)	150	0	–
Vanilla	1 can	160	0	–
Vanilla Diet	1 can	0	0	0
Prism				
Green Tea Soda Cola	8 oz	105	0	–
Lemon Lime	8 oz	117	0	–
Qibla				
Diet Cola	1 bottle (18 oz)	1	0	0

FOOD	PORTION	CALS	CHOL	FIBER
Red Flash				
Soda	8 oz	105	0	–
Santa Cruz				
Organic Cherry	1 can	140	0	–
Organic Concord Grape	1 can	150	0	–
Organic Ginger Ale	1 can	150	0	–
Organic Lemon Lime	1 can	130	0	–
Organic Orange Mango	1 can	130	0	–
Organic Root Beer	1 can	150	0	–
Organic Vanilla Creme	1 can	160	0	–
Schweppes				
Ginger Ale	8 oz	120	0	0
Seagram's				
Ginger Ale	1 can (12 oz)	130	0	–
Sex Kola				
All Flavors	1 bottle (12 oz)	0	0	0
Diet All Flavors	1 bottle (12 oz)	0	0	0
Sierra Mist				
Lemon Lime	1 can (12 oz)	140	0	0
Ski				
Citrus	1 bottle (10 oz)	150	0	–
Snow				
Sparkling Mint	8 oz	75	0	–
Souix City				
Cream	1 bottle (12 oz)	180	0	–
Orange Cream	1 bottle (12 oz)	200	0	–
Root Beer	1 bottle (12 oz)	170	0	–
Sarsaparilla	1 bottle (12 oz)	170	0	–
Sprite				
Diet Zero	8 oz	0	0	–
ReMix Aruba Jam	8 oz	97	0	–
ReMix Berryclear	8 oz	97	0	–
Soda	8 oz	96	0	–
Steap				
Green Tea Soda Orange	8 oz	90	0	–
Green Tea Soda Root Beer	8 oz	90	0	–
Organic Green Tea Soda Raspberry	8 oz	90	0	–
Stewart's				
Cream	1 bottle (12 oz)	180	0	–

FOOD	PORTION	CALS	CHOL	FIBER
Diet Cream	1 bottle (12 oz)	0	0	0
Root Beer	1 bottle (12 oz)	160	0	–
Stirrings				
Club	1 bottle (6.3 oz)	0	0	0
Ginger Ale	1 bottle (6.3 oz)	100	0	0
Tonic Water	1 bottle (6.3 oz)	85	0	0
Sunkist				
Diet Orange	8 oz	0	0	0
Orange	8 oz	130	0	0
Tab				
Soda	8 oz	1	0	–
Thomas Kemper				
Black Cherry	1 bottle	177	0	–
Old Fashion Birch	1 bottle	170	0	–
Orange Cream	1 bottle	180	0	–
Pure Draft Honey Cola	1 bottle	140	0	–
Pure Draft Root Beer	1 bottle	160	0	–
Vanilla Cream	1 bottle	170	0	–
Three Drinks				
Citrus	12 oz	12	0	–
Tommyknocker				
Almond Creme	1 bottle (12 oz)	150	0	–
Key Lime Creme	1 bottle (12 oz)	180	0	–
Orange Creme	1 bottle (12 oz)	180	0	–
Root Beer	1 bottle (12 oz)	150	0	–
Root Beer Float	1 bottle (12 oz)	110	0	–
Strawberry Creme	1 bottle (12 oz)	150	0	–
Uno Mas				
All Flavors	1 can (12 oz)	130	0	0
Vermont Sweetwater				
Country Apple Jack	1 bottle	180	0	0
Kickin'Cow Cola	1 bottle	129	0	0
Mango Moonshine	1 bottle	180	0	0
Maple	1 bottle	101	0	0
Raspberry Rhubarb Ramble	1 bottle	180	0	0
Tangerine Cream Twister	1 bottle	180	0	0
Vermont Maple Seltzer	1 bottle	53	0	0
Vignette				
Wine Country All Flavors	1 bottle (12 oz)	130	0	–

FOOD	PORTION	CALS	CHOL	FIBER
Virgil's				
Micro Brewed Root Beer	1 bottle (12 oz)	160	0	–
White Rock				
Organics Raspberry Creme	1 can (12.4 oz)	120	0	–
Organics Red Peach	1 can (12.4 oz)	120	0	–
White T				
All Flavors	1 bottle (12 oz)	128	0	0
Diet All Flavors	1 bottle (12 oz)	0	0	0
Windy City				
Root Beer	1 bottle (12 oz)	170	0	0
Yoo-Hoo				
Original	9 oz	150	0	tr
Z Cola				
No Artifical Sweeteners	8 oz	0	0	0
SOLE				
cooked	1 fillet (4.5 oz)	148	86	–
cooked	3 oz	99	58	–
TAKE-OUT				
breaded & fried	3.2 oz	211	31	–
SORGHUM				
sorghum	1 cup (6.7 oz)	651	0	–
SOUFFLE				
lemon chilled	1 cup	176	2	–
raspberry chilled	1 cup	173	3	–
spinach	1 cup	233	160	1
Atkins				
Broccoli Cheddar & Bacon	1 serv	200	205	1
SOUP				
CANNED				
clam chowder new england as prep w/ milk	1 cup	163	22	–
Amy's				
Organic Barley	1 cup	50	0	2
Organic Black Bean Vegetable	1 cup	110	0	5
Organic Cream Of Mushroom	1 cup	120	5	2
Organic Cream Of Tomato	1 cup	100	10	4

FOOD	PORTION	CALS	CHOL	FIBER
Organic Lentil	1 cup	130	0	9
Organic Minestrone	1 cup	90	0	3
Organic No Chicken Noodle Soup	1 cup	90	0	2
Organic Vegetable	1 cup	35	0	1
Boston Market				
Chicken Broth Reduced Sodium	1 cup	15	0	0
Butterball				
Chicken Broth Reduced Sodium 99% Fat Free	1 cup	10	0	0
Campbell's				
98% Fat Free Cream Of Chicken as prep	1 cup	70	10	1
98% Fat Free Cream Of Mushroom	1 cup	70	5	1
Cheddar Cheese	1 cup	110	5	1
Chicken Broth	½ cup	20	<5	0
Chicken Gumbo as prep	1 cup	55	5	1
Chicken Noodle	1 cup	70	15	tr
Chicken Vegetable as prep	1 cup	74	9	1
Chunky Beef Barley	1 cup	160	25	2
Chunky Beef w/ Country Vegetables	1 cup	150	20	5
Chunky Chicken & Dumplings	1 cup	190	30	3
Chunky Chicken Corn Chowder	1 cup	230	20	3
Chunky Chili Roadhouse Beef & Bean	1 cup	220	1	7
Chunky Classic Chicken Noodle	1 cup	120	20	2
Chunky New England Clam Chowder	1 cup	240	15	2
Chunky Old Fashioned Vegetable Beef	1 cup	130	15	4
Chunky Sirloin Burger w/ Country Vegetables	1 cup	180	15	4
Chunky Vegetable	1 cup	130	0	4

FOOD	PORTION	CALS	CHOL	FIBER
Clam Chowder New England as prep	1 cup	89	3	1
Classics Beef Noodle	1 cup	70	15	1
Classics Chicken Rice	1 cup (8.4 oz)	80	5	1
Classics Minestrone	1 cup	90	<5	3
Classics Old Fashioned Vegetable	1 cup	90	<5	2
Classics Vegetarian Vegetable as prep	1 cup	90	0	2
Consomme as prep	1 cup	24	tr	tr
Cream Of Asparagus as prep	1 cup	72	2	1
Cream Of Celery as prep	1 cup	107	2	1
Cream Of Chicken	1 cup	120	10	2
Cream Of Chicken w/ Herbs	1 cup	90	10	1
Cream Of Mushroom as prep	1 cup	108	2	2
Double Noodle	1 cup	90	10	2
Fiesta Tomato as prep	1 cup	72	1	1
Garden Vegetable as prep	1 cup	69	3	1
Green Pea as prep	1 cup	173	1	4
Healthy Request Chicken Noodle as prep	1 cup	70	15	0
Healthy Request Chicken Rice as prep	1 cup	60	10	tr
Healthy Request Cream Of Chicken as prep	1 cup	80	10	1
Healthy Request Cream Of Chicken & Broccoli as prep	1 cup	78	6	1
Healthy Request Hearty Pasta w/ Vegetables	1 cup	87	1	2
Healthy Request Tomato as prep	1 cup	91	1	2
Healthy Request Vegetable as prep	1 cup	84	1	2
Italian Tomato as prep	1 cup	105	1	4
Kitchen Classics Bean w/ Bacon	1 cup	180	5	8
Kitchen Classics Chicken Noodle	1 cup	90	15	2
Kitchen Classics Chicken w/ White & Wild Rice	1 cup	100	10	2

FOOD	PORTION	CALS	CHOL	FIBER
Kitchen Classics Lentil	1 cup	120	5	5
Low Sodium Chicken w/ Noodles	1 can (10.75 oz)	162	40	2
Low Sodium Cream Of Mushroom	1 can (10.75 oz)	200	12	2
Low Sodium Green Pea	1 can (10.75 oz)	235	4	6
Low Sodium Tomato w/ Pieces	1 can (10.75 oz)	170	6	3
Ready To Serve Bean w/ Bacon 'N Ham	1 can (10.5 oz)	274	13	11
Ready To Serve Chicken w/ Rice	1 can (10.5 oz)	122	11	2
Savory Tomato & Dill as prep	1 cup	99	tr	2
Select Beef w/ Portobello Mushrooms & Rice	1 cup	110	15	2
Select Blended Red Pepper Black Bean	1 cup	110	<5	4
Select Chicken & Pasta w/ Roasted Garlic	1 cup (8.4 oz)	100	10	2
Select Chicken Rice	1 cup	100	5	2
Select Chicken w/ Egg Noodles	1 cup	90	20	2
Select Creamy Potato w/ Roasted Garlic	1 cup	180	10	2
Select Fiesta Vegetable	1 cup (8.4 oz)	120	0	3
Select Herbed Chicken w/ Roasted Vegetables	1 cup	90	15	1
Select Honey Roasted Chicken w/ Golden Potatoes	1 cup	110	15	3
Select Italian Style Wedding	1 cup	110	15	2
Select Mexican Chicken Tortilla	1 cup	140	10	3
Select Roasted Chicken w/ Long Grain & Wild Rice	1 cup	130	10	1
Select Roasted Chicken w/ Rotini & Penne Pasta	1 cup	90	10	2
Soup At Hand Chicken & Stars	1 pkg	70	5	2
Soup At Hand Chicken w/ Mini Noodles	1 pkg (10.75 oz)	80	10	2

FOOD	PORTION	CALS	CHOL	FIBER
Soup At Hand Cream Of Broccoli	1 pkg (10.75 oz)	160	5	3
Soup At Hand Creamy Chicken	1 pkg (10.75 oz)	130	5	4
Soup At Hand Creamy Tomato	1 pkg	180	<5	4
Soup At Hand Italian Style Wedding	1 pkg	90	10	2
Soup At Hand Vegetable Medley	1 pkg (10.75 oz)	110	5	3
Soup At Hand Velvety Potato	1 pkg (10.75 oz)	160	<5	4
Vegetable Beef as prep	1 cup	68	8	2
College Inn				
Beef Broth 99% Fat Free	1 cup	20	0	0
Beef Broth Fat Free Lower Sodium	1 cup	15	0	0
Chicken Broth Light & Fat Free	1 cup	5	0	0
Gold's				
Borscht Low Calorie	1 cup	20	0	1
Borscht Unsalted	1 cup	70	0	tr
Hungarian Cabbage	6 oz	70	0	2
Schav	1 cup	15	15	1
Healthy Choice				
Bean & Ham	1 cup	170	10	6
Beef & Potato	1 cup	110	10	2
Broccoli Cheddar	1 cup (8.4 oz)	116	4	2
Chicken & Dumplings	1 cup	130	20	7
Chicken & Pasta	1 cup	110	5	2
Chicken Corn Chowder	1 cup	140	5	3
Chicken Fiesta	1 cup	100	5	3
Chicken w/ Roasted Garlic	1 cup	120	10	2
Chicken w/ Rice	1 cup	90	15	2
Chili Beef	1 cup	170	15	6
Clam Chowder	1 cup	110	15	4
Country Vegetable	1 cup	110	0	4
Cream Of Mushroom	1 cup (8.8 oz)	77	tr	1
Cream Of Chicken Vegetable	1 cup (8.9 oz)	127	10	1
Creamy Tomato	1 cup	100	0	2
Garden Vegetable	1 cup	120	0	4

FOOD	PORTION	CALS	CHOL	FIBER
Hearty Chicken	1 cup	120	20	3
Italian Bean & Pasta	1 cup	100	0	3
Old Fashioned Chicken Noodle	1 cup	110	20	3
Roasted Italian Style Chicken	1 cup	120	15	4
Split Pea w/ Ham	1 cup	170	5	4
Turkey w/ Rice	1 cup	90	10	3
Vegetable Beef	1 cup	130	15	3
Vegetable Clam Chowder	1 cup	230	0	3
Zesty Gumbo	1 cup	100	20	3
Imagine				
Lobster Bisque	1 cup	130	15	–
Organic Creamy Butternut Squash	1 cup	90	0	2
Organic Creamy Chicken	1 cup	70	0	1
Organic Creamy Sweet Corn	1 cup	120	0	3
Organic Sweet Potato	1 cup	110	0	1
Organic Bistro Cuban Black Bean Bisque	1 cup	170	0	6
Organic Broth Beef	1 cup	20	5	0
Organic Broth Free Range Chicken	1 cup	10	0	0
Organic Broth Vegetable	8 oz	20	0	0
Lunch Bucket				
Chicken Noodle	1 pkg (7.25 oz)	80	10	0
Country Vegetable	1 pkg (7.25 oz)	60	0	3
Manischewitz				
Clear Chicken Condensed	½ cup	15	0	2
Pacific Foods				
Beef Broth	1 cup	20	0	0
Creamy Butternut Squash	1 cup	90	0	4
Creamy Roasted Carrot	1 cup	100	0	2
Creamy Roasted Red Pepper & Tomato	1 cup	100	10	1
Hearty Beef Barley	1 cup	110	10	2
Hearty Chicken Noodle	1 cup	80	20	1
Hearty Chicken Tortilla	1 cup	130	5	5
Hearty Roasted Red Pepper & Corn Chowder	1 cup	210	45	3
Organic Creamy Tomato	1 cup	100	10	1

FOOD	PORTION	CALS	CHOL	FIBER
Organic Free Range Chicken Broth	1 cup	10	0	–
Organic French Onion	1 cup	35	0	tr
Organic Low Sodium Chicken Broth	1 cup	10	0	–
Organic Mushroom Broth	1 cup	5	0	–
Organic Vegetarian Broth	1 cup	15	0	tr
Progresso				
50% Less Sodium Chicken Noodle	1 cup	90	20	1
50% Less Sodium Minestrone	1 cup	120	0	4
99% Fat Free Beef Barley	1 cup	130	10	4
99% Fat Free Chicken Rice w/ Vegetables	1 cup (8.4 oz)	110	10	1
99% Fat Free Lentil	1 cup (8.5 oz)	130	0	6
99% Fat Free Minestrone	1 cup (8.5 oz)	130	0	4
99% Fat Free Vegetable	1 cup (8.4 oz)	70	0	2
99% Fat Free White Cheddar Potato	1 cup (8.6 oz)	140	5	2
Bean & Ham	1 cup (8.4 oz)	160	10	8
Carb Monitor Chicken Vegetable	1 cup	70	15	1
Cheese & Herb Tortellini Tomato	1 cup (8.6 oz)	140	<5	2
Chicken Barley	1 cup (8.5 oz)	110	15	3
Chicken Broth	1 cup (8.2 oz)	20	0	0
Chicken Minestrone	1 cup (8.4 oz)	110	15	2
Chicken Rice w/ Vegetable	1 cup	100	10	1
Chicken Vegetable	1 cup (8.4 oz)	90	15	2
Clam & Rotini Chowder	1 cup (8.8 oz)	190	10	0
Escarole In Chicken Broth	1 cup (8.1 oz)	25	<5	1
Hearty Black Bean	1 cup (8.5 oz)	170	<5	10
Hearty Penne In Chicken Broth	1 cup (8.4 oz)	80	0	tr
Herb Rotini Vegetable	1 cup (9.1 oz)	120	0	4
Italian Herb Shells Minestrone	1 cup (9.1 oz)	120	0	4
Manhattan Clam Chowder	1 cup (8.4 oz)	110	10	3
Meatballs & Pasta Pearls	1 cup (8.3 oz)	140	15	0

FOOD	PORTION	CALS	CHOL	FIBER
Minestrone Parmesan	1 cup (8.3 oz)	100	0	3
New England Clam Chowder	1 cup (8.4 oz)	190	15	1
Oregano Penne Italian Style Vegetable	1 cup (8.7 oz)	90	0	1
Peppercorn Penne Vegetable	1 cup (9.1 oz)	100	0	2
Potato Broccoli & Cheese	1 cup (8.8 oz)	160	<5	1
Potato Ham & Cheese	1 cup (8.6 oz)	170	10	1
Rich & Hearty Beef Pot Roast	1 cup	130	20	2
Rich & Hearty Chicken & Homestyle Noodles	1 cup	110	25	1
Rich & Hearty Chicken Pot Pie	1 cup	170	15	2
Rich & Hearty Sirloin Steak & Vegetables	1 cup	130	20	2
Roasted Garlic Pasta Lentil	1 cup (9.3 oz)	120	0	5
Rotisserie Seasoned Chicken	1 cup (8.5 oz)	100	15	2
Spicy Chicken & Penne	1 cup (8.5 oz)	110	15	1
Tomato	1 cup (8.5 oz)	100	0	1
Tomato Basil	1 cup (8.8 oz)	100	0	1
Tomato Vegetable	1 cup (8.5 oz)	90	0	4
Tortellini In Chicken Broth	1 cup (8.3 oz)	70	10	2
Traditional Beef & Vegetable	1 cup	100	15	2
Traditional Beef Barley	1 cup	140	15	2
Traditional Chicken & Herb Dumplings	1 cup	110	30	1
Traditional Chicken & Wild Rice	1 cup	100	15	1
Traditional Chicken Noodle	1 cup	100	25	1
Traditional Hearty Chicken & Rotini	1 cup	100	15	1
Traditional Italian Style Wedding	1 cup	130	15	1
Traditional Split Pea w/ Ham	1 cup	140	5	4
Turkey Noodle	1 cup	90	20	1
Turkey Rice w/ Vegetables	1 cup (8.5 oz)	110	15	1
Vegetable Classics French Onion	1 cup	50	<5	1
Vegetable Classics Green Split Pea w/ Bacon	1 cup	170	<5	5

FOOD	PORTION	CALS	CHOL	FIBER
Vegetable Classics Hearty Tomato	1 cup	110	0	3
Vegetable Classics Lentil	1 cup	150	0	4
Vegetable Classics Macaroni & Bean	1 cup	160	<5	6
Vegetable Classics Minestrone	1 cup	110	0	4
Vegetable Classics Tomato Rotini	1 cup	140	0	2
Vegetable Classics Vegetable	1 cup	80	0	2
Rienzi				
Chicken & Rice	1 cup	110	5	2
Italian Wedding Bell	1 cup	130	15	tr
Snow's				
Clam Chowder	1 cup	200	15	1
Streit's				
Hearty Vegetarian Vegetable	1 cup	90	0	3
Mushroom Barley	1 cup	100	0	3
Swanson				
Beef Broth 100% Fat Free Lower Sodium	1 cup	15	<5	–
Beef Broth 99% Fat Free	1 cup	15	0	–
Beef Broth Onion Seasoned	1 cup (8.4 oz)	20	0	tr
Chicken Broth 100% Fat Free 33% Less Sodium	1 cup	15	0	–
Chicken Broth 99% Fat Free	1 cup	15	<5	–
Vegetable Broth	1 cup	19	1	0
Valley Fresh				
Chicken Broth	1 cup	30	<5	–
Chicken Broth 40% Less Sodium	1 cup	15	<5	–
Walnut Acres				
Organic Country Corn Chowder	1 cup (8.8 oz)	150	10	2
Wolfgang Puck				
Chicken Parmesan w/ Pasta	1 cup	300	0	1
Hearty Lentil & Vegetable	1 cup	170	<5	6

FOOD	PORTION	CALS	CHOL	FIBER
FROZEN				
Nature's Entree				
Chowder	1 pkg (12 oz)	230	15	5
Tortellini Minestone	1 pkg (12 oz)	360	10	5
Phillips Seafood				
Cream Of Crab	1 cup	310	130	–
Shrimp Bisque	1 cup	280	195	–
MIX				
beef broth cube	1 cube (3.6 g)	6	tr	–
chicken broth cube	1 cube (4.8 g)	9	1	–
A Taste Of Thai				
Coconut Ginger	2 tsp	15	0	0
Alpine Aire				
Low Carb Bay Shrimp Bisque	1 pkg	150	35	1
Low Carb Beefy Vegetable	1 pkg	100	30	1
Low Carb Broccoli Cheddar	1 pkg	140	35	2
Low Carb Mushroom & Chicken w/ Roasted Garlic	1 pkg	130	35	1
Annie Chun's				
Noodle Bowl Chicken Noodle	1 pkg	260	0	2
Noodle Bowl Hot & Sour	1 pkg	280	0	2
Noodle Bowl Korean Kimchi	½ pkg	140	0	1
Noodle Bowl Miso	1 pkg	230	0	2
Noodle Bowl Thai Tom Yum	½ pkg	150	0	1
Noodle Bowl Udon	1 pkg	220	0	1
Azumaya				
Asian Style Thin Noodle	1 cup	120	0	tr
Asian Style Wide Noodle	1 cup	120	0	tr
Bean Cuisine				
13 Bean Bouillabasse	1 cup	220	0	5
Island Black Bean	1 cup	210	0	7
Lots of Lentil	1 cup	230	0	5
Mesa Maize	1 cup	160	0	6
White Bean Provencal	1 cup	250	0	11
Fantastic				
Noodle Bowl Hot & Sour as prep	2 cups	138	0	1

FOOD	PORTION	CALS	CHOL	FIBER
Noodle Bowl Miso w/ Tofu as prep	1 cup	100	0	tr
Noodle Bowl Sesame Miso as prep	2 cups	90	0	tr
Noodle Bowl Spring Vegetable as prep	2 cups	90	0	tr
Noodle Soup Cup Spicy Thai as prep	2 cups	110	0	1
Noodle Soup Cup Vegetarian Chicken as prep	1 cup	90	0	1
Soup Cup Italian Tomato as prep	2 cups	130	0	2
Soup Cup Mandarin Broccoli as prep	2 cups	110	0	2
MiniCarb				
Miso w/ Tofu & Shitake	1 pkg	33	0	1
Szechuan Beef	1 pkg	24	0	0
Thai Coconut Cream	1 pkg	100	3	1
Miso-Cup				
Golden Vegetable as prep	1 cup	30	0	tr
Miso Reduced Sodium as prep	1 cup	25	0	tr
Organic Miso as prep	1 cup	35	0	tr
Savory Seaweed as prep	1 cup	30	0	tr
Nissin				
Chicken Vegetable as prep	1 pkg	290	<5	2
White Cheddar as prep	1 pkg	290	0	2
Nueva Cocina				
Frijoles Negros Con Chipotle Chile	1 cup	140	0	9
Sopa De Calabaza	1 cup	180	15	1
Sopa De Frijoles Colorados	1 cup	140	0	7
Sopa De Frijoles Negros	1 cup	140	0	9
Sopa De Maiz	1 cup	150	5	2
Sopa De Tortilla	1 cup	140	0	2
Ramen Noodle				
Beef as prep	1 pkg (2.2 oz)	280	tr	3
Beef Low Fat as prep	1 pkg (2.2 oz)	216	1	2
Chicken as prep	1 pkg (2.2 oz)	279	1	6
Chicken Low Fat as prep	1 pkg (2.2 oz)	216	tr	2

FOOD	PORTION	CALS	CHOL	FIBER
Oriental Low Fat as prep	1 pkg (2.2 oz)	217	0	2
Shrimp as prep	1 pkg (2.2 oz)	294	1	3
Shrimp Low Fat as prep	1 pkg (2.2 oz)	218	5	3
Tomato as prep	1 pkg (2.2 oz)	295	tr	2
Simply Asia				
Soy Noodle Bowl	1 pkg	70	0	3
Slim-Fast				
Creamy Broccoli	1 pkg	210	20	5
Creamy Chicken	1 pkg	220	20	5
Creamy Potato Cheddar & Chive	1 pkg	220	15	5
Thai Kitchen				
Instant Rice Noodle Bangkok Curry	1 pkg	192	0	0
Rice Noodle Bowl Roasted Garlic	1 bowl	170	0	0
Rice Noodle Bowl Spring Onion	1 bowl	170	0	0
Uncle Ben's				
Black Bean & Rice as prep	1 cup	150	0	7
Broccoli Cheese & Rice as prep	1 cup	110	5	1
SHELF-STABLE				
TastyBite				
Tom Yum	½ pkg (5.3 oz)	92	0	1
TAKE-OUT				
beef stew soup	1 cup (8.8 oz)	221	60	–
black bean turtle soup	1 cup	241	0	10
broccoli cheese	1 cup	165	14	2
brunswick stew soup	1 cup (8.5 oz)	232	71	–
caldo de res beef soup	1 cup	143	22	2
chinese velvet corn	1¼ cup	135	1	–
corn & cheese chowder	¾ cup	215	66	3
egg drop	1 cup	73	102	0
gazpacho	1 cup	46	0	–
greek lemon	¾ cup	63	83	2
hot & sour	1 serv (14 oz)	173	87	1
matzo ball soup	1 cup	118	63	1
minestrone	1 cup	233	9	4
miso w/ tofu	1 cup	84	0	2

FOOD	PORTION	CALS	CHOL	FIBER
onion soup gratinee	1 serv	492	77	4
oxtail	1 cup	68	2	1
pasta e fagioll	1 cup (8.8 oz)	194	3	–
ratatouille	1 cup (7.5 oz)	266	0	–
shrimp bisque	1 cup	263	129	tr
sopa de albondigas	1 cup	171	50	1
sopa de feijao portuguese bean & sausage	1 cup	220	10	6
thai lemon grass	1 bowl	100	65	–
vietnamese pho beef noodle	1 serv (7.8 oz)	480	46	1
wonton soup	1 cup	183	53	1
zupa koprowa polish dill soup	1 bowl	54	55	–

SOUR CREAM

FOOD	PORTION	CALS	CHOL	FIBER
sour cream	1 tbsp (0.4 oz)	26	5	–
sour cream	1 cup (8 oz)	493	102	–
Breakstone's				
Sour Cream	2 tbsp (1 oz)	60	20	0
Cabot				
Light	2 tbsp	35	10	0
No Fat	2 tbsp	20	0	0
Sour Cream	2 tbsp	50	15	0
Crowley				
Sour Cream	2 tbsp	60	20	0
Daisy				
No Fat	2 tbsp	20	0	0
Sour Cream	2 tbsp	60	0	0
Hood				
Fat Free	2 tbsp	20	0	0
Low Fat	2 tbsp	35	5	0
Sour Cream	2 tbsp	60	20	0
Horizon Organic				
Lowfat	2 tbsp	35	10	0
Sour Cream	2 tbsp	60	20	0
Land O Lakes				
Fat Free	2 tbsp (1.1 oz)	25	<5	0
Light	2 tbsp (1 oz)	40	10	0
Sour Cream	2 tbsp (1 oz)	60	15	0

FOOD	PORTION	CALS	CHOL	FIBER
SOUR CREAM SUBSTITUTES				
nondairy	1 cup	479	0	–
SOURSOP				
fresh	1	416	0	–
fresh cut up	1 cup	150	0	–
SOY (*see also* CHEESE SUBSTITUTES, ICE CREAM AND FROZEN DESSERTS, MILK SUBSTITUTES, MISO, SMOOTHIES, SOY SAUCE, SOYBEANS, TEMPEH, TOFU, YOGURT FROZEN)				
lecithin	1 tbsp	104	0	0
soy milk	1 cup	79	0	–
Fearn				
Granules	¼ cup	110	0	8
Powder	¼ cup	100	0	4
GeniSoy				
Soy Nuts Deep Sea Salted	1 oz	120	0	5
Soy Nuts Old Hickory Smoked	1 oz	120	0	5
Soy Nuts Praline	55 pieces (1 oz)	120	0	2
Soy Nuts Unsalted	1 oz	120	0	5
Soy Nuts Zesty Barbeque	1 oz	120	0	5
Good Sense				
Soynuts Honey Roasted	⅓ cup	140	0	4
Soynuts Roasted & Salted	⅓ cup	140	0	5
Soynuts Roasted w/o Salt	⅓ cup	140	0	5
Health Trip				
Soynut Butter Honey Sweet	2 tbsp	170	0	1
Soynut Butter Original	2 tbsp	180	0	1
Soynut Butter Unsalted	2 tbsp	180	0	1
I.M. Healthy				
SoyNut Butter Chocolate	2 tbsp (1.1 oz)	190	0	4
SoyNut Butter Honey Creamy	2 tbsp (1.1 oz)	170	0	2
SoyNut Butter Original Creamy	2 tbsp (1.1 oz)	170	0	1
SoyNut Butter Unsweetened Chunky	2 tbsp (1.1 oz)	160	0	5
SoyNut Butter Unsweetened Creamy	2 tbsp (1.1 oz)	160	0	5

FOOD	PORTION	CALS	CHOL	FIBER
Revival				
Shake Chocolate Daydream Fructose	1 pkg	240	0	2
Shake Strawberry Smile Fructose	1 pkg	225	0	0
Shake Strawberry Smile Splenda	1 pkg	130	0	0
Shake Strawberry Smile Unsweetened	1 pkg	130	0	0
Soy Shake Plain	1 pkg	110	0	0
Soy Shake Vanilla Pleasure	1 pkg	220	0	0
Soy Shake Vanilla Pleasure Splenda	1 pkg	120	0	0
Soy Shake Vanilla Pleasure Unsweetened	1 pkg	120	0	0
Soynuts Chocolate Covered	⅙ cup	70	2	tr
Soynuts Hot Jalapeno & Cheddar	⅙ cup	78	0	2
Soynuts Unsalted	⅙ cup	78	0	2
Soynuts Yogurt Covered	⅙ cup	720	0	tr
Soy Juicy				
All Flavors	8 oz	160	0	1
Soy Wonder				
Creamy	2 tbsp	170	0	1
Crunchy	2 tbsp	170	0	1

SOY DRINKS (*see* MILK SUBSTITUTES, SMOOTHIES)

SOY SAUCE

FOOD	PORTION	CALS	CHOL	FIBER
shoyu	1 tbsp	9	0	–
soy sauce	1 tbsp	7	0	–
tamari	1 tbsp	11	0	–
Chun King				
Lite	1 tbsp (0.5 oz)	15	0	0
Soy Sauce	1 tbsp (0.6 oz)	11	0	0
Eden				
Organic Shoyu	1 tbsp	15	0	0
Organic Tamari	1 tbsp	15	0	0
House Of Tsang				
Ginger Soy Sauce	1 tbsp	20	0	0
Less Sodium	1 tbsp	5	0	0

FOOD	PORTION	CALS	CHOL	FIBER
Just Rite				
Soy Sauce	1 tbsp (0.5 oz)	11	0	0
Kikkoman				
Lite	1 tbsp (0.5 oz)	10	0	–
Soy Sauce	1 tbsp (0.5 oz)	10	0	0
La Choy				
Lite	1 tbsp (0.5 oz)	15	0	0
Soy Sauce	1 tbsp (0.6 oz)	11	0	0
San-J				
Shoyu Organic	1 tbsp	15	0	–
Tamari	1 tbsp	15	0	–
Tamari Reduced Sodium	1 tbsp	20	0	–
Tamari Organic Wheat Free	1 tbsp	15	0	–
Tamari Organic Wheat Free Reduced Sodium	1 tbsp	20	0	–
Tree Of Life				
Shoyu	1 tbsp (0.5 oz)	15	0	–
Tamari Wheat Free	1 tbsp (0.5 oz)	15	0	–
SOYBEANS				
dried cooked	1 cup	298	0	–
dry roasted	½ cup	387	0	–
green cooked	½ cup	127	0	4
roasted	½ cup	405	0	–
roasted & toasted	1 cup	490	0	–
roasted & toasted salted	1 cup	490	0	–
sprouts raw	½ cup	43	0	–
sprouts steamed	½ cup	38	0	–
sprouts stir fried	1 cup	125	0	–
Arrowhead				
Organic not prep	¼ cup	180	0	10
C&W				
In the Pod	½ cup	110	0	9
Eden				
Organic Blacksoy	½ cup	120	0	7
Frieda's				
Edamame	½ cup (2.6 oz)	100	0	3
Seapoint Farms				
Edamame Organic	½ cup (2.6 oz)	100	0	4
Edamame In Pods frzn	½ cup (2.6 oz)	100	0	4

FOOD	PORTION	CALS	CHOL	FIBER
Edamame Rice Bowl Kung Pao Vegetable	1 pkg (12 oz)	420	0	6
Edamame Rice Bowl Szechwan Vegetables	1 pkg (12 oz)	420	0	6
Edamame Rice Bowl Teriyaki Vegetable	1 pkg (12 oz)	430	0	5
Edamame Rice Bowl Vegetable Fried Rice	1 pkg (11 oz)	220	40	1
Edamame Shelled	½ cup (2.6 oz)	100	0	4

SPAGHETTI (see PASTA, PASTA DINNERS, PASTA SALAD, SPAGHETTI SAUCE)

SPAGHETTI SAUCE
JARRED
Amy's

FOOD	PORTION	CALS	CHOL	FIBER
Family Marinara	½ cup	50	0	3
Garlic Mushroom	½ cup	120	5	3
Puttanesca	½ cup	40	0	1
Tomato Basil	½ cup	80	0	3
Wild Mushroom	½ cup	60	0	2
Barilla				
Arrabbiata Tomato & Spicy Pepper	½ cup	90	0	3
Basilico Tomato & Basil	½ cup	70	0	3
Boscaiola Mushrooms & Garlic	½ cup	90	0	3
Campagnola Roasted Garlic & Onion	½ cup	60	0	3
Restaurant Creations Cheese & Tomatoes	¼ cup	110	3	1
Restaurant Creations Garlic Herbs & Tomatoes	¼ cup	100	3	2
Restaurant Creations Pesto & Tomatoes	¼ cup	150	3	2
Rustica Sweet Peppers & Garlic	½ cup	70	0	3
Catelli				
Garden Select Country Mushroom	½ cup	80	0	3
Garden Select Diced Diced Tomatoes & Basil	½ cup	80	0	3

FOOD	PORTION	CALS	CHOL	FIBER
Garden Select Fine Herbs	½ cup	80	0	3
Garden Select Garlic & Onion	½ cup	80	0	3
Garden Select Parmesan & Romano	½ cup	80	0	4
Garden Select Zucchini Primavera	½ cup	80	0	4
Classico				
Italian Sausage	½ cup	90	5	2
Tomato & Basil	½ cup	60	0	2
Colavita				
Garden Style	½ cup (4.4 oz)	60	0	3
Del Monte				
Chunky Garlic & Herb	½ cup	60	0	tr
Chunky Italian Herb	½ cup	60	0	1
Garlic & Onion	½ cup	80	0	2
Tomato & Basil	½ cup	70	0	3
W/ Four Cheese	½ cup	70	0	3
With Green Peppers & Mushrooms	½ cup	80	0	3
With Meat	½ cup	60	2	3
With Mushrooms	½ cup	60	0	2
Eden				
Organic	½ cup	80	0	3
Organic No Salt	½ cup	80	0	3
Organic Pizza Pasta Sauce	½ cup	65	0	5
Emeril's				
Homestyle Marinara	½ cup	90	0	3
Sicilian Gravy	½ cup	90	0	1
Vodka	½ cup	130	10	2
Francesco Rinaldi				
Alfredo	¼ cup (2.1 oz)	70	15	0
Chunky Garden Mushroom & Onion	½ cup (4.4 oz)	80	0	3
Chunky Garden Mushroom & Peppers	½ cup (4.4 oz)	80	0	3
Chunky Garden Tomato Garlic & Onion	½ cup	70	0	tr
Dolce Super Mushroom	½ cup (4.4 oz)	110	0	3
Dolce Sweet & Tasty Tomato	½ cup (4.4 oz)	110	0	3

FOOD	PORTION	CALS	CHOL	FIBER
Hearty Diavolo	½ cup (4.4 oz)	70	0	3
Hearty Mushroom Pepper & Onion	½ cup (4.4 oz)	80	0	3
Hearty Tomato & Basil	½ cup (4.4 oz)	80	0	4
Puttanesca	½ cup (4.3 oz)	70	0	tr
Three Cheese	½ cup	80	0	tr
Tomato Alfredo	¼ cup (2.1 oz)	60	10	0
Traditional Meat Flavored	½ cup (4.4 oz)	90	4	3
Traditional Mushroom	½ cup (4.4 oz)	90	0	3
Traditional No Salt Added	½ cup (4.4 oz)	70	0	tr
Traditional Original	½ cup (4.4 oz)	90	0	3
Traditional Original	½ cup (4.4 oz)	90	0	3
Vodka Sauce	¼ cup (2.1 oz)	60	10	0
Healthy Choice				
Chunky Italian Vegetable	½ cup (4.4 oz)	40	0	2
Chunky Mushroom	½ cup (4.4 oz)	42	0	2
Garlic & Herbs	½ cup (4.4 oz)	49	0	2
Garlic Lovers Garlic & Mushroom	½ cup (4.4 oz)	44	0	2
Garlic Lovers Roasted Garlic	½ cup (4.4 oz)	52	0	3
Garlic Lovers Roasted Garlic & Sun Dried Tomato	½ cup (4.4 oz)	52	0	3
Super Chunky Mushroom & Sweet Peppers	½ cup (4.4 oz)	43	0	2
Super Chunky Tomato Mushroom & Garlic	½ cup (4.4 oz)	45	0	2
Super Chunky Vegetable Primavera	½ cup (4.4 oz)	43	0	2
Traditional	½ cup (4.4 oz)	48	0	2
With Mushrooms	½ cup (4.4 oz)	48	0	2
Hunt's				
Basil Garlic & Oregano	¼ cup	15	0	tr
Cheese & Garlic	½ cup	50	0	2
Chunky Vegetable	½ cup	50	0	3
Diced In Tomato Sauce	½ cup	30	0	1
Family Favorites Lasagna	¼ cup	30	0	1
Four Cheese	½ cup	50	0	3
Italian Sausage	½ cup	60	0	3
Light	½ cup	45	0	3

FOOD	PORTION	CALS	CHOL	FIBER
Meat	½ cup	68	0	3
No Added Sugar	½ cup	45	0	3
Roasted Garlic & Onion	½ cup	50	0	3
Traditional	½ cup	50	0	2
With Mushrooms	½ cup	45	0	3
Joey Pots & Pans				
Arrabbiata	½ cup	100	0	1
Marinara	½ cup	50	0	1
Vodka Sauce	½ cup	110	30	1
Muir Glen				
Organic Balsamic Roasted Onion	½ cup (4.4 oz)	50	0	0
Organic Cabernet Marinara	½ cup (4.4 oz)	50	0	0
Organic Chunky Herb	½ cup (4.4 oz)	50	0	0
Organic Garden Vegetable	½ cup (4.4 oz)	50	0	0
Organic Garlic & Onion	½ cup (4.4 oz)	55	0	0
Organic Garlic Roasted Garlic	½ cup (4.4 oz)	50	0	0
Organic Green Olive	½ cup (4.4 oz)	60	0	0
Organic Italian Herb	½ cup (4.4 oz)	55	0	0
Organic Mushroom Marinara	½ cup (4.4 oz)	45	0	0
Organic Portabello Mushroom	½ cup (4.4 oz)	50	0	0
Organic Sun Dried Tomato	½ cup (4.4 oz)	55	0	1
Organic Tomato Basil	½ cup (4.4 oz)	50	0	0
Newman's Own				
Bambolina	½ cup	90	0	tr
Cabernet Marinara	½ cup	70	0	2
Five Cheese	½ cup	80	5	tr
Italian Sausage & Peppers	½ cup	90	10	tr
Marinara	½ cup	70	0	tr
Marinara w/ Mushrooms	½ cup	70	0	tr
Pesto & Tomato Sauce	½ cup	80	0	tr
Roasted Garlic & Green Peppers	½ cup	70	0	4
Sockarooni	½ cup	70	0	tr
Tomato & Roasted Garlic	½ cup	70	0	tr
Vodka Sauce	½ cup	110	5	0

FOOD	PORTION	CALS	CHOL	FIBER
Pomi				
Marinara	½ cup	80	0	3
Prego				
Pasta Bake Sauce Tomato Garlic & Basil	1 serv (3.4 oz)	80	0	2
Traditional	½ cup (4.2 oz)	140	0	2
Progresso				
Marinara	½ cup (4.3 oz)	80	<5	2
Meat Flavored	½ cup (4.4 oz)	100	5	3
Sauce	½ cup (4.4 oz)	100	<5	2
Ragu				
Chunky Garden Style Tomato Garlic & Onion	½ cup (4.5 oz)	110	0	2
Seeds Of Change				
Balsamic Olive & Onion	½ cup	80	0	2
Garden Vegetable	½ cup	70	0	2
Mushroom & Onion	½ cup	70	0	2
Three Cheese Marinara	½ cup	70	5	2
Traditional Herb	½ cup	70	0	2
Tree Of Life				
Pasta Sauce	½ cup (4 oz)	50	0	–
Pasta Sauce Fat Free Classic	½ cup (3.9 oz)	40	0	0
Pasta Sauce Fat Free Mushroom & Basil	½ cup (3.9 oz)	30	0	0
Pasta Sauce Fat Free Onion & Garlic	½ cup (3.9 oz)	30	0	0
Pasta Sauce Fat Free Sweet Pepper	½ cup (3.9 oz)	30	0	0
Pasta Sauce No Salt Added	½ cup (3.9 oz)	50	0	–
Tuttorosso				
Pasta Sauce Meat	½ cup	90	0	3
Walden Farms				
Alfredo Sauce Calorie Free	¼ cup	0	0	0
Marinara Calorie Free	⅓ cup	0	0	0
MIX				
McCormick				
Alfredo Pasta Blend as prep	½ cup	60	10	0
Pasta Rosa Blend	1 tbsp (10 g)	40	<5	0

FOOD	PORTION	CALS	CHOL	FIBER
REFRIGERATED				
Buitoni				
Alfredo	¼ cup	140	35	0
Alfredo Portabello Mushroom	¼ cup	100	20	0
Alfredo Light	¼ cup	80	20	0
Marinara	½ cup	80	0	2
Marinara Roasted Garlic	½ cup	60	0	1
Pesto	¼ cup	330	20	6
Pesto w/ Basil	¼ cup	300	20	2
Pesto w/ Basil Reduced Fat	¼ cup	230	15	2
Pesto w/ Sun Dried Tomatoes	¼ cup	210	5	2
Tomato Herb Parmesan	½ cup	120	10	2
SPANISH FOOD				
CANNED				
Derby				
Tamales	3 (6.5 oz)	253	23	4
Gebhardt				
Enchiladas	2 (5.7 oz)	258	25	3
Tamales	2 (5.7 oz)	268	28	3
Tamales Jumbo	2 (6.9 oz)	332	34	3
Rosarita				
Enchilada Sauce Mild	¼ cup (2.1 oz)	23	0	0
Van Camp's				
Tamales	2 (5 oz)	210	20	3
FROZEN				
Amy's				
Black Bean Vegetable Enchilada	1 (4.75 oz)	130	0	2
Bowls Santa Fe Enchilada	1 pkg (10 oz)	340	5	10
Burrito Bean & Cheese	1 (6 oz)	280	10	6
Burrito Bean & Rice Non-Dairy	1 (6 oz)	270	0	5
Burrito Black Bean Vegetable	1 (6 oz)	320	0	4
Burrito Breakfast	1 (6 oz)	210	0	5
Cheese Enchilada	1 (4.75 oz)	210	35	2
Mexican Tamale Pie	1 (8 oz)	150	0	4
Banquet				
Chimichanga Meal	1 meal (9.5 oz)	500	20	9

FOOD	PORTION	CALS	CHOL	FIBER
Enchilada Beef	1 pkg (11 oz)	370	20	6
Enchilada Beef & Tamale Combo	1 pkg (11 oz)	450	30	9
Enchilada Cheese	1 pkg (11 oz)	360	20	6
Enchilada Chicken	1 pkg (11 oz)	350	25	9
Mexican Style Enchilada Combo	1 meal (11 oz)	360	20	9
Cedarlane				
Burrito Beans Rice & Cheese	1 (6 oz)	260	0	7
Contessa				
Fajitas Shrimp	2 (8 oz)	230	45	5
Paella w/ Chicken & Seafood	1½ cups	200	50	2
Seafood Veracruz not prep	1¾ cups	180	35	6
El Monterey				
Quesadillas Chicken Breast & Cheese	1 (5 oz)	280	60	tr
Health Is Wealth				
Burrito Munchees	10 (5 oz)	310	5	6
Mexican Munchees	2 (1 oz)	49	0	1
Healthy Choice				
Chicken Enchiladas	1 pkg	360	30	8
Enchilada Chicken	1 pkg	300	40	6
Jose Ole				
Burrito Beef & Cheese	1 (5 oz)	300	25	2
Burrito Chicken Monterey	1 (5 oz)	270	15	2
Chimichanga Chicken & Cheese	1 (5 oz)	330	20	2
Chimichanga Shredded Beef	1 (5 oz)	350	25	2
Mini Burrito Chicken & Cheese	3	200	10	1
Mini Chimichanga Beef & Cheddar	3	240	10	1
Mini Quesadilla Grilled Chicken	3	220	20	1
Mini Tacos Beef & Cheese	4	200	20	3
Mini Taquitos Beef & Cheese	4	180	5	2
Soft Taco Beef & Cheese	1 (5 oz)	280	25	1
Taquitos Beef & Cheese Flour Tortilla	2	220	10	1
Taquitos Buffalo Chicken Flour Tortilla	2	200	15	tr

FOOD	PORTION	CALS	CHOL	FIBER
Taquitos Chicken Flour Tortilla	3	180	10	2
Taquitos Chicken & Cheese Flour Tortilla	2	220	15	1
Taquitos Pepperoni Pizza Flour Tortilla	2	240	15	1
Taquitos Shredded Beef Corn Tortilla	3	180	<5	2
Lean Cuisine				
One Dish Favorites Chicken Enchilada	1 pkg (9 oz)	280	20	3
Patio				
Beef & Cheese Enchiladas Chili 'N Beans	1 meal (15.5 oz)	670	60	12
Beef Enchiladas Chili 'N Beans	1 meal (15.5 oz)	540	50	12
Burrito Bean & Cheese	1 (5 oz)	280	5	5
Burrito Beef & Bean Hot	1 (5 oz)	320	25	4
Burrito Beef & Bean Medium	1 (5 oz)	300	<5	5
Burrito Beef & Bean Red Chili Pepper Red Hot	1 (5 oz)	320	20	4
Burrito Chicken	1 (5 oz)	280	15	2
Enchilada Beef	1 meal (12 oz)	320	25	9
Enchilada Cheese	1 meal (12 oz)	370	25	7
Enchilada Chicken	1 meal (12 oz)	400	35	8
Fiesta	1 meal (12 oz)	350	25	7
Mexican Style	1 meal (13.25 oz)	470	20	10
READY-TO-EAT				
taco shell corn	1 (6.5 inch)	98	0	2
taco shell flour	1 (7 inch)	173	0	1
Gebhardt				
Taco Shells	3 (1.1 oz)	155	0	3
La Mexicana				
Flour Burritos	1 (1.6 oz)	160	0	2
Ortega				
Tostada Shells	2 (1 oz)	140	0	1
Rosarita				
Taco Shells	3 (1.1 oz)	155	0	3
Tostada Shells	2 (1 oz)	125	37	0

FOOD	PORTION	CALS	CHOL	FIBER
SHELF-STABLE				
Fantastic				
Spanish Paella	1 pkg (8 oz)	280	0	4
TAKE-OUT				
burrito w/ beans	1 med (5 oz)	295	6	7
burrito w/ beans & rice	1 (3.5 oz)	221	2	4
burrito w/ beef	1 sm (3.4 oz)	297	49	1
burrito w/ beef & beans	1 med (5 oz)	331	34	6
burrito w/ beef beans & cheese	1 med (5 oz)	379	57	5
burrito w/ chicken & beans	1 med (5 oz)	295	37	5
burrito w/ pork & beans	1 med (5 oz)	320	34	6
chiles rellenos meat & cheese filled	1 (5 oz)	213	109	2
chimichanga w/ bean cheese lettuce & tomato	1 (4.1 oz)	271	17	3
chimichanga w/ beef & rice	1 (10 oz)	634	35	5
chimichanga w/ beef beans lettuce & tomato	1 (4.1 oz)	254	15	3
chimichanga w/ beef cheese lettuce & tomato	1 (4.1 oz)	337	37	1
chimichanga w/ chicken sour cream lettuce & tomato	1 (4 oz)	277	30	1
enchilada w/ beans	1 (4.1 oz)	179	4	6
enchilada w/ beans & cheese	1 (4.6 oz)	233	21	5
enchilada w/ beef	1 (4 oz)	214	30	3
enchilada w/ beef & beans	1 (4 oz)	195	15	4
frijoles	1 cup	278	0	9
frijoles w/ cheese	1 cup	225	37	–
nachos w/ beans & cheese	1 serv (9.4 oz)	616	56	13
nachos w/ beef beans cheese & sour cream	1 serv (19 oz)	1620	171	19
pupusa meat filled	1 (3.6 oz)	187	20	3
quesadilla w/ cheese	1 (5 oz)	498	60	3
quesadilla w/ meat & cheese	1 (6.5 oz)	605	98	2
taco de jueye w/ crab meat	1 (4.2 oz)	266	79	2
taco w/ beans lettuce tomato & salsa	1 (2.8 oz)	117	2	4
taco w/ chicken lettuce tomato & salsa	1 (2.5 oz)	114	22	1

FOOD	PORTION	CALS	CHOL	FIBER
taco w/ fish lettuce tomato & salsa	1 (2.7 oz)	101	39	1
tostada w/ beef lettuce tomato & salsa	1 (2.7 oz)	143	21	2

SPICES (see individual names, HERBS/SPICES)

SPINACH
CANNED
drained	1 cup	49	0	5
Del Monte				
Whole Leaf	½ cup	30	0	2
Popeye				
Spinach	½ cup	45	0	3
FRESH				
baby raw	2 cups	20	0	3
cooked	1 cup	41	0	4
malabar cooked	1 cup	10	0	1
mustard cooked	1 cup	29	0	4
new zealand cooked	1 cup	22	0	–
raw	1 cup	7	0	1
Fresh Express				
Baby Spinach	3 cups	20	0	2
Spicy Spinach	3 cups (3 oz)	10	0	6
Ready Pac				
Baby	2 cups	20	0	3
Microwave Spinach as prep	½ cup	20	0	tr
FROZEN				
chopped cooked	1 cup	30	0	4
Amy's Organic				
Snacks Spinach Feta	5-6 pieces	170	15	2
C&W				
Baby Chopped	1 cup	30	0	1
Creamed	½ cup	100	20	4
Green Giant				
Creamed Low Fat Sauce	½ cup	80	0	1
No Sauce	½ cup	25	0	1
Health Is Wealth				
Spinach Munchees	2 (1 oz)	60	0	1
Spinach Feta Munchees	2 (1 oz)	70	5	1

FOOD	PORTION	CALS	CHOL	FIBER
Taverna				
Spinach Pie	1 piece (4.8 oz)	190	55	5
Tree Of Life				
Organic	1 cup (3 oz)	20	0	2
SHELF-STABLE				
TastyBite				
Kashmir Spinach	½ pkg (5 oz)	170	35	3
TAKE-OUT				
indian saag	1 serv	28	0	1
spanakopita spinach pie	1 serv (3 oz)	148	60	1

SPINACH JUICE

FOOD	PORTION	CALS	CHOL	FIBER
juice	7 oz	14	0	–

SPORTS DRINKS (see ENERGY DRINKS)

SPROUTS

FOOD	PORTION	CALS	CHOL	FIBER
kidney bean	½ cup	27	0	–
lentil sprouts	½ cup	40	0	–
mung bean	½ cup	16	0	–
mung bean cooked	½ cup	13	0	–
pea	½ cup	77	0	–
radish	½ cup	8	0	–
Brassica				
Broccoli Sprouts	½ cup (1 oz)	16	0	1
Chun King				
Bean Sprouts	1 cup (3 oz)	11	0	1
Fresh Alternatives				
Salad Blend	½ cup (1 oz)	10	0	tr
Sandwich Blend	½ cup (1 oz)	5	0	tr
La Choy				
Bean Sprouts	1 cup (2.9 oz)	11	0	1
TAKE-OUT				
mung bean stir fried	½ cup	31	0	–

SQUAB

FOOD	PORTION	CALS	CHOL	FIBER
boneless baked	1 (4 oz)	242	129	0

SQUASH (see also SQUASH SEEDS, ZUCCHINI)

FOOD	PORTION	CALS	CHOL	FIBER
CANNED				
crookneck sliced	½ cup	14	0	–
Farmer's Market				
Organic Butternut	½ cup	50	0	2

FOOD	PORTION	CALS	CHOL	FIBER
FRESH				
acorn cooked mashed	½ cup	41	0	3
acorn cubed baked	½ cup	57	0	2
butternut baked	½ cup	41	0	2
crookneck sliced cooked	½ cup	18	0	1
hubbard baked	½ cup	51	0	3
hubbard cooked mashed	½ cup	35	0	3
scallop sliced cooked	½ cup	14	0	1
spaghetti cooked	½ cup	23	0	2
Frieda's				
Acorn	¾ cup (3 oz)	35	0	2
Baby Crookneck	⅔ cup (3 oz)	15	0	1
Baby Scallop	⅔ cup (3 oz)	15	0	1
Eight Ball	2 (4.4 oz)	18	0	1
Hubbard	¾ cup (3 oz)	35	0	2
Mini Pumpkin	¾ cup (3 oz)	20	0	2
Spaghetti	¾ cup (3 oz)	30	0	1
Star Spangled	⅔ cup (3 oz)	20	0	1
Turban	¾ cup (3 oz)	30	0	1
Glory				
Yellow Sliced	¾ cup	20	0	1
Martin Farms				
Butternut Fresh Cut	½ cup	40	0	1
FROZEN				
butternut cooked mashed	½ cup	47	0	3
crookneck sliced cooked	½ cup	24	0	–
C&W				
Butternut	½ cup	45	0	1
TAKE-OUT				
fritter	1 (0.8 oz)	81	15	1
SQUASH SEEDS				
roasted	1 oz	148	0	–
salted & roasted	1 oz	148	0	–
seeds dried	1 oz	154	0	–
seeds whole roasted	1 oz	127	0	–
SQUID				
baked	1 cup	192	393	0
canned in its own ink	1 can (4 oz)	122	308	0
dried	1 sm (1.5 oz)	147	371	0

FOOD	PORTION	CALS	CHOL	FIBER
pickled	1 oz	26	63	0
steamed	1 cup	147	374	0
Contessa				
Calamari + Sauce	13 pieces + 2 tbsp sauce	160	55	1
Margaritaville				
Captain's Calamari Strips + Sauce	⅓ pkg	330	85	0
TAKE-OUT				
arroz con calamares	1 cup	400	150	1
calamari breaded & fried	1 cup	296	378	1

SQUIRREL
FOOD	PORTION	CALS	CHOL	FIBER
roasted	3 oz	147	103	–

STARFRUIT
FOOD	PORTION	CALS	CHOL	FIBER
fresh	1	42	0	–
Frieda's				
Dried	⅓ cup (1.4 oz)	120	0	1

STRAWBERRIES
FOOD	PORTION	CALS	CHOL	FIBER
CANNED				
in heavy syrup	½ cup	117	0	–
DRIED				
Frieda's				
Dried	½ cup (1.4 oz)	150	0	3
FRESH				
strawberries	1 cup	45	0	4
strawberries	1 pint	97	0	–
FROZEN				
sweetened sliced	1 cup	245	0	–
sweetened sliced	1 pkg (10 oz)	273	0	–
unsweetened	1 cup	52	0	–
whole sweetened	1 pkg (10 oz)	223	0	–
whole sweetened	1 cup	200	0	–
C&W				
Ultimate Sliced	⅔ cup	50	0	1
Europe's Best				
Sliced	¾ cup	40	0	3
Tree Of Life				
Organic	¾ cup (5 oz)	50	0	2

FOOD	PORTION	CALS	CHOL	FIBER
STRAWBERRY JUICE				
Adina				
California Kiss Hibiscus Strawberry	8 oz	80	0	–
Ceres				
Strawberry	8 oz	115	0	1
Giant Berry Farms				
Just Strawberries	1 bottle (12 oz)	140	0	2
Hi-C				
Blast	8 oz	120	0	–
Squeezit				
Strawberry	1 bottle (7 oz)	110	0	0
STUFFING/DRESSING				
Kellogg's				
Stuffing Mix as prep	1 cup	240	0	1
Pepperidge Farm				
Herb Seasoned	¾ cup (1.5 oz)	170	0	3
One Step Chicken	½ cup (1.2 oz)	140	<5	tr
One Step Southwestern Corn Bread	½ cup (1.2 oz)	150	0	tr
One Step Turkey	½ cup (1.2 oz)	150	<5	tr
Tofurky				
Wild Rice & Mushroom	½ cup	110	0	1
TAKE-OUT				
bread	1 cup	352	0	2
cornbread	½ cup	179	0	3
oyster	1 cup	304	23	2
sausage	½ cup	292	12	1
STURGEON				
broiled	3 oz	115	65	0
smoked	1 oz	49	23	0
TAKE-OUT				
breaded & fried	4 oz	252	85	1
SUCKER				
white baked	3 oz	101	45	0
SUGAR				
brown packed	1 cup (7.7 oz)	828	0	–
brown unpacked	1 cup (5.1 oz)	547	0	0

FOOD	PORTION	CALS	CHOL	FIBER
brown organic	1 tsp	17	0	0
cinnamon sugar	1 tsp	16	0	tr
maple	1 piece (1 oz)	99	0	0
powdered	1 tbsp (0.3 oz)	31	0	–
powdered unsifted	1 cup (4.2 oz)	467	0	–
raw	1 pkg (5 g)	19	0	0
sugarcane stem	3 oz	54	0	3
white	1 tsp (4 g)	15	0	–
white	1 cup (7 oz)	773	0	–
white	1 packet (3 g)	12	0	0
Billington's				
Muscovado Light Brown	1 tsp	15	0	–
Domino				
Dark Brown	1 tsp	15	0	–
Light Brown	1 tsp	15	0	–
Organic Cane Sugar	1 tsp	15	0	–
White	1 tsp	15	0	–
Gluco Burst				
Artic Cherry	1 pkg (1.3 oz)	70	0	–
Maui Brand				
Raw Sugar	1 tsp	15	0	–
Princess Of Yum				
Citrus Lemon	2.5 tsp	40	0	–
French Vanilla	2.5 tsp	40	0	–

SUGAR SUBSTITUTES
Equal

Flavor Sticks	1 pkg	0	0	–
Packet	1 pkg	0	0	–
Spoonful	1 tsp	0	0	–
Sugar Lite	1 tsp	8	0	0
Fran Gare's				
Miracle Sweet	1 tsp	10	0	0
Keto				
Sweet	½ tsp	0	0	0
Lo Han				
Sweet	2 scoops	2	0	tr
SomerSweet				
Sweetener	¼ tsp	0	0	tr

FOOD	PORTION	CALS	CHOL	FIBER
Splenda				
Flavor Blends All Flavors	1 pkg	0	0	0
No Calorie Granules	1 tsp	0	0	0
Sugar Blend For Baking	½ tsp	10	0	–
Sweetener	1 pkg	0	0	0
Steel's				
Brown	1 tsp	10	0	0
Sugar Substitute	1 tsp	10	0	0
Stevita				
Spoonable	⅓ tsp	0	0	0
Sugar Twin				
Packets	1	0	0	–
Spoonable Brown	1 tsp	0	0	0
Spoonable White	1 tsp	0	0	0
Sweet Simplicity				
Sweetener	1 pkg	0	0	–
SweetLeaf				
SteviaPlus	1 pkg	0	0	1
Whey Low				
Gold	1 tsp	4	0	0
Granular	1 tsp	4	0	0
Powder	1 tsp	4	0	0
SUGAR-APPLE				
fresh	1	146	0	–
fresh cut up	1 cup	236	0	–
SUNCHOKE				
fresh raw sliced	½ cup	57	0	–
Frieda's				
Sunchock	½ cup (3 oz)	70	0	1
SUNFISH				
pumpkinseed baked	3 oz	97	73	0
SUNFLOWER				
seeds dry roasted w/ salt	¼ cup	185	0	–
seeds dry roasted w/o salt	¼ cup	186	0	3
seeds w/ hulls dried	¼ cup	66	0	1
David				
Kernals Original	¼ cup	200	0	2

FOOD	PORTION	CALS	CHOL	FIBER
Seeds BBQ	¼ cup	190	0	2
Seeds BBQ Sizzlin	¼ cup	190	0	2
Seeds Jalapeno	¼ cup	190	0	2
Seeds Nacho Cheese	¼ cup	180	0	2
Seeds Original	¼ cup	190	0	2
Seeds Ranch	¼ cup	190	0	2
Seeds Reduced Sodium	¼ cup	190	0	2
Frito Lay				
Seeds	3 tbsp	180	0	2
Good Sense				
Nuts Honey Roasted	¼ cup	190	0	2
Nuts Raw	¼ cup	170	0	4
Nuts Roasted & Salted	¼ cup	190	0	2
Seeds In Shell Roasted & Salted	½ cup	150	0	13
Sunflower Nuts Roasted w/o Salt	¼ cup	190	0	2
Maranatha				
Tamari Seeds	¼ cup	160	0	2
SunButter				
Creamy	2 tbsp	200	0	4
Organic	2 tbsp	220	0	2
SunGold				
Seeds Roasted Salted	1 oz	172	0	2

SUSHI
TAKE-OUT

FOOD	PORTION	CALS	CHOL	FIBER
california roll	1 piece (0.8 oz)	28	1	–
fresh salmon rolls	4 pieces	250	20	3
sashimi	1 serv (6 oz)	198	63	–
tuna roll	1 piece (0.7 oz)	23	3	–
vegetable roll	1 piece (1.2 oz)	27	0	–
vinegared ginger	⅓ cup (1.6 oz)	48	0	–
wasabi	2 tsp (0.3 oz)	5	0	–
yellowtail roll	1 piece (0.6 oz)	25	0	–

SWAMP CABBAGE

FOOD	PORTION	CALS	CHOL	FIBER
chopped cooked w/o salt	1 cup	20	0	2

SWEET POTATO (*see also* YAM)

FOOD	PORTION	CALS	CHOL	FIBER
baked w/ skin	1 (3 ½ oz)	118	0	3

FOOD	PORTION	CALS	CHOL	FIBER
canned in syrup	½ cup	106	0	–
canned pieces	1 cup	183	0	–
frzn cooked	½ cup	88	0	–
leaves cooked	½ cup	11	0	–
mashed	½ cup	172	0	3
Framer's Market				
Organic Puree	½ cup	96	0	2
Glory				
Casserole	½ cup	180	0	2
Cut Fresh	1 serv (5 oz)	140	0	4
Sweet Potatoes	⅔ cup	160	0	2
Princella				
In Light Syrup	⅔ cup	160	0	3
Royal Prince				
Orange Pineapple	½ cup	160	0	2
TAKE-OUT				
candied	3.5 oz	144	0	–

SWEETBREAD (PANCREAS)

beef braised	3 oz	230	223	0
lamb braised	3 oz	199	340	0
pork braised	3 oz	186	268	0
testicles cooked	1 pair (6.8 oz)	241	673	0

SWISS CHARD

cooked	½ cup	18	0	–
raw chopped	½ cup	3	0	–
Frieda's				
Bright Lights	1 cup (3 oz)	15	0	1

SWORDFISH

cooked	3 oz	132	43	0
raw	3 oz	103	33	–

SYRUP

corn dark & light	¼ cup	240	0	0
maple	1 tbsp	52	0	–
maple	1 cup (11.1 oz)	824	0	–
raspberry	1 oz	76	0	–
sorghum	1 cup (11.6 oz)	957	0	–
sorghum	1 tbsp (0.7 oz)	61	0	–
sugar syrup	¼ cup	76	0	0

FOOD	PORTION	CALS	CHOL	FIBER
Cary's				
Maple	¼ cup	210	0	–
DaVinci Gourmet				
Sugar Free All Flavors	1 tbsp	0	0	0
Eden				
Organic Barley Malt	1 tbsp	60	0	0
Estee				
Blueberry	¼ cup	30	0	–
Hershey's				
Strawberry	2 tbsp	100	0	–
Karo				
Corn Syrup Dark	2 tbsp	120	0	–
Corn Syrup Light	2 tbsp	120	0	–
Nesquik				
Strawberry Calcium Fortified	2 tbsp	100	0	1
Pacifica Culinaria				
Pomegranate	1 tbsp	60	0	–
Watermelon	1 tbsp	60	0	–
Quik				
Strawberry	2 tbsp (1.5 oz)	110	0	0
Smucker's				
Blackberry	¼ cup	210	0	–
Blueberry	¼ cup	210	0	–
Boysenberry	¼ cup	210	0	–
Red Raspberry	¼ cup	210	0	–
Strawberry	¼ cup	210	0	–
Sundae Syrup Butterscotch	2 tbsp	100	0	–
Sundae Syrup Caramel	2 tbsp	100	0	–
Spectrum				
Balsamic Organic	1 tbsp	35	0	0

TAHINI (*see* SESAME)

TAMARILLOS
Frieda's

Gold Or Red	2 (4.2 oz)	40	0	4

TAMARIND

dried sweetened pulpitas	1 piece (0.8 oz)	56	0	1
dried sweetened pulpitas	½ cup	279	0	5

FOOD	PORTION	CALS	CHOL	FIBER
fresh	1 (2 g)	5	0	tr
fresh cut up	1 cup	143	0	3

TAMARIND JUICE
nectar	1 cup	143	0	1
Teptip				
Drink	1 can (11.2 oz)	210	0	0

TANGERINE
CANNED
in light syrup	1 cup	154	0	2
juice pack	1 cup	92	0	2

FRESH
fresh	1 sm (2.7 oz)	40	0	1
fresh	1 lg (4.2 oz)	64	0	2
fresh	1 med (3.1 oz)	47	0	2
sections	1 cup	103	0	4
Chiquita				
Tangerine	1 med (3.5 oz)	50	0	2
Noble				
Florida	1 (3.8 oz)	50	0	3
Sunkist				
Fresh	1 (3.8 oz)	50	0	3

TANGERINE JUICE
canned sweetened	1 cup	124	0	1
fresh	1 cup	106	0	1
Fresh Samantha				
Fresh Juice	1 cup (8 oz)	110	0	0
Italian Volcano				
Organic	1 serv (6.75 oz)	94	0	tr
Naked Juice				
Tangerine Scream	8 oz	110	0	0
Odwalla				
Juice	8 oz	110	0	0

TAPIOCA
pearl dry	¼ cup (1.3 oz)	136	0	tr

TARO
chips	10 (0.8 oz)	115	0	–
leaves cooked	½ cup	18	0	–

FOOD	PORTION	CALS	CHOL	FIBER
raw sliced	½ cup	56	0	–
shoots sliced cooked	½ cup	10	0	–
sliced cooked	½ cup (2.3 oz)	94	0	–
tahitian sliced cooked	½ cup	30	0	–
Frieda's				
Taro Root	⅔ cup (3 oz)	90	0	3

TARRAGON

FOOD	PORTION	CALS	CHOL	FIBER
ground	1 tsp	5	0	–

TEA/HERBAL TEA (see also ICED TEA)
HERBAL

FOOD	PORTION	CALS	CHOL	FIBER
chamomile brewed	1 cup	2	0	0
Celestial Seasonings				
Chamomile	1 cup	0	0	0
Dessert Tea English Toffee	1 cup	0	0	0
Moroccan Pomegranate Red	1 cup	0	0	0
Peppermint	1 cup	0	0	0
Red Safari Spice	1 cup	0	0	0
Roastaroma Herb	1 cup	0	0	–
Wellness Tea Ginseng Energy	1 tea bag	0	0	0
Zinger Acai Mango	1 cup	0	0	0
Zinger Lemon	1 cup	0	0	0
Eden				
Organic Genmaicha Tea	1 tea bag	0	0	0
Organic Kukicha Tea	1 tea bag	0	0	0
Guayaki				
Yerba Mate Magical Mint	1 tea bag	5	0	–
Yerba Mate Organic Chai Spice	1 tea bag	5	0	–
Yerba Mate Organic Chocolatte	1 tea bag	5	0	–
Yerba Mate Organic Orange Blossom	1 tea bag	5	0	–
Yerba Mate Organic Rooiboost	1 tea bag	5	0	–
Yerba Mate Organic Traditional	1 tea bag	5	0	–
Lipton				
Cinnamon Apple	1 tea bag	0	0	–
Ginger Twist	1 tea bag	0	0	0

FOOD	PORTION	CALS	CHOL	FIBER
Honey Lemon	1 tea bag	0	0	–
Lemon	1 tea bag	0	0	–
Mango	1 tea bag	0	0	–
Orange	1 tea bag	0	0	–
Peach	1 tea bag	0	0	–
Peppermint	1 tea bag	0	0	–
Quietly Chamomile	1 tea bag	0	0	–
Raspberry	1 tea bag	0	0	–
Silk				
Chai	1 cup	140	0	0
Tetley				
Chamomile	1 cup	0	0	0
Orange & Peach	1 cup	0	0	0
Peppermint	1 cup	0	0	0
REGULAR				
brewed tea	6 oz	2	0	0
Activitea				
Green Tea	1 cup	36	0	–
Celestial Seasonings				
Black Fast Lane	1 cup	0	0	0
Black Decafe Victorian Earl Grey	1 cup	0	0	–
Chai White Honey Vanilla	1 tea bag	0	0	0
Green Antioxidant	1 cup	0	0	0
Green Tropical Acai	1 cup	0	0	0
Green Tea	1 cup	0	0	0
Morning Thunder	1 cup	0	0	0
TeaHouse Chai Cinnamon Spice as prep	1 serv	110	0	–
White Tea Antioxidant Plum	1 tea bag	0	0	0
DaVinci Gourmet				
Sugar Free Tea Concentrate Green	2 tbsp	0	0	0
Sugar Free Tea Concentrate Lemon	2 tbsp	0	0	0
Sugar Free Tea Concentrate Spiced Chai	1.5 tbsp	0	0	0
Eden				
Organic Bancha Green Tea	1 tea bag	0	0	0
Organic Hojicha Tea	1 tea bag	0	0	0

FOOD	PORTION	CALS	CHOL	FIBER
General Foods				
International Tea Chai Latte	1 serv	70	0	–
Guayaki				
Yerba Mate Organic Greener Green Tea	1 tea bag	5	0	–
Lipton				
Black Tea as prep	1 teabag	0	0	0
Black Tea French Vanilla	1 tea bag	0	0	–
Black Tea Honey & Lemon	1 tea bag	0	0	–
Black Tea Mint	1 tea bag	0	0	–
Black Tea Orange & Spice	1 tea bag	0	0	–
Black Tea Spiced Chai	1 tea bag	0	0	–
Decaffeinated Black Tea as prep	1 serv	0	0	0
Earl Grey	1 tea bag	0	0	0
English Breakfast	1 tea bag	0	0	0
English Estate	1 tea bag	0	0	–
Green Tea as prep	1 tea bag	0	0	–
Green Tea Citrus Blossom	1 tea bag	5	0	–
Green Tea Decaffeinated	1 tea bag	0	0	–
Green Tea Lemon Ginseng	1 tea bag	0	0	–
Green Tea Mint	1 tea bag	0	0	–
Raspberry Truffle	1 teabag	0	0	–
Vanilla Hazelnut	1 tea bag	0	0	–
Low Carb Creations				
Chai as prep	1 cup	25	0	0
Oregon				
Chai Latte Cider	½ cup	110	0	–
Chai Latte Java	½ cup	42	0	–
Chai Latte Kashmir Green Tea	½ cup	81	0	–
Chai Latte Nog	½ cup	90	0	–
Chai Latte The Original	½ cup	78	0	–
Pacific Chai				
All Flavors as prep	1 serv	93	0	0
Paradise				
Tropical Tea	8 oz	1	0	0
Tropical Tea Decafe	8 oz	1	0	0
Tropical Tea Passion Fruit	8 oz	1	0	0

FOOD	PORTION	CALS	CHOL	FIBER
Red Rose				
Black Tea Teabag	1	0	0	0
Decaffeinated	1 cup	0	0	0
English Breakfast Teabag	1 cup	0	0	0
Salada				
Green Tea	1 cup	0	0	0
Green Tea Decaffeinated	1 tea bag	0	0	–
Original Blend Black Tea	1 tea bag	0	0	0
Tea Tech				
Instant Green Tea All Flavors	1 tube	0	0	–
XtraGreen Tea Mix All Flavors	1 tube	0	0	–
Tetley				
British Blend Round Teabags	1 cup	0	0	0
Chai Black Tea	1 cup	0	0	0
Decaffeinated Tea Bag as prep	1	0	0	0
Earl Grey	1 cup	0	0	0
English Breakfast	1 cup	0	0	0
Honey Lemon Green Tea	1 cup	0	0	0
TAKE-OUT				
chai spiced latte decaf	1 cup	130	0	0
TEMPEH				
tempeh	½ cup	165	0	–
Lightlife				
Garden Veggie	1 serv (4 oz)	230	0	10
Organic Flax	1 serv (4 oz)	230	0	11
Organic Grilles Lemon	1 patty (2.7 oz)	140	0	0
Organic Grilles Tamari	1 patty (2.7 oz)	130	0	0
Organic Soy	1 serv (4 oz)	210	0	10
Organic Three Grain	1 serv (4 oz)	240	0	8
Organic Wild Rice	1 serv (4 oz)	280	0	10
Tofurky				
Edamame Veggie	3 oz	145	0	7
Five Grain	3 oz	190	0	6
Soy	3 oz	160	0	7
Turtle Island				
Five Grain	3 oz	190	0	6
Low Fat Millet	3 oz	130	0	3

FOOD	PORTION	CALS	CHOL	FIBER
Soy	3 oz	160	0	7
Wild Rice Rhapsody	3 oz	160	0	7
White Wave				
Five Grain	⅓ block	140	0	4
Organic Original Soy	⅓ block	150	0	6
Organic Sea Veggie	⅓ block	120	0	8
Soy Rice	⅓ block	140	0	5

TESTICLES (see SWEETBREAD)

THYME

ground	1 tsp	4	0	–

TILAPIA

Beacon Light

Farm Raised Fillets	3 oz	85	50	0

TAKE-OUT

battered & fried	1 filet (4 oz)	206	109	tr
breaded & fried	1 filet (4 oz)	300	142	1
broiled	1 filet (3.4 oz)	128	101	0

TOFU

firm	¼ block (3 oz)	118	0	1
firm	½ cup	183	0	2
fresh fried	1 piece (0.5 oz)	35	0	tr
fuyu salted & fermented	1 block (0.33 oz)	13	0	tr
koyadofu dried frozen	1 piece (0.5 oz)	82	0	tr
okara	½ cup	47	0	1
regular	¼ block (4 oz)	88	0	1
regular	½ cup	94	0	1
Azumaya				
Extra Firm	1 serv (2.8 oz)	70	0	1
Firm	1 serv (2.8 oz)	70	0	tr
Lite Silken	1 serv (3.2 oz)	40	0	0
Lite Extra Firm	1 serv (2.8 oz)	60	0	1
Seasoned Oriental Spice	1 serv (3 oz)	90	0	1
Seasoned Zesty Garlic & Onion	1 serv (3 oz)	90	0	1
Silken	1 serv (3.2 oz)	40	0	tr
Eden				
Dried	1 piece (0.4 oz)	50	0	2

FOOD	PORTION	CALS	CHOL	FIBER
Hinoichi				
Firm	1 in slice (3 oz)	60	0	1
Nasoya				
Chinese Spice	¼ pkg (3 oz)	90	0	1
Extra Firm	⅕ pkg (2.8 oz)	80	0	1
Firm	⅕ pkg (2.8 oz)	70	0	tr
Garlic & Onion	¼ pkg (3 oz)	90	0	1
Lite Firm	⅕ pkg (2.8 oz)	40	0	tr
Lite Silken	⅕ pkg (3.2 oz)	30	0	tr
Seasoned Ginger Sesame	½ (5.5 oz)	210	0	2
Seasoned Sweet & Sour	½ (5.5 oz)	190	0	1
Seasoned Teriyaki	½ (5.5 oz)	190	0	2
Seasoned Thai Peanut	½ pkg (5.5 oz)	240	0	2
Silken	⅕ pkg (3.2 oz)	45	0	0
Soft	⅕ pkg (2.8 oz)	60	0	tr
TofuMate Breakfast Scramble	¼ pkg	15	0	–
TofuMate Eggless Salad	¼ pkg	15	0	–
TofuMate Mandarin Stirfry	¼ pkg	25	0	–
TofuMate Mediterranean Herb	¼ pkg	15	0	–
TofuMate Szechwan StirFry	¼ pkg	25	0	–
TofuMate Texas Taco	¼ pkg	15	0	0
Pete's Tofu				
Dessert Peach Mango	1 serv (6 oz)	120	0	0
Dessert Very Berry	1 serv (6 oz)	120	0	0
Medium Firm	3 oz	70	0	0
Soft	3 oz	56	0	0
Super Firm Italian Herb	3 oz	120	0	tr
Super Frim	3 oz	130	0	0
Tofu 2 Go Lemon Pepper	2 pieces + sauce	160	0	2
Tofu 2 Go Santa Fe	2 pieces + sauce	150	0	2
Tofu 2 Go Sesame Ginger	2 pieces + sauce	160	0	2
Tofu 2 Go Thai Tango	2 pieces + sauce	165	0	2
Tree Of Life				
30% Reduced Fat Firm	⅕ block (3.2 oz)	90	0	2
Easymeal Pasta Primavera as prep	1 serv	460	10	3

FOOD	PORTION	CALS	CHOL	FIBER
Easymeal Southwest Medley as prep	1 serv	380	0	3
Easymeal Teriyaki Stir Fry as prep	1 serv	270	0	6
Easymeal Thai Stir Fry as prep	1 serv	270	0	6
Organic Baked	⅓ block (2.7 oz)	150	0	0
Organic Baked Island Spice	⅓ pkg (2.7 oz)	130	0	0
Organic Baked Oriental	⅓ pkg (2.7 oz)	130	0	0
Organic Baked Savory	⅓ block (2.7 oz)	140	0	0
Organic Firm	⅕ block (3.2 oz)	100	0	0
Raw Firm	⅕ block (3.2 oz)	100	0	0
White Wave				
Baked Garlic Herb Italian	1 piece	120	0	1
Baked Hickory Smoke BBQ	1 piece	75	0	1
Baked Roma Italian Basil	1 piece	100	0	2
Baked Teriyaki Oriental	1 piece	120	0	1
Baked Thai Style	1 piece	120	0	1
Baked Zesty Lemon Pepper	1 piece	120	0	1
Extra Firm	¼ block	80	0	1
Organic Extra Firm	⅕ block	90	0	1
Organic Soft	⅕ block	90	0	1
Reduced Fat	⅕ block	90	0	2
TAKE-OUT				
soy sauce marinated & grilled	1 serv (4 oz)	181	0	1

TOMATILLO
fresh	1 (1.2 oz)	11	0	–
fresh chopped	½ cup	21	0	–
Las Palmas				
Tomatillos Crushed	½ cup	45	0	2

TOMATO
CANNED
paste	½ cup	110	0	6
puree	1 cup	102	0	6
puree w/o salt	1 cup	102	0	6
red whole	½ cup	24	0	–
sauce	½ cup	37	0	2
sauce spanish style	½ cup	40	0	2

FOOD	PORTION	CALS	CHOL	FIBER
sauce w/ mushrooms	½ cup	42	0	–
sauce w/ onion	½ cup	52	0	–
stewed	½ cup	34	0	–
w/ green chiles	½ cup	18	0	–
wedges in tomato juice	½ cup	34	0	–
Big R				
Cajun Stewed	½ cup (4.2 oz)	25	0	1
Diced w/ Chilies	½ cup (4.2 oz)	25	0	1
Cento				
Crushed	¼ cup	35	0	2
Paste	2 tbsp	30	0	1
Puree	¼ cup	25	0	1
Claussen				
Halves	1 serv (1 oz)	5	0	tr
Contadina				
Crushed w/ Italian Herbs	¼ cup	20	0	tr
Italian Pasta	2 tbsp	35	0	1
Italian Paste Roasted Garlic	2 tbsp	35	0	1
Paste	2 tbsp (1.2 oz)	30	0	1
Petite Cut Diced	½ cup	25	0	2
Puree	¼ cup (2.2 oz)	20	0	tr
Stewed	½ cup	35	0	1
Stewed w/ Celery & Green Peppers	½ cup	35	0	1
Del Monte				
Chunky Pasta Style	½ cup	45	0	2
Diced No Salt Added	½ cup	25	0	2
Diced w/ Garlic & Onion	½ cup	40	0	1
Diced w/ Green Pepper & Onion	½ cup	40	0	2
Diced Zesty Chili Style	½ cup	30	0	2
Diced Zesty w/ Mild Green Chilies	½ cup	30	0	1
Garden Select Petite Diced	½ cup	15	0	tr
Organic Diced w/ Basil Garlic & Oregano	½ cup	50	0	tr
Organic Diced	½ cup	25	0	2
Organic Tomato Paste	2 tbsp	30	0	1
Petite Cut	½ cup	25	0	2
Petite Cut Garlic & Olive Oil	½ cup	45	0	1

FOOD	PORTION	CALS	CHOL	FIBER
Sauce	¼ cup	20	0	tr
Stewed Cajun Recipe	½ cup	35	0	2
Stewed Italian Recipe	½ cup	30	0	2
Stewed Mexican Recipe	½ cup	35	0	2
Stewed No Salt Added	½ cup	35	0	2
Stewed Original	½ cup	35	0	2
Wedges	½ cup	35	0	2
Eden				
Organic Crushed	¼ cup	20	0	1
Organic Diced	½ cup	30	0	2
Organic Whole Roma	½ cup	30	0	1
Hunt's				
Crushed	½ cup	30	0	2
Diced Original	½ cup	20	0	tr
Diced w/ Basil Garlic & Oregano	½ cup	25	0	1
Diced w/ Green Pepper Celery & Onions	½ cup	45	0	1
Diced w/ Mild Green Chilies	½ cup	30	0	2
Diced w/ Roasted Garlic	½ cup	30	0	1
Diced w/ Sweet Onion	½ cup	45	0	tr
Family Favorites Meatloaf	¼ cup	30	0	2
Paste	2 tbsp	25	0	2
Paste No Salt Added	2 tbsp	30	0	2
Paste w/ Basil Garlic & Oregano	2 tbsp	25	0	2
Petite Diced	½ cup	20	0	1
Petite Diced w/ Mushrooms	½ cup	40	0	tr
Puree	½ cup	30	0	2
Sauce	¼ cup	15	0	tr
Sauce Garlic & Herb	½ cup	40	0	3
Sauce No Salt Added	2 tbsp	30	0	2
Sauce Roasted Garlic	¼ cup	15	0	tr
Stewed	½ cup	35	0	1
Stewed No Salt Added	½ cup	40	0	1
Whole No Salt Added	¼ cup	20	0	1
Muir Glen				
Diced Fire Roasted	¼ cup	30	0	1
Diced w/ Green Chilies	½ cup (4.5 oz)	25	0	1
Organic Chunky Sauce	¼ cup (2.3 oz)	20	0	1

FOOD	PORTION	CALS	CHOL	FIBER
Organic Crushed Fire Roasted	¼ cup	20	0	1
Organic Diced	½ cup (4.5 oz)	25	0	1
Organic Diced No Salt Added	½ cup (4.5 oz)	25	0	1
Organic Diced w/ Basil & Garlic	½ cup (4.5 oz)	25	0	1
Organic Diced w/ Italian Herbs	½ cup (4.4 oz)	25	0	1
Organic Ground Peeled	¼ cup (2.3 oz)	10	0	1
Organic Paste	2 tbsp (1.2 oz)	30	0	1
Organic Puree	¼ cup (2.2 oz)	20	0	1
Organic Sauce	¼ cup (2.2 oz)	20	0	1
Organic Sauce No Salt Added	¼ cup (2.2 oz)	20	0	1
Organic Stewed	½ cup (4.5 oz)	30	0	tr
Organic Whole Peeled	½ cup (4.6 oz)	30	0	1
Whole Peeled w/ Basil	½ cup (4.6 oz)	30	0	1
Pomi				
Chopped	½ cup	20	0	3
Progresso				
Crushed w/ Added Puree	¼ cup (2.1 oz)	20	0	0
Italian Style Peeled	½ cup (4.2 oz)	20	0	1
Paste	2 tbsp (1.2 oz)	30	0	1
Puree	¼ cup (2.2 oz)	25	0	1
Puree Thick Style	¼ cup (2.2 oz)	20	0	1
Sauce	¼ cup (2.1 oz)	20	0	1
Whole Peeled	½ cup (4.2 oz)	25	0	1
Redpack				
Chunky Style In Puree	½ cup	30	0	1
Crushed In Puree	¼ cup	20	0	1
Diced In Juice	½ cup	25	0	1
Paste	2 tbsp	0	0	1
Rienzi				
Paste	2 tbsp	25	0	1
Ro-Tel				
Diced In Sauce	½ cup	40	0	tr
Mexican Festival	½ cup	30	0	1
Original	½ cup	20	0	1

FOOD	PORTION	CALS	CHOL	FIBER
Tillen Farms				
Sunnyside Tomatoes	3 pieces (1 oz)	40	0	1
Tuttorosso				
Puree	¼ cup	20	0	1
DRIED				
sun dried	1 cup	140	0	–
sun dried	1 piece	5	0	–
sun dried in oil	1 piece (3 g)	6	0	–
sun dried in oil	1 cup (4 oz)	235	0	–
Frieda's				
Red Chopped	⅓ cup (1.1 oz)	100	0	2
FRESH				
bruschetta	¼ cup	50	0	tr
cooked	½ cup	32	0	–
grape tomatoes	20	30	0	1
green	1	30	0	–
red	1 (4.5 oz)	26	0	2
red chopped	1 cup	35	0	2
Chiquita				
Tomato	1 med (5.2 oz)	35	0	1
Earthbound Farm				
Organic Roma	1 med (5.2 oz)	35	0	1
Eurofresh				
Tomatoes On The Vine	1 med (5.2 oz)	35	0	1
Foxy				
Roma	1 med (5 oz)	35	0	1
Frieda's				
Baby Roma	⅔ cup (3 oz)	120	0	1
Tear Drop	⅔ cup (3 oz)	20	0	1
TAKE-OUT				
bruschetta on toasted italian bread	1 slice	106	0	tr
stewed	1 cup	80	0	–
TOMATO JUICE				
beef broth & tomato	1 can (5.5 oz)	62	0	tr
tomato juice	6 oz	32	0	–
tomato juice	½ cup	21	0	–
Campbell's				
Juice	8 oz	50	0	2

FOOD	PORTION	CALS	CHOL	FIBER
Del Monte				
Juice	8 oz	50	0	1
Hunt's				
Juice	1 can (6 oz)	22	0	1
No Salt Added	8 oz	34	0	2
Kagome				
Sweet Summer	8 oz	50	0	1
Luvli Juices				
Smashing Tomato	1 bottle (10 oz)	125	0	4
Spicy Tomato	1 bottle (10 oz)	125	0	4
Mott's				
Tomato Juice	8 oz	40	0	–
Muir Glen				
Organic	5.5 oz	40	0	4
TONGUE				
beef simmered	3 oz	241	112	0
lamb braised	3 oz	234	161	0
pork braised	3 oz	230	124	0
veal braised	3 oz	172	202	0
TORTILLA				
corn	1 (6 in diam)	56	0	1
corn w/o salt	1 (6 in diam) 0.9 oz	56	0	1
flour w/o salt	1 (8 in diam) 1.2 oz	114	0	1
Alvarado Street Bakery				
Sprouted Wheat Burrito Size	1 (2.2 oz)	170	0	1
CarbOle				
Low-Carb	1 (2 oz)	100	0	9
Food For Life				
Sprouted Corn	2 (1.7 oz)	120	0	4
La Mexicana				
Corn	1 (0.8 oz)	50	0	1
Flour	1 (0.8 oz)	80	0	1
Tortillas de Trigo	1 (1 oz)	140	0	1
Manny's				
Burrito Tortilla	1 (2.1 oz)	180	0	4
Fajita Tortilla	1 (2 oz)	170	0	4
Fat Free	1 (1 oz)	65	0	1
Low Carb	1 (1.7 oz)	140	0	6
Soft Taco Tortilla	1 (1 oz)	80	0	tr

FOOD	PORTION	CALS	CHOL	FIBER
Tortilla Wrap Tomato Basil	1 (1.4 oz)	100	tr	2
White Corn Gluten Free	1 (2 oz)	60	0	tr
Whole Wheat	1 (2 oz)	170	0	3
Super Bakery				
Organic	1 (2.5 oz)	210	0	13
Tumaro's				
Low In Carb Green Onion	1 (8 in)	130	0	11
Low In Carb Multi-grain	1 (8 in)	146	0	12
Low In Carb Salsa	1 (8 in)	130	0	12
Low In Carbs Garden Vegetable	1 (8 in)	100	0	8

TREE FERN
chopped cooked	½ cup	28	0	–

TRIPE
beef simmered	3 oz	80	133	0
TAKE-OUT				
mondongo w/ potatoes	1 cup	300	148	6

TRITICALE
dry	½ cup (3.4 oz)	323	0	–

TROUT
baked	3 oz	162	63	0
rainbow cooked	3 oz	129	62	0
seatrout baked	3 oz	113	90	0

TRUFFLES
fresh	0.5 oz	4	0	2

TUNA (see also TUNA DISHES)
CANNED				
light in oil	3 oz	169	15	0
light in oil	1 can (6 oz)	399	30	0
light in water	3 oz	99	25	0
light in water	1 can (5.8 oz)	192	49	0
white in oil	1 can (6.2 oz)	331	55	0
white in oil	3 oz	158	26	0
white in water	1 can (6 oz)	234	72	0
white in water	3 oz	116	35	0
Bumble Bee				
Chunk Light In Oil	¼ cup	110	20	0

FOOD	PORTION	CALS	CHOL	FIBER
Chunk Light In Water	2 oz	60	30	0
Chunk Light Touch Of Lemon In Water	¼ cup	60	30	0
Chunk White In Oil	¼ cup	100	25	0
Chunk White In Water	¼ cup	60	25	0
Chunk White In Water Very Low Sodium	¼ cup	70	25	0
Light In Oil	¼ cup	110	30	0
Solid White In Oil	¼ cup	90	25	0
Solid White In Water	2 oz	70	25	0
Tonno In Olive Oil	¼ cup	120	0	0
Chicken Of The Sea				
Albacore Solid In Water	2 oz	70	25	0
Chunk Light In Oil	2 oz	110	30	0
Chunk Light In Water	¼ cup (2 oz)	60	30	0
Chunk White Low Sodium In Spring Water	1 can (3 oz)	80	35	0
Chunk White In Spring Water	½ can	60	25	0
Premium Albacore Pouch	2 oz	60	25	0
Coral				
Light In Water	¼ cup	60	30	0
Progresso				
In Olive Oil drained	¼ cup (2 oz)	160	30	0
StarKist				
Chunk Light In Water	¼ cup (2 oz)	60	30	0
Chunk Light No Drain Package	¼ cup (2 oz)	60	30	0
Low Sodium Chunk White In Water	2 oz	60	25	0
Solid White Albacore In Water	¼ cup	70	25	0
Tuna Fillet In Spring Water	¼ cup (2 oz)	60	30	0
FRESH				
bluefin cooked	3 oz	157	42	0
bluefin raw	3 oz	122	32	0
skipjack baked	3 oz	112	51	0
yellowfin baked	3 oz	118	49	0
MIX				
Chicken Of The Sea				
Salad Kit	1 serv (3.5 oz)	380	22	1

FOOD	PORTION	CALS	CHOL	FIBER
Tuna Salad Kit Single Mayo & Onion	1 pkg	380	55	1
StarKist				
Lunch To-Go	1 pkg	310	40	tr
Ready-Mixed Tuna Salad Kit	1 pkg (3.5 oz)	190	5	2
Tuna Salad Lunch Kit	1 pkg (4.3 oz)	230	35	1
Tuna Helper				
AuGratin 50% Less Fat Recipe as prep	1 cup	240	15	1
AuGratin as prep	1 cup	300	20	1
Cheesy Broccoli as prep	1 cup	290	20	1
Cheesy Broccoli 50% Less Fat Recipe as prep	1 cup	240	15	1
Cheesy Pasta as prep	1 cup	280	20	tr
Cheesy Pasta 50% Less Fat Recipe as prep	1 cup	230	15	tr
Creamy Broccoli 50% Less Fat Recipe as prep	1 cup	240	15	1
Creamy Pasta as prep	1 cup	300	20	1
Creamy Pasta 50% Less Fat Recipe as prep	1 cup	230	15	1
Fettuccine Alfredo as prep	1 cup	310	15	1
Fettuccine Alfredo 50% Less Fat Recipe as prep	1 cup	240	15	1
Garden Cheddar as prep	1 cup	290	20	1
Garden Cheddar 50% Less Fat Recipe as prep	1 cup	240	15	1
Pasta Salad as prep	⅔ cup	380	10	1
Pasta Salad Low Fat Recipe as prep	⅔ cup	230	10	1
Tetrazzini as prep	1 cup	300	20	1
Tetrazzini 50% Less Fat Recipe as prep	1 cup	230	20	1

FOOD	PORTION	CALS	CHOL	FIBER
Tuna Melt as prep	1 cup	300	20	1
Tuna Melt Reduced Fat Recipe as prep	1 cup	240	15	1
Tuna Pot Pie as prep	1 cup	440	110	1
Tuna Romanoff as prep	1 cup	280	20	1
Tuna Romanoff 50% Less Fat Recipe as prep	1 cup	240	20	1
SHELF-STABLE				
Bumble Bee				
Steak Entrees Ginger & Soy	1 pkg (4 oz)	170	40	0
Steak Entrees Lemon & Cracked Pepper	1 pkg (4 oz)	160	50	0
Steak Entrees Mesquite Grilled	1 pkg (4 oz)	150	40	0
TAKE-OUT				
tuna salad	1 cup	383	27	–
TURKEY (*see also* TURKEY DISHES, TURKEY SUBSTITUTES)				
CANNED				
Valley Fresh				
Chunk White	2 oz	80	55	0
FRESH				
back w/ skin roasted	½ back (9 oz)	637	238	0
breast w/ skin roasted	4 oz	212	83	0
dark meat w/ skin roasted	3.6 oz	230	93	0
dark meat w/o skin roasted	1 cup (5 oz)	262	119	0
dark meat w/o skin roasted	3 oz	170	78	0
ground cooked	3 oz	188	57	–
leg w/ skin roasted	1 (1.2 lbs)	1133	466	0
leg w/ skin roasted	2.5 oz	147	61	0
light meat w/ skin roasted	4.7 oz	268	103	0
light meat w/ skin roasted	from ½ turkey (2.3 lbs)	2069	794	0
light meat w/o skin roasted	4 oz	183	81	0
neck simmered	1 (5.3 oz)	274	186	0
skin roasted	from ½ turkey (9 oz)	1096	281	0
skin roasted	1 oz	141	36	0
w/ skin roasted	½ turkey (4 lbs)	3857	1514	0

FOOD	PORTION	CALS	CHOL	FIBER
w/ skin roasted	8.4 oz	498	196	0
w/ skin neck & giblets roasted	½ turkey (8.8 lbs)	4123	1920	–
w/o skin roasted	1 cup (5 oz)	238	107	0
w/o skin roasted	7.3 oz	354	159	0
wing w/ skin roasted	1 (6.5 oz)	426	150	0
Jennie-O				
Ground	4 oz	160	80	0
Perdue				
Breast Tenderloins Butter Garlic	3 oz	100	45	–
Burger Cooked	1 (4 oz)	160	85	0
Dark Cooked	3 oz	180	85	–
Drumsticks Cooked	1 (2.2 oz)	110	80	0
Ground Cooked	3 oz	160	85	–
Tenderloins Black Pepper Cooked	3 oz	90	45	–
Thighs Cooked	1 (3.2 oz)	240	115	0
White Cooked	3 oz	150	65	0
Shady Brook				
Breast Tenderloin	4 oz	130	70	0
Breast Tenderloin Creamy Dijon Mustard	4 oz	140	50	0
Breast Tenderloin Teriyaki	4 oz	140	50	0
Breast Cutlets	4 oz	110	60	0
Ground 85% Lean	4 oz	220	75	–
Ground 93% Lean	4 oz	160	80	0
Ground 99% Lean	4 oz	120	70	0
Marinated Strips Asian Grill	4 oz	160	55	0
Marinated Strips Mild Herb	4 oz	130	60	0
Necks	4 oz	150	90	0
Tenderloins Turkey Breast Homestyle	4 oz	130	55	0
Thigh	4 oz	145	75	0
Whole Turkey	4 oz	180	85	–
Wing	4 oz	210	110	0
Turkey Store				
Lean Ground Italian Style	4 oz	190	80	–
Wampler				
Boneless Breast Roast	4 oz	160	35	0

FOOD	PORTION	CALS	CHOL	FIBER
Breast Half	4 oz	160	35	0
Breast Steaks	4 oz	120	70	0
Drumsticks	4 oz	180	75	0
Ground	4 oz	210	100	–
Ground Breast	4 oz	130	70	0
Ground Lean	4 oz	160	90	0
Thighs	4 oz	170	80	0
Wings	4 oz	220	80	0
Woodfire Grill Burger	1 (3 oz)	180	65	–
FROZEN				
roast boneless seasoned light & dark meat roasted	1 pkg (1.7 lbs)	1213	413	–
Jennie-O				
Burger	1 (4 oz)	160	100	0
Wampler				
Burger BBQ	1 (4 oz)	240	140	–
Burgers Cracked Peppercorn & Garlic	1 (3 oz)	170	65	0
Seasoned Burgers Cracker Peppercorn & Garlic	1 (3 oz)	170	65	0
READY-TO-EAT				
bologna	1 slice (1 oz)	59	21	tr
breast	1 slice (0.75 oz)	23	9	0
prebasted breast w/ skin roasted	½ breast (1.9 lbs)	1087	359	0
prebasted breast w/ skin roasted	1 breast (3.8 lbs)	2175	718	0
prebasted thigh w/ skin roasted	1 thigh (11 oz)	494	194	0
roll light & dark meat	1 oz	42	16	–
roll light meat	1 oz	42	12	–
salami cooked beef	1 slice (0.9 oz)	67	18	0
turkey loaf breast meat	1 pkg (6 oz)	187	69	0
turkey loaf breast meat	2 slices (1.5 oz)	47	17	0
turkey salad sandwich spread	¼ cup	104	15	0
Alpine Lace				
Breast Fat Free	2 oz	45	25	0
Boar's Head				
Breast 50% Lower Sodium Skin On	2 oz	60	25	0

FOOD	PORTION	CALS	CHOL	FIBER
Breast Cracked Pepper Smoked	2 oz	60	30	0
Breast Hickory Smoked Black Forest	2 oz	60	25	0
Breast Maple Glazed Honey Coat	2 oz	70	30	0
Breast Ovengold	2 oz	60	35	0
Breast Ovengold Skinless	2 oz	60	20	0
Breast Roasted Mesquite Smoked Skinless	2 oz	60	25	0
Breast Roasted Salsalito	2 oz	60	25	0
Carl Buddig				
Lean Slices Honey Roasted Breast	1 pkg (2.5 oz)	70	30	–
Lean Slices Oven Roasted Breast	1 pkg (2.5 oz)	70	30	–
Lean Slices Smoked Breast	1 pkg (2.5 oz)	70	30	–
Oven Roasted Breast	1 pkg (2.5 oz)	110	40	–
Smoked Breast	1 pkg (2.5 oz)	110	40	–
Turkey Ham	1 pkg (2.5 oz)	100	40	–
Healthy Choice				
Smoked Breast	4 slices (1.8 oz)	60	25	0
Hebrew National				
98% Fat Free Oven Roasted	5 slices (2 oz)	50	20	–
98% Fat Free Smoked Breast	5 slices (2 oz)	60	25	0
Jennie-O				
Turkey Breast Golden Roast	3 oz	100	35	–
Jordan's				
Fat Free Turkey Breast	1 slice (1 oz)	25	10	–
Oscar Mayer				
Lunchables Turkey Bagels	1 pkg	420	35	2
Smoked Turkey Breast	2 oz	60	20	0
Smoked White	3 slices (3 oz)	90	30	–
Turkey Bologna	3 slices (3 oz)	160	55	–
Turkey Cotto Salami	3 slices (3 oz)	130	65	–
Perdue				
Breast Sliced Cajun Style	2 oz	50	20	–
Breast Sliced Honey Smoked	2 oz	50	20	–
Breast Sliced Pan Roasted	2 oz	70	30	–
Ham Hickory Smoked	2 oz	60	40	–

FOOD	PORTION	CALS	CHOL	FIBER
Healthsense Breast Sliced Oven Roasted	2 oz	60	20	–
Pastrami Hickory Smoked	2 oz	70	40	–
Sara Lee				
Breast Cracked Pepper	2 oz	50	15	0
Breast Honey Roasted	2 slices (1.6 oz)	50	20	0
Shady Brook				
Breast Bone-In Oven Roasted	3 oz	160	60	–
Hickory Smoked Breast Fat Free	2 oz	50	25	–
Turkey Ham Smoked	2 oz	60	30	0
Whole Oven Roasted	3 oz	160	65	–
Wampler				
Bologna	2 oz	130	50	–
Dark Cured	2 oz	80	30	–
Deli Roast Classic Spiced Breast	2 oz	70	25	–
Deli Roast Peppered Breast	21 oz	40	20	–
Deli Roast Rotisserie Breast	2 oz	50	20	–
Pastrami	2 oz	90	40	–
Salami	2 oz	90	55	–
Turkey Ham	2 oz	60	40	0

TURKEY DISHES
FROZEN
Banquet

FOOD	PORTION	CALS	CHOL	FIBER
Homestyle Gravy & Sliced Turkey	2 slices + gravy	130	45	1
Sandwich Toppers Gravy & Sliced Turkey	1 pkg (5 oz)	160	30	0

READY-TO-EAT
Jennie-O

FOOD	PORTION	CALS	CHOL	FIBER
Stuffed Breast Cheddar Cheese & Broccoli	1 serv (6 oz)	240	85	0
Stuffed Turkey Breast Pepper Cheese & Rice	1 piece (6 oz)	250	70	0
Turkey Breast Roast In Homestyle Gravy	1 serv (5 oz)	110	40	0

FOOD	PORTION	CALS	CHOL	FIBER
Mosey's				
Turkey Breast w/ Gravy	1 serv (5 oz)	140	90	0
Wampler				
Turkey Ham Salad	⅓ cup	150	30	–
TAKE-OUT				
boneless breast w/ cranberry apple stuffing	1 serv (5 oz)	260	80	1

TURKEY SUBSTITUTES
Lightlife

FOOD	PORTION	CALS	CHOL	FIBER
Smart Deli Roast Turkey	4 slices (2 oz)	80	0	1
Tofurky				
Deli Slices Cranberry	3 slices (1.8 oz)	98	0	3
Deli Slices Hickory Smoked	3 slices (1.8 oz)	100	0	3
Deli Slices Italian	3 slices (1.8 oz)	103	0	4
Deli Slices Original	3 slices (1.8 oz)	103	0	3
Deli Slices Peppered	3 slices (1.8 oz)	103	0	3
Deli Slices Philly Steak	3 slices (1.8 oz)	110	0	3
Roast	1 serv (4 oz)	190	0	2
Worthington				
Turkee Slices	3 slices (3.3 oz)	180	0	0
Yves				
Veggie Turkey Deli Slices	1 serv (2.2 oz)	85	0	1

TURMERIC

FOOD	PORTION	CALS	CHOL	FIBER
ground	1 tsp	8	0	–

TURNIPS

FOOD	PORTION	CALS	CHOL	FIBER
canned greens	½ cup	17	0	–
cooked mashed	½ cup (4.2 oz)	47	0	–
cubed cooked	½ cup (3 oz)	33	0	–
frzn greens cooked	½ cup	24	0	2
greens chopped cooked	½ cup	15	0	2
greens raw chopped	½ cup	7	0	1
raw cubed	½ cup (2.4 oz)	25	0	–
Allens				
Green Seasoned Southern Style	½ cup	30	0 ●	2
Glory				
Greens Fresh	2 cups	20	0	3
Greens Seasoned canned	½ cup	35	0	2

FOOD	PORTION	CALS	CHOL	FIBER
Root Cut Fresh	½ cup	20	0	1
Sensibly Seasoned Greens	½ cup	20	0	2

VANILLA
vanilla extract	1 tsp	17	0	0
Steel's				
Sugar Free	1 tbsp	24	0	0
Virginia Dare				
Extract	1 tsp	10	0	–

VEAL (see also VEAL DISHES)
breast braised	3 oz	226	96	0
chop cooked	1 med (6.5 oz)	230	109	0
chop breaded fried	1 med (6.5 oz)	290	142	tr
cubed braised	3 oz	160	123	0
cutlet cooked	3 oz	141	83	0
ground broiled	3 oz	146	88	0
leg roasted	3 oz	136	88	0
loin roasted	3 oz	184	88	0
patty breaded fried	1 (2.8 oz)	211	80	tr
shank braised	3 oz	162	105	0

VEAL DISHES
TAKE-OUT
cordon bleu	1 serv (8 oz)	490	172	1
parmigiana	1 serv (6.4 oz)	362	146	2
scallopini	1 slice + sauce (3.4 oz)	238	64	tr
stew	1 serv (8.8 oz)	192	50	3
veal marengo	1 serv (8.8 oz)	274	118	1
veal marsala	1 slice + sauce (3.4 oz)	268	69	tr
veal paprikash	1 serv (8.6 oz)	280	138	1
veal picatta	1 piece + sauce (3.5 oz)	154	72	tr

VEGETABLE JUICE
vegetable juice cocktail	6 oz	34	0	–
vegetable juice cocktail	½ cup	22	0	–
Hunt's				
Cocktail	1 can (6 oz)	20	0	2
Muir Glen				
Organic	5.5 oz	50	0	2
V8				
Lemon Twist	1 bottle (12 oz)	70	0	3

FOOD	PORTION	CALS	CHOL	FIBER
VEGETABLES MIXED				
CANNED				
mixed vegetables	½ cup	39	0	–
peas & carrots	½ cup	48	0	–
peas & carrots low sodium	½ cup	48	0	–
peas & onions	½ cup	30	0	–
succotash	½ cup	102	0	–
Chun King				
Chow Mein Vegetables	⅔ cup (3 oz)	14	0	1
Del Monte				
Mixed	½ cup	40	0	2
Mixed Vegetables w/ Potatoes	½ cup	45	0	2
Peas And Carrots	½ cup	60	0	2
Savory Sides Homestyle Vegetable Medley	½ cup	70	0	2
Savory Sides Rio Grande Vegetables	½ cup	70	0	2
La Choy				
Chop Suey Vegetables	½ cup (2.2 oz)	10	0	1
S&W				
Mixed	½ cup (4.4 oz)	35	0	2
Peas & Carrots	½ cup (4.5 oz)	60	0	2
Peas & Onions	½ cup (4.3 oz)	40	0	3
Veg-All				
Cajun Mixed	½ cup	50	0	3
Original Mixed	½ cup	40	0	2
FRESH				
Mann's				
California Stir Fry	1 serv (3 oz)	30	0	2
River Ranch				
Broccoli & Carrots	1 cup	25	0	2
Broccoli & Cauliflower	1 cup	25	0	2
Stir Fry Blend	1 cup	30	0	2
Vegetable Medley	1 cup	25	0	2
FROZEN				
mixed vegetables cooked	½ cup	54	0	2
peas & carrots cooked	½ cup	38	0	–
peas & onions cooked	½ cup	40	0	–
succotash cooked	½ cup	79	0	–

FOOD	PORTION	CALS	CHOL	FIBER
Birds Eye				
Broccoli & Cauliflower	1 cup	30	0	2
Steamfresh Asian Medley	1 cup	50	0	2
Steamfresh Broccoli Cauliflower & Carrots	¾ cup	30	0	2
Steamfresh Broccoli Carrots Sugar Snap Peas & Water Chestnuts	¾ cups	35	0	2
Steamfresh Mixed Vegetables	⅔ cup	40	0	2
C&W				
Early Harvest Peas & Baby Carrots	⅔ cup	60	0	3
Petite Peas & Pearl Onions	⅔ cup	60	0	3
Europe's Best				
Zen Garden	¾ cup	60	0	3
Green Giant				
Alfredo Vegetables	¾ cup	70	5	2
Cheese Sauce Broccoli Cauliflower Carrots	1 cup (4.1 oz)	60	5	2
Seasoned Broccoli & Carrots w/ Garlic & Herbs	½ cup	45	0	3
Health Is Wealth				
Veggie Munchees	2 (1 oz)	50	0	1
La Choy				
Fancy Chinese Mixed Vegetables	½ cup (2.9 oz)	9	0	1
Lean Cuisine				
Cafe Classics Roasted Potatoes w/ Broccoli & Cheddar Cheese Sauce	1 pkg (10.25 oz)	230	15	5
McKenzie's				
Gumbo Mixture	1 serv (2.9 oz)	35	0	2
Okra Tomatoes w/ Onions	1 serv (2.8 oz)	20	0	2
Pictsweet				
Peas & Carrots	⅔ cup	50	0	3
Roast Works				
Flame Roasted Redskins & Vegetables	1 serv (3 oz)	90	0	3

FOOD	PORTION	CALS	CHOL	FIBER
Tree Of Life				
Mixed	½ cup (3 oz)	65	0	3
SHELF-STABLE				
TastyBite				
Curry Bangkok Red	½ pkg (5.3 oz)	88	0	1
Curry Patong Yellow	½ pkg (5.3 oz)	118	0	1
Curry Siam Green	½ pkg (5.3 oz)	63	0	1
Jaipur Vegetables	½ pkg (5 oz)	220	25	7
Malabar Mixed	½ pkg (5 oz)	67	0	1
TAKE-OUT				
buddha's delight	1 serv (16 oz)	174	35	3
caponata	¼ cup	28	0	–
gyoza potstickers vegetable	8 (4.9 oz)	210	0	5
ratatouille	1 serv (3.5 oz)	96	0	4
samosa	2 (4 oz)	170	0	3
succotash	½ cup	111	0	–
tapenade grilled vegetables	¼ cup	40	0	tr
VENISON				
roasted	4 oz	215	127	0
VINEGAR				
balsamic	1 tbsp	14	0	–
cider	1 tbsp	3	0	0
white	1 tbsp	3	0	0
Carapelli				
Balsamic	1 tbsp	15	0	0
Red Wine	1 tbsp	5	0	0
White Wine	1 tbsp	5	0	0
Eden				
Organic Apple Cider	1 tbsp	0	0	0
Organic Brown Rice	1 tbsp	2	0	0
Red Wine	1 tbsp	0	0	0
Ume Plum	1 tsp	0	0	0
Heinz				
White	2 tbsp	2	0	0
Newman's Own				
Organic Balsamic	1 tbsp	20	0	0
Pacifica Culinaria				
Balsamic Dark Sweet Cherry	1 tbsp	15	0	–
Pear Pomegranate	1 tbsp	10	0	–

FOOD	PORTION	CALS	CHOL	FIBER
Progresso				
Balsamic	2 tbsp (0.5 oz)	10	0	0
Regina				
Red Wine	1 tbsp	0	0	–
Spectrum				
Apple Cider Organic	1 tbsp	7	0	0
Balsamic Organic	1 tbsp	6	0	0
Brown Rice Organic	1 tbsp	10	0	0
Golden Balsamic Organic	1 tbsp	6	0	0
Red Wine Organic	1 tbsp	0	0	0
White Organic	1 tbsp	2	0	0
White Wine Organic	1 tbsp	0	0	0
White House				
White	1 tbsp (0.5 oz)	0	0	–
Wild Thyme Farms				
Balsamic Red Raspberry	1 tbsp	13	0	–

WAFFLES
FROZEN

FOOD	PORTION	CALS	CHOL	FIBER
Eggo				
Buttermilk	2	180	15	1
Homestyle	2	190	20	1
Homestyle Minis	12	250	30	1
Nutri-Grain Low Fat Whole Wheat	2	140	0	3
Special K	3	190	0	1
Waf-Fulls Strawberry	1	150	10	tr
EnviroKidz				
Organic Gorilla Banana	2 (2.7 oz)	230	0	2
Kashi				
Heart To Heart Honey Oat	2 (3 oz)	160	0	3
Van's				
Belgian 7 Grain	2	230	0	7
Belgian Blueberry	2	184	0	2
Belgian Original	2	172	0	2
Carb Manager Flax	2	200	0	6
Carb Manager Homestyle	2	200	65	6
Gourmet 97% Fat Free	2	230	0	4
Gourmet Blueberry	2	190	0	5
Gourmet Buckwheat	2	145	0	2

FOOD	PORTION	CALS	CHOL	FIBER
Gourmet Flax	2	157	0	2
Gourmet Multi Grain	2	260	0	6
Gourmet Original	2	180	0	5
Hearty Oat Berry Boost	2	200	0	4
Hearty Oat Maple Fusion	2	210	0	4
Hearty Oat Oats 'N Honey	2	200	0	4
Mini Blueberry	4	110	0	2
Mini Chocolate Chip	4	119	0	2
Mini Homestyle	4	116	0	2
Organic Blueberry	2	240	0	4
Organic Original	2	190	0	6
Organic Soy Flax	2	230	0	6
Wheat Free Blueberry	2	201	0	5
Wheat Free Cinnamon Apple	2	189	0	5
Wheat Free Flax	2	230	0	5
Wheat Free Mini	4	160	0	tr
Wheat Free Original	2	189	0	5
MIX				
plain as prep	1 (7 in diam) 2.6 oz	218	39	1
READY-TO-EAT				
Gol D Lite				
Low Carb Belgian	1 (0.9 oz)	100	0	5
Low Carb Belgian Chocolate Covered	1 (1.1 oz)	130	0	1
Kashi				
GoLean Blueberry	2 (3 oz)	170	0	6
GoLean Original	2 (3 oz)	170	0	6
Thomas'				
Buttermilk	1 (1.6 oz)	130	0	tr
Homestyle	1 (1.6 oz)	140	0	tr
TAKE-OUT				
plain	1 (7 in diam)	218	52	–
WALNUTS				
black dried chopped	1 cup	759	0	–
english dried	1 oz	182	0	1
english dried chopped	1 cup	770	0	6
halves	14 (1 oz)	190	0	2
Emerald				
Glazed	¼ cup	140	0	1

FOOD	PORTION	CALS	CHOL	FIBER
Organic				
Raw Walnuts	¼ cup	210	0	3
Sweet Delights				
Walnut Roasters	⅓ pkg (1 oz)	210	0	2

WASABI (see HORSERADISH)

WATER

FOOD	PORTION	CALS	CHOL	FIBER
ice cubes	3	0	0	0
tap water	8 oz	0	0	0
Absopure				
Natural Spring	8 oz	0	0	0
Aloe Splash				
All Flavors	8 oz	0	0	0
Aquafina				
Essentials Daily C Citrus	8 oz	40	0	–
Sparkling Berry Burst	8 oz	0	0	0
Sparkling Citrus Twist	8 oz	0	0	0
Water	8 oz	0	0	–
Aquess				
Purified Water w/ Soluble Fiber	1 bottle (18 oz)	30	0	5
Aroma Water				
All Flavors	8 oz	0	0	–
Base Energy + Water				
All Flavors	8 oz	28	0	–
Blu Italy				
Sparkling Lemon	8 oz	0	0	0
Calabria				
Mineral	8 oz	0	0	0
Carpe Diem				
Botanic Water All Flavors	8 oz	35	0	–
Castellina				
Sparkling Spring	8 oz	0	0	0
Clearly Canadian				
Sparkling Blackberry	8 oz	90	0	–
Sparkling Cherry	8 oz	85	0	–
Sparkling Raspberry	8 oz	75	0	–
Sparkling Strawberry	8 oz	85	0	–
Zero Sparkling All Flavors	8 oz	0	0	–

FOOD	PORTION	CALS	CHOL	FIBER
Crystal Geyser				
Spring Water	8 oz	0	0	0
Dasani				
Purfied Water	8 oz	0	0	-
w/ Lemon	8 oz	2	0	-
w/ Raspberry	8 oz	1	0	-
Eden				
Springs Artesian	8 oz	0	0	0
Evamor				
Artesian Water	8 oz	0	0	0
Evian				
Spring Water	1 bottle (11.5 oz)	0	0	0
Ferrarelle				
Sparkling	8 oz	0	0	1
Fiji				
Natural Artesian	1 bottle (16.9 oz)	0	0	0
FlavH20				
All Flavors	1 can (12.3 oz)	80	0	-
Fruit 2 0				
Grape	8 oz	0	0	0
Natural Berry	8 oz	0	0	0
Watermelon Kiwi	8 oz	0	0	0
Fruit Refreshers				
Lemonade	8 oz	0	0	0
Gerolsteiner				
Sparling Mineral	8 oz	0	0	0
Glaceau Vitamin Water				
Balance Cran Grapefruit	8 oz	50	0	-
Defense	8 oz	50	0	-
Endurance Peach Mango	8 oz	50	0	-
Energy Tropical Citrus	8 oz	40	0	-
Essential Orange Orange	8 oz	40	0	-
Focus Kiwi Strawberry	8 oz	40	0	-
Formula 50	8 oz	50	0	-
Multi-V Lemonade	8 oz	40	0	-
Perform Lemon Lime	8 oz	50	0	-
Power-C Dragonfruit	8 oz	40	0	-
Rescue Green Tea	8 oz	40	0	-
Revive Fruit Punch	8 oz	50	0	-
Stress-B Lemon Lime	8 oz	40	0	-

FOOD	PORTION	CALS	CHOL	FIBER
Hansen's				
Energy Water Lemon	8 oz	10	0	–
Hint				
All Flavors	1 bottle (15 oz)	0	0	0
Flavored Water All Flavors	1 bottle (15 oz)	0	0	0
Iceland Spring				
Spring Water	1 liter	0	0	0
Meridian				
Clear All Flavors	8 oz	100	0	–
Metromint				
Peppermint or Spearmint Water	8 oz	0	0	0
Multi Vitamin Enhanced Water				
All Flavors	8 oz	50	0	–
No Carb All Flavors	8 oz	0	0	0
Nestle				
Pure Life Splash All Flavors	8 oz	0	0	0
O Waters				
All Flavors	8 oz	0	0	0
Paradiso				
Slightly Sparkling	8 oz	0	0	0
Pellegrino				
Mineral Water	8 oz	0	0	0
Pink2O				
Fortified	1 bottle (20 oz)	0	0	0
Propel				
Fitness Water All Flavors	1 bottle (23.7 oz)	30	0	–
Rapid				
Hydra-Cell Water	1 bottle (16.9 oz)	0	0	0
Reebok				
Fitness Water Berry	1 bottle (24 oz)	30	0	0
Fitness Water Natural	1 bottle (24 oz)	0	0	0
Replenish				
Elements Enhanced Water Orange	8 oz	40	0	–
San Benedetto				
Nautral Mineral Water	1 liter	0	0	0
Sanfaustino				
Mineral	8 oz	0	0	0

FOOD	PORTION	CALS	CHOL	FIBER
Saratoga				
Spring	8 oz	0	0	0
SoBe				
All Flavors	8 oz	50	0	–
Spa				
Mineral Water Reine	1 bottle (17.5 oz)	0	0	0
Special K2O				
Protein Water All Flavors	1 bottle (16.6 oz)	50	0	–
Speedo Sportswater				
All Flavors	8 oz	10	0	–
Splash				
All Flavors	8 oz	0	0	0
Stacker 2				
Protein Water All Flavors	1 bottle (19.44 oz)	80	0	0
Sulinka				
Sparkling Mineral	8 oz	0	0	0
TalkingRain				
Ice All Flavors	8 oz	5	0	0
Tao Tea				
Lychee Water	8 oz	67	0	–
Thorpedo				
Ultra Low GI Energy Water	8 oz	45	0	0
Tipperary				
Mineral Water	1 liter	0	0	0
Trinity				
Energize	8 oz	50	0	–
Multi-Esstential	8 oz	50	0	–
Revive	8 oz	50	0	–
Strength	8 oz	50	0	–
Think	8 oz	50	0	–
Ty Nant				
Mineral Water	1 liter	0	0	0
Vasa				
Natural Spring	8 oz	0	0	0
Veryfine				
Fruit 2 O Lemon	8 oz	0	0	–
Fruit 2 O Lemon Lime	8 oz	0	0	–
Fruit 2 O Orange	8 oz	0	0	–
Fruit 2 O Raspberry	8 oz	0	0	–
VitaZest				
All Flavors	8 oz	0	0	0

FOOD	PORTION	CALS	CHOL	FIBER
Vittel				
Mineral Water	1 bottle (18 oz)	0	0	0
Volvic				
Mineral Water	1 liter	0	0	0
Natural Lemon	8 oz	0	0	0
Natural Orange	8 oz	30	0	0
Voss				
Artesian	8 oz	0	0	0
W20 For Women				
All Flavors	8 oz	40	0	0
Wateroos				
All Flavors	1 box (8 oz)	0	0	0
WaterPlus				
Antioxidants Acai Berry	8 oz	50	0	–
Electrolytes Fruit Punch	8 oz	50	0	–
Extra-C Orange Tangerine	8 oz	50	0	0
Vitamins Dragonfruit Kiwi	8 oz	50	0	–
Wild Waters				
All Flavors	8 oz	50	0	–
WATER CHESTNUTS				
chinese sliced canned	½ cup	35	0	–
fresh sliced	½ cup	66	0	–
Chun King				
Sliced	2 tbsp (0.8 oz)	11	0	1
Whole	2 (0.7 oz)	10	0	1
La Choy				
Chopped	2 tbsp (0.6 oz)	9	0	1
Sliced	2 tbsp (0.8 oz)	11	0	1
Whole	2 (0.7 oz)	10	0	1
WATERCRESS				
fresh chopped	½ cup	2	0	tr
garden fresh	½ cup	8	0	–
garden fresh cooked	½ cup	16	0	–
Frieda's				
Watercress	1 cup	10	0	2
WATERMELON				
cut up	1 cup	46	0	1
seeds dried	¼ cup	150	0	–
wedge	1 med (10 oz)	86	0	1

FOOD	PORTION	CALS	CHOL	FIBER
wedge	1 sm (2.5 oz)	21	0	tr
wedge	1 lg (20 oz)	172	0	2
whole melon	1 (9 lb)	1227	0	16
Dulcinea				
Fresh Mini Seedless	2 cups	88	0	2
Frieda's				
Yellow Seedless	½ cup (3 oz)	25	0	0
Sundia				
Fresh	2 cups	80	0	2

WATERMELON JUICE

FOOD	PORTION	CALS	CHOL	FIBER
juice	8 oz	71	0	1
Snapple				
What-A-Melon	8 oz	90	0	–
Sundia				
100% Natural	8 oz	110	0	1
Tang				
Watermelon Wallop	1 box (7 oz)	90	0	0

WHEAT

FOOD	PORTION	CALS	CHOL	FIBER
sprouted	1 cup (3.8 oz)	214	0	1
Bob's Red Mill				
Vital Wheat Gluten	¼ cup	120	0	0
Hodgson Mill				
Vital Wheat Gluten	4 tsp	40	0	1
Near East				
Pilaf Mix Wheat as prep	1 cup	220	9	9
Taboule Salad Mix as prep	⅔ cup	110	0	5
NOW				
Wheat Gluten Flour	¼ cup	125	0	–

WHEAT GERM

FOOD	PORTION	CALS	CHOL	FIBER
plain	¼ cup	108	0	4
Hodgson Mill				
Untoasted	2 tbsp	55	0	4
Kretschmer				
Original Toasted	2 tbsp	50	0	2
Mother's				
Toasted	2 tbsp	50	0	2

WHEY

FOOD	PORTION	CALS	CHOL	FIBER
acid dry	1 tbsp	10	0	0

FOOD	PORTION	CALS	CHOL	FIBER
sweet dry	1 tbsp	26	0	0
sweet fluid	½ cup	33	2	0

WHIPPED TOPPINGS

FOOD	PORTION	CALS	CHOL	FIBER
cream pressurized	1 cup (2.1 oz)	154	46	–
cream pressurized	1 tbsp (3 g)	8	2	–
nondairy frzn	1 tbsp	13	0	–
nondairy powdered as prep w/ whole milk	1 cup	151	8	–
nondairy pressurized	1 tbsp (4 g)	11	0	–
nondairy pressurized	1 cup	184	0	–
Cabot				
Whipped Cream	2 tbsp	15	<5	0
Estee				
Whipped Topping as prep	1 serv	10	0	0
Hood				
Light Sugar Free Whipped Cream	2 tbsp	10	<5	0
Whipped Light Cream	2 tbsp	20	5	0
Reddiwip				
Chocolate	2 tbsp	15	<5	0
Extra Creamy	2 tbsp	15	5	0
Fat Free	2 tbsp	5	0	0
Original	2 tbsp	15	<5	0
Soyatoo				
Soy Whip	2 tbsp	10	0	0

WHITE BEANS

FOOD	PORTION	CALS	CHOL	FIBER
canned	1 cup	306	0	–
dried regular cooked	1 cup	249	0	–
dried small cooked	1 cup	253	0	–
Progresso				
Cannellini	½ cup (4.6 oz)	100	0	5

WHITEFISH

FOOD	PORTION	CALS	CHOL	FIBER
baked	3 oz	146	65	0
smoked	1 oz	39	9	0
smoked	3 oz	92	28	0

WHITING

FOOD	PORTION	CALS	CHOL	FIBER
cooked	3 oz	98	71	0
raw	3 oz	77	57	0

FOOD	PORTION	CALS	CHOL	FIBER
WILD RICE				
cooked	1 cup (5.7 oz)	166	0	3
Gourmet House				
Cracked not prep	¼ cup	170	0	2
Hand Harvested not prep	¼ cup	170	0	2
Quick Cooking not prep	½ cup	170	0	2
White & Wild not prep	¼ cup	170	0	1
Wild & Rice Garden Blend no prep	¼ cup	190	0	1
WINE				
cooking	1 oz	15	0	0
dessert dry	1 glass (4 oz)	179	0	0
haiku	1 serv	93	0	0
japanese plum	3 oz	139	0	0
japanese sake	1 oz	33	0	0
kir	1 serv	78	0	0
red	1 glass (4 oz)	85	0	0
rosé	1 glass (4 oz)	84	0	0
sake screwdriver	1 serv	175	0	tr
sangria	1 serv	88	0	tr
sangria blanco	1 serv	155	0	3
sherry	2 oz	84	0	–
sweet dessert	1 glass (4 oz)	189	0	0
vermouth dry	3.5 oz	105	0	–
vermouth sweet	3.5 oz	167	0	–
wassail wine	1 serv	142	0	2
white	1 glass (4 oz)	80	0	0
wine cooler	1 serv	218	0	0
wine spritzer	1 serv	60	0	0
Eden				
Mirin Rice Cooking Wine	1 tbsp	25	0	–
WINGED BEANS				
dried cooked	1 cup	252	0	–
WRAPS (*see* BREAD, SANDWICHES)				
XANTHAN GUM				
Bob's Red Mill				
Xanthan Gum	1 tbsp	8	0	8

FOOD	PORTION	CALS	CHOL	FIBER
YAM (*see also* SWEET POTATO)				
CANNED				
Bruce's				
In Syrup	⅔ cup	150	0	3
Glory				
Candied	½ cup	210	0	1
S&W				
Candied	½ cup (4.9 oz)	170	0	4
FRESH				
mountain yam hawaii cooked	½ cup	59	0	–
yam cubed cooked	½ cup	79	0	–
Earthbound Farm				
Organic	1 med (4.6 oz)	130	0	4
Frieda's				
Name	¾ cup	100	0	3
YARDLONG BEANS				
sliced cooked w/o salt	1 cup	49	0	–
YEAST				
baker's compressed	1 cake (0.6 oz)	18	0	1
baker's dry	1 tbsp	35	0	3
baker's dry	1 pkg (7 g)	21	0	2
brewer's dry	1 tbsp	35	0	3
Hodgson Mill				
Active Dry	1 tsp	30	0	1
Fast Rise	1 tsp (9 g)	25	0	1
YELLOW BEANS				
fresh cooked w/o salt	1 cup	44	0	4
fresh raw	1 cup	34	0	4
Del Monte				
Wax Beans	½ cup	20	0	2
S&W				
Wax Beans Cut	½ cup (4.2 oz)	20	0	2
YELLOWTAIL				
baked	4 oz	199	75	0
YOGURT (*see also* YOGURT DRINKS, YOGURT FROZEN)				
plain low fat	8 oz	143	14	0

FOOD	PORTION	CALS	CHOL	FIBER
plain nonfat	8 oz	127	5	0
plain whole milk	8 oz	138	30	0
tofu yogurt	1 cup	246	0	1
Axelrod				
Fat Free Lemon	1 pkg (6 oz)	90	<5	0
Fat Free Raspberry	6 oz	90	<5	0
Fat Free Vanilla	1 pkg (6 oz)	90	<5	0
Breyers				
Vanilla 98% Fat Free	½ cup	90	5	4
Cabot				
Non Fat	8 oz	100	0	0
Non Fat Berry Banana	8 oz	130	5	0
Non Fat Blueberry	8 oz	130	5	0
Non Fat French Vanilla	8 oz	130	10	0
Non Fat Lemon	8 oz	130	5	0
Non Fat Raspberry	8 oz	130	5	0
Non Fat Very Berry	8 oz	130	5	0
Colombo				
Fat Free Plain	8 oz	100	10	0
Fat Free Vanilla	8 oz	160	5	0
French Vanilla	8 oz	180	15	0
Fruit On The Bottom Strawberry Banana	8 oz	230	15	0
Lowfat Plain	8 oz	130	15	0
Multipack Blended All Flavors	4 oz	110	5	0
Strawberry	8 oz	190	15	–
Dannon				
Activia Blueberry	1 pkg (4 oz)	110	5	0
Activia Mixed Berry	1 pkg (4 oz)	110	5	0
Activia Peach	1 pkg (4 oz)	110	10	0
Activia Prune	1 pkg (4 oz)	110	10	0
Activia Strawberry	1 pkg (4 oz)	110	5	0
Activia Vanilla	1 pkg (4 oz)	110	10	0
Chunky Fruit Nonfat Apple Cinnamon	6 oz	160	5	0
Chunky Fruit Nonfat Blueberry	6 oz	160	5	0
Chunky Fruit Nonfat Cherry Vanilla	6 oz	160	5	0

FOOD	PORTION	CALS	CHOL	FIBER
Chunky Fruit Nonfat Peach	6 oz	160	5	0
Chunky Fruit Nonfat Strawberry	6 oz	160	5	0
Chunky Fruit Nonfat Strawberry Banana	6 oz	160	5	0
Creamy Fruit Blends Raspberry	6 oz	170	10	tr
Danimals Lowfat Blueberry	4.4 oz	130	5	0
Danimals Lowfat Grape Lemonade	4.4 oz	120	5	0
Danimals Lowfat Lemon Ice	4.4 oz	120	5	0
Danimals Lowfat Orange Banana	4.4 oz	130	5	0
Danimals Lowfat Strawberry	4.4 oz	130	5	0
Danimals Lowfat Tropical Punch	4.4 oz	130	5	0
Danimals Lowfat Vanilla	4.4 oz	120	5	0
Danimals Lowfat Wild Raspberry	4.4 oz	120	5	0
Double Delights Banana Creme Strawberry	6 oz	160	10	0
Double Delights Bavarian Creme Raspberry	6 oz	170	10	0
Double Delights Cheesecake Cherry	6 oz	170	10	0
Double Delights Cheesecake Strawberry	6 oz	170	10	0
Double Delights Chocolate Cheesecake	6 oz	220	10	0
Double Delights Chocolate Dipped Strawberry	6 oz	210	10	0
Double Delights Chocolate Eclair	6 oz	220	10	0
Double Delights Vanilla Strawberry	6 oz	170	10	0
Double Delights Vanilla Peach & Apricot	6 oz	170	10	0
Fruit On The Bottom Lowfat Apple Cinnamon	8 oz	240	15	1

FOOD	PORTION	CALS	CHOL	FIBER
Fruit On The Bottom Lowfat Blueberry	8 oz	240	15	1
Fruit On The Bottom Lowfat Boysenberry	8 oz	240	15	1
Fruit On The Bottom Lowfat Cherry	8 oz	240	15	1
Fruit On The Bottom Lowfat Minipack Mixed Berry	4.4 oz	130	10	tr
Fruit On The Bottom Lowfat Minipack Strawberry	4.4 oz	130	10	tr
Fruit On The Bottom Lowfat Mixed Berries	8 oz	240	15	1
Fruit On The Bottom Lowfat Orange	8 oz	240	15	0
Fruit On The Bottom Lowfat Peach	8 oz	240	15	1
Fruit On The Bottom Lowfat Strawberry	8 oz	240	15	1
Fruit On The Bottom Lowfat Strawberry Banana	8 oz	240	15	1
La Creme Strawberry	1 pkg (4 oz)	140	20	–
La Creme Vanilla	1 pkg (4 oz)	140	20	–
Light Duets Cherry Cheesecake	6 oz	90	0	0
Light Duets Raspberry Royale	6 oz	90	0	0
Light Duets Strawberry Cheesecake	6 oz	90	0	0
Light 'N Crunchy Mint Chocolate Chip	8 oz	140	5	0
Light 'N Crunchy Nonfat Caramel Apple Crunch	8 oz	140	<5	0
Light 'N Crunchy Nonfat Lemon Blueberry Cobbler	8 oz	140	<5	0
Light 'N Crunchy Nonfat Mocha Cappuccino	8 oz	140	<5	0
Light 'N Crunchy Nonfat Raspberry w/ Granola	8 oz	140	<5	2
Light 'N Crunchy Nonfat Vanilla Chocolate Crunch	8 oz	130	<5	0

FOOD	PORTION	CALS	CHOL	FIBER
Light 'N Fit Vanilla	6 oz	90	<5	–
Light Nonfat Banana Cream Pie	8 oz	100	<5	0
Light Nonfat Blueberry	8 oz	100	<5	0
Light Nonfat Cappuccino	8 oz	100	5	0
Light Nonfat Cherry Vanilla	8 oz	100	<5	0
Light Nonfat Coconut Cream Pie	8 oz	100	5	0
Light Nonfat Creme Caramel	8 oz	100	<5	0
Light Nonfat Lemon Chiffon	8 oz	100	5	0
Light Nonfat Mint Chocolate Cream Pie	8 oz	100	<5	0
Light Nonfat Peach	8 oz	100	<5	0
Light Nontat Raspberry	8 oz	100	<5	0
Light Nonfat Strawberry	8 oz	100	<5	0
Light Nonfat Strawberry Banana	8 oz	100	<5	0
Light Nonfat Strawberry Kiwi	8 oz	100	5	0
Light Nonfat Tangerine Chiffon	8 oz	100	5	0
Light'N Fit w/ Fiber Blueberry	4 oz	70	<5	3
Lowfat Cranberry Raspberry	8 oz	210	15	0
Lowfat Lemon	8 oz	210	15	0
Lowfat Vanilla	8 oz	210	15	0
Minipack Blended Nonfat Cherry	4.4 oz	110	5	0
Sprinkl'ins Cherry Vanilla	1 (4.1 oz)	130	5	0
Sprinkl'ins Strawberry	1 (4.1 oz)	130	5	0
Sprinkl'ins Strawberry Banana	1 (4.1 oz)	130	5	0
Sprinkl'ins Vanilla w/ Cherry Crystals	1 (4.1 oz)	110	5	0
Sprinkl'ins Vanilla w/ Orange Crystals	1 (4.1 oz)	110	5	0
Fage				
Sheep & Goat's Milk	1 pkg (7 oz)	190	35	0

FOOD	PORTION	CALS	CHOL	FIBER
Horizon Organic				
Fat Free Peach	1 pkg (6 oz)	140	<5	1
Fat Free Vanilla	1 cup	180	5	0
Kids Strawberry	1 pkg (4 oz)	110	5	1
Lowfat Blended Blueberry	1 pkg (6 oz)	160	10	2
Tube Lowfat Blueberry	1 (2 oz)	70	5	0
Whole Milk Plain	1 cup	160	30	0
LeCarb				
YoCarb Plain	1 pkg (4 oz)	50	10	–
Oberweis				
Peach	1 pkg (8 oz)	210	15	0
Pascual				
Nonfat Cherries & Berries	1 pkg (4.4 oz)	100	0	5
Nonfat Peach	1 pkg (4.4 oz)	100	0	5
Redwood Hill Farm				
Goat Milk Apricot Mango	1 cup	180	15	2
Goat Milk Cranberry Orange	1 cup	180	15	2
Goat Milk Plain	1 cup	130	20	1
Goat Milk Strawberry	1 cup	180	15	2
Goat Milk Vanilla	1 cup	190	25	2
Silk				
Organic Soy Strawberry	1 pkg (6 oz)	160	0	1
Soy Apricot Mango	1 pkg	160	0	1
Soy Banana Strawberry	1 pkg	160	0	1
Soy Black Cherry	1 pkg	160	0	1
Soy Blueberry	1 pkg	160	0	1
Soy Key Lime	1 pkg	170	0	1
Soy Lemon	1 pkg	160	0	1
Soy Lemon Kiwi	1 pkg	150	0	1
Soy Peach	1 pkg	170	0	1
Soy Plain	8 oz	120	0	1
Soy Raspberry	1 pkg	160	0	1
Soy Vanilla	1 pkg (8 oz)	120	0	1
Spega				
La Natura Low Fat	1 pkg (5.2 oz)	80	5	0
Stonyfield Farm				
Kids' Lowfat BaNilla	1 pkg (4 oz)	110	5	2
Light Black Cherry	1 pkg (6 oz)	100	0	3

FOOD	PORTION	CALS	CHOL	FIBER
Light Blueberry	1 pkg (4 oz)	100	0	3
Light Peach	1 pkg (6 oz)	100	0	3
Light Strawberry	1 pkg (4 oz)	100	0	3
Nonfat French Vanilla	1 pkg	90	0	2
Nonfat Strawberry	1 pkg	140	0	2
O'Soy Chocolate	1 pkg (6 oz)	160	0	4
O'Soy Peach	1 pkg (4 oz)	100	0	3
Squeezers Lowfat Strawberry	1 tube (2 oz)	60	5	tr
Whole Milk French Vanilla	1 pkg (6 oz)	190	25	3
Total				
Greek Yogurt 0% Fat	1 pkg (5.3 oz)	80	0	0
Greek Yogurt 2% Fat	1 pkg (7 oz)	130	10	0
Greek Yogurt Classic	1 pkg (7 oz)	180	35	0
Greek Yogurt Light	1 pkg (5.3 oz)	130	20	0
Honey	1 pkg (3.5 oz)	250	20	0
WholeSoy & Co.				
Organic Soy Apricot Mango	1 pkg (6 oz)	160	0	2
Organic Soy Lemon	1 pkg (6 oz)	160	0	2
Organic Soy Plain	1 pkg (6 oz)	150	0	2
Organic Soy Raspberry	1 pkg (6 oz)	170	0	2
Organic Soy Vanilla	1 pkg (6 oz)	150	0	2
Yoplait				
Go-Gurt All Fruit Flavors	1 pkg (2.25 oz)	80	5	0
Grande 99% Fat Free All Flavors	1 cup	250	15	0
Grande Fat Free Plain	1 cup	90	5	0
Kids Banana Vanilla	1 pkg (4 oz)	100	10	1
Kids Strawberry Vanilla	1 pkg (4 oz)	100	5	1
Light All Fruit Flavors	1 pkg (6 oz)	180	<5	0
Light All Indulgent Flavors	1 pkg (6 oz)	110	<5	0
Light Thick & Creamy All Fruit Flavors	1 pkg (6 oz)	100	50	–
Original All Fruit Flavors	1 pkg (6 oz)	170	10	0
Original Coconut Cream	1 pkg (6 oz)	190	10	0
Original Lemon Burst	1 pkg (6 oz)	180	10	0
Original Pina Colada	1 pkg (6 oz)	170	10	0
Trix All Fruit Flavors	1 pkg (4 oz)	120	5	0

FOOD	PORTION	CALS	CHOL	FIBER
YOGURT DRINKS (see also SMOOTHIES)				
Dannon				
DanActive	1 bottle (3.5 oz)	90	5	–
Frusion Smoothie Peach Passion Fruit	1 bottle (10 oz)	270	15	0
Frusion Smoothie Tropical Fruit	1 bottle (10 oz)	270	15	0
Stonyfield Farm				
Kids' Juice Smoothie Orange Strawberry Banana Wave	1 bottle (6 oz)	160	5	2
Smoothie Light Strawberry	1 bottle (10 oz)	130	5	3
Smoothie Lowfat Strawberry	1 bottle (10 oz)	250	10	4
Yo-Goat				
Blueberry	8 oz	150	30	–
Yoplait				
Nouriche All Fruit Flavors	1 bottle (11 oz)	260	10	5
YOGURT FROZEN				
chocolate soft serve	1 cup	230	7	3
vanilla soft serve	1 cup	236	3	0
Breyers				
Chocolate	½ cup	150	15	tr
Vanilla	½ cup	140	15	0
Vanilla No Sugar Added	½ cup	100	20	0
Dannon				
Light'N Fit w/ Fiber Strawberry	4 oz	70	<5	3
Edy's				
Black Cherry Vanilla Swirl	½ cup	90	0	–
Caramel Praline Crunch	½ cup	100	0	–
Chocolate	½ cup	90	0	–
Strawberry	½ cup	100	0	–
Vanilla	½ cup	90	0	–
Vanilla Chocolate Swirl	½ cup	90	0	–
Haagen-Dazs				
Lowfat Dulce De Leche	½ cup	190	5	0
Nonfat Chocolate	½ cup	140	<5	tr
Nonfat Coffee	½ cup	140	<5	0
Nonfat Strawberry	½ cup	140	<5	0
Nonfat Vanilla	½ cup	140	<5	0

FOOD	PORTION	CALS	CHOL	FIBER
Nonfat Vanilla Raspberry Swirl	½ cup	130	<5	tr
Nonfat Vanilla Fudge	½ cup	160	<5	0
Hood				
Fat Free Old Fashioned Vanilla	½ cup	110	0	tr
Fat Free Strawberry	½ cup	100	0	tr
Vanilla Swiss Almond	½ cup	150	10	tr
Turkey Hill				
Black Raspberry	½ cup	110	10	–
Caramel Cashew Crunch	½ cup	160	25	–
Chocolate Chip Cookie Dough	½ cup	140	10	0
Clark Bar	½ cup	140	10	–
Fat Free Chocolate Cherry Cordial	½ cup	100	0	0
Fat Free Chocolate Marshmallow	½ cup	130	0	0
Fat Free Mint Cookie 'N Cream	½ cup	110	0	0
Fat Free Neapolitan	½ cup	100	0	0
Fat Free Orange Swirl	½ cup	100	0	–
Fat Free Vanilla Fudge	½ cup	110	0	0
Peach Raspberry	½ cup	110	10	0
Tin Roof Sundae	½ cup	140	10	0
Vanilla & Chocolate	½ cup	110	10	0
Vanilla Bean	½ cup	110	10	0
WholeSoy & Co.				
Organic All Flavors	½ cup	120	0	1

ZUCCHINI

FOOD	PORTION	CALS	CHOL	FIBER
baby raw	1 (0.5 oz)	3	0	tr
canned italian style	1 cup	66	0	–
fresh	1 sm (4.1 oz)	19	0	1
pickled	¼ cup	16	0	1
raw sliced	1 cup	19	0	1
sliced cooked w/o salt	1 cup	29	0	3
C&W				
Yellow & Green	⅔ cup	20	0	tr

FOOD	PORTION	CALS	CHOL	FIBER
Frieda's				
Baby	⅔ cup (3 oz)	20	0	0
Progresso				
Italian Style	½ cup (4.2 oz)	50	0	2
TAKE-OUT				
breaded & fried	6 slices (3 oz)	141	2	1
indian paalkora	1 serv	46	1	2
sticks breaded & fried	6 (2 oz)	90	2	1

PART TWO

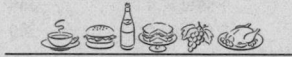

Restaurant Chains

YOU SHOULD KNOW—

Most restaurant meals are high in fat and cholesterol and the portion sizes are often too much for 1 person.

Split a meal with a friend.

Order an appetizer, half size, or lunch portion for your entrée.

Take the extra home for another meal.

FOOD	PORTION	CALS	CHOL	FIBER
A&W				
BEVERAGES				
Coke	1 sm (11 oz)	145	0	0
Diet Coke	1 sm (11 oz)	0	0	0
Diet Root Beer	1 sm (15 oz)	0	0	0
Diet Root Beer Float	1 sm (14.4 oz)	170	40	0
Root Beer Float	1 sm (14.4 oz)	330	40	0
Root Beet	1 sm (15 oz)	220	0	0
MAIN MENU SELECTIONS				
Cheese Curds	1 serv	570	105	2
Cheese Dog	1	320	40	1
Cheeseburger	1	470	70	2
Cheeseburger Deluxe	1	510	80	2
Cheeseburger Deluxe Bacon	1	570	90	2
Cheeseburger Deluxe Bacon Double	1	800	165	2
Cheeseburger Deluxe Double	1	720	150	2
Coney Chili Dog	1	310	40	2
Coney Chili Dog Cheese	1	350	45	2
Fries	1 lg	430	30	6
Fries Cheese	1 serv	380	5	4
Fries Chili	1 serv	370	10	5
Fries Chili & Cheese	1 serv	400	10	5
Fries Kids	1 serv	310	0	4
Hamburger	1	430	55	3
Hamburger Deluxe	1	460	65	2
Hot Dog Plain	1	280	35	1
Onion Rings	1 serv	350	5	2
Sandwich Crispy Chicken	1	580	65	5
Sandwich Grilled Chicken	1	430	80	4
Sauce BBQ	1 serv (1 oz)	40	0	0
Sauce Honey Mustard	1 serv (1 oz)	100	0	0
Sauce Ranch	1 serv (1 oz)	160	15	1
Sauce Sweet & Sour	1 serv (1 oz)	45	0	0

FOOD	PORTION	CALS	CHOL	FIBER
APPLEBEE'S				
DESSERTS				
Apple Betty Cobbler Ala Mode	1 serv	598	31	2
Fudge Brownie Sundae	1 serv	739	66	6
Low Fat Bikini Banana Strawberry Shortcake	1 serv	248	8	2
Low Fat Brownie Sundae	1 serv	415	3	3
Low Fat Marble Cheesecake	1 serv	261	10	4
MAIN MENU SELECTIONS				
Applebee's Burger w/ Fries	1 serv	1274	263	7
Basic Hamburger w/ Fries	1 serv	980	118	6
Beef Fajita Quesadilla	1 serv	1205	159	6
Bourbon Street Steak w/ Fried New Potatoes	1 serv	1115	168	–
Low Fat Asian Chicken Salad	1 serv (5 oz)	623	76	14
Low Fat Asian Chicken Salad	1 med (2.5 oz)	370	40	7
Low Fat Blacked Chicken Salad	1 serv (5 oz)	411	82	11
Low Fat Blacked Chicken Salad	1 med (2.5 oz)	287	43	6
Low Fat Garlic Chicken Pasta	1 serv	587	39	9
Low Fat Lemon Chicken Pasta	1 serv	528	50	8
Low Fat Quesadilla Chicken Fajita	1 serv	518	35	2
Low Fat Quesadilla Veggie	1 serv	344	8	3
Mozzarella Stix	8 pieces	963	64	1
Quesadillas	1 serv	684	99	4
Riblet Basket w/ Fries	1 serv	1317	219	7
Salad Dinner w/o Dressing	1 serv	303	277	3
Salad Santa Fe Chicken	1 med	724	96	7
Sandwich Bacon Cheese Chicken Grill w/o Fries	1	746	133	1
Sandwich Gyro	1	880	15	3
Stir Fry Chicken	1 serv	566	76	5

FOOD	PORTION	CALS	CHOL	FIBER
ARBY'S				
BEVERAGES				
Chocolate Shake	1 (14 oz)	480	45	0
Hot Chocolate	1 serv (8.6 oz)	110	0	0
Jamocha Shake	1 (14 oz)	470	45	0
Milk	1 serv (8 oz)	120	20	0
Orange Juice	1 serv (10 oz)	140	0	0
Strawberry Shake	1 (14 oz)	500	15	0
Vanilla Shake	1 (14 oz)	470	45	0
BREAKFAST SELECTIONS				
Add Egg	1 serv (2 oz)	110	175	0
Add Swiss Cheese Slice	1 slice (0.5 oz)	45	10	0
Biscuit w/ Bacon	1 (3.2 oz)	320	10	1
Biscuit w/ Butter	1 (2.9 oz)	280	0	1
Biscuit w/ Ham	1 (4.3 oz)	330	30	1
Biscuit w/ Sausage	1 (4.2)	460	30	1
Croissant w/ Bacon	1 (2.5 oz)	300	30	0
Croissant w/ Ham	1 (3.7 oz)	310	50	0
Croissant w/ Sausage	1 (3.6 oz)	420	50	0
French Toast Syrup	1 serv (0.5 oz)	130	0	0
Sourdough w/ Bacon	1 (5 oz)	380	10	2
Sourdough w/ Ham	1 (4 oz)	220	30	1
Sourdough w/ Sausage	1 (4 oz)	330	30	1
Toastix w/o Syrup	1 serv (4.4 oz)	370	0	4
DESSERTS				
Apple Turnover Iced	1 (4.5 oz)	420	0	2
Cherry Turnover Iced	1 (4.5 oz)	410	0	1
MAIN MENU SELECTIONS				
Arby's Sauce	1 serv (0.5 oz)	15	0	0
Au Jus Sauce	1 serv (3 oz)	5	0	tr
Baked Potato Broccoli'N Cheddar	1 (14 oz)	540	50	7
Baked Potato Deluxe	1 (13 oz)	650	90	6
Baked Potato w/ Butter & Sour Cream	1 (11.2 oz)	500	55	6
BBQ Dipping Sauce	1 serv (1 oz)	40	0	0
Bronco Berry Sauce	1 serv (1.5 oz)	90	0	0
Chicken Finger 4-Pak	1 serv (6.77 oz)	640	70	0
Chicken Finger Snack w/ Curly Fries	1 serv (6.4 oz)	580	35	3

FOOD	PORTION	CALS	CHOL	FIBER
Curly Fries	1 sm (3.8 oz)	310	0	3
Curly Fries	1 med (4.5 oz)	400	0	4
Curly Fries	1 lg (7 oz)	620	0	7
Curly Fries Cheddar	1 serv (6 oz)	460	5	4
German Mustard	1 pkg (0.25 oz)	5	0	0
Homestyle Fries	1 sm (4 oz)	300	0	3
Homestyle Fries	1 med (5 oz)	370	0	4
Homestyle Fries	1 lg (7.5 oz)	560	0	6
Homestyle Fries Child-Size	1 serv (3 oz)	220	0	3
Honey Mustard	1 serv (1 oz)	130	10	0
Horsey Sauce	1 pkg (0.5 oz)	60	5	0
Jalapeno Bites	1 serv (4 oz)	330	40	2
Ketchup	1 pkg (0.3 oz)	10	0	0
Marinara Sauce	1 serv (1.5 oz)	35	0	0
Mayonnaise	1 pkg (0.4 oz)	90	10	0
Mayonnaise Light Cholesterol Free	1 pkg (0.4 oz)	20	0	0
Mozzarella Sticks	4 (4.8 oz)	470	60	2
Onion Petals	1 serv (4 oz)	410	0	2
Potato Cakes	2 (3.5 oz)	250	0	3
Sandwich Chicken Bacon'N Swiss	1 (7.4 oz)	610	110	2
Sandwich Chicken Breast Fillet	1 (7.2 oz)	540	90	2
Sandwich Chicken Cordon Bleu	1 (8.4 oz)	630	120	2
Sandwich Grilled Chicken Deluxe	1 (8.7 oz)	450	110	2
Sandwich Hot Ham 'N Swiss	1 (5.9 oz)	340	90	1
Sandwich Market Fresh Roast Beef & Swiss	1 (12.5 oz)	810	130	5
Sandwich Market Fresh Roast Beef Ranch & Bacon	1 (13.5 oz)	880	155	5
Sandwich Market Fresh Roast Chicken Caesar	1 (12.7 oz)	820	140	5
Sandwich Market Fresh Roast Ham & Swiss	1 (12.5 oz)	730	125	5
Sandwich Market Fresh Roast Turkey & Swiss	1 (12.5 oz)	760	130	5

FOOD	PORTION	CALS	CHOL	FIBER
Sandwich Market Fresh Ultimate BLT	1 (10.5 oz)	820	110	5
Sandwich Roast Beef Arby-Q	1 (6.4 oz)	360	70	2
Sandwich Roast Beef Beef'N Cheddar	1 (6.9 oz)	480	90	2
Sandwich Roast Beef Big Montana	1 (11 oz)	630	155	3
Sandwich Roast Beef Giant	1 (7.9 oz)	480	110	3
Sandwich Roast Beef Junior	1 (4.4 oz)	310	70	2
Sandwich Roast Beef Melt w/ Cheddar	1 (5.2 oz)	340	70	2
Sandwich Roast Beef Regular	1 (5.4 oz)	350	85	2
Sandwich Roast Beef Super	1 (8.5 oz)	470	85	3
Sandwich Roast Chicken Club	1 (8.4 oz)	520	115	2
Sub Sandwich French Dip	1 (10 oz)	440	100	2
Sub Sandwich Hot Ham'N Swiss	1 (9.7 oz)	530	110	3
Sub Sandwich Italian	1 (11 oz)	780	120	3
Sub Sandwich Pilly Beef'N Swiss	1 (10.8 oz)	700	130	4
Sub Sandwich Roast Beef	1 (11.6 oz)	760	130	3
Sub Sandwich Roast Beef	1 (11.6 oz)	760	130	3
Sub Sandwich Turkey	1 (10.6 oz)	630	100	2
Tangy Southwest Sauce	1 serv (1.5 oz)	250	30	0
SALAD DRESSINGS				
Bleu Cheese	1 serv (2 oz)	300	45	0
Buttermilk Ranch	1 serv (2 oz)	290	25	0
Buttermilk Ranch Light	1 serv (2 oz)	100	0	1
Caesar	1 serv (2 oz)	310	60	0
Honey French	1 serv (2 oz)	290	0	tr
Italian Reduced Calorie	1 serv (2 oz)	25	0	tr
Italian Parmesan	1 serv (2 oz)	240	0	0
Thousand Island	1 serv (2 oz)	290	35	0
SALADS				
Caesar Side Salad	1 (5 oz)	45	5	2
Caesar Salad w/o Dressing	1 serv (8 oz)	90	10	3
Chicken Finger w/o Dressing	1 serv (13 oz)	570	65	3
Croutons Seasoned	1 serv (0.25 oz)	30	0	1

FOOD	PORTION	CALS	CHOL	FIBER
Garden Salad	1 (12.3 oz)	70	0	6
Grilled Chicken	1 serv (16.3 oz)	210	65	6
Grilled Chicken Caesar w/o Dressing	1 serv (12 oz)	230	80	3
Roast Chicken	1 serv (14.8 oz)	160	40	6
Side Salad	1 (5.7 oz)	25	0	2
Turkey Club Salad w/o Dressing	1 serv (12 oz)	350	90	3

AU BON PAIN
BAKED SELECTIONS

FOOD	PORTION	CALS	CHOL	FIBER
Bagel Cinnamon Crisp	1 (6 oz)	540	0	4
Baguette	1 loaf (10.6 oz)	680	0	6
Bread Stick	1 (2.3 oz)	200	0	2
Cinnamon Roll	1 (4 oz)	300	20	2
Cookie Chocolate Chip	1 (2 oz)	230	20	1
Cookie Chocolate Chunk Macadamia	1 (2 oz)	250	25	1
Cookie Gingerbread Man w/ Raisins & Icing	1 (2.7 oz)	280	30	tr
Cookie Oatmeal Raisin	1 (2 oz)	210	20	2
Cookie Peanut Butter	1 (2 oz)	240	20	2
Cookie Shortbread	1 (2.3 oz)	240	15	1
Cookie Walnut Raisin	1 (2 oz)	250	20	2
Cookie English Toffee	1 (2 oz)	230	35	tr
Creme De Fleur	1 serv (5.55 oz)	470	70	2
Croissant Almond	1 (4.7 oz)	480	95	3
Croissant Apple	1 (3.5 oz)	200	20	2
Croissant Chocolate	1 (3.1 oz)	330	20	3
Croissant Cinnamon Raisin	1 (3.8 oz)	300	20	2
Croissant Raspberry Cheese	1 (3.6 oz)	290	45	1
Croissant Sweet Cheese	1 (3.6 oz)	320	60	1
Danish Cranberry	1 (4.5 oz)	350	45	2
Danish Lemon	1 (4.3 oz)	340	45	5
Danish Sweet Cheese	1 (4.2 oz)	390	70	1
Focaccia	1 piece (5.4 oz)	430	0	3
Four Grain Bread	1 serv (4.7 oz)	400	0	3
French Roll	1 (4.2 oz)	260	0	2
French Roll Roast Beef	1 (11 oz)	540	80	3
Hearth Roll	1 (3 oz)	210	0	2

FOOD	PORTION	CALS	CHOL	FIBER
Holiday Cookie w/ w/ Icing & Sprinkles	1 (1.6 oz)	150	10	0
Loaf Multigrain	1 slice (1.8 oz)	130	0	1
Muffin Banana Walnut	1 (5.4 oz)	430	45	2
Muffin Blueberry	1 (5.6 oz)	470	90	2
Muffin Bran Raisin	1 (5.5 oz)	400	50	8
Muffin Carrot	1 (5.8 oz)	520	55	4
Muffin Corn	1 (5.7 oz)	390	60	2
Muffin Cranberry Walnut	1 (5.4 oz)	500	50	3
Muffin Milk Chocolate Chunk	1 (5.3 oz)	530	65	3
Muffin Pumpkin	1 (6 oz)	510	65	3
Muffin Low Fat 3 Berry	1 (4.4 oz)	270	25	2
Muffin Low Fat Chocolate Cake	1 (4.2 oz)	470	0	0
Parisienne Loaf	1 loaf (19 oz)	1210	0	11
Petit Pain	1 (2.9 oz)	180	0	2
Roll Braided w/ Topping	1 (10 oz)	430	40	3
Roll Pecan	1 (6 oz)	620	15	3
Sandwich Loaf Country White	1 serv (1.75 oz)	110	0	1
Sandwich Loaf Tomato Herb	1 serv (1.75 oz)	120	0	1
Scone Chocolate Walnut	1 (4 oz)	420	55	3
Scone Cranberry Orange Almond	1 (4 oz)	400	77	3
Scone Maple Oat Pecan Date	1 (4 oz)	410	60	3
Scone Orange	1 (4.2 oz)	370	115	2
Shortbread Heart ½ Chocolate	1 (2.7 oz)	290	20	1
Shortbread Heart w/ Red Sugar	1 (2.5 oz)	270	15	1
Sourdough Bagel Asiago Cheese	1 (4.8 oz)	340	15	2
Sourdough Bagel Cheddar Scallion	1 (4.1 oz)	310	10	2
Sourdough Bagel Cinnamon Crisp	1 (4.6 oz)	360	0	3
Sourdough Bagel Cinnamon Raisin	1 (4.5 oz)	300	0	3

FOOD	PORTION	CALS	CHOL	FIBER
Sourdough Bagel Cranberry Nut	1 (4.7 oz)	400	0	6
Sourdough Bagel Double Cheddar Jalapeno	1 serv (4.1 oz)	320	20	2
Sourdough Bagel Dutch Apple	1 (4.7 oz)	380	0	4
Sourdough Bagel Everything	1 (4.4 oz)	330	0	3
Sourdough Bagel Focaccia	1 (4.1 oz)	320	0	3
Sourdough Bagel Honey 9 Grain	1 (4.8 oz)	310	0	6
Sourdough bagel Onion	1 (4.4 oz)	320	0	3
Sourdough Bagel Plain	1 (4 oz)	300	0	3
Sourdough Bagel Poppy Seed	1 (4.4 oz)	330	0	3
Sourdough Bagel Sesame	1 (4.4 oz)	340	0	3
Sourdough Bagel Wild Blueberry	1 (4.1 oz)	280	0	3
Streudel Apple	1 serv (4.35 oz)	400	0	tr
Streudel Cherry	1 serv (4 oz)	380	0	tr
SALADS				
Caesar w/o Dressing	1 serv (7.8 oz)	240	30	4
Chef's	1 serv (10.3 oz)	290	65	3
Chicken Caesar	1 serv (10.2 oz)	380	85	4
Chicken Oriental	1 serv (8.6 oz)	220	60	5
Chicken Pesto Salad	1 serv (8 oz)	400	105	2
Garden	1 serv (9.3 oz)	160	0	5
Garden Side	1 serv (5.1 oz)	90	0	3
Gorgonzola & Walnut	1 serv (5 oz)	330	25	5
Mozzarella & Red Pepper Salad	1 serv (10.5 oz)	360	90	2
Tuna	1 serv (13.2 oz)	440	35	5
SANDWICHES AND FILLINGS				
Club Hot Roasted Turkey	1 (11.7 oz)	630	80	3
Cream Cheese Plain	1 serv (2 oz)	190	55	0
Cream Cheese Reduced Fat Honey Walnut	1 serv (2 oz)	150	35	0
Cream Cheese Reduced Fat Sundried Tomato	1 serv (2 oz)	140	40	0

FOOD	PORTION	CALS	CHOL	FIBER
Cream Cheese Reduced Fat Veggie	1 serv (2 oz)	140	40	0
Croissant Spinach & Cheese	1 (3.6 oz)	220	35	2
Croque Madame	1 (11 oz)	570	75	3
Croque Monsieur	1 (11 oz)	590	85	3
Egg On A Bagel	1 serv (7.1 oz)	500	120	4
Egg On A Bagel w/ Bacon	1 serv (7.6 oz)	580	130	4
Egg On A Bagel w/ Cheese	1 serv (7.85 oz)	590	145	4
Egg On A Bagel w/ Cheese & Bacon	1 serv (8.35 oz)	670	155	4
Focaccia Chicken & Mozzarella	1 serv (13.75 oz)	800	125	6
Focaccia Chicken Tarragon w/ Field Greens	1 (12.5 oz)	870	115	4
Focaccia Garden Vegetable Goat Cheese w/ Artichoke Spread	1 (14.25 oz)	570	25	5
Focaccia Hickory Smoked Ham & Brie	1 (13.3 oz)	620	100	5
Focaccia Smoked Turkey & Swiss w/ Cilantro	1 (13.25 oz)	810	90	4
Fo-Ca-Cha-Cha Chicken	1 serv (11.15 oz)	730	110	9
French Roll Ham	1 (11 oz)	390	65	3
French Roll Hot Grilled Chicken	1 (11 oz)	620	100	3
French Roll Hot Roast Turkey	1 (11 oz)	500	55	3
French Roll Tuna	1 (10.6 oz)	550	35	4
Hot Croissant Spinach & Cheese	1 (4 oz)	290	45	1
Pane Bagniate	1 (12 oz)	670	30	6
Sandwich Arizona Chicken	1 (12 oz)	600	120	4
Sandwich Cheese	1 (7.2 oz)	590	60	2
Sandwich Fresh Mozzarella Tomato & Pesto	1 (11 oz)	790	100	3
Sandwich Honey Dijon Chicken	1 (13.6 oz)	750	145	3
Sandwich Thai Chicken	1 (11.4 oz)	550	95	3
Wrap Chicken Caesar	1 (10.5 oz)	640	115	5
Wrap Fields & Feta	1 (13.5 oz)	620	15	14

FOOD	PORTION	CALS	CHOL	FIBER
Wrap Honey Smoked Turkey	1 (15 oz)	520	35	11
Wrap Roast Beef & Brie	1 (14 oz)	570	125	6
SOUPS				
Autumn Pumpkin	1 serv (8 oz)	170	20	5
Black Bean	1 serv (8 oz)	180	0	18
Chicken Florentine	1 serv (8 oz)	140	30	1
Chicken Noodle	1 serv (8 oz)	100	15	1
Clam Chowder	1 serv (8 oz)	220	35	1
Corn & Gree Chili Bisque	1 serv (8 oz)	200	30	2
Corn Chowder	1 serv (8 oz)	270	40	2
Curried Rice & Lentil	1 serv (8 oz)	140	0	5
French Moroccan Tomato Lentil	1 serv (8 oz)	130	0	7
Garden Vegetable	1 serv (8 oz)	50	0	2
Low Sodium Mediterranean Pepper	1 serv (12 oz)	280	0	10
Low Sodium Southwest Vegetable	1 serv (12 oz)	220	0	6
Old Fashioned Tomato	1 serv (8 oz)	140	10	2
Pasta E Fagioli	1 serv (8 oz)	240	5	7
Potato Cheese	1 serv (8 oz)	190	5	1
Potato Leek	1 serv (8 oz)	200	45	2
Red Beans & Rice	1 serv (8 oz)	200	10	12
Soup Bread Bowl	1 (9.25 oz)	600	0	5
Southern Black Eyed Pea	1 serv (8 oz)	320	5	20
Split Pea	1 serv (8 oz)	160	5	9
Tomato Florentine	1 serv (8 oz)	120	5	2
Tuscan Vegetable	1 serv (8 oz)	140	5	3
Vegetable Beef Barley	1 serv (8 oz)	110	10	3
Vegetarian Lentil	1 serv (8 oz)	120	0	8
Vegetarian Chili	1 serv (8 oz)	170	0	15
Wild Mushroom Bisque	1 serv (8 oz)	140	5	2

AUNTIE ANNE'S
BEVERAGES

FOOD	PORTION	CALS	CHOL	FIBER
Dutch Ice Blue Raspberry	1 (14 oz)	165	0	0
Dutch Ice Grape	1 (14 oz)	180	0	0
Dutch Ice Kiwi Banana	1 (14 oz)	190	0	0
Dutch Ice Lemonade	1 (14 oz)	315	0	0
Dutch Ice Mocha	1 (14 oz)	400	0	0

FOOD	PORTION	CALS	CHOL	FIBER
Dutch Ice Orange Creme	1 (14 oz)	280	0	0
Dutch Ice Pina Colada	1 (14 oz)	220	0	0
Dutch Ice Strawberry	1 (14 oz)	220	0	0
Dutch Ice Wild Cherry	1 (14 oz)	210	0	0
Dutch Shake Chocolate	1 (14 oz)	580	105	0
Dutch Shake Coffee	1 (14 oz)	590	105	0
Dutch Shake Strawberry	1 (14 oz)	610	105	0
Dutch Shake Vanilla	1 (14 oz)	510	105	0
Dutch Smoothie Blue Raspberry	1 (14 oz)	230	30	0
Dutch Smoothie Grape	1 (14 oz)	230	30	0
Dutch Smoothie Kiwi Banana	1 (14 oz)	240	30	0
Dutch Smoothie Lemonade	1 (14 oz)	300	30	0
Dutch Smoothie Mocha	1 (14 oz)	330	30	0
Dutch Smoothie Orange Creme	1 (14 oz)	280	30	0
Dutch Smoothie Pina Colada	1 (14 oz)	260	30	0
Dutch Smoothie Strawberry	1 (14 oz)	250	30	0
Dutch Smoothie Wild Cherry	1 (14 oz)	250	30	0
Lemonade	1 (22 oz)	180	0	0
Lemonade Strawberry	1 (22 oz)	190	0	0
DIPPING SAUCES				
Caramel Dip	1 serv (1.5 oz)	135	5	0
Cheese Sauce	1 serv (1.25 oz)	100	10	0
Chocolate Dip	1 serv (1.25 oz)	130	2	1
Cream Cheese Light	1 serv (1.25 oz)	70	25	0
Cream Cheese Strawberry	1 serv (1.25 oz)	110	35	0
Hot Salsa Cheese	1 serv (1.25 oz)	100	10	0
Marinara Sauce	1 serv (1.25 oz)	10	0	0
Sweet Mustard	1 serv (1.25 oz)	60	40	0
PRETZELS				
Almond	1	400	20	2
Almond w/o Butter	1	350	0	2
Cinnamon Raisin w/o Butter	1	350	0	2
Cinnamon Sugar	1	450	25	3
Garlic	1	350	10	2
Garlic w/o Butter	1	320	0	2

FOOD	PORTION	CALS	CHOL	FIBER
Glazin' Raisin	1	510	10	4
Glazin' Raisin w/o Butter	1	470	0	3
Jalapeno	1	310	10	2
Jalapeno w/o Butter	1	270	0	2
Maple Crumb	1	550	10	3
Maple Crumb w/o Butter	1	520	0	3
Original	1	370	10	2
Original w/o Butter	1	340	0	3
Parmesan Herb	1	440	30	9
Parmesan Herb w/o Butter	1	390	10	4
Sesame	1	410	15	7
Sesame w/o Butter	1	350	0	3
Sour Cream & Onion w/o Butter	1	310	0	2
Sour Cream & Onion	1	340	10	2
Stixs	4	247	7	2
Stixs w/o Butter	4	227	0	2
Whole Wheat	1	370	10	7
Whole Wheat w/o Butter	1	350	0	7

BAJA FRESH
MAIN MENU SELECTIONS

FOOD	PORTION	CALS	CHOL	FIBER
Baja Burrito Chicken	1 serv	820	130	11
Baja Burrito Steak	1 serv	920	155	9
Black Beans	1 serv	360	5	26
Burrito Bean & Cheese Chicken	1 serv	1000	145	21
Burrito Bean & Cheese Steak	1 serv	1100	170	20
Burrito Bean & Cheese Vegetarian	1 serv	870	70	20
Burrito Dos Manos Chicken	1 full serv	1480	130	28
Burrito Dos Manos Steak	1 full serv	1580	160	26
Burrito Mexicano Chicken	1 serv	830	75	20
Burrito Mexicano Steak	1 serv	920	100	19
Burrito Ultimo Chicken	1 serv	860	130	10
Burrito Ultimo Steak	1 serv	950	155	8
Cebollitas	1 serv	40	0	3
Chips & Salsa Baja	1 serv	1100	0	17
Enchiladas Cheese	1 serv	850	90	19
Enchiladas Chicken	1 serv	780	100	20

FOOD	PORTION	CALS	CHOL	FIBER
Enchiladas Steak	1 serv	890	125	20
Enchiladas Verde Cheese	1 serv	840	90	19
Enchiladas Verde Chicken	1 serv	770	100	20
Enchiladas Verde Vegetarian	1 serv	720	50	21
Fajitas Chicken Corn Tortillas	1 serv	1200	155	36
Fajitas Chicken Flour Tortillas	1 serv	1360	155	32
Fajitas Steak Corn Tortillas	1 serv	1360	205	33
Fajitas Steak Flour Tortillas	1 serv	1530	205	30
Grilled Vegetarian	1 serv	770	60	16
Mini Quesa-Dita Cheese	1 serv	620	45	15
Mini Quesa-Dita Chicken	1 serv	670	70	16
Mini Quesa-Dita Steak	1 serv	700	80	15
Mini Tosta-Dita Chicken	1 serv	570	55	13
Mini Tosta-Dita Steak	1 serv	630	75	12
Nachos Cheese	1 serv	1880	175	33
Nachos Chicken	1 serv	2010	245	34
Nachos Steak	1 serv	2100	275	33
Pinto Beans	1 serv	320	5	21
Quesadilla	1 serv	1180	175	12
Quesadilla Cheese	1 serv	1130	170	9
Quesadilla Chicken	1 serv	1260	245	10
Quesadilla Steak	1 serv	1350	270	9
Rice	1 serv	280	0	4
Taco Baja Style Chicken	1 serv	190	25	4
Taco Baja Style Steak	1 serv	220	30	3
Taco Baja Style Wild Gulf Shrimp	1 serv	190	90	3
Taco Chilito Chicken	1 serv	320	40	9
Taco Chilito Steak	1 serv	340	45	8
Taco Fish	1 serv	270	15	3
Taco Mahi Mahi	1 serv	260	20	6
Taquitos Chicken w/ Beans	1 serv	750	85	9
Taquitos Chicken w/ Rice	1 serv	710	80	9
Taquitos Steak w/ Beans	1 serv	820	105	20
Taquitos Steak w/ Rice	1 serv	790	105	10
Tostada Chicken	1 serv	1140	120	30
Tostada Steak	1 serv	1230	145	28
Tostada Vegetarian	1 serv	1010	45	28

FOOD	PORTION	CALS	CHOL	FIBER
SALAD DRESSINGS				
Fat Free Salsa Verde	1 serv (2.6 oz)	15	0	0
Guacamole	2 oz	70	0	4
Olive Oil Vinaigrette	1 serv (2.6 oz)	230	0	0
Pico De Gallo	1 serv	50	0	3
Pronto Guacamole	1 serv	550	0	11
Ranch	1 serv (2.6 oz)	220	15	0
Salsa Baja	1 serv	70	0	4
Salsa Roja	1 serv	70	0	4
Salsa Verde	1 serv	50	0	3
Sour Cream	1 oz	60	15	0
SALADS				
Baja Ensalada Chicken	1 serv	310	110	7
Baja Ensalada Fish	1 serv	360	70	10
Baja Ensalada Steak	1 serv	460	150	5
Side Salad	1 serv	70	5	3

BASKIN-ROBBINS

FOOD	PORTION	CALS	CHOL	FIBER
FROZEN YOGURT				
Cafe Mocha Truly Free Soft Serve	1 reg	140	5	–
Chocolate Nonfat Soft Serve	1 reg	190	5	–
Lowfat Maui Brownie Madness	1 reg	250	20	–
ICE CREAM				
Cappuccino Blast w/ Whipped Cream	1 reg	340	70	–
Chocolate	1 reg	270	55	–
Chocolate Chip	1 reg	270	60	–
Espresso'n Cream Lowfat	1 reg	180	10	–
Jamoca Almond Fudge	1 reg	280	45	–
Peach Crumb Pie No Sugar Added	1 reg	180	10	–
Pralines'n Cream	1 reg	280	50	–
Shake Chocolate	16 oz	750	115	–
Shake Vanilla	16 oz	630	170	–
Smoothie Very Strawberry w/ Soft Serve Ice Cream	1 reg	320	5	–
Thin Mint No Sugar Added	1 reg	160	10	–
Vanilla	1 reg	270	80	–

FOOD	PORTION	CALS	CHOL	FIBER
ICES				
Daiquiri Ice	1 reg	130	0	–
Sherbet Rainbow	1 reg	160	10	–
Sorbet Peachy Keen	1 reg	110	0	–
BEAR ROCK CAFE				
BAKED SELECTIONS				
Almond French Horn	1	491	5	4
Bear Claw	1	260	20	1
Cinnamon Roll w/ Cream Cheese Icing	1	540	25	2
English Muffin	1	120	0	1
Pecan Sticky Bun	1	555	25	2
SALAD DRESSINGS				
Balsamic Vinaigrette	1 serv (1.5 oz)	156	0	0
Blue Cheese	1 serv (1.5 oz)	230	25	0
Caesar	1 serv (1.5 oz)	198	21	0
Creamy Italian	1 serv (1.5 oz)	180	0	0
Fat Free Ranch	1 serv (1.5 oz)	40	0	1
Fat Free Vidalia Onion	1 serv (1.5 oz)	56	0	tr
Honey Mustard	1 serv (1.5 oz)	184	21	0
Oil & Vinegar	1 serv (1.5 oz)	250	0	0
Ranch	1 serv (1.5 oz)	213	7	0
Red Wine Vinaigrette	1 serv (1.5 oz)	198	0	0
Sesame Oriental	1 serv (1.5 oz)	128	0	0
Sweet Vidalia Onion	1 serv (1.5 oz)	170	0	0
Thousand Island	1 serv (1.5 oz)	184	21	0
SALADS				
Almond Citrus Chicken w/o Dressing	1 serv	443	85	4
BLT Chicken w/o Dressing	1 serv	394	124	4
BLT w/o Dressing	1 sm	146	34	2
BLT w/o Dressing	1 lg	285	68	4
Caesar Chicken w/ Dressing	1 serv	580	107	3
Caesar w/ Dressing	1 sm	236	26	2
Caesar w/ Dressing	1 lg	451	51	3
Dusk Mountain Blackened Chicken w/o Dressing	1 serv	304	85	3
Fruit Salad	1 serv (4 oz)	61	0	1
Lodge	1 sm	55	0	2

FOOD	PORTION	CALS	CHOL	FIBER
Lodge w/o Dressing	1 lg	82	0	3
Low Carb BLT	1 serv	721	92	4
Low Carb Side Salad w/ Dressing	1 serv	316	9	2
Low Carb w/ Chicken w/ Dressing	1 serv	567	70	3
Low Fat Grilled Chicken w/o Dressing	1 serv	151	56	3
Mount Fuji w/ Dressing	1 serv	554	56	4
SANDWICHES				
Bagel & Cream Cheese	1	378	30	2
Bear Cristo	1	310	91	6
BLT	1	585	61	2
Coop's Chicken Salad Croissant	1	439	44	5
Fajita Chicken	1	659	95	2
Fireside Jack	1	699	98	6
Garden	1	390	44	2
Giant Panda Wrap	1	556	58	23
Grilled Cheese	1	480	52	1
Ham & Swiss On Rye	1	394	76	2
Hoot Owl	1	641	92	2
Italian Asiago Focaccia	1	901	107	3
Low Carb Wrap	1	308	56	19
Low Fat Ham	1	309	50	2
Low Fat Turkey	1	280	40	3
Mountain Bird	1	691	98	6
Peanut Butter & Jelly	1	387	0	3
Reuben's Peak	1	540	76	3
Rising Sunflower	1	591	93	2
Roast Turkey & Bacon	1	522	71	2
Rockside Focaccia	1	958	129	3
Sasquash	1.	408	19	3
The Early Bear Bagel + Bacon	1	530	254	2
The Early Bear English Muffin + Bacon	1	344	248	1
The Early Bear English Muffin + Sausage	1	514	288	1
The Moose	1	976	142	7

FOOD	PORTION	CALS	CHOL	FIBER
Turkey On Whole Wheat	1	602	102	2
SOUPS				
Aztec Black Bean	1 serv	162	0	9
Baked Potato Mountain Chowder	1 serv	352	27	4
Chicken & Dumpling	1 serv	249	73	4
Chicken Gumbo	1 serv	123	14	3
Chicken Noodle	1 serv	165	28	1
Chicken w/ Wild Rice	1 serv	313	41	3
Cream Of Broccoli w/ Cheddar	1 serv	264	21	4
French Onion	1 serv	121	0	2
Grande Chili	1 serv	351	35	19
In Bread Bowl Aztec Black Bean	1 serv	545	0	12
In Bread Bowl Baked Potato Mountain Chowder	1 serv	735	27	7
In Bread Bowl Chicken & Dumplings	1 serv	632	73	7
In Bread Bowl Chicken Gumbo	1 serv	506	14	5
In Bread Bowl Chicken Noodle	1 serv	548	28	4
In Bread Bowl Chicken w/ Wild Rice	1 serv	696	41	5
In Bread Bowl Cream Of Broccoli w/ Cheddar	1 serv	647	21	7
In Bread Bowl French Onion	1 serv	504	0	4
In Bread Bowl Grande Chili	1 serv	734	35	22
In Bread Bowl New England Clam Chowder	1 serv	653	15	4
In Bread Bowl Normandy Vegetable Cheddar	1 serv	728	38	4
In Bread Bowl Tomato Florentine	1 serv	533	5	4
New England Clam Chowder	1 serv	270	15	1
Normandy Vegetable Cheddar	1 serv	345	38	2
Tomato Florentine	1 serv	150	5	2

FOOD	PORTION	CALS	CHOL	FIBER
BEN & JERRY'S				
Sugar Cone	1	48	0	tr
FROZEN YOGURT				
Black Raspberry Low Fat	½ cup	140	15	tr
Cherry Garcia	½ cup	170	20	0
Chocolate Fudge Brownie	½ cup	190	15	1
Half Baked	½ cup	210	20	tr
Phish Food	½ cup	230	15	1
ICE CREAM				
Brownie Batter	½ cup	310	70	1
Butter Pecan	½ cup	290	70	1
Cherry Garcia	½ cup	250	70	0
Chocolate Chip Cookie Dough	½ cup	280	70	0
Chocolate Chocolate Cookie	½ cup	280	35	2
Chocolate For A Change	½ cup	270	55	2
Chocolate Fudge Brownie	½ cup	280	40	2
Chubby Hubby	½ cup	330	60	1
Chunky Monkey	½ cup	300	60	1
Coffee For A Change	½ cup	240	75	0
Coffee Heath Bar Crunch	½ cup	310	65	0
Everything But The	½ cup	320	60	1
Fudge Central	½ cup	300	55	1
Half Baked	½ cup	280	60	1
Karamel Sutra	½ cup	290	55	1
Makin' Whoopie Pie	½ cup	270	40	2
Mint Chocolate Cookie	½ cup	270	70	tr
New York Super Fudge Chunk	½ cup	270	40	2
Oatmeal Cookie Chunk	½ cup	280	55	1
One Sweet Whirled	½ cup	280	60	1
Organic Chocolate Fudge Brownie	½ cup	260	35	2
Organic Strawberry	½ cup	200	55	0
Organic Sweet Cream & Cookies	½ cup	240	60	0
Organic Vanilla	½ cup	220	65	0
Peanut Butter Cup	½ cup	380	70	2
Peanut Butter Me Up	½ cup	330	50	2
Phish Food	½ cup	280	35	2

FOOD	PORTION	CALS	CHOL	FIBER
Pistachio Pistachio	½ cup	280	70	0
Uncanny Cashew	½ cup	290	70	0
Vanilla Almond	1 bar (3.7 oz)	340	65	2
Vanilla Heath Bar Crunch	½ cup	300	70	0
Vanilla For A Change	½ cup	240	75	0
SORBETS				
Berry Berry Extraordinary	½ cup	100	0	tr
Mango Lime	½ cup	100	0	0
Strawberry Kiwi	½ cup	100	0	tr

BIG APPLE BAGELS

FOOD	PORTION	CALS	CHOL	FIBER
BAGELS				
Apple Cinnamon	1	332	0	4
Banana Nut	1	340	0	4
Blueberry	1	330	0	4
Cheddar Herb	1	352	16	2
Chocolate Chip	1	348	0	4
Cinnamon Raisin	1	336	0	4
Cinnamon Sugar	1	175	0	2
Cranberry Walnut	1	352	0	4
Egg	1	328	4	2
Everything	1	336	0	4
Garlic	1	330	0	4
Honey Oat	1	320	0	2
Jalapeno	1	350	16	2
Onion	1	336	0	4
Pizzah Bagel	1	481	16	5
Plain	1	334	0	4
Poppy	1	344	0	4
Pumpernickel	1	332	0	4
Salt	1	324	0	2
Sesame	1	358	0	4
Spinach	1	356	0	4
Strawberry	1	342	0	4
Tomato Basil	1	322	0	4
Vegetable	1	318	0	4
Wheat	1	330	0	4
SANDWICHES				
All American Duo	1	762	107	4
Big Apple Club	1	797	110	4

FOOD	PORTION	CALS	CHOL	FIBER
Breakfast BLT	1	704	91	4
Chicken Caesar	1	611	64	4
Classic Turkey	1	552	66	4
Enchilada Bagellata	1	522	30	4
Grilled Chicken	1	571	55	4
Hoely Guacamole	1	476	61	4
Kick-N Roast Beef	1	579	74	4
Lox & Cream Cheese	1	602	58	4
Mediterranean Veg-Out	1	506	0	8
Morning Classic	1	486	256	3
Northern Omelette	1	699	296	3
Roma Italian	1	764	109	4
Toasted Cafe Chicken Melt	1	815	133	4
Toasted Deli Style Turkey	1	732	115	4
Toasted Roast Beef Parmesan Grinder	1	583	66	4
Toasted Spicy Italian Sub	1	770	109	4
Toasted Tuna Melt	1	641	54	4
Turkey Club	1	782	113	4

BILLY'S BURGER HUT
BEVERAGES

Shake Chocolate	1 (20 oz)	420	30	0
Shake Vanilla	1 (20 oz)	320	25	0

MAIN MENU SELECTIONS

Big Billy's Roast Beef Sub	1	843	151	3
Billyburger	1	426	63	3
Billyburger w/ Cheese	1	498	57	4
Billy's Best Red Potato Salad	1 serv	190	80	3
Billy's Biggest Burger ½ Pounder w/ Everything	1	852	140	4
Billy's Famous 7 Layer Salad	1 serv	558	119	2
Billy's Seafood Sandwich	1	399	42	3
Caesar Side Salad	1 serv	360	70	4
Chili w/ Cheese & Onion	1 serv	380	64	7
Cowboy Cobb Salad	1 serv	735	239	9
Cowboy Coleslaw	1 serv	180	10	3
French Fries	1 reg	230	0	1
Onion Rings	1 serv	250	0	1
Super Billy Burger w/ Bacon	1	663	98	4

FOOD	PORTION	CALS	CHOL	FIBER
BLIMPIE				
COOKIES				
Chocolate Chunk	1	200	15	1
Macadamia White Chunk	1	210	20	1
Oatmeal Raisin	1	190	10	1
Peanut Butter	1	220	15	1
Sugar	1	330	30	0
SALAD DRESSINGS AND TOPPINGS				
Caesar Dressing	1 serv (1.5 oz)	208	10	0
Cracked Peppercorn Dressing	1 serv (1.5 oz)	237	15	0
Frank's Red Hot Buffalo Sauce	1 serv (1 oz)	13	0	tr
French's Honey Mustard	1 tbsp	5	0	0
GourMayo Chipotle Chili	1 tbsp	50	10	0
GourMayo Sun Dried Tomato	1 tbsp	50	10	0
GourMayo Wasabi Horseradish	1 tbsp	50	10	0
Guacamole	1 serv (1.5 oz)	194	tr	1
Oil & Vinegar	1 serv	36	0	0
Pesto Dressing	1 serv (1 oz)	132	0	0
SALADS				
Antipasto	1 reg serv	244	69	3
Chef	1 reg serv	212	66	3
Chili Ole	1 reg serv	480	45	3
Grilled Chicken w/ Caesar Dressing	1 reg serv	347	45	3
Grilled Chicken w/o Dressing	1 serv	139	35	3
Roast Beef 'N Blue	1 reg serv	390	70	0
Seafood	1 reg serv	122	19	3
Tuna	1 reg serv	261	50	3
Zesto Pesto Turkey	1 reg serv	370	40	0
SANDWICHES				
6 Inch Hot Sub BLT	1	588	41	3
6 Inch Hot Sub Buffalo Chicken	1	400	61	3
6 Inch Hot Sub Buffalo Chicken w/o Cheese	1	320	61	3

FOOD	PORTION	CALS	CHOL	FIBER
6 Inch Hot Sub ChiliMax	1	511	0	8
6 Inch Hot Sub Grilled Chicken	1	373	35	3
6 Inch Hot Sub Meatball	1	572	58	2
6 Inch Hot Sub MexiMelt	1	425	0	7
6 Inch Hot Sub Pastrami	1	507	74	3
6 Inch Hot Sub Steak & Onion Melt	1	440	68	3
6 Inch Hot Sub VegiMax	1	395	0	8
6 Inch Sub Blimpie Best	1	476	69	2
6 Inch Sub Club	1	440	66	3
6 Inch Sub Ham & Cheese	1	436	59	3
6 Inch Sub Roast Beef	1	468	71	3
6 Inch Sub Roast Beef w/o Cheese	1	388	51	3
6 Inch Sub Seafood	1	355	19	4
6 Inch Sub Tuna	1	493	50	3
6 inch Sub Turkey	1	424	62	3
6 Inch Sub Turkey w/o Cheese	1	344	42	3
Cheddar	1 slice	52	10	0
Grilled Subs Beef Turkey & Cheddar	1	600	69	3
Grilled Subs Cuban	1	462	67	3
Grilled Subs Pastrami	1	462	44	3
Grilled Subs Reuben	1	630	46	2
Provolone	1 slice	80	20	0
Swiss	1 slice	80	20	0
Wraps Beef & Cheddar	1	714	78	3
Wraps Chicken Caesar	1	646	45	3
Wraps Southwestern	1	674	56	3
Wraps Steak & Onions	1	716	78	3
Wraps Ultimate BLT	1	831	78	3
Wraps Zesty Italian	1	638	62	3
SIDE ORDERS				
Cole Slaw	1 serv (5 oz)	180	<5	1
Macaroni Salad	1 serv (5 oz)	360	10	1
Mustard Potato Salad	1 serv (5 oz)	160	5	1
Potato Chips Cheddar & Sour Cream	1 bag	210	<5	1

FOOD	PORTION	CALS	CHOL	FIBER
Potato Chips Jalapeno	1 bag	210	0	2
Potato Chips Lea & Perrins Barbecue	1 bag	210	0	2
Potato Chips Regular	1 bag	210	0	2
Potato Chips Romano & Garlic	1 bag	210	<5	2
Potato Chips Sour Cream & Onion	1 bag	210	<5	1
Potato Salad	1 serv (5 oz)	270	10	1
SOUPS				
Chicken w/ White & Wild Rice	1 serv (8 oz)	230	30	2
Cream Of Broccoli & Cheese	1 serv (8 oz)	190	15	3
Cream Of Potato	1 serv (8 oz)	190	<5	3
Garden Vegetable	1 serv (8 oz)	80	0	3
Grande Chili w/ Beans & Beef	1 serv (8 oz)	250	40	18
Homestyle Chicken Noodle	1 serv (8 oz)	120	20	1
Tomato Basil w/ Raviolini	1 serv (8 oz)	110	10	tr
Vegetable Beef	1 serv (8 oz)	80	5	2

BOB EVANS
BAKED SELECTIONS

FOOD	PORTION	CALS	CHOL	FIBER
Biscuit	1	277	0	–
Bread Apple Walnut	1 slice	142	2	–
Bread Banana Nut	1 slice	186	7	–
Bread Garlic	1 slice	218	0	–
Bread Sourdough	1	130	0	–
Bun Kaiser	1	167	0	–
Bun Mini	1	105	0	–
English Muffin	1	139	0	–
Roll Cinnamon Swirl Frosted	1	607	9	–
Roll Cinnamon Swirl Unfrosted	1	510	5	–
Roll Dinner	1	201	9	–
Texas Toast	1 slice	120	0	–
BEVERAGES				
Coca-Cola	12.5 oz	145	0	–
Coffee Decafe	7 oz	5	0	

FOOD	PORTION	CALS	CHOL	FIBER
Coffee Regular	7 oz	2	0	0
Creamer Half & Half	0.5 oz	40	15	3
Creamer Non-Dairy	0.5 oz	19	0	–
Diet Coke	12.5 oz	4	0	0
Dr Pepper	12.5 oz	145	0	–
Hot Chocolate	1 serv (8.8 oz)	142	2	–
Hot Tea	7 oz	2	0	–
Iced Tea	9.4 oz	3	0	–
Iced Tea Blackberry	9.4 oz	92	0	–
Iced Tea Strawberry	9.4 oz	120	0	–
Kool Aid Ice Blue Raspberry Lemonade	1 kids cup (8 oz)	70	0	–
Lemonade	12 oz	136	0	–
Lemonade Blackberry	12 oz	214	0	–
Lemonade Strawberry	12 oz	242	0	–
Root Beer	12.5 oz	145	0	–
Sprite	12.5 oz	142	0	–
Strawberry Splash	12.5 oz	218	0	–
BREAKFAST SELECTIONS				
Bacon	1 piece	36	5	–
Belgian Waffle	1	351	0	–
Canadian Bacon	1 piece	21	9	–
Country Biscuit Breakfast	1 serv	841	267	–
Egg Hardboiled	1	60	190	–
Egg Over Easy	1	93	213	–
Eggs Scrambled	1 serv	170	482	–
Eggs Benedict	1 serv	514	484	–
French Toast	1 slice	135	25	–
Fruit Cup	1 serv	164	0	–
Grits	1 serv	187	0	–
Ham Smoked	1 slice	66	39	–
Home Fries	1 serv	193	0	–
Hotcake Blueberry	1	192	0	–
Hotcake Buttermilk	1	176	0	–
Hotcake Cinnamon	1	166	8	–
Hotcake Multigrain	1	208	10	–
Lite Sausage Breakfast	1 serv	479	42	–
Mush	1 serv	73	0	–
Oatmeal Plain	1 serv	185	0	–
Omelette Border	1	847	571	–

FOOD	PORTION	CALS	CHOL	FIBER
Omelette Cheese	1	457	530	–
Omelette Farmer's Market	1	634	558	–
Omelette Garden Harvest	1 serv	437	508	–
Omelette Ham & Cheese	1 serv	486	546	–
Omelette Sausage & Cheese	1 serv	729	567	–
Omelette Southwestern Chicken	1 serv	641	590	–
Omelette Western	1 serv	503	546	–
Pot Roast Hash Breakfast	1 serv	698	529	–
Sausage	1 link	117	21	0
Sausage Lite	1 link	100	37	–
Skillet Chicken Cordon Bleu	1 serv	880	612	–
Skillet Sunshine	1 serv	754	536	–
Strawberry Yogurt	1 serv	145	5	–
CHILDREN'S MENU SELECTIONS				
Colorful Cool Cakes	1 serv	542	1	–
Garden Salad	1 kid serv	41	7	–
Hot Diggety Dog Plain	1	446	55	–
L'il Homesteader	1 serv	414	262	–
Mac & Cheese	1 serv	330	20	–
Mini Cheeseburger	1 serv	252	25	–
Pizza Pizzazz	1 serv	520	31	–
Plenty O Pancakes	1 serv	515	0	–
Quesadilla Chicken	1 serv	542	73	–
Smiley Face Potatoes	1 serv	335	0	–
Spaghetti & Meatballs	1 serv	523	51	–
Sundae Fudge Blast	1 serv	254	30	–
Sundae Oreo Cookies 'n' Cream	1 serv	315	21	–
Sundae Rainbow	1 serv	320	30	–
Sundae Reese's I'm Smiling	1 serv	325	31	–
DESSERTS ·				
A La Mode Vanilla Ice Cream	1 serv	159	34	–
Cake Hershey's Hot Fudge	1 slice	688	34	–
Cake Pineapple Upside Down	1 slice	500	64	–
Oreo Cheesecake	1 slice	625	125	–
Peach Cobbler	1 serv	499	11	–
Pie Apple Dumpling	1 slice	682	7	–

FOOD	PORTION	CALS	CHOL	FIBER
Pie Banana Cream	1 slice	456	8	–
Pie Coconut Cream	1 slice	461	11	–
Pie French Silk	1 slice	653	128	–
Pie Lemon Meringue	1 slice	536	20	–
Pie Reese's Peanut Butter Cup	1 slice	1130	22	–
Pie Strawberry Supreme	1 slice	589	58	–
Pie No Sugar Added Apple	1 slice	483	0	–
Sundae Fudge	1	501	64	–
Sundae Reese's	1 serv	769	67	–
MAIN MENU SELECTIONS				
Applesauce	1 serv	101	0	–
Baked Potato Loaded	1	427	54	–
Baked Potato Plain	1	207	0	–
Broccoli Florets	1 serv	156	0	–
Broccoli Florets Cheddar	1 serv	230	20	–
Carrots Glazed	1 serv	188	0	–
Catfish Grilled New Orleans	1 piece	255	58	–
Cheeseburger Bacon Plain	1	1005	153	–
Cheeseburger Plain	1	691	104	–
Chicken Quesadilla	1 serv	502	61	–
Chicken & Broccoli Alfredo	1 serv	826	112	–
Chicken Fried	1 piece	291	154	–
Chicken Grilled	1 piece	229	98	–
Chicken Pot Pie	1 serv	758	209	–
Chicken Tenders Grilled	1 piece	103	33	–
Chicken-N-Noodle	1 serv	407	115	–
Coleslaw	1 serv	198	12	–
Corn Buttered	1 serv	225	0	–
Cottage Cheese	1 serv	122	36	–
Country Fried Steak w/ Gravy	1 serv	535	60	–
Country Fried Steak w/o Gravy	1 serv	481	60	–
Dressing Bread & Celery	1 serv	362	5	–
Fish Market Halibut	1 piece	209	32	–
French Fries	1 serv	217	0	–
Green Beans w/ Ham	1 serv	83	11	–
Grilled Garden Vegetables	1 serv	290	0	–
Hamburger Patty	1	388	82	–

FOOD	PORTION	CALS	CHOL	FIBER
Hamburger Plain	1	585	82	–
Hamburger Shroomin' Onion Plain	1	695	104	–
Home Fries	1 serv	193	0	–
Mashed Potatoes	1 serv	171	18	–
Meat Loaf	1 serv	626	157	–
Mushrooms Grilled	1 serv	152	0	–
Onion Rings	1 serv	460	0	–
Open Faced Roast Beef Dinner	1 serv	633	118	–
Pork Chop Dinner	1 serv	466	129	–
Pork Chop Dinner w/ Garlic Herb Butter	1 serv	624	130	–
Pork Chop Dinner w/ Wildfire Barbecue Sauce	1 serv	645	129	–
Rice Pilaf	1 serv	163	0	–
Salmon	1 serv	334	109	–
Salmon w/ Garlic Herb Butter	1 serv	491	110	–
Salmon w/ Wildfire Barbecue Sauce	1 serv	512	109	–
Sandwich Bob's BLT	1	795	276	–
Sandwich Chicken Salad	1	694	62	–
Sandwich Fish Market Haddock	1	570	32	–
Sandwich Fried Chicken	1	508	77	–
Sandwich Fried Chicken Club	1	994	155	–
Sandwich Grilled Cheese	1	391	30	–
Sandwich Grilled Chicken	1	447	98	–
Sandwich Grilled Chicken Club	1	993	194	–
Sandwich Pot Roast	1	728	113	–
Sandwich Turkey Bacon Melt	1	872	166	–
Seniors Chicken & Broccoli Alfredo	1 serv	513	77	–
Seniors Chicken Pot Pie	1 serv	758	209	–
Seniors Spaghetti & Meatballs	1 serv	617	69	–

FOOD	PORTION	CALS	CHOL	FIBER
Seniors Steak Tips & Noodles	1 serv	550	134	–
Seniors Stir-Fry Grilled Chicken	1 serv	479	66	–
Spaghetti & Marinara Sauce	1 serv	619	15	–
Spaghetti w/ Meatballs	1 serv	1087	107	–
Steak Monterey	1 serv	584	126	–
Steak Tips & Noodles	1 serv	985	266	–
Stir-Fry Grilled Chicken	1 serv	728	98	–
Stir-Fry Grilled Shrimp	1 serv	713	334	–
Stir-Fry Vegetable	1 serv	497	0	–
T-Bone Steak Plain	1 serv	1335	261	–
T-Bone Steak w/ Garlic Herb Butter	1 serv	1492	262	–
Turkey & Dressing	1 serv	542	105	–
SALAD DRESSINGS AND TOPPINGS				
Dressing Bleu Cheese	1 serv (1.5 oz)	220	22	–
Dressing Colonial	1 serv (1.5 oz)	232	0	–
Dressing French	1 serv (1.5 oz)	219	14	–
Dressing Honey Mustard	1 serv (1.5 oz)	192	21	–
Dressing Hot Bacon	1 serv (1.5 oz)	106	4	–
Dressing Lite Italian	1 serv (1.5 oz)	82	0	–
Dressing Oriental	1 serv (1.5 oz)	194	0	–
Dressing Ranch	1 serv (1.5 oz)	156	14	–
Dressing Ranch Lite	1 serv (1.5 oz)	103	11	–
Dressing Raspberry Vinaigrette	1 serv (1.5 oz)	155	0	–
Dressing Thousand Island	1 serv (1.5 oz)	212	21	–
Dressing Wildfire Ranch	1 serv (1.5 oz)	212	8	–
Gravy Chicken	1 serv (3 oz)	60	4	–
Gravy Chicken	1 serv (3 oz)	29	1	–
Gravy Country	1 serv (3 oz)	54	0	–
Gravy Sausage	1 serv (7 oz)	244	23	–
Syrup	1 serv (3 oz)	213	0	–
Syrup Sugar Free	1 serv (3 oz)	47	0	–
Topping Oregon Berry	1 serv (3 oz)	49	0	–
Topping Strawberry	1 serv (3 oz)	50	0	–
Whipped Topping	1 serv	69	0	–
SALADS				
Chicken Salad Plate	1 serv	789	87	–

FOOD	PORTION	CALS	CHOL	FIBER
Cobb Salad w/ Grilled Chicken	1 serv	778	373	–
Country Spinach w/ Grilled Chicken	1 serv	532	282	–
Frisco Salad w/ Fried Chicken	1 serv	672	98	–
Frisco Salad w/ Grilled Chicken	1 serv	599	154	–
Fruit & Yogurt	1 serv	414	5	–
Raspberry Grilled Chicken	1 serv	637	155	–
Speciality Side	1 serv	174	22	–
Wildfire Fried Chicken Salad	1 serv	806	66	–
Wildfried Grilled Chicken Salad	1 serv	733	123	–
SOUPS				
Bean	1 cup	125	10	–
Cheddar Baked Potato	1 cup	307	49	–
Vegetable Beef	1 cup	198	17	–
BOJANGLES				
Biscuit	1	243	2	2
Biscuit + Bacon	1	290	10	1
Biscuit + Bacon Egg Cheese	1	550	160	1
Biscuit + Cajun Filet	1	454	41	1
Biscuit + Country Ham	1	270	20	1
Biscuit + Egg	1	400	120	1
Biscuit + Sausage	1	350	20	1
Biscuit + Smoked Sausage	1	380	20	1
Biscuit + Steak	1	649	34	1
Botato Rounds	1 serv	235	13	3
Buffalo Bites	1 serv	180	105	0
Cajun Pintos	1 serv	110	0	6
Cajun Spiced Breast	1 serv	278	75	tr
Cajun Spiced Leg	1 serv	284	96	tr
Cajun Spiced Thigh	1 serv	310	67	tr
Cajun Spiced Wing	1 serv	355	94	tr
Chicken Supremes	1 serv	337	58	1
Corn On The Cob	1 serv	140	0	2
Dirty Rice	1 serv	166	10	1
Green Beans	1 serv	25	0	2

FOOD	PORTION	CALS	CHOL	FIBER
Macaroni & Cheese	1 serv	198	26	tr
Marinated Cole Slaw	1 serv	136	0	3
Potatoes w/o Gravy	1 serv	80	0	1
Sandwich Cajun Filet w/o Mayo	1	337	45	3
Sandwich Cajun Filet w/ Mayo	1	437	55	3
Sandwich Grilled Filet w/ Mayo	1	335	61	2
Sandwich Grilled Filet w/o Mayo	1 serv	235	51	2
Seasoned Fries	1 serv	344	13	4
Southern Style Breast	1 serv	261	76	tr
Southern Style Leg	1 serv	254	94	tr
Southern Style Thigh	1 serv	308	78	tr
Southern Style Wing	1 serv	337	86	tr
Sweet Biscuit Bo Berry	1	220	tr	1
Sweet Biscuit Cinnamon	1	320	tr	1

BOSTON MARKET
DESSERTS

FOOD	PORTION	CALS	CHOL	FIBER
Apple Pie	1 slice	550	0	3
Brownie Caramel Pecan	1	900	120	6
Brownie Chocolate	1	580	95	6
Chocolate Cake	1 serv	290	60	2
Chocolate Mania	1 serv	290	55	1
Cookie Chocolate Chip	1	390	15	2
Cookie Oatmeal Scotchie	1	390	30	2
Cornbread	1 piece	120	5	0
Strawberry Bliss	1 serv	100	40	0

MAIN MENU SELECTIONS

FOOD	PORTION	CALS	CHOL	FIBER
½ Spicy Tuscan Rotisserie Chicken	1 serv	630	295	1
½ Sweet Garlic Rotisserie Chicken w/ Skin	1 serv	590	290	0
¼ Dark Spicy Tuscan Rotisserie Chicken	1 serv	340	160	1
¼ Dark Sweet Rotisserie Chicken No Skin	1 serv	190	115	0

FOOD	PORTION	CALS	CHOL	FIBER
¼ Dark Sweet Rotisserie Chicken w/ Skin	1 serv	320	155	0
¼ White Spicy Tuscan Rotisserie Chicken	1 serv	200	95	1
¼ White Sweet Garlic Rotisserie Chicken No Skin Or Wing	1 serv	170	85	0
¼ White Sweet Rotisserie Chicken w/ Skin & Wing	1 serv	280	135	0
Butternut Squash	1 serv	150	20	6
Carver Meatloaf w/ Cheese	1	1070	190	7
Carver Chicken w/ Cheese & Sauce	1	670	90	5
Carver Turkey w/ Cheese & Sauce	1	690	130	5
Coleslaw	1 serv	310	20	10
Cranberry	1 serv	120	1	tr
Creamed Spinach	1 serv	260	55	2
Crispy Baked Country Chicken w/ Gravy	1 serv	440	35	5
Double Sauced Angus Meatloaf	1 serv	510	140	2
Garlic Dill New Potatoes	1 serv	130	0	2
Green Bean Casserole	1 serv	80	5	2
Green Beans	1 serv	70	0	2
Homestyle Mashed Potatoes & Gravy	1 serv	230	25	3
Honey Glazed Ham	1 serv	210	75	0
Hot Cinnamon Apples	1 serv	250	0	3
Macaroni & Cheese	1 serv	280	30	1
Mashed Potatoes	1 serv	210	25	2
Meatloaf Double Sauce Angus & Chunky Tomato	1 serv	550	140	3
Meatloaf Double Sauced Angus & Beef Gravy	1 serv	580	140	2
Pot Pie Pastry Topped	1	750	110	2
Poultry Gravy	1 serv	15	0	0
Roasted Sirloin	5 oz	270	125	0

FOOD	PORTION	CALS	CHOL	FIBER
Rotisserie Turkey Hand Carved	1 serv	170	100	0
Savory Stuffing	1 serv	190	5	2
Seasonal Fruit Salad	1 serv	70	0	1
Squash Casserole	1 serv	330	70	3
Steamed Vegetable Medley	1 serv	30	0	2
Sweet Corn	1 serv	180	0	2
Sweet Potato Casserole	1 serv	280	10	2
SALADS				
Asian Rotisserie Chicken Salad No Dressing or Noodles	1 serv	270	85	7
Asian Rotisserie Chicken Salad w/ Dressing & Noodles	1 serv	540	85	8
Caesar	1 entree	470	35	3
Caesar Rotisserie Chicken	1 serv	640	120	3
Caesar Side Salad	1 serv	300	15	tr
Southwest Chicken Salad	1 serv	750	100	6
SOUPS				
Chicken Tortilla + Toppings	1 serv	170	25	2
Hearty Chicken Noodle	1 cup	130	6	0
Tortilla Soup No Toppings	1 serv	80	15	1
BREWSTER'S COFFEE				
Americano	1 serv (16 oz)	12	0	0
Black Forest Coffee	1 serv (16 oz)	198	16	1
Cafe Caramello	1 serv (16 oz)	212	26	0
Cappuccino 2% Milk	1 serv (16 oz)	195	26	0
Cappuccino Fat Free Milk	1 serv (16 oz)	133	7	0
Italiano 2% Milk	1 serv (16 oz)	131	18	0
Italiano Fat Free Milk	1 serv (16 oz)	89	5	0
Jittery Monkey 2% Milk	1 serv (16 oz)	482	39	1
Jittery Monkey Fat Free Milk	1 serv (16 oz)	429	22	1
Latte 2% Milk	1 serv (16 oz)	212	28	0
Latte Cinnamon Toast 2% Milk	1 serv	299	25	0
Latte Cinnamon Toast Fat Free Milk	1 serv (16 oz)	240	6	0

FOOD	PORTION	CALS	CHOL	FIBER
Latte Creme Caramel 2% Milk	1 serv (16 oz)	303	25	0
Latte Creme Caramel Fat Free Milk	1 serv (16 oz)	244	6	0
Latte Fat Free Milk	1 serv (16 oz)	145	7	0
Latte Oregon Chai Tea 2% Milk	1 serv (16 oz)	274	18	0
Latte Oregon Chai Tea Fat Free Milk	1 serv (16 oz)	231	5	0
Latte Raspberry Cheesecake 2% Milk	1 serv (16 oz)	319	25	0
Latte Raspberry Cheesecake Fat Free Milk	1 serv (16 oz)	259	6	0
Mocha w/ Whipped Cream 2% Milk	1 serv (16 oz)	454	42	2
Mocha w/ Whipped Cream Fat Free Milk	1 serv (16 oz)	392	23	2

BROWN'S CHICKEN & PASTA

FOOD	PORTION	CALS	CHOL	FIBER
Breadsticks Garlic	1	50	tr	–
Breast	3 oz	284	67	–
Cheezy Potatoes	1 serv (12 oz)	188	19	1
Coleslaw	3 oz	131	6	–
Corn Fritters	3 oz	415	4	–
Corn On Cob	1 ear (3 inch)	126	1	–
French Fries	3 oz	503	1	–
Gizzard	3 oz	387	88	–
Leg	3 oz	287	52	–
Liver	3 oz	341	147	–
Mostaccioli Meatless Sauce	1 serv (12 oz)	792	0	–
Mostaccioli w/ Meat Sauce	1 serv (12 oz)	835	17	–
Mushrooms	3 oz	289	1	–
Potato Salad	3 oz	94	11	–
Ravioli Meatless Sauce	1 serv (12 oz)	822	0	–
Ravioli w/ Meat Sauce	1 serv (12 oz)	865	17	–
Shrimp	3 oz	277	31	–
Spaghetti w/ Meat Sauce	1 serv (12 oz)	835	17	–
Spaghetti w/ Meatless Sauce	1 serv (12 oz)	792	0	–
Thigh	3 oz	355	63	–
Wing	3 oz	385	81	–

FOOD	PORTION	CALS	CHOL	FIBER
BRUEGGER'S BAGELS				
BAGELS				
Blueberry	1	330	0	4
Chocolate Chip	1	310	0	4
Cinnamon Raisin	1	320	0	4
Cinnamon Sugar	1	340	0	6
Everything	1	310	0	4
Garlic	1	310	0	4
Honey Grain	1	330	0	5
Jalapeno Bagel	1	310	0	4
Onion	1	310	0	4
Orange Cranberry	1	330	0	4
Plain	1	300	0	4
Poppy Seed	1	310	0	4
Pumpernickel	1	320	0	5
Rosemary Olive Oil	1	350	0	4
Salt	1	300	0	4
Sesame	1	320	0	4
Sun Dried Tomato	1	320	0	4
DESSERTS				
Blondies	1	370	25	2
Brownie Chocolate Chunk	1	330	55	2
Brownie Mint	1	300	40	0
Bruegger Bar	1	420	15	3
Cappuccino Bar	1	420	60	1
Luscious Lemon Bar	1	350	85	0
Oatmeal Cranberry Mountains	1	430	60	3
Raspberry Sammies	1	270	35	1
SANDWICH FILLINGS				
Atlantic Smoked Salmon	2 oz	90	30	0
Cream Cheese Bacon Scallion	2 tbsp	100	30	0
Cream Cheese Chive	2 tbsp	100	30	0
Cream Cheese Garden Veggie	2 tbsp	90	25	0
Cream Cheese Garden Veggie Light	2 tbsp	60	15	0
Cream Cheese Herb Garlic Light	2 tbsp	70	15	0

FOOD	PORTION	CALS	CHOL	FIBER
Cream Cheese Honey Walnut	2 tbsp	110	25	0
Cream Cheese Jalapeno	2 tbsp	100	30	0
Cream Cheese Light Strawberry	2 tbsp	70	15	0
Cream Cheese Olive Pimento	2 tbsp	100	30	0
Cream Cheese Plain	2 tbsp	90	25	0
Cream Cheese Plain Light	2 tbsp	70	15	0
Cream Cheese Smoked Salmon	2 tbsp	100	25	0
Cream Cheese Wildberry	2 tbsp	100	25	0
Hummus	2 tbsp	60	0	2
Tuna Salad	1 serv (2.5 oz)	180	20	0
SANDWICHES				
Atlantic Smoked Salmon	1	470	55	4
Chicken Breast	1	440	60	4
Chicken Fajita	1	500	85	5
Chicken Salad w/ Mayo	1	460	55	4
Deli-Style Ham w/ Honey Mustard	1	440	30	4
Egg Cheese	1	480	190	4
Egg Cheese Sausage	1	680	235	4
Egg Cheese Bacon	1	560	200	4
Egg Cheese Ham	1	520	205	4
Garden Veggie	1	390	0	7
Herby Turkey	1	530	55	4
Leonardo Da Veggie	1	460	40	4
Santa Fe Turkey	1	480	55	4
Turkey w/ Mayo	1	480	35	4

BURGER KING
BEVERAGES

Aquafina Water	1 bottle	0	0	0
Coffee Black	1 sm	0	0	0
Coffee Black	1 lg	10	0	0
Coke Classic	1 sm	160	0	0
Coke Classic	1 lg	330	0	0
Coke Classic frzn	1 sm	370	0	0
Diet Coke	1 sm	0	0	0

FOOD	PORTION	CALS	CHOL	FIBER
Dr Pepper	1 sm	160	0	0
Dr Pepper	1 lg	410	0	0
Milk 1%	1	100	10	0
Minute Maid Cherry frzn	1 sm	370	0	0
Minute Maid Orange Juice	1 serv	140	0	0
Shake Chocolate	1 sm	620	95	2
Shake Strawberry	1 sm	620	95	1
Shake Vanilla	1 sm	560	95	1
Sprite	1 sm	160	0	0
Sprite	1 lg	320	0	0
BREAKFAST SELECTIONS				
Croissan'wich Bacon Egg & Cheese	1	360	195	tr
Croissan'wich Egg & Cheese	1	320	185	tr
Croissan'wich Ham Egg & Cheese	1	360	200	tr
Croissan'wich Sausage Egg & Cheese	1	520	210	1
Croissan'wich w/ Sausage & Cheese	1	420	45	tr
French Toast Sticks	5 pieces	390	0	2
Hash Browns	1 sm	230	0	2
Hash Browns	1 lg	390	0	4
Sourdough Breakfast Sandwich Bacon Egg & Cheese	1	380	190	2
Sourdough Breakfast Sandwich Ham Egg & Cheese	1	380	195	2
Sourdough Breakfast Sandwich Sausage Egg & Cheese	1	540	210	2
DESSERTS				
Chocolate Chip Cookies	2	440	20	0
Hershey Sundae Pie	1	300	10	1
MAIN MENU SELECTIONS				
Bacon Cheeseburger	1	400	60	2
Bacon Double Cheeseburger	1	580	110	2

FOOD	PORTION	CALS	CHOL	FIBER
Baguette Santa Fe Fire Grilled Chicken	1	350	45	4
Baguette Savory Mustard Fire Grilled Chicken	1	350	45	3
Baguette Smokey BBQ Fire Grilled Chicken	1	350	45	4
Baja BBQ Sauce	1 serv	14	0	tr
BK Veggie Burger	1	340	0	4
Cheeseburger	1	360	50	2
Chicken Tenders	5 pieces	210	30	tr
Chicken Tenders	8 pieces	340	50	tr
Chili	1 serv	190	25	5
Dipping Sauce Sweet And Sour	1 serv	40	0	0
Double Cheeseburger	1	540	100	2
Double Hamburger	1	450	75	2
Double Whopper	1	980	160	4
Double Whopper w/ Cheese	1	1070	185	4
Dutch Apple Pie	1 serv	340	0	1
French Fries No Salt Added	1 sm	230	0	2
French Fries No Salt Added	1 lg	500	0	5
French Fries Salted	1 sm	230	0	2
French Fries Salted	1 lg	500	0	5
Hamburger	1	310	40	2
Onion Rings	1 sm	180	0	2
Onion Rings	1 lg	480	<5	5
Sandwich BK Fish Filet	1	520	55	2
Sandwich Grilled Chicken Caesar Club	1	540	65	3
Sandwich Original Chicken	1	560	60	3
Sandwich Whopper	1	580	75	4
Whopper	1	710	85	4
Whopper Jr.	1	390	45	2
Whopper Jr. w/ Cheese	1	440	55	2
Whopper w/ Cheese	1	800	110	4
SALAD DRESSINGS AND TOPPINGS				
Breakfast Syrup	1 serv	80	0	0
Dipping Sauce Barbecue	1 serv	35	0	0
Dipping Sauce Honey	1 serv	90	0	0

FOOD	PORTION	CALS	CHOL	FIBER
Dipping Sauce Honey Mustard	1 serv	90	10	0
Dipping Sauce Ranch	1 serv	140	<5	–
Dipping Sauce Zesty Onion Ring	1 serv	150	15	tr
Dressing Kraft Catalina	1 serv	180	0	0
Dressing Kraft Fat Free Ranch	1 serv	60	0	0
Dressing Kraft Ranch	1 serv	220	10	0
Dressing Light Done Right Light Italian	1 serv	50	0	0
Dressing Signature Creamy Caesar	1 serv	140	10	0
Fire Roasted Sauce	1 serv	9	0	tr
Grape Jam	1 serv	30	0	0
Peppers & Onions Flame Roasted	1 serv	18	0	2
Savory Mustard Sauce	1 serv	21	2	tr
Strawberry Jam	1 serv	30	0	0
SALADS				
Chicken Caesar w/o Dressing And Croutons	1 serv	230	60	3
Side Salad w/o Dressing	1 serv	25	0	2

BURGERVILLE
BEVERAGES

FOOD	PORTION	CALS	CHOL	FIBER
Milkshake Black Forest	1 (16 oz)	600	75	–
Milkshake Blackberry	1 (16 oz)	610	100	–
Milkshake Caramel Apple	1 (16 oz)	540	110	–
Milkshake Chocolate	1 (16 oz)	520	95	–
Milkshake Fresh Strawberry	1 (16 oz)	560	85	–
Milkshake Mocha Perk	1 (16 oz)	590	100	–
Milkshake Pumpkin	1 (16 oz)	460	90	–
Milkshake Vanilla	1 (16 oz)	500	85	–
Smoothies Chocolate Monkey	1 (16 oz)	470	0	–
Smoothies Fresh Blackberry	1 (16 oz)	420	0	–
Smoothies Fresh Raspberry	1 (16 oz)	470	0	–
Smoothies Fresh Strawberry	1 (16 oz)	390	0	–

FOOD	PORTION	CALS	CHOL	FIBER
Smoothies Strawberry Splash	1 (16 oz)	310	0	–
Smoothies Triple Berry Blast	1 (16 oz)	360	0	–
BREAKFAST SELECTIONS				
American Cheese	2 slices	90	20	–
Bagel Bacon Egg	1	450	250	–
Bagel Cheese	1	290	10	–
Bagel Ham Egg	1	450	260	–
Bagel Plain	1	310	0	–
Bagel Sausage Egg	1	640	280	–
Biscuit Bacon Egg	1	400	250	–
Biscuit Ham Egg	1	400	260	–
Biscuit Sausage Egg	1	590	280	–
Tillamook Cheese	1 slice	120	40	–
MAIN MENU SELECTIONS				
Cheeseburger	1	370	45	–
Cheeseburger Double Beef	1	470	75	–
Cheeseburger Pepper Bacon	1	680	75	–
Cheeseburger Tillamook	1	630	65	–
Cheeseburger Walla Walla Onion	1	679	80	–
Chicken Strips	5 pieces	550	20	–
Colossal	1	530	35	–
Gardenburger	1	460	30	–
Gardenburger Spicy Black Bean	1	550	40	–
Halibut	3 pieces	230	15	–
Hamburger	1	320	35	–
Onion Rings Walla Walla	3 pieces	485	0	–
Roasted Turkey Salad w/o Hazelnuts	1 serv	375	65	–
Rogue River Blue Cheese Bacon Burger	1	510	70	–
Sandwich Crispy Chicken	1	450	40	–
Sandwich Deluxe Crispy Chicken	1	610	85	–
Sandwich Grilled Chicken	1	350	5	–
Sandwich Halibut	1	490	35	–
Sandwich Turkey Club	1	490	55	–
Side Salad w/o Dressing	1 serv	70	10	–

FOOD	PORTION	CALS	CHOL	FIBER
Smoked Salmon Salad w/o Hazelnuts	1 serv	370	55	–
Sweet Potato Fries	1 serv	530	0	–
Turkey Burger	1	470	75	–

CAPTAIN D'S SEAFOOD

Baked Chicken Dinner	1 serv	350	60	5
Baked Fish Dinner	1 serv	390	10	5
Baked Potato	1 serv	190	0	4
Baked Salmon Dinner	1 serv	470	30	5
Carb Counter Chicken Dinner	1 serv	320	70	6
Carb Counter Fish Dinner	1 serv	350	70	6
Cole Slaw	1 serv	150	5	1
Corn On The Cob	1 serv	150	0	2
Fresh Steamed Broccoli	1 serv	25	0	3
Green Beans	1 serv	90	5	4
Rice Pilaf	1 serv	160	0	1
Shrimp Scampi Dinner	1 serv	370	170	5
Side Salad w/o Dressing	1	30	0	2
Tuscan Style Vegetables	1 serv	30	0	2

CARL'S JR.
BAKED SELECTIONS

Cheese Danish	1	400	15	1
Cheesecake Strawberry Swirl	1 serv	290	55	2
Chocolate Cake	1 serv	300	30	1
Chocolate Chip Cookie	1	350	20	1
Muffin Blueberry	1	340	40	1
Muffin Bran Raisin	1	370	45	6

BEVERAGES

Coca-Cola Classic	1 reg (21 oz)	220	0	0
Coffee	1 reg (12 oz)	2	0	0
Diet Coke	1 reg (21 oz)	tr	0	0
Dr Pepper	1 reg (21 oz)	200	0	0
Hot Chocolate	1 serv (12 oz)	120	0	1
Iced Tea	1 reg (12 oz)	5	0	0
Lemonade Minute Maid Orange	1 reg (21 oz)	200	0	0
Milk 1%	1 (10 fl oz)	150	15	0

FOOD	PORTION	CALS	CHOL	FIBER
Minute Maid Orange Soda	1 reg (21 oz)	200	0	0
Nestea Raspberry	1 reg (21 oz)	160	0	0
Orange Juice	1 (10 oz)	150	0	0
Ramblin' Root Beer	1 reg (21 oz)	220	0	0
Shake Chocolate	1 reg (32 oz)	770	65	tr
Shake Strawberry	1 reg (32 oz)	750	65	0
Shake Vanilla	1 reg (32 oz)	700	70	0
Sprite	1 reg (21 oz)	200	0	0
BREAKFAST SELECTIONS				
Bacon	2 strips	45	10	0
Breakfast Burrito	1	560	495	1
Breakfast Quesadilla	1	370	240	1
English Muffin w/ Margarine	1	210	0	2
French Toast Dips w/o Syrup	1 serv	370	0	1
Grape Jelly	1 serv (0.5 oz)	40	0	0
Hash Brown Nuggets	1 serv	330	0	2
Sausage	1 patty	190	40	0
Scrambed Eggs	1 serv	180	455	0
Sourdough Breakfast	1 serv	410	275	1
Strawberry Jam	1 serv (0.5 oz)	40	0	0
Sunrise Sandwich w/o Meat	1	360	245	tr
Table Syrup	1 serv (1 oz)	90	0	0
MAIN MENU SELECTIONS				
American Cheese	1 sm	50	10	0
BBQ Sauce	1 serv (1.1 oz)	50	0	0
Breadstick	1 (0.3 oz)	35	0	tr
Carl's Famous Star	1	590	70	3
Chicken Stars	6 pieces	260	40	tr
CrissCut Fries	1 serv	410	0	4
Croutons	1 serv (0.5 oz)	30	0	0
Double Sourdough Bacon Cheeseburger	1	880	165	2
Double Western Bacon Cheeseburger	1	920	155	3
Famous Bacon Cheeseburger	1	700	95	3
French Fries	1 kid serv	250	0	2
French Fries	1 med	460	0	5
Hamburger	1	280	35	1
Honey Sauce	1 serv (1 oz)	90	0	0

FOOD	PORTION	CALS	CHOL	FIBER
Mustard Sauce	1 serv (1 oz)	50	0	0
Onion Rings	1 serv	430	0	3
Potato Bacon & Cheese	1	640	40	6
Potato Broccoli & Cheese	1 serv	530	15	6
Potato Plain w/o Margarine	1	290	0	6
Potato Sour Cream & Chives	1	430	10	6
Salsa	1 serv (0.9 oz)	10	0	0
Sandwich Bacon Swiss Crispy Chicken	1	760	90	3
Sandwich Carl's Catch Fish	1	530	80	2
Sandwich Charbroiled Sirloin Stead	1	550	80	2
Sandwich Chargrilled Chicken Club	1	470	95	2
Sandwich Chargrilled Santa Fe Chicken	1	540	95	2
Sandwich Chargrilled BBQ Chicken	1	290	60	2
Sandwich Ranch Crispy Chicken	1	660	70	3
Sandwich Southwest Spicy Chicken	1	620	65	2
Sandwich Spicy Chicken	1	480	40	2
Sandwich Western Bacon Crispy Chicken	1	750	80	3
Sourdough Bacon Cheeseburger	1	640	95	2
Sourdough Ranch Bacon Cheeseburger	1	720	95	3
Super Star	1	790	130	3
Sweet N'Sour Sauce	1 serv (1 oz)	50	0	0
Swiss Cheese	1 serv	50	15	0
Western Bacon Cheeseburger	1	660	85	3
Zucchini	1 serv	320	0	2
SALAD DRESSINGS				
1000 Island	1 serv (2 oz)	230	20	0
Blue Cheese	1 serv (2 oz)	320	25	0
French Fat Free	1 serv (2 oz)	60	0	tr

FOOD	PORTION	CALS	CHOL	FIBER
House	1 serv (2 oz)	220	25	0
Italian Fat Free	1 serv (2 oz)	15	0	0
SALADS				
Salad-To-Go Charbroiled Chicken	1 serv	200	75	4
Salad-To-Go Garden	1	50	5	2

CARVEL
BEVERAGES

FOOD	PORTION	CALS	CHOL	FIBER
Carvelanche w/ Topping	1 (16 oz)	600	95	tr
Regular Fizzlers	1 (16 oz)	340	10	1
Thick Shake Chocolate	1 (16 oz)	720	115	0
Thick Shake Reduced Fat Chocolate	1 (16 oz)	520	35	tr
Thick Shake Reduced Fat Vanilla	1 (16 oz)	460	35	tr
ICE CREAM				
Cake Butterscotch Dream	1 slice (4 oz)	260	25	0
Cake Celebration	1 slice (4 oz)	200	25	tr
Cake Cookies & Cream	1 serv (4 oz)	240	25	1
Cake Fudge Drizzle	1 slice (4 oz)	240	20	1
Cake Game Ball	1 slice (4 oz)	330	40	1
Cake Holiday	1 slice (4 oz)	200	25	tr
Cake Lil'Love	1 piece (4 oz)	200	25	tr
Cake Lil'Love All Vanilla	1 piece (4.4 oz)	330	35	tr
Cake Sinfully Chocolate	1 slice (4 oz)	240	20	1
Cake Strawberries & Cream	1 slice (4 oz)	270	30	1
Chocolate	4 oz	190	25	0
Chocolate No Fat	4 oz	120	0	0
Flying Saucer 98% Fat Free Black Raspberry	1	170	5	tr
Flying Saucer 98% Fat Free Chocolate	1	170	0	1
Flying Saucer 98% Fat Free Coffee	1	190	5	tr
Flying Saucer 98% Fat Free Maple	1	190	5	tr
Flying Saucer 98% Fat Free Mint	1	190	5	tr

FOOD	PORTION	CALS	CHOL	FIBER
Flying Saucer 98% Fat Free Pistachio	1	190	5	tr
Flying Saucer 98% Fat Free Strawberry	1	190	5	1
Flying Saucer 98% Fat Free Vanilla	1	190	5	tr
Flying Saucer Chocolate	1	230	30	2
Flying Saucer Vanilla	1	240	30	tr
Vanilla	4 oz	200	40	0
Vanilla No Fat	4 oz	120	0	0
Vanilla No Sugar Added	4 oz	130	15	0
ICES				
Italian Ice Blue Raspberry	4 oz	70	0	0
Italian Ice Bubble Gum	4 oz	70	0	0
Italian Ice Cherry	4 oz	100	0	0
Italian Ice Chocolate Ice Cream	4 oz	90	7	0
Italian Ice Cotton Candy	4 oz	70	0	0
Italian Ice Lemon	4 oz	70	0	0
Italian Ice Mango	4 oz	70	0	0
Italian Ice Orange	4 oz	70	0	0
Italian Ice Vanilla Ice Cream	4 oz	90	7	0
Italian Ice Watermelon	4 oz	70	0	0
Sherbet All Flavors	4 oz	140	5	0

CHICK-FIL-A
BEVERAGES

FOOD	PORTION	CALS	CHOL	FIBER
Coca-Cola Classic	1 sm	110	0	0
Diet Coke	1 sm	0	0	0
Diet Lemonade	1 sm	25	0	0
Iced Tea Sweetened	1 sm	80	0	0
Iced Tea Unsweetened	1 sm	0	0	0
Lemonade	1 sm	170	0	0
BREAKFAST SELECTIONS				
Bagel Chicken Egg & Cheese	1	500	290	3
Bagel Wheat	1	220	0	2
Biscuit Bacon	1	300	5	1
Biscuit Bacon & Egg	1	390	250	1
Biscuit Bacon Egg Cheese	1	440	265	1
Biscuit Buttered	1	270	0	1

FOOD	PORTION	CALS	CHOL	FIBER
Biscuit Chicken	1	420	35	2
Biscuit Chicken w/ Cheese	1	470	50	2
Biscuit Egg	1	350	240	1
Biscuit Egg Cheese	1	400	255	1
Biscuit Sausage	1	410	20	1
Biscuit Sausage Egg	1	500	265	1
Biscuit Sausage Egg Cheese	1	550	280	1
Biscuit w/ Gravy	1	330	5	1
Burrito Chicken	1	420	270	2
Burrito Sausage	1	460	270	2
Chick-N-Minis	1 serv	270	50	1
Hashbrowns	1 serv	260	5	3
DESSERTS				
Cheesecake	1 slice	340	90	2
Fudge Nut Brownie	1	330	20	2
Icedream Cone	1 sm	160	15	0
Lemon Pie	1 slice	390	30	1
MAIN MENU SELECTIONS				
Carrot & Raisin Salad	1 sm	170	10	2
Chicken Filet	1	230	60	0
Chicken Filet Chargrilled	1	100	65	0
Chick-N-Strips	4	290	65	1
Cole Slaw	1 sm	260	25	2
Cool Wrap Chargrilled Chicken	1	390	65	3
Cool Wrap Chicken Caesar	1	460	80	3
Cool Wrap Spicy Chicken	1	380	60	3
Fruit Cup	1 serv	60	0	2
Hearty Breast of Chicken Soup	1 cup	140	23	1
Nuggets	8	260	70	tr
Polynesian Sauce	1 pkg	110	0	0
Sandwich Chargrilled Chicken	1	270	65	3
Sandwich Chicken	1	410	60	1
Sandwich Chicken Deluxe	1	420	60	2
Sandwich Chicken Salad On Wheat Bread	1	350	65	5
Waffle Fries w/o Salt	1 sm	280	15	4
Waffle Potato Fries	1 sm	270	0	4

FOOD	PORTION	CALS	CHOL	FIBER
SALAD DRESSINGS AND SAUCES				
Barbecue Sauce	1 pkg	45	0	0
Blue Cheese	2 tbsp	150	20	0
Buffalo Sauce	1 pkg	15	0	0
Buttermilk Ranch	2 tbsp	160	5	0
Buttermilk Ranch Sauce	1 pkg	110	5	0
Caesar	2 tbsp	160	30	0
Fat Free Honey Mustard	2 tbsp	60	0	0
Honey Mustard	1 pkg	45	0	0
Honey Roasted BBQ Sauce	1 pkg	60	5	0
Light Italian	2 tbsp	15	0	0
Raspberry Vinaigrette Reduced Fat	2 tbsp	80	0	0
Spicy	2 tbsp	140	5	0
Thousand Island	2 tbsp	150	10	0
SALADS				
Chargrilled Chicken Garden Salad	1 serv	180	65	3
Chick-N-Strips Salad	1 serv	390	80	4
Croutons Garlic & Butter	1 pkg	50	0	0
Honey Roasted Sunflower Kernels	1 pkg	80	0	1
Side Salad	1 serv	60	10	2
Southwest Chargrilled Salad	1 serv	240	60	5
Tortilla Strips	1 pkg	70	0	1
CHIPOTLE				
Barbacoa	1 serv (5 oz)	285	74	–
Black Beans	1 serv (4 oz)	130	0	–
Carnitas	1 serv (4 oz)	227	66	–
Cheese	1 serv (1 oz)	110	30	0
Chicken	1 serv (4 oz)	219	96	–
Chips	1 serv (4 oz)	490	0	5
Crispy Taco Shells	4	240	0	2
Fajita Vegetables	1 serv (3 oz)	100	0	1
Flour Tortilla	1 (6 in)	300	0	2
Flour Tortilla	1 (13 in)	340	0	2
Guacamole	1 serv (4 oz)	170	0	5
Lettuce	1 serv (1 oz)	5	0	tr
Pinto Beans	1 serv (4 oz)	138	0	–

FOOD	PORTION	CALS	CHOL	FIBER
Rice	1 serv (5 oz)	240	0	tr
Salsa Corn	1 serv (4 oz)	100	0	3
Salsa Tomato	1 serv (4 oz)	25	0	1
Sour Cream	1 serv (2 oz)	120	40	0
Steak	1 serv (4 oz)	230	51	–
Tomatillo Green	1 serv (2 oz)	15	0	–
Tomatillo Red	1 serv (2 oz)	28	0	–

CHURCH'S CHICKEN
DESSERTS

Apple Pie	1 pie	280	<5	1
Edward's Double Lemon Pie	1 pie	300	25	0
Edward's Strawberry Cream Cheese Pie	1 pie	280	15	2

MAIN MENU SELECTIONS

Breast	1 serv	200	65	0
Cajun Rice	1 reg	130	5	tr
Chicken Fried Steak w/ White Gravy	1 serv	470	65	1
Cole Slaw	1 reg	92	0	2
Collard Greens	1 reg	25	0	2
Corn On The Cob	1 ear	139	0	9
French Fries	1 reg	210	0	2
Honey Butter Biscuit	1	250	<5	1
Jalapeno Cheese Bombers	4 pieces	240	28	3
Krispy Tender Strips	1 piece	137	25	tr
Leg	1 serv	140	45	0
Macaroni & Cheese	1 reg	210	15	1
Mashed Potatoes & Gravy	1 reg	90	0	1
Okra	1 reg	210	0	4
Sweet Corn Nuggets	1 reg	250	0	2
Tender Crunchers	6-8 pieces	411	74	1
Thigh	1 serv	230	80	0
Whole Jalapeno Peppers	2	10	0	1
Wing	1 serv	250	60	0

SAUCES

BBQ	1 pkg	29	0	0
Creamy Jalapeno	1 pkg	102	10	0
Honey Mustard	1 pkg	111	10	0
Purple Pepper	1 pkg	21	0	0
Sweet & Sour	1 pkg	31	0	0

FOOD	PORTION	CALS	CHOL	FIBER
COLD STONE CREAMERY				
Waffle Cone Dipped	1	310	5	2
Waffle Cone Dipped w/ Candy	1	390	5	2
Waffle Cone Or Bowl	1	160	5	0
FROZEN YOGURT				
Cheesecake	1 serv (6 oz)	170	<5	0
Low Fat Chocolate	1 serv (6 oz)	230	<5	3
Nonfat Coffee	1 serv (6 oz)	220	<5	0
Nonfat Sweet Cream	1 serv (6 oz)	220	<5	0
ICE CREAM				
Amaretto	1 serv (6 oz)	390	95	0
Banana	1 serv (6 oz)	370	85	0
Black Cherry	1 serv (6 oz)	390	90	0
Butter Pecan	1 serv (6 oz)	390	95	0
Cake A Cheesecake Named Desire	1 slice (5 oz)	410	50	0
Cake Batter	1 serv (6 oz)	410	85	0
Cake Butterfinger Bonanza	1 slice (5 oz)	450	50	tr
Cake Celebration Sensation	1 slice (4.5 oz)	350	50	tr
Cake Chocolate Chipper	1 slice (4.6 oz)	450	50	3
Cake Coffeehouse Crunch	1 slice (5 oz)	530	45	2
Cake Cookie Dough Delirium	1 slice (4.8 oz)	420	55	tr
Cake Cookies & Creamery	1 slice (4.5 oz)	390	50	1
Cake Midnight Delight	1 slice (5.3 oz)	510	50	4
Cake Mmmmmmint Chip	1 slice (4.5 oz)	380	45	2
Cake Peanut Butter Playground	1 slice (5 oz)	490	45	4
Cake Raspberry Truffle Temptation	1 slice (5 oz)	480	50	4
Cake Snicker's Supreme	1 slice (5 oz)	510	50	3
Cake Strawberry Passion	1 slice (5 oz)	380	50	1
Cake Zebra Stripes	1 slice (4.8 oz)	400	55	1
Candy Cane	1 serv (6 oz)	420	85	0
Caramel Latte	1 serv (6 oz)	400	85	0
Carrot Cake Batter	1 serv (6 oz)	450	80	0
Cheesecake	1 serv (6 oz)	390	85	0
Chocolate	1 serv (6 oz)	390	90	1
Cinnamon	1 serv (6 oz)	400	95	tr

FOOD	PORTION	CALS	CHOL	FIBER
Coconut	1 serv (6 oz)	390	90	0
Coffee	1 serv (6 oz)	400	95	0
Cookie Batter	1 serv (6 oz)	450	80	0
Cotton Candy	1 serv (6 oz)	390	90	0
Dark Chocolate Peppermint	1 serv (6 oz)	410	90	2
Egg Nog	1 serv (6 oz)	400	90	0
Expresso	1 serv (6 oz)	350	85	0
French Vanilla	1 serv (6 oz)	400	120	0
Irish Cream	1 serv (6 oz)	390	95	0
Macadamia Nut	1 serv (6 oz)	390	95	0
Mango	1 serv (6 oz)	370	85	0
Mint	1 serv (6 oz)	400	90	0
Mocha	1 serv (6 oz)	390	90	1
Oatmeal Batter	1 serv (6 oz)	400	90	0
Orange Dreamsicle	1 serv (6 oz)	380	90	0
Peanut Butter	1 serv (6 oz)	440	85	tr
Pecan Praline	1 serv (6 oz)	400	85	0
Pistachio	1 serv (6 oz)	390	95	0
Pumpkin	1 serv (6 oz)	390	90	0
Raspberry	1 serv	390	90	0
Sinless Sans Fat Sweet Cream	1 serv (6 oz)	160	<5	tr
Strawberry	1 serv (6 oz)	380	90	0
Sweet Cream	1 serv (6 oz)	390	95	0
Vanilla Bean	1 serv (6 oz)	400	90	0
White Chocolate	1 serv (6 oz)	390	90	0
MIX-INS AND TOPPINGS				
Almond Joy	1 piece	180	0	2
Apple Pie Filling	0.75 oz	60	0	1
Banana	½	60	0	1
Black Cherries	0.75 oz	80	0	0
Blackberries	0.75 oz	10	0	1
Blueberries	0.75 oz	10	0	0
Brownies	1 piece	180	5	1
Butterfinger	½ bar	140	0	1
Caramel Topping	1 oz	110	0	0
Cashews	1 oz	170	0	1
Chocolate Chips	1 oz	130	0	0
Cinnamon	⅛ tsp	15	0	3
Coconut	1 oz	80	0	1

FOOD	PORTION	CALS	CHOL	FIBER
Cookie Dough	1 piece	180	10	1
Fat Free Butterscotch	1 oz	80	0	0
Fat Free Caramel	1 oz	80	0	0
Fat Free Fudge	1 oz	80	0	0
Fudge Topping	1 oz	110	0	0
Granola	1 oz	120	0	2
Gumballs	1 oz	120	0	0
Gummi Bears	1 oz	120	0	0
Heath Candy	1 bar	110	0	0
Honey	1 oz	90	0	0
Kit Kat	½ bar	100	0	0
Krackel Candy	½ bar	130	<5	1
M&M's	1 oz	170	<5	1
M&M's Peanut	1 oz	150	<5	1
Macadamia Nuts	1 oz	180	0	2
Maraschino Cherry	1	5	0	0
Marshmallow Creme	1 oz	100	0	0
Marshmallows	1 oz	100	0	0
Nestle Crunch	½ bar	130	<5	1
Nilla Wafers	3	70	5	0
Oreo Cookies	2	120	0	1
Peach Pie Filling	1 oz	60	0	1
Peanut Butter	0.75 oz	150	0	1
Peanuts	1 oz	200	0	3
Pecan Pralines	1 oz	210	0	2
Pecans	1 oz	140	0	1
Pie Crust Graham Cracker	1 oz	110	0	1
Pie Crust Oreo	1 oz	180	0	0
Pistachio Nuts	1 oz	210	0	4
Raisins	1 oz	80	0	1
Raspberries	0.75 oz	15	0	1
Red Hot Candy	1 oz	130	0	0
Reese's Peanut Butter Cup	1 piece	190	0	1
Reese's Pieces	1 oz	170	0	1
Roasted Almonds	1 oz	190	0	3
Sliced Almonds	1 oz	210	0	4
Snickers	½ bar	170	<5	1
Sprinkles Chocolate	1 oz	25	0	0
Sprinkles Rainbow	1 oz	25	0	0
Strawberries	0.75 oz	20	0	1

FOOD	PORTION	CALS	CHOL	FIBER
Toasted Coconut	1 oz	180	0	1
Walnuts	1 oz	130	0	1
Whip Topping	1 serv	50	0	0
White Chocolate Chips	1 oz	160	<5	0
Whoppers	1 oz	100	0	0
Yellow Sponge Cake	1 piece	70	25	0
York Peppermint Patties	2 pieces	120	0	1
SORBET				
Sinless Lemon	1 serv	180	0	0
Sinless Raspberry	1 serv (6 oz)	200	0	0
Sinless Tangerine	1 serv (6 oz)	200	0	0

COLOMBO FROZEN YOGURT

Strawberry Lowfat	½ cup	110	10	0
Strawberry Nonfat	½ cup	100	<5	0

COSI
BEVERAGES

Arctic Double Chi	1 tall (12 oz)	621	72	1
Arctic Latte	1 tall (12 oz)	396	37	0
Arctic Mocha	1 tall (12 oz)	623	0	0
Arctic Raspberry Chai	1 tall (12 oz)	300	26	0
Arctic Thai as prep	1 tall (12 oz)	432	27	0
Caramel Mocha	1 tall (9 oz)	344	78	1
Chai Tea Latte	1 tall (8 oz)	109	16	0
Hot Chocolate	1 tall (12 oz)	436	111	1
Kefir Blueberry	1 (12 oz)	278	15	4
Lemonade	1 (15 oz)	112	0	0
Lemonade Strawberry	1 tall (12 oz)	290	55	1
Smoothie Mango Mania	1 tall (12 oz)	186	33	tr
Smoothie Peach	1 tall (12 oz)	186	33	tr
Smoothie Strawberry Banana	1 tall (12 oz)	186	33	tr
Smores Latte	1 tall (11 oz)	401	71	1
Wildberry Blast	1 tall (12 oz)	186	33	tr
BREAKFAST SELECTIONS				
Bagel Asiago Cheese	1 (6 oz)	327	3	2
Bagel Cinnamon Raisin	1 (6 oz)	438	3	5
Bagel Cranberry Orange	1 (6 oz)	372	3	2
Bagel Everything	1 (5.5 oz)	353	3	3
Bagel Plain	1 (5.5 oz)	326	0	2

FOOD	PORTION	CALS	CHOL	FIBER
Bagel Poppy Seed	1 (5.5 oz)	346	3	3
Cream Cheese Honey Pecan	1 serv (2 oz)	159	53	0
Cream Cheese Plain	1 serv (2 oz)	182	51	0
Cream Cheese Plain Low Fat	1 serv (2 oz)	121	40	0
Cream Cheese Veggie Low Fat	1 serv (2 oz)	113	28	0
Croissant Almond	1	340	35	2
Croissant Butter	1	330	45	1
Croissant Chocolate	1	370	35	2
Fruit Salad	1 serv	216	0	5
Granola Cereal	1 serv	564	16	8
Granola Parfait Peach	1 serv	389	13	3
Granola Parfait Strawberry	1 serv	426	13	4
Muffin Banana Nut	1	480	80	3
Muffin Blueberry	1	440	70	2
Muffin Carrot Raisin	1	470	85	3
Muffin Corn	1	450	75	3
Muffin Lowfat Bran	1	351	40	8
Scones Blueberry	1	410	50	2
DESSERTS				
Apple Tart	1 serv	396	10	4
Blondie Brownie	1	570	65	2
Cheesecake	1 serv	567	62	0
Cheesecake Brownie	1 serv	470	95	1
Cinnamon Apple Pie	1 serv	960	73	4
Cookie Chocolate Chunk	1	480	40	0
Cookie Oatmeal Raisin	1	440	40	0
Ice Cream Double Scoop	1 serv	225	38	0
Sundae	1 med	408	76	1
SALAD DRESSINGS				
Caesar	1 serv (2 oz)	301	77	0
Cosi Vinaigrette	1 serv (2 oz)	357	0	0
Fat Free Balsamic Vinaigrette	1 serv (2 oz)	45	0	0
Lowfat Ginger Soy	1 serv (2 oz)	74	0	1
Pepperanch	1 serv (2 oz)	262	17	0
Reduced Fat Roasted Shallot Sherry Vinaigrette	1 serv (2 oz)	85	0	0
Roasted Shallot Sherry Vinaigrette	1 serv (2 oz)	308	0	0

FOOD	PORTION	CALS	CHOL	FIBER
SALADS				
Bombay Chicken No Dressing	1 serv	176	50	4
Caesar No Dressing	1 serv	182	<5	2
Caesar w/ Grilled Chicken No Dressing	1 serv	340	72	3
Cosi Cobb No Dressing	1 serv	419	135	4
Greek No Dressing	1 serv	236	30	4
Mixed Greens No Dressing	1 serv	46	0	4
Shanghai Chicken No Dressing	1 serv	221	61	5
Signature No Dressing	1 serv	375	38	7
SANDWICHES				
Buffalo Blue	1	649	130	5
Cosi Club	1	729	81	4
Green Market	1	555	16	7
Grilled Chicken T.B.M.	1	791	95	6
Hummus & Fresh Veggies	1	432	0	8
Italiano	1	834	107	4
Melts Bacon Turkey Cheddar	1	682	98	4
Melts Chicken T.B.M.	1	926	182	8
Melts Grilled Chicken Parmesan	1	701	116	8
Melts Pesto Chicken	1	809	150	7
Melts Tomato Basil & Mozzarella	1	666	79	7
Melts Tuna	1	1012	122	4
Polpette Rustica	1	553	38	5
Roasted Turkey & Brie	1	772	111	3
Sesame Ginger Chicken	1	508	81	6
Shrimp Salad	1	471	112	4
Smoked Ham & Brie	1	639	90	3
T.B.M.	1	729	21	6
Tondoori Chicken	1	633	67	4
Tuna Cheddar	1	956	109	4
Turkey Light	1	476	51	4
Turkey Rustica	1	619	101	4
Tuscan Pesto Chicken	1	571	108	6
Vegi Muffaletta	1	824	24	4
Wasabi Roast Beef	1	626	78	5

FOOD	PORTION	CALS	CHOL	FIBER
SOUPS				
Cajun Gumbo	1 serv (10 oz)	251	29	1
Chicken Gumbo	1 serv (6 oz)	151	17	1
Chicken Noodle	1 serv (10 oz)	116	11	1
Grilled Chicken Corn Chowder	1 serv (10 oz)	305	72	2
Lentil	1 serv (10 oz)	199	0	7
Minestrone	1 serv (10 oz)	174	6	4
New England Clam Chowder	1 serv (10 oz)	440	133	1
Three Bean Chili	1 serv (10 oz)	162	0	10
DAIRY QUEEN				
FOOD SELECTIONS				
Chicken Strip Basket	4 pieces	520	40	7
Chili Cheese Dog	1	330	45	2
DQ Homestyle Bacon Double Cheeseburger	1	610	130	2
DQ Homestyle Burger	1	290	45	2
DQ Homestyle Cheeseburger	1	340	55	2
DQ Homestyle Double Cheeseburger	1	540	115	2
DQ Ultimate Burger	1	670	135	2
French Fries	1 sm	300	0	3
Grillburger ½ Lb	1	800	130	2
Grillburger ½ Lb w/ Cheese	1	930	160	2
Grillburger ¼ Lb FlameThrower	1	850	130	1
Grillburger Bacon Cheddar	1	710	105	1
Grillburger California	1	630	75	1
Grillburger Classic	1	540	65	2
Grillburger Classic w/ Cheese	1	610	85	2
Grillburger Mushroom Swiss	1	700	90	1
Hot Dog	1	240	25	1
Onion Rings	1 reg	470	0	3
Salad Crispy Chicken No Dressing	1 serv	350	40	6

FOOD	PORTION	CALS	CHOL	FIBER
Salad Grilled Chicken No Dressing	1 serv	240	65	4
Sandwich Crispy Chicken	1	590	40	5
Sandwich Grilled Chicken	1	340	55	2
Side Salad	1 serv	60	5	2
ICE CREAM				
Banana Split	1	510	30	3
Blizzard Banana Split	1 sm	460	40	tr
Blizzard Chocolate Chip Cookie Dough	1 sm	720	50	0
Blizzard Oreo Cookies	1 sm	570	40	tr
Blizzard Reese's Peanut Butter Cup	1 sm	600	40	0
Blizzard Strawberry Cheesecake	1 sm	530	85	tr
Brownie Earthquake	1	740	50	0
Buster Bar	1	500	15	2
Cake 8 Inch Round	⅛ cake	370	25	tr
Cake Blizzard Oreo Cookie	⅛ cake	490	30	1
Cake Blizzard Reese's Peanut Butter Cup	⅛ cake	490	30	1
Cone Chocolate	1 sm	240	20	0
Cone Vanilla	1 sm	230	20	0
Cone Dipped	1 sm	340	20	1
Dilly Bar Chocolate	1	220	15	0
DQ Fudge Bar No Sugar Added	1	50	0	0
DQ Sandwich	1	200	10	1
DQ Soft Serve Chocolate	½ cup	150	15	0
DQ Soft Serve Vanilla	½ cup	140	15	0
DQ Vanilla Orange Bar No Sugar Added	1	60	0	0
Malt Chocolate	1 sm	640	55	1
MooLatte Cappuccino	1 (16 oz)	490	30	0
MooLatte Caramel	1 (16 oz)	630	35	0
MooLatte French Vanilla	1 (16 oz)	570	30	0
MooLatte Mocha	1 (16 oz)	590	30	1
Peanut Buster Parfait	1	730	35	2
Shake Chocolate	1 sm	560	50	1
Slush Artic Rush	1 sm	220	0	0

FOOD	PORTION	CALS	CHOL	FIBER
Starkiss	1	80	0	0
Sundae Chocolate	1 sm	280	20	0
Sundae Strawberry	1 sm	240	20	0
SALAD DRESSINGS				
Blue Cheese	1 serv (2 oz)	210	5	0
Honey Mustard	1 serv (2 oz)	260	20	0
italian Fat Free	1 serv (2 oz)	10	0	0
Ranch	1 serv (2 oz)	310	25	0

D'ANGELO'S SANDWICH SHOP
CHILDREN'S MENU SELECTIONS

FOOD	PORTION	CALS	CHOL	FIBER
D'Lite Turkey	1 kidz	217	14	3
Sub Cheeseburger	1 kidz	294	43	3
Sub Ham & Cheese	1 kidz	214	27	1
Sub Meatball	1 kidz	330	37	4
Sub Tuna	1 kidz	450	35	1
SALAD DRESSINGS AND TOPPINGS				
Bacon	1 serv	64	15	0
Bleu Cheese	1 serv (1 oz)	152	15	0
Buffalo Sauce	1 serv (1 oz)	10	0	0
Caesar	1 serv (1 oz)	140	15	0
Caesar Fat Free	1 serv (1 oz)	20	0	0
Creamy Italian	1 serv (1 oz)	122	0	0
Cucumbers	3 slices	2	0	tr
Greek Dressing w/ Feta	1 serv (3 oz)	227	14	0
Honey Mustard Dressing	1 serv (1 oz)	150	0	0
Hot Peppers	1 serv	0	0	0
Mayonnaise	2 tbsp	236	21	0
Mayonnaise Fat Free	1 pkg	10	0	0
Mustard Honey Dijon	2 tbsp	60	0	0
Mustard Yellow	2 tbsp	20	0	1
Olive Oil Vinaigrette	1 serv (3 oz)	170	0	0
Olive Oil Blend	2 tbsp	239	0	0
Ranch Lite	1 serv (3 oz)	240	20	1
Sesame Ginger	1 serv (1 oz)	170	0	0
SALADS				
Antipasto Salad w/o Dressing	1 serv	275	38	6
Asian Chicken w/o Dressing	1 serv	224	59	6
Caesar w/ Dressing	1 serv	474	29	3

FOOD	PORTION	CALS	CHOL	FIBER
Chef w/o Dressing	1 serv	273	48	4
Chicken Caesar w/ Dressing	1 serv	532	86	3
Chicken Stir Fry w/o Dressing	1 serv	166	59	4
Cobb w/o Dressing	1 serv	289	76	4
Greek w/o Dressing	1 serv	298	50	4
Lobster w/o Dressing	1 serv	385	101	4
Roast Beef w/o Dressing	1 serv	146	49	4
Tossed Garden w/o Dressing	1 serv	47	0	4
Turkey w/o Dressing	1 serv	157	22	4
SANDWICHES				
D'Lite Chicken Stir Fry	1 sm	426	73	7
D'Lite Fresh Veggie	1	348	13	7
D'Lite Grilled Chicken Breast	1 sm	387	67	6
D'Lite Ham & Cheese	1 sm	351	46	2
D'Lite Roast Beef	1 sm	353	49	6
D'Lite Turkey	1 sm	364	22	6
D'Lite Turkey Cranberry	1 sm	460	22	6
Pokket BLT & Cheese	1 sm	421	50	2
Pokket Caesar Salad	1 sm	643	29	2
Pokket Capacola & Cheese	1 sm	426	50	6
Pokket Cheeseburger	1 sm	481	85	1
Pokket Chicken Caesar Salad	1 sm	701	88	2
Pokket Chicken Club	1 sm	559	97	1
Pokket Chicken Honey Dijon	1 sm	527	108	1
Pokket Chicken Salad	1 sm	705	129	1
Pokket Chicken Stir Fry	1 sm	425	88	1
Pokket Classic Veggie No Cheese	1 sm	238	0	4
Pokket Greek	1 sm	812	50	3
Pokket Grilled Chicken	1 sm	328	67	1
Pokket Ham & Cheese	1 sm	349	60	1
Pokket Ham & Salami	1 sm	412	60	1
Pokket Hamburger	1 sm	422	72	1
Pokket Italian	1 sm	574	88	1
Pokket Lobster	1 sm	568	102	1
Pokket Meatball	1 sm	600	73	3

FOOD	PORTION	CALS	CHOL	FIBER
Pokket Mortadella & Cheese	1 sm	505	73	1
Pokket Seafood Salad	1 sm	532	29	2
Pokket Steak	1 sm	335	59	0
Pokket Steak & Cheese	1 sm	407	74	0
Pokket Tuna	1 sm	791	71	1
Sub Cheeseburger	1 sm	542	86	5
Sub Chicken Club	1 sm	619	97	6
Sub Chicken Honey Dijon	1 sm	587	108	6
Sub Chicken Salad	1 sm	769	130	6
Sub Chicken Stir Fry	1 sm	487	88	6
Sub Classic Veggie	1 sm	465	34	8
Sub Grilled Chicken	1 sm	387	67	6
Sub Ham & Cheese	1 sm	412	60	2
Sub Ham & Salami	1 sm	474	60	2
Sub Hamburger	1 sm	482	73	5
Sub Italian	1 sm	637	88	3
Sub Lobster	1 sm	628	102	5
Sub Meatball	1 sm	663	73	8
Sub Mortadella & Cheese	1 sm	568	73	6
Sub Number 9	1 sm	475	74	5
Sub Pastrami	1 sm	526	91	5
Sub Pepperoni	1 sm	614	76	6
Sub Roast Beef	1 sm	350	49	5
Sub Salad	1 sm	298	0	9
Sub Salami & Cheese	1 sm	597	75	6
Sub Seafood Salad	1	595	29	7
Sub Steak	1 sm	383	59	4
Sub Steak & Cheese	1 sm	455	74	4
Sub Steak Tip	1 sm	486	57	3
Sub Stuffed Turkey	1 sm	1036	36	10
Sub Tuna	1 sm	853	71	2
Sub Turkey	1 sm	361	22	5
Sub Turkey Club	1 sm	360	54	3
Wrap Asian Chicken Salad	1	914	59	9
Wrap BLT & Cheese	1	500	50	3
Wrap Buffalo Chicken Salad	1	778	101	3
Wrap Caesar Salad	1	669	29	4
Wrap Capacola & Cheese	1	451	50	3
Wrap Cheese	1	631	74	3
Wrap Cheeseburger	1	569	86	3

FOOD	PORTION	CALS	CHOL	FIBER
Wrap Chef	1	832	72	5
Wrap Chicken Caesar Salad	1	788	88	4
Wrap Chicken Cobb	1	855	102	4
Wrap Chicken Filet & Bacon	1	643	97	3
Wrap Chicken Honey Dijon	1	619	106	4
Wrap Chicken Salad	1	780	128	3
Wrap Chicken Stir Fry	1	511	88	3
Wrap Classic Veggie	1	490	34	6
Wrap Greek	1	761	50	4
Wrap Grilled Chicken	1	420	67	4
Wrap Ham & Cheese	1	436	60	3
Wrap Ham & Salami	1	499	60	3
Wrap Hamburger	1	509	74	3
Wrap Italian	1	654	88	3
Wrap Lobster	1	766	112	3
Wrap Meatball	1	687	73	5
Wrap Mortadella & Cheese	1	592	73	3
Wrap Number 9	1	494	74	3
Wrap Pastrami	1	550	91	2
Wrap Pepperoni	1	638	76	3
Wrap Roast Beef	1	374	49	3
Wrap Salad	1	322	0	6
Wrap Salami & Cheese	1	605	72	3
Wrap Seafood Salad	1	619	29	4
Wrap Steak	1	402	59	2
Wrap Steak & Cheese	1	474	74	2
Wrap Steak Tip	1	374	57	2
Wrap Tuna	1	881	71	3
Wrap Turkey	1	385	22	3
Wrap Turkey Club	1	435	54	3
SOUPS				
#9 Steak & Cheese	1 sm	280	65	1
Chicken Noodle	1 sm	130	50	1
Hearty Vegetable	1 sm	40	0	2
Lobster Bisque	1 sm	360	105	0
New England Clam Chowder	1 sm	270	70	1
Santa Fe Chipotle Vegetable	1 sm	130	0	8
Shrimp & Roasted Corn	1 sm	250	65	2
Thanksgiving Everyday	1 sm	250	55	2

FOOD	PORTION	CALS	CHOL	FIBER
DELTACO				
BEVERAGES				
Barq's Root Beer	1 sm	278	0	0
Classic Coke	1 sm	248	0	0
Diet Coke	1 sm	2	0	0
Iced Tea	1 sm	0	0	0
Light Lemonade Minute Maid	1 sm	13	0	0
Milk 2% Low Fat	1 serv	152	24	0
Mr. Pibb Xtra	1 sm	243	0	0
Orange Juice	1 serv	140	0	1
Shake Chocolate	1 (15 oz)	680	45	1
Shake Strawberry	1 (15 oz)	540	40	1
Shake Vanilla	1 (15 oz)	550	50	0
Sprite	1 sm	243	0	0
BREAKFAST SELECTIONS				
Burrito Breakfast	1	250	160	1
Burrito Egg & Cheese	1	450	530	3
Burrito Macho Bacon & Egg	1	1030	790	6
Burrito Steak & Egg	1	580	560	3
Hash Brown Sticks	5 pieces	250	0	0
Quesadilla Bacon & Egg	1	450	260	2
Side of Bacon	2 strips	50	10	0
MAIN MENU SELECTIONS				
Beans 'n Cheese Cup	1 serv	260	5	16
Bun Taco	1	440	65	4
Burrito Del Beef	1	550	90	3
Burrito Del Classic Chicken	1	560	70	3
Burrito Del Combo	1	530	55	11
Burrito Deluxe Combo	1	570	60	12
Burrito Deluxe Del Beef	1	590	95	4
Burrito Green Bean & Cheese	1	280	15	6
Burrito Green Half Pound	1	430	20	13
Burrito Macho Beef	1	1170	190	7
Burrito Macho Chicken	1	930	100	16
Burrito Macho Combo	1	1050	115	17
Burrito Red Bean & Cheese	1	270	15	6
Burrito Red Half Pound	1	430	20	13
Burrito Spicy Chicken	1	480	40	8

FOOD	PORTION	CALS	CHOL	FIBER
Burrito Works Chicken	1	520	65	4
Burrito Works Steak	1	590	70	5
Burrito Works Veggie	1	490	25	9
Burritos Crispy Fish	1	497	48	2
Cheeseburger	1	330	35	3
Cheeseburger Double Del	1	560	85	4
Cheeseburger Double Del Bacon	1	610	95	4
Chips & Salsa	1 sm	156	0	1
Del Cheeseburger	1	430	45	4
Fries	1 sm	350	0	3
Fries Chili Cheese	1 serv	670	45	5
Fries Deluxe Chili Cheese	1 serv	710	50	6
Hamburger	1	280	25	3
Nachos	1 serv	380	5	2
Nachos Macho	1 serv	1100	55	15
Quesadilla Cheddar	1	500	75	2
Quesadilla Spicy Jack	1	490	75	2
Quesadilla Spicy Jack Chicken	1	570	105	2
Quesadillas Chicken Cheddar	1	580	104	2
Rice Cup	1 serv	140	2	1
Taco	1	160	20	1
Taco Big Fat	1	320	35	3
Taco Big Fat Chicken	1	340	45	3
Taco Big Fat Steak	1	390	45	3
Taco Came Asada	1	237	25	2
Taco Crispy Fish	1	290	20	2
Taco Del Carbon Chicken	1	170	30	2
Taco Del Carbon Steak	1	220	30	2
Taco Macho	1	504	107	5
Taco Soft	1	160	20	1
Taco Soft Chicken	1	210	30	1
SALADS				
Deluxe Chicken Salad	1 serv	740	70	15
Taco Salad	1 serv	350	45	2
Taco Salad Deluxe	1	780	80	14

FOOD	PORTION	CALS	CHOL	FIBER
DENNY'S				
BEVERAGES				
2% Milk	10 oz	151	22	0
Apple Juice	1 reg	126	0	0
Cappuccino French Vanilla	8 oz	100	0	1
Cappuccino Original	8 oz	100	0	0
Chocolate Milk	10 oz	235	37	0
Grapefruit	1 serv (10 oz)	162	0	0
Hot Chocolate	8 oz	100	0	1
Lemonade	16 oz	150	0	0
Malted Milk Shake Chocolate Or Vanilla	12 oz	583	100	tr
Orange Juice	10 oz	126	0	0
Raspberry Ice Tea	16 oz	78	0	0
Tomato Juice	1 serv (10 oz)	56	0	2
BREAKFAST SELECTIONS				
All American Slam	1 serv	816	828	1
Applesauce	1 serv	60	0	1
Bacon	4 strips	162	36	0
Bagel Dry	1	235	0	0
Banana	1	110	0	4
Belgian Waffle	1	619	274	0
Breakfast Dagwood	1 serv	1446	765	1
Buttermilk Hotcakes	3	466	47	2
Cantaloup	¼	32	0	1
Chicken Fajita Skillet	1 serv	855	515	11
Corned Beef Hash Slam	1 serv	668	535	1
Country Fish Potatoes	1 serv	394	9	10
Egg	1	120	210	0
English Muffin Dry	1	125	0	1
Fabulous French Toast	1 serv	1146	297	3
Farmer's Slam	1 serv	1200	704	3
French Slam	1 serv	1119	705	3
Fruit Mix	1 serv	36	0	1
Grand Slam Slugger	1 serv	927	476	3
Grapefruit	½	60	0	6
Grapes	1 serv	55	0	1
Grits	1 serv	80	0	0
Ham & Cheddar Omelette	1 serv	595	783	0

FOOD	PORTION	CALS	CHOL	FIBER
Ham & Cheese Omelette w/ Eggbeaters	1 serv	468	58	0
Ham Slice	1	94	23	0
Hashed Browns	1 serv	197	0	2
Hashed Browns Covered	1 serv	280	23	2
Hashed Browns Covered & Smothered	1 serv	493	29	3
Honeydew	¼	31	0	1
Lumberjack Slam w/ Hash Browns	1 serv	1035	589	3
Meat Lover's Skillet	1 serv	1031	528	10
Moon Over My Hammy	1 serv	841	580	2
Oatmeal	1 serv	100	0	3
Oatmeal Deluxe	1 serv	460	11	7
Original Grand Slam	1 serv	665	515	2
Ready To Eat Cereal	1 serv	100	0	1
Sausage	4 links	354	64	0
Scram Slam	1 serv	827	801	1
Senior Belgian Waffle Slam	1 serv	399	302	0
Senior Omelette	1 serv	429	515	2
Sirloin Steak & Eggs	1 serv	675	643	1
Slim Slam	1 serv	438	50	2
T-Bone Steak & Eggs	1 serv	991	657	1
Toast Dry	1 slice	92	0	1
Two Egg Breakfast w/ Hash Browns	1 serv	825	538	2
Ultimate Omelette	1 serv	611	756	3
Veggie Cheese Omelette	1 serv	494	747	2
CHILDREN'S MENU SELECTIONS				
Burgerlicious	1 serv	296	28	1
Burgerlicious w/ Cheese	1 serv	341	40	1
Dennysaur Chicken Nuggets	1 serv	190	30	0
Frenchtastic Slam	1 serv	452	311	1
Junior Fish & Chips	1 serv	698	46	4
Junior Grand Slam	1 serv	397	230	1
Junior Shrimps Ahoy!	1 serv	411	66	4
Oreo Blender Blaster	1 serv	580	87	1
Pizza Party	1 serv	400	10	7
Smiley-Face Hotcakes w/ Meat	1 serv	463	38	2

FOOD	PORTION	CALS	CHOL	FIBER
Smiley-Face Hotcakes w/o Meat	1 serv	344	13	2
The Big Cheese	1 serv	334	24	2
DESSERTS				
Apple Pie	1 serv	470	0	1
Banana Split	1	894	78	6
Carrot Cake	1 serv	799	125	2
Cheesecake	1 serv	580	174	0
Chocolate Topping	1 serv	317	0	0
Chocolate Peanut Butter Pie	1 serv	653	27	3
Double Scoop Sundae	1 serv	375	74	0
Float Rootbeer or Coke	12 oz	280	39	0
Hot Fudge Brownie A La Mode	1 serv	997	14	6
Milkshake Vanilla Or Chocolate	12 oz	560	100	tr
Oreo Blender Blaster	1 serv	895	135	2
Single Scoop Sundae	1 serv	188	37	0
MAIN MENU SELECTIONS				
Albacore Tuna Melt	1 serv	640	109	3
Applesauce	1 serv	60	0	1
Bacon Lettuce & Tomato	1	610	35	2
Baked Potato Plain	1	220	0	5
BBQ Chicken Sandwich	1 serv	1089	103	5
Bread Stuffing Plain	1 serv	100	0	1
Buffalo Chicken Sandwich	1 serv	708	74	5
Buffalo Chicken Strips	5 pieces	734	96	0
Buffalo Wings	12 pieces	856	500	1
Burger Bacon Cheddar	1	875	163	5
Burger BBQ	1 serv	953	136	4
Burger Boca	1 serv	601	14	9
Burger Classic	1	694	100	4
Burger Classic w/ Cheese	1	852	140	4
Burger Mushroom Swiss	1 serv	880	137	5
Carrots In Honey Glaze	1 serv	80	0	3
Chicken Strips	5 pieces	720	95	0
Chicken Ranch Melt	1 serv	758	105	3
Chicken Strips	1 serv	635	95	0
Club Sandwich	1	718	75	3
Coleslaw	1 serv	274	37	2

FOOD	PORTION	CALS	CHOL	FIBER
Corn In Butter Sauce	1 serv	120	5	5
Cottage Cheese	1 serv	72	10	0
Country Fried Steak	1 serv	644	89	11
Fish & Chips Dinner	1 serv	955	97	6
French Fries Unsalted	1 serv	423	0	5
Fried Shrimp Dinner	1 serv	219	133	1
Fried Shrimp & Shrimp Scampi	1 serv	346	241	1
Green Beans w/ Bacon	1 serv	60	5	3
Grilled Cheese Sandwich	1	510	54	3
Grilled Chicken Dinner	1 serv	130	67	0
Grilled Chicken Sandwich	1	469	77	4
Ham & Swiss On Rye	1	417	57	5
Herb Toast	1 serv	170	tr	1
Hoagie Chicken Melt	1	751	93	2
Hoagie Philly Melt	1 serv	874	114	5
Mashed Potatoes Plain	1 serv	168	8	2
Mozzarella Sticks	8 pieces	710	48	6
Onion Rings	1 serv	381	6	1
Patty Melt	1	798	127	4
Pot Roast Dinner w/ Gravy	1 serv	292	87	0
Roast Turkey & Stuffing w/ Gravy	1 serv	388	116	2
Sampler	1 serv	1405	75	4
Seasoned Fries	1 serv	261	0	0
Senior Chicken Strip Dinner	1 serv	285	37	0
Senior Club	1 serv	540	89	3
Senior Country Fried Steak	1 serv	341	44	6
Senior Fish & Chips	1 serv	756	67	6
Senior French Slam	1 serv	820	432	1
Senior Fried Shrimp Dinner	1 serv	129	66	1
Senior Grilled Chicken Breast	1 serv	200	67	1
Senior Pot Roast	1 serv	160	48	0
Senior Starter	1 serv	544	245	2
Senior Turkey & Stuffing	1 serv	220	60	1
Shrimp Scampi Skillet Dinner	1 serv	289	192	tr
Sirloin Steak Dinner	1 serv	337	687	1
Sliced Tomatoes	3 slices	13	0	1

FOOD	PORTION	CALS	CHOL	FIBER
Smoothered Cheese Fries	1 serv	767	78	0
Steak & Shrimp Dinner	1 serv	645	150	2
T-Bone Steak Dinner	1 serv	860	196	0
The Super Bird Sandwich	1	620	60	2
Turkey Breast On Multigrain w/o Mayo	1	277	15	5
SALAD DRESSINGS AND TOPPINGS				
BBQ Sauce	1.5 oz	47	0	0
Bleu Cheese	1 oz	163	20	0
Blueberry Topping	1 serv	71	0	0
Caesar	1 oz	133	2	0
Cherry Topping	1 serv	57	0	0
Cream Cheese	1 oz	100	31	0
French	1 oz	106	7	0
Fudge Topping	1 serv	201	3	1
Gravy Brown	1 serv	13	0	0
Gravy Chicken	1 serv	14	2	0
Gravy Country	1 serv	17	0	0
Honey Mustard	1 serv	160	20	0
Low Calorie Italian	1 oz	15	0	0
Marinara Sauce	1 serv	48	0	1
Ranch	1 oz	129	8	0
Ranch Fat Free	1 serv	25	0	0
Sour Cream	1.5 oz	91	19	0
Strawberry Topping	1 serv	77	0	1
Syrup	3 tbsp	143	0	0
Syrup Sugar Free	1 serv	23	0	0
Tartar Sauce	1 serv	225	15	0
Thousand Island	1 oz	118	15	0
Thousand Island	2 tbsp	170	15	0
Whipped Margarine	1 serv	87	0	0
Whipped Cream	2 tbsp	23	7	0
SALADS				
Garden Salad w/ Albacore Tuna	1 serv	444	81	4
Garden Salad w/ Fried Chicken Strips	1 serv	438	78	4
Garden Salad w/ Grilled Chicken Breast	1 serv	264	89	4

FOOD	PORTION	CALS	CHOL	FIBER
Grilled Chicken Caesar Salad w/ Dressing	1 serv	600	101	4
Side Caesar w/ Dressing	1 serv	362	23	3
Side Garden Salad w/o Dressing	1 serv	113	0	3
SOUPS				
Chicken Noodle	1 serv	60	10	0
Clam Chowder	1 serv	624	5	4
Cream Of Broccoli	1 serv	574	0	2
Vegetable Beef	1 serv	79	5	2

DESERT MOON CAFE
CHILDREN'S MENU SELECTIONS

FOOD	PORTION	CALS	CHOL	FIBER
Burrito Bean & Cheese	1 serv	650	30	6
Kids Nachos	1 serv	500	25	2
Kids Taco w/ Chicken	1	280	30	2
Kids Taco w/ Steak	1	290	30	2
Kidsadilla	1 serv	630	50	1
MAIN MENU SELECTIONS				
Alamo Burger	1	810	160	3
Burrito Adobe Moon w/ Chicken	1	730	65	4
Burrito Adobe Moon w/ Steak	1	750	70	4
Burrito Black Bean w/ Chicken	1	770	85	5
Burrito Black Bean w/ Steak	1	790	85	5
Burrito Full Moon w/ Chicken	1	620	70	7
Burrito Full Moon w/ Steak	1	640	75	7
Burrito Get It Smothered	1	120	30	0
Burrito Harvest Wrap w/ Chicken	1	620	65	6
Burrito Harvest Wrap w/ Steak	1	300	70	6
Enchilada Mesa	1	710	105	4
Enchilada Queso	1	730	105	4
Enchilada Shrimp	1	830	110	4
Fajita Platter w/ Chicken	1 serv	1160	165	13

FOOD	PORTION	CALS	CHOL	FIBER
Fajita Platter w/ Shrimp	1 serv	1060	175	13
Fajita Platter w/ Steak	1	1190	165	13
Hell Canyon Chili	1 serv	260	45	3
Mucho Nachos	1 serv	800	80	5
Mucho Nachos w/ Chicken	1 serv	900	130	5
Mucho Nachos w/ Steak	1 serv	920	130	5
Pizza Texas BBQ	1	330	125	2
Quesadilla Baja Chicken	1	650	150	2
Quesadilla Coyote w/ Chicken	1	660	105	2
Quesadilla Coyote w/ Steak	1	680	105	2
Quesadilla Sonoran	1	660	50	5
Rice Bowl Black Bean w/ Chicken	1 serv	790	75	4
Rice Bowl Black Bean w/ Steak	1 serv	820	80	4
Rice Bowl Chili w/ Chicken	1 serv	760	90	2
Rice Bowl Chili w/ Steak	1 serv	790	95	2
Rice Bowl Shrimp Creole	1 serv	910	300	3
Shrimp Dippers	1 serv	430	85	4
Soup Black Bean	1 serv	360	15	10
Soup Tortilla	1 serv	330	15	5
Taco Acapulco Shrimp	1	230	35	2
Taco Classic w/ Chicken	1	190	35	2
Taco Classic w/ Steak	1	200	35	2
Taco Fajita w/ Chicken	1	200	35	2
Taco Fajita w/ Steak	1	210	35	2
SALAD DRESSINGS AND SAUCES				
BBQ Sauce	1 serv (1 oz)	50	0	0
Buffalo Wing Sauce	1 serv (1 oz)	45	0	0
Dressing Bleu Cheese	1 serv (2 oz)	300	30	0
Dressing Creamy Caesar	1 serv (2 oz)	320	30	0
Dressing Honey Dijon Fat Free	1 serv (2 oz)	80	0	2
Dressing Lite Ranch	1 serv (2 oz)	150	10	0
Dressing Lite Raspberry Vinaigrette	1 serv (2 oz)	150	0	0
Dressing Poblano	1 serv (1 oz)	150	10	1
Guacamole	1 serv (2 oz)	100	0	3
Pepper Cream Sauce	1 serv (2 oz)	100	30	0

FOOD	PORTION	CALS	CHOL	FIBER
Pico De Gallo	1 serv (2 oz)	15	0	1
Salsa Black Bean	1 serv (2 oz)	20	0	1
Salsa Fruit	1 serv (2 oz)	60	0	0
Salsa Mild Tomato	1 serv (2 oz)	15	0	1
Salsa Rattlesnake	1 serv (2 oz)	15	0	1
SALADS W/O TORTILLA BOWL				
Caesar	1 serv	530	50	4
Caesar w/ Chicken	1 serv	640	100	4
Caesar w/ Shrimp	1 serv	570	110	4
Chopped Chicken	1 serv	520	95	5
Taco w/ Chicken	1 serv	310	95	3
Taco w/ Steak	1 serv	340	95	3
DOMINO'S PIZZA				
12 INCH MEDIUM PIZZAS				
Deep Dish Cheese Only	2 slices	482	30	3
Hand Tossed America's Favorite Feast	1 serv	508	49	4
Hand Tossed Bacon Cheeseburger Feast	2 slices	549	60	3
Hand Tossed Barbeque Feast	2 slices	506	46	3
Hand Tossed Cheese Only	2 slices	375	23	3
Hand Tossed Deluxe Feast	2 slices	465	40	3
Hand Tossed ExtravaganZZa Feast	2 slices	576	64	4
Hand Tossed Hawaiian Feast	2 slices	450	41	3
Hand Tossed MeatZZa Feast	2 slices	560	64	3
Hand Tossed Pepperoni Feast	2 slices	534	57	3
Hand Tossed Vegi Feast	2 slices	439	34	4
Thin Crust Cheese	¼ pie	273	23	2
Toppings Pineapple	1 serv	12	0	tr
DESSERTS				
Cinna Stix	1 serv	111	0	1
Sweet Icing	1 serv	283	0	0
MAIN MENU SELECTIONS				
Breadstick	1	116	0	1

FOOD	PORTION	CALS	CHOL	FIBER
Buffalo Chicken Kickers	1 piece	47	9	tr
Buffalo Wings Barbeque	1 piece	50	25	tr
Buffalo Wings Hot	1 piece	45	26	tr
Cheesy Bread	1 piece	142	6	1
TOPPINGS				
Blue Cheese	1 serv	223	20	tr
Hot Sauce	1 serv	14	0	tr
Medium Pizza Anchovies	1 serv	34	14	0
Medium Pizza Bacon	1 serv	102	15	0
Medium Pizza Banana Peppers	1 serv	5	0	0
Medium Pizza Beef	1 serv	78	15	tr
Medium Pizza Cheddar Cheese	1 serv	57	15	0
Medium Pizza Extra Cheese	1 serv	49	11	tr
Medium Pizza Green Olives	1 serv	19	0	tr
Medium Pizza Green Peppers	1 serv	4	0	tr
Medium Pizza Ham	1 serv	23	9	0
Medium Pizza Italian Sausage	1 serv	77	16	tr
Medium Pizza Mushrooms	1 serv	6	0	tr
Medium Pizza Onion	1 serv	5	0	tr
Medium Pizza Pepperoni	1 serv	74	15	tr
Medium Pizza Ripe Olives	1 serv	21	0	1
Ranch	1 serv	197	9	tr

DONATOS PIZZA

PIZZA

FOOD	PORTION	CALS	CHOL	FIBER
Dessert Apple	¼ pie	722	21	15
Dessert Cherry	¼ pie	818	20	13
Original	¼ pie	660	54	6
Original Chicken Vegy Medley	¼ pie	500	80	11
Original Chicken Vegy Medley No Cheese	¼ pie	392	56	11
Original Founders	¼ pie	737	134	10
Original Hawaiian	¼ pie	620	60	4
Original Hawaiian No Cheese	¼ pie	411	46	11

FOOD	PORTION	CALS	CHOL	FIBER
Original Mariachi Beef	¼ pie	613	81	11
Original Mariachi Chicken	¼ pie	580	94	11
Original Serious Cheese	¼ pie	640	140	6
Original Serious Meat	¼ pie	817	136	10
Original Vegy	¼ pie	564	60	12
Original Vegy No Cheese	¼ pie	370	21	12
Original Works	¼ pie	729	106	12
Traditional Chicken Vegy Medley	¼ pie	647	62	4
Traditional Founders	¼ pie	900	112	3
Traditional Hawaiian	¼ pie	794	74	4
Traditional Mariachi Beef	¼ pie	797	68	4
Traditional Mariachi Chicken	¼ pie	770	79	4
Traditional Original	¼ pie	928	121	9
Traditional Serious Cheese	¼ pie	830	123	12
Traditional Serious Meat	¼ pie	977	118	3
Traditional Vegy	¼ pie	752	49	5
Traditional Works	¼ pie	892	90	5
SALAD DRESSINGS				
Italian	1 serv (1.5 oz)	230	0	0
Italian Lite	1 serv (1.5 oz)	20	0	0
SALADS				
Grilled Chicken w/o Dressing	1 serv	314	71	5
Italian Chef w/o Dressing	1 serv	338	72	5
Side w/o Dressing	1 serv	106	16	2
SIDE ORDERS				
Breadsticks	2	220	0	0
Chicken Wings Hot	5	449	286	tr
Chicken Wings Mild	5	451	286	tr
Three Cheese Garlic Bread	1 bun	605	38	3
SUBS				
Big Don Italian	1 serv	705	85	3
Big Don Lite Italian	1 serv	631	84	3
Grilled Chicken	1 serv	786	71	3
Ham & Cheese Italian	1 serv	609	86	3
Ham & Cheese Lite Italian	1 serv	534	85	3
Southwest Turkey	1 serv	710	70	3
Steak & Cheese	1 serv	929	111	3

FOOD	PORTION	CALS	CHOL	FIBER
Vegy Italian	1 serv	730	38	6
Vegy Lite Italian	1 serv	661	38	6

DUNKIN' DONUTS
BAGELS AND CREAM CHEESE

FOOD	PORTION	CALS	CHOL	FIBER
Bagel Blueberry	1	330	0	2
Bagel Cinnamon Raisin	1	330	0	3
Bagel Everything	1	370	0	3
Bagel Harvest	1	350	0	7
Bagel Onion	1	320	0	3
Bagel Plain	1	320	0	2
Bagel Poppyseed	1	370	0	3
Bagel Reduced Carb w/ Cheese	1	380	20	14
Bagel Salsa	1	310	0	2
Bagel Salt	1	370	0	2
Bagel Sesame	1	380	0	3
Bagel Wheat	1	330	0	4
Cream Cheese Chive	2 oz	170	45	2
Cream Cheese Garden Vegetable	2 oz	170	45	0
Cream Cheese Lite	2 oz	110	30	0
Cream Cheese Plain	2 oz	190	55	0
Cream Cheese Salmon	2 oz	170	45	0
Cream Cheese Strawberry	2 oz	190	45	0

BAKED SELECTIONS

FOOD	PORTION	CALS	CHOL	FIBER
Apple Fritter	1	300	0	1
Biscuit	1	250	0	1
Bismark Chocolate Iced	1	340	0	1
Coffee Roll	1	270	0	1
Coffee Roll Chocolate Frosted	1	290	0	1
Coffee Roll Maple Frosted	1	290	0	1
Coffee Roll Vanilla Frosted	1	290	0	1
Cookie Chocolate Chunk	2	220	35	1
Cookie Chocolate Chunk w/ Walnuts	2	230	35	1
Cookie Oatmeal Raisin Pecan	2	220	30	1

FOOD	PORTION	CALS	CHOL	FIBER
Cookie White Chocolate Chunk	2	230	35	1
Croissant Plain	1	330	5	0
Danish Apple	1	330	30	1
Danish Cheese	1	340	35	1
Danish Strawberry Cheese	1	320	30	1
Donut Apple Crumb	1	230	0	1
Donut Apple Crumb Cake	1	290	15	1
Donut Apple N' Spice	1	200	0	1
Donut Bavarian Kreme	1	210	0	1
Donut Black Raspberry	1	210	0	1
Donut Blueberry	1	290	10	1
Donut Blueberry Crumb	1	240	0	1
Donut Boston Kreme	1	240	0	1
Donut Bow Tie	1	300	0	1
Donut Chocolate Coconut	1	300	0	1
Donut Chocolate Frosted	1	360	25	1
Donut Chocolate Glazed	1	290	0	1
Donut Chocolate Kreme Filled	1	270	0	1
Donut Cinnamon	1	330	25	1
Donut Double Chocolate	1	310	0	2
Donut Frosted Lemon	1	240	0	0
Donut Glazed	1	180	0	1
Donut Glazed Ginerbread	1	260	20	1
Donut Glazed Lemon	1	240	0	0
Donut Jelly Filled	1	210	0	1
Donut Lemon Burst	1	300	0	3
Donut Maple Frosted	1	210	0	1
Donut Marble Frosted	1	200	0	1
Donut Old Fashioned	1	300	25	1
Donut Powdered	1	330	25	1
Donut Strawberry	1	210	0	1
Donut Strawberry Frosted	1	210	0	1
Donut Sugar Raised	1	170	0	1
Donut Vanilla Kreme Filled	1	270	0	1
Donut Whole Wheat Glazed	1	310	0	2
Eclair	1	270	0	1
English Muffin	1	160	0	2
French Cruller	1	150	20	1

FOOD	PORTION	CALS	CHOL	FIBER
Fritter Glazed	1	260	0	1
Muffin Banana Walnut	1	540	65	3
Muffin Blueberry	1	470	60	2
Muffin Chocolate Chip	1	630	70	2
Muffin Coffee Cake	1	580	65	1
Muffin Corn	1	510	75	1
Muffin Cranberry Orange	1	440	65	3
Muffin Honey Bran Raisin	1	480	60	5
Muffin Reduced Fat Blueberry	1	400	60	3
Munchkins Chocolate Glazed	3	200	0	1
Munchkins Cinnamon	4	270	25	1
Munchkins Glazed	3	280	20	1
Munchkins Jelly Filled	5	210	0	1
Munchkins Lemon Filled	4	170	0	0
Munchkins Plain	4	270	25	1
Munchkins Powdered	4	270	25	1
Munchkins Sugar Raised	7	220	0	1
Stick Cinnamon	1	450	35	1
Stick Glazed	1	490	35	1
Stick Glazed Chocolate	1	470	0	2
Stick Jelly	1	530	35	1
Stick Plain	1	420	35	1
Stick Powdered	1	450	35	1
BEVERAGES				
Cappuccino	1 (10 oz)	60	20	0
Cappuccino w/ Soy Milk	1 (10 oz)	70	0	1
Cappuccino w/ Soy Milk Sugar	1 (10 oz)	120	0	1
Cappuccino w/ Sugar	1 (10 oz)	130	15	0
Coffee Blueberry	1 (10 oz)	20	0	0
Coffee Caramel	1 (10 oz)	20	0	0
Coffee Chocolate	1 (10 oz)	20	0	0
Coffee Cinnamon	1 (10 oz)	20	0	0
Coffee Coconut	1 (10 oz)	20	0	0
Coffee French Vanilla	1 (10 oz)	20	0	0
Coffee Hazelnut	1 (10 oz)	20	0	0
Coffee Marshmallow	1 (10 oz)	20	0	0
Coffee Regular	1 (10 oz)	15	0	0

FOOD	PORTION	CALS	CHOL	FIBER
Coffee Toasted Almond	1 (10 oz)	20	0	0
Coffee w/ Cream	1 (10 oz)	70	20	0
Coffee w/ Cream Sugar	1 (10 oz)	120	20	0
Coffee w/ Milk	1 (10 oz)	35	5	0
Coffee w/ Milk Sugar	1 (10 oz)	80	5	0
Coffee w/ Skim Milk	1 (10 oz)	25	0	0
Coffee w/ Skim Milk Sugar	1 (10 oz)	70	0	0
Coffee w/ Sugar	1 (10 oz)	60	0	0
Coolatta Lemonade	1 (16 oz)	240	0	0
Coolatta Strawberry Fruit	1 (16 oz)	290	0	1
Coolatta Tropicana Orange	1	370	0	3
Coolatta Vanilla Bean	1 (16 oz)	440	0	1
Coolatta Coffee w/ 2% Milk	1 (16 oz)	190	10	0
Coolatta Coffee w/ Cream	1 (16 oz)	350	75	0
Coolatta Coffee w/ Milk	1 (16 oz)	210	15	0
Coolatta Coffee w/ Skin Milk	1 (16 oz)	170	0	0
Dunkaccino	1 (10 oz)	230	5	0
Expresso	1 (2 oz)	0	0	0
Expresso w/ Sugar	1 (2 oz)	30	0	0
Hot Chocolate	1 (10 oz)	220	0	2
Iced Coffee	1 (16 oz)	15	0	0
Iced Coffee w/ Cream	1 (16 oz)	70	20	0
Iced Coffee w/ Cream Sugar	1 (16 oz)	120	20	0
Iced Coffee w/ Milk	1 (16 oz)	35	5	0
Iced Coffee w/ Milk Sugar	1 (16 oz)	80	5	0
Iced Coffee w/ Skim Milk	1 (16 oz)	25	0	0
Iced Coffee w/ Skim Milk Sugar	1 (16 oz)	70	0	0
Iced Coffee w/ Sugar	1 (16 oz)	60	0	0
Iced Latte	1 (16 oz)	120	25	0
Iced Latte Caramel Creme	1 (16 oz)	260	20	0
Iced Latte Caramel Swirl	1 (16 oz)	240	25	0
Iced Latte Caramel Swirl w/ Skim Milk	1 (16 oz)	180	0	0
Iced Latte Lite	1 (16 oz)	80	0	0
Iced Latte Mocha Almond	1 (16 oz)	290	20	1
Iced Latte Mocha Swirl	1 (16 oz)	240	25	1
Iced Latte Mocha Swirl w/ Skim Milk	1 (16 oz)	180	0	1
Iced Latte w/ Skim Milk	1 (16 oz)	70	0	0

FOOD	PORTION	CALS	CHOL	FIBER
Iced Latte w/ Skim Milk Sugar	1 (16 oz)	120	0	0
Iced Latte w/ Sugar	1 (16 oz)	170	25	0
Latte	1 (10 oz)	120	25	0
Latte Caramel Creme	1 (10 oz)	260	20	0
Latte Caramel Swirl	1 (10 oz)	230	25	0
Latte Caramel Swirl w/ Soy Milk	1 (10 oz)	210	0	1
Latte Lite	1 (10 oz)	70	0	0
Latte Mocha Almond	1 (10 oz)	290	20	1
Latte Mocha Swirl	1 (10 oz)	230	25	1
Latte Mocha Swirl w/ Soy Milk	1 (10 oz)	210	0	2
Latte w/ Soy Milk	1 (10 oz)	90	0	1
Latte w/ Soy Milk Sugar	1 (10 oz)	150	0	1
Latte w/ Sugar	1 (10 oz)	160	25	0
Smoothie Mango Passion Fruits	1 (16 oz)	360	10	2
Smoothie Strawberry Banana	1 (16 oz)	360	10	2
Smoothie Wildberry	1 (16 oz)	360	10	1
Tea Regular Or Decaffeinated	1 (10 oz)	0	0	0
Tea w/ Milk	1 (10 oz)	25	5	0
Tea w/ Milk Sugar	1 (10 oz)	70	5	0
Tea w/ Skim Milk	1 (10 oz)	25	0	0
Tea w/ Skim Milk Sugar	1 (10 oz)	60	0	0
Tea w/ Sugar	1 (10 oz)	50	0	0
Turbo Ice	1 (16 oz)	120	20	0
Vanilla Chai	1 (10 oz)	230	5	0
SANDWICHES				
Bagel Bacon Egg Cheese	1	540	200	2
Bagel Egg Cheese	1	470	190	2
Bagel Ham Egg Cheese	1	510	200	2
Bagel Sausage Egg Cheese	1	660	225	3
Biscuit Egg Cheese	1	410	190	1
Biscuit Sausage Egg Cheese	1	610	235	1
Croissant Bacon Egg Cheese	1	520	205	0
Croissant Egg Cheese	1	550	320	0
Croissant Ham Egg Cheese	1	520	215	0

FOOD	PORTION	CALS	CHOL	FIBER
Croissant Sausage Egg Cheese	1	490	230	0
English Muffin Bacon Egg Cheese	1	360	200	1
English Muffin Egg Cheese	1	280	140	1
English Muffin Ham Egg Cheese	1	310	160	1
English Muffin Sausage Egg Cheese	1	530	235	1
Panini Meatball	1	480	40	3
Panini Southwestern Chicken	1	420	45	3
Panini Steak	1	450	45	3

EDDIE'S PIZZA

FOOD	PORTION	CALS	CHOL	FIBER
Bar Pie	1 pie	350	41	8
Bar Pie No Fat Cheese	1 pie	270	10	8

EINSTEIN BROS BAGELS
BAGELS AND BREADS

FOOD	PORTION	CALS	CHOL	FIBER
Bagel Asiago Cheese	1	360	5	2
Bagel Cranberry Special	1	350	0	3
Bagel Egg	1	340	35	2
Bagel Honey Whole Wheat	1	320	0	3
Bagel Jalapeno	1	330	0	2
Bagel Lucky Gree	1	320	0	2
Bagel Mango	1	360	0	2
Bagel Marble Rye	1	340	0	3
Bagel Potato	1	350	0	2
Bagel Power	1	410	0	4
Bagel Power w/ Peanut Butter	1	750	0	7
Bagel Pumpkin	1	330	0	3
Bagel Roasted Red Pepper & Pesto	1	410	15	2
Bagel Six Cheese	1	390	15	2
Bagel Spicy Nacho	1	450	20	3
Bagel Spinach Florentine	1	410	20	3
Bagel Croutons	¼ cup	25	0	0
Bagel Twist	1	220	5	1
Bread Ciabatta	1 serv	320	0	3
Chocolate Chip	1	370	0	3

FOOD	PORTION	CALS	CHOL	FIBER
Chopped Garlic	1	380	0	4
Chopped Onion	1	330	0	2
Cinnamon Raisin Swirl	1	350	0	2
Cinnamon Sugar	1	330	0	2
Dark Pumpernickel	1	320	0	3
Everything	1	340	0	2
Focaccia Cheese Pizza	1 serv	500	35	3
Focaccia Margherita	1 serv	400	5	3
Focaccia Pepperoni Pizza	1 serv	590	55	3
Nutty Banana	1	360	0	2
Plain	1	320	0	2
Poppy Dip'd	1	350	0	2
Roll Challah	1	300	40	2
Salt	1	330	0	2
Sesame Dip'd	1	300	0	3
Sun Dried Tomato	1	320	0	3
Wild Blueberry	1	350	0	3
BEVERAGES				
Americano	1 reg	1	0	0
Cafe Latte	1 reg	140	20	0
Cafe Latte Nonfat	1 reg	100	5	0
Cappuccino	1 reg	90	15	0
Cappuccino Nonfat	1 reg	60	5	0
Chai 2% Milk	1 reg	210	10	0
Chai Skim Milk	1 reg	190	0	0
Coffee	1 reg	0	0	0
Espresso	1 reg	1	0	0
Half & Half	2 tbsp	40	15	–
Hot Chocolate	1 reg	290	20	0
Hot Chocolate Lower Fat	1 reg	260	5	0
Hot Tea All Flavors	1 cup	0	0	0
Iced Americano	1 serv	1	0	0
Iced Coffee	1 serv	0	0	0
Iced Latte	1 serv	120	20	0
Iced Latte Nonfat	1 serv	90	5	0
Iced Mocha	1 serv	210	15	0
Iced Mocha Low Fat	1 serv	180	5	0
Mocha	1 reg	230	15	0
Mocha Low Fat	1 reg	190	5	0

FOOD	PORTION	CALS	CHOL	FIBER
DESSERTS				
Brownie Iced	1	550	35	3
Brownie Iced w/ Walnuts	1	600	35	4
Cherry Figure 8	1	400	40	1
Cinnamon Roll	1	810	45	4
Cookie Chocolate Chunk	1	640	50	3
Cookie Oatmeal Raisin	1	600	50	2
Cookie Peanut Butter	1	640	55	3
Muffin Banana Nut	1	640	80	2
Muffin Blueberry	1	540	95	1
Muffin Chocolate Chip	1	620	90	3
Pound Cake Lemon Iced	1 slice	540	155	0
Pound Cake Marble	1 slice	460	150	1
Rice Krispy Bar	1	420	0	1
Scone Blueberry w/ Icing	1	450	55	2
Scone Lemon Currant	1	430	40	4
Strudel Cinnamon Walnut	1 piece	550	30	3
Sweetie Pie	1	620	5	1
SALAD DRESSINGS				
Asian Sesame	2 tbsp	80	0	0
Caesar	2 tbsp	150	10	0
Chipotle Vinaigrette	2 tbsp	110	0	0
Horseradish Sauce	2 tbsp	170	20	0
Raspberry Vinaigrette	2 tbsp	160	0	0
Thousand Island	2 tbsp	110	10	0
SALADS				
Asian Chicken Salad	1 serv (14.5 oz)	550	55	5
Bros Bistro	1 serv (9.5 oz)	520	25	2
Chicken Caesar	1 serv (12.5 oz)	750	90	2
Chicken Chipotle Salad	1 serv	710	80	13
Chicken Salad On Greens	1 serv (10.5 oz)	210	55	3
Egg Salad	1 serv (4 oz)	200	310	0
Fresh Fruit Cup	1 serv (8 oz)	110	0	2
Mixed Greens	1 serv (3.5 oz)	228	0	1
Potato	½ cup	290	15	2
Tuna Salad On Greens	1 serv (10.5 oz)	170	35	3
SANDWICHES				
12 Grain Bread Deli Chicken Salad	1	440	55	6

FOOD	PORTION	CALS	CHOL	FIBER
12 Grain Bread Deli Egg Salad	1	490	315	5
12 Grain Bread Deli Ham	1	560	75	5
12 Grain Bread Deli Roast Beef	1	560	80	5
12 Grain Bread Deli Smoked Turkey	1	530	70	5
12 Grain Bread Deli Tuna Salad	1	440	55	6
12 Grain Bread Deli Turkey Pastrami	1	540	70	5
12 Grain Bread Ultimate Toasted Cheese w/ Tomato	1	870	110	2
Bagel Chicken Salad	1	500	55	4
Bagel Egg Bacon	1	580	285	2
Bagel Egg Ham	1	530	295	2
Bagel Egg Salad	1	560	315	3
Bagel Egg Sausage	1	550	295	2
Bagel Ham	1	450	45	3
Bagel Holey Cow	1	900	105	3
Bagel Hummus & Feta	1	540	15	5
Bagel New York Lox	1	660	85	3
Bagel Original	1	480	270	2
Bagel Roast Beef	1	460	45	3
Bagel Rueben Deli	1	660	65	4
Bagel Salmon & Shmear	1	650	310	2
Bagel Sante Fe	1	650	300	2
Bagel Smoked Turkey	1	420	30	3
Bagel Tasty Turkey	1	570	80	4
Bagel The Veg Out	1	490	30	3
Bagel Tuna Salad	1	470	35	4
Bagel Turkey Pastrami	1	440	40	3
Challah Club Mex	1	750	135	2
Challah Cobbie	1	630	110	4
Challah Deli Chicken Salad	1	480	95	4
Challah Deli Egg Salad	1	430	345	2
Challah Deli Pastrami	1	480	100	2
Challah Deli Roast Beef	1	500	110	2
Challah Deli Smoked Turkey	1	470	100	2

FOOD	PORTION	CALS	CHOL	FIBER
Challah Deli Tuna Salad	1	370	60	2
Challah Deli Turkey Ham	1	500	105	2
Challah EBBQ Chicken	1	380	80	2
Challah Roasted Chicken & Smoked Gouda	1	440	110	2
Chicago Bagel Dog Asiago	1	740	80	2
Chicago Bagel Dog Chili Cheese	1	810	105	4
Chicago Bagel Dog Everything	1	730	70	3
Chicago Bagel Dog Onion w/o Cheese	1	680	70	2
Country White Deli Chicken Salad	1	540	55	4
Country White Deli Egg Salad	1	590	315	3
Country White Deli Ham	1	660	15	3
Country White Deli Roast Beef	1	660	80	3
Country White Deli Smoked Turkey	1	630	70	3
Country White Deli Tuna Salad	1	510	35	4
Country White Deli Turkey Pastrami	1	640	70	3
Country White Ultimate Toasted Cheese w/ Tomato	1	870	110	2
Panini Cali Club	1	730	75	9
Panini Cuban Ham	1	700	90	4
Panini Denver Omelet Breakfast	1	740	310	3
Panini Italian Chicken	1	770	85	4
Panini Taos Turkey	1	740	80	9
Panini Ultimate Toasted Cheese	1	900	110	7
Roll Ups Albuquerque Turkey	1	790	85	5
Roll Ups Thai Vegetable	1	630	0	5

FOOD	PORTION	CALS	CHOL	FIBER
Roll Ups Thai Vegetable w/ Chicken	1	670	40	4
SOUPS				
Broccoli Sharp Cheddar	1 cup	230	40	1
Chicken & Wild Rice	1 cup	190	15	2
Chicken Noodle	1 cup	220	60	2
Clam Chowda	1 cup	160	35	0
Minestroni Low Fat	1 cup	180	0	5
Tomato Bisque	1 cup	190	15	3
Tortilla	1 cup	90	0	2
Turkey Chili	1 cup	140	20	2
SPREADS				
Butter	1 tbsp	100	30	0
Butter & Margarine Blend	1 tbsp	60	0	0
Cream Cheese Blueberry	1 tbsp	70	15	0
Cream Cheese Cappuccino	2 tbsp	70	15	0
Cream Cheese Garden Vegetable	2 tbsp	60	15	0
Cream Cheese Honey Almond Reduced Fat	2 tbsp	70	15	0
Cream Cheese Jalapeno Salsa	1 tbsp	60	15	0
Cream Cheese Maple Walnut Raisin	2 tbsp	60	15	0
Cream Cheese Onion & Chive	2 tbsp	70	20	0
Cream Cheese Plain	2 tbsp	60	20	0
Cream Cheese Plain Reduced Fat	2 tbsp	60	15	0
Cream Cheese Pumpkin	2 tbsp	100	25	0
Cream Cheese Smoked Salmon	2 tbsp	60	15	0
Cream Cheese Strawberry	2 tbsp	70	15	0
Cream Cheese Sun Dried Tomato & Basil	2 tbsp	60	15	0
Fruit Spread Apricot	1 serv	75	0	0
Fruit Spread Grape	1 serv (1 oz)	75	0	0
Fruit Spread Strawberry	1 serv (1 oz)	75	0	0
Honey Butter	1 tbsp	90	15	0
Hummus	1 serv	110	0	2

FOOD	PORTION	CALS	CHOL	FIBER
Mayo Ancho Lime	1 tbsp	50	5	0
Mustard French Dijon	1 tsp	10	0	0
Mustard Grain Dijon	1 tsp	5	0	0
Mustard Honey	1 tsp	15	0	0
Mustard Raspberry	2 tbsp	50	2	0
Mustard Yellow	1 tbsp	5	0	0
Peanut Butter	2 tbsp	190	0	2
Salsa Ancho Lime	¼ cup	20	0	0

EL POLLO LOCO
DESSERTS

FOOD	PORTION	CALS	CHOL	FIBER
Churro	1	179	5	1
Fosters Freeze Soft Serve	1 cup	180	20	0

MAIN MENU SELECTIONS

FOOD	PORTION	CALS	CHOL	FIBER
Bowl Chicken Caesar	1 serv	535	50	4
Bowl Pollo	1 serv	545	40	12
Bowl Veggie	1 serv	570	10	16
Bowl Veggie w/o Cheese	1 serv	529	0	16
Burrito Classic Chicken	1	580	108	6
Burrito Twice Grilled	1 serv	835	150	2
Burrito BRC	1 serv	530	15	6
Burrito Caesar	1 serv	895	100	4
Burrito Chicken Lover's	1 serv	525	100	2
Burrito Spicy	1 serv	555	70	9
Burrito Ultimate Chicken	1 serv	685	65	6
Chicken Breast	1 piece	153	95	0
Chicken Leg	1 piece	86	80	0
Chicken Thigh	1 piece	120	82	0
Chicken Wing	1	83	58	0
Cole Slaw	1 serv	206	11	2
Corn Cobbette	1 serv	80	0	1
French Fries	1 serv	444	0	0
Fresh Vegetables	1 serv	70	0	4
Gravy	1 serv (1 oz)	107	8	0
Mashed Potatoes	1 serv	97	0	2
Nachos Chicken	1 serv	1420	161	15
Pinto Beans	1 serv	165	0	10
Popcorn Chicken	1 serv	226	53	0
Potato Salad	1 serv	256	15	3
Quesadilla Cheese	1 serv	495	53	2

FOOD	PORTION	CALS	CHOL	FIBER
Quesadilla Chicken	1 serv	593	107	0
Smokey Black Beans	1 serv	306	13	5
Spanish Rice	1 serv	165	0	1
Taco Al Carbon Chicken	1 serv	135	30	1
Taco Soft Chicken	1	237	74	0
Taquitos Chicken	2	370	25	3
Tortilla Chips	1 serv	426	0	4
Tortilla Corn	1 (4.5 in)	40	0	1
Tortilla Corn	1 (6 in)	70	0	1
Tortilla Flour	1 (6.5 in)	110	0	0
Tortilla Flour	1 (12 in)	325	0	2
Tortilla Spicy Tomato	1 (12 in)	270	0	2
Tostada Salad	1 serv	700	65	10
SALAD DRESSINGS AND TOPPINGS				
Bleu Cheese	1 serv (1.5 oz)	230	30	0
Buttermilk Ranch	1 serv (1.5 oz)	220	10	0
Creamy Chipotle	1 (0.5 oz)	75	5	0
Creamy Cilantro	1 serv (0.5 oz)	80	5	0
Guacamole	1 serv (1 oz)	30	0	0
Hot Sauce Jalapeno	1 pkg (0.5 oz)	5	0	0
Light Italian	1 serv (1.5 oz)	20	0	0
Salsa Avocado	1 serv (1 oz)	20	0	0
Salsa House	1 serv (1 oz)	6	0	0
Salsa Pico De Gallo	1 serv (1 oz)	10	0	0
Salsa Spicy Chipotle	1 serv (1 oz)	7	0	0
Sour Cream	1 serv (1 oz)	60	20	0
Thousand Island	1 serv (1.5 oz)	220	30	0
SALADS				
Caesar	1 serv	565	70	3
Ceasar w/o Dressing	1 serv	250	55	3
Fiesta Salad	1 serv	755	105	4
Fiesta Salad w/o Dressing	1 serv	450	95	4
Garden Salad	1 serv	110	15	2
Macaroni & Cheese	1 serv	381	65	2
Tostada Salad w/o Shell	1 serv	360	65	6

FAZOLI'S
DESSERTS

Cheesecake	1 slice	290	950	0
Cheesecake Turtle	1 slice	420	100	2

FOOD	PORTION	CALS	CHOL	FIBER
Cookie Milk Chocolate Chunk	1	360	30	0
Lemon Ice	1 serv	190	0	0
Specialty Cheesecake	1 serv	300	85	1
Strawberry Topping	1 serv	35	0	0
MAIN MENU SELECTIONS				
Baked Chicken Parmesan	1 serv	740	65	6
Baked Spaghetti Parmesan	1 serv	700	60	5
Baked Ziti	1 sm	490	35	4
Baked Ziti	1 reg	750	55	6
Breadstick	1	140	0	1
Breadstick Dry	1	90	0	1
Broccoli Fettuccine Alfredo	1 sm	560	15	6
Broccoli Fettuccine Alfredo	1 reg	830	20	6
Cheese Ravioli w/ Marinara Sauce	1 serv	480	65	4
Cheese Ravioli w/ Meat Sauce	1 serv	510	70	4
Classic Sampler	1 serv	710	85	6
Fettuccine Alfredo	1 sm	530	15	3
Fettuccine Alfredo	1 reg	800	20	5
Fettuccine w/ Shrimp & Scallop	1 serv	590	95	3
Homestyle Lasagna	1 serv	440	145	4
Homestyle Lasagna w/ Broccoli	1 serv	420	140	5
Minestrone Soup	1 serv	120	0	8
Peppery Chicken Alfredo	1 serv	610	50	3
Pizza Cheese	1 serv	460	40	2
Pizza Combination Double Slice	1 serv	570	60	3
Pizza Pepperoni	1 serv	530	53	2
Pizza Baked Spaghetti	1 serv	750	75	5
Spaghetti w/ Marinara Sauce	1 sm	420	0	5
Spaghetti w/ Marinara Sauce	1 reg	620	0	7
Spaghetti w/ Meat Sauce	1 sm	450	10	5
Spaghetti w/ Meat Sauce	1 reg	670	10	8
Spaghetti w/ Meatballs	1 sm	730	60	6
Spaghetti w/ Meatballs	1 reg	1020	80	8

FOOD	PORTION	CALS	CHOL	FIBER
SALAD DRESSINGS				
Honey French	1 serv	150	0	0
House Italian	1 serv	110	0	0
Ranch	1 serv	150	3	0
Reduced Calorie Italian	1 serv	50	0	0
Thousand Island	1 serv	130	15	0
SALADS				
Caesar Side Salad	1	220	5	3
Chicken & Pasta Caesar Salad	1	500	55	4
Chicken Caesar Salad	1	420	45	4
Chicken Finger Salad	1	190	45	2
Chicken Finger Salad w/ Bacon & Honey Mustard	1	400	50	2
Garden Salad	1	25	0	1
Garden Salad w/ Balsamic Vinaigrette	1	120	0	1
Italian Chef Salad	1	260	45	3
Pasta Salad	1 serv	590	20	5
SANDWICHES				
Panini Chicken Caesar Club	1	660	110	3
Panini Chicken Pesto	1	510	60	3
Panini Four Cheese & Tomato	1	720	75	3
Panini Ham & Swiss	1	600	70	2
Panini Italian Club	1	670	85	3
Panini Italian Deli	1	660	90	4
Panini Smoked Turkey	1	710	110	3
Submarinos Club	half	1100	120	7
Submarinos Ham & Swiss	1	1000	75	7
Submarinos Meatball	half	1260	125	8
Submarinos Orignal	half	1160	105	8
Submarinos Pepperoni Pizza	half	1060	95	6
Submarinos Turkey	half	990	90	7
FRESHENS				
PRETZELS				
Bites	1 serv (3 oz)	255	0	2
Gourmet	1 (6 oz)	510	0	4
SMOOTHIES				
Berry Berry	1 serv (21 oz)	280	tr	–

FOOD	PORTION	CALS	CHOL	FIBER
Blueberry Breeze	1 serv (21 oz)	396	14	-
Caribbean Craze	1 serv (21 oz)	315	tr	-
Cayman Cooler	1 serv (21 oz)	320	tr	-
Club Trim	1 serv (21 oz)	291	0	-
Fitness Fuel	1 serv (21 oz)	521	24	-
Immune Support	1 serv (21 oz)	377	10	-
Jamaican Jammer	1 serv (21 oz)	378	14	-
Maui Mango	1 serv (21 oz)	354	tr	-
Mocha Coffee	1 serv (21 oz)	385	15	-
Mystic Mango	1 serv (21 oz)	407	10	-
Orange Shooter	1 serv (21 oz)	330	10	-
Orange Sunrise	1 serv (21 oz)	367	10	-
Peach Sunset	1 serv (21 oz)	388	tr	-
Peachy Pineapple	1 serv (21 oz)	415	14	-
Peanut Butter Chocolate	1 serv (21 oz)	312	45	-
Pina Colada	1 serv (21 oz)	451	14	-
Pineapple Passion	1 serv (21 oz)	389	tr	-
Raspberry Royale	1 serv (21 oz)	346	tr	-
Rockin' Raspberry	1 serv (21 oz)	332	14	-
Strawberry Shooter	1 serv (21 oz)	251	tr	-
Strawberry Squeeze	1 serv (21 oz)	313	14	-
Vanilla Coffee	1 serv (21 oz)	438	15	-
Vanilla Fudge	1 serv (21 oz)	275	45	-

FRUITFULL
BREADS

FOOD	PORTION	CALS	CHOL	FIBER
Almond Cherry	½ slice	226	23	1
Apple Spice	½ slice	186	19	1
Banana	½ slice	165	22	1
Cappuccino Chocolate Chip	½ slice	229	25	1
Carrot	½ slice	190	24	0
Chocolate	½ slice	120	0	2
Lemon Blueberry	½ slice	120	0	1
Old Fashion Pound Cake	½ slice	227	51	0
Orange Cranberry	½ slice	130	0	0
Pumpkin	½ slice	150	0	0
Sweet Potato	½ slice	176	19	1
Zucchini	½ slice	190	22	1

DIPS

FOOD	PORTION	CALS	CHOL	FIBER
Banana Cream	1 serv (4.5 oz)	250	5	-

FOOD	PORTION	CALS	CHOL	FIBER
Banana Split	1 serv (4.5 oz)	290	10	–
Cherry Cream	1 serv (4.5 oz)	280	15	–
Coconut Cream	1 serv (4.5 oz)	300	10	–
Mud Pie	1 serv (4.5 oz)	380	15	–
Strawberry Cream	1 serv (4.5 oz)	270	10	–
FROZEN BARS				
Cream Banana	1	110	20	–
Cream Coconut	1	130	15	–
Cream Peaches 'n' Cream	1	150	25	–
Cream Pina Colada	1	90	10	–
Cream Raspberry Cream	1	110	10	–
Cream Strawberry Cream	1	110	15	–
Happy Indulgence Berry Cobbler	1	200	20	–
Happy Indulgence Key Lime Pie	1	220	35	–
Happy Indulgence Peach Cobbler	1	170	20	–
Juice Fuzzy Navel	1	70	0	–
Juice Green Tea Melon	1	90	0	–
Juice Guava	1	70	0	–
Juice Lemon	1	90	0	–
Juice Lime	1	80	0	–
Juice Passionate Cherry	1	80	0	–
Juice Pineapple	1	80	0	–
Juice Raspberry	1	70	0	–
Juice Strawberry	1	70	0	–
Juice Tamarind	1	90	0	–
Juice Tropical Splash	1	80	0	–
Juice Watermelon	1	60	0	–
Yogurt Blueberry	1	120	0	–
Yogurt Chocolate	1	160	0	–
Yogurt Vanilla	1	140	0	–
SMOOTHIES				
Berry Berry Best	1 (4 oz)	160	5	–
Make Mine Mango	4 oz	160	0	–
Strawberry Ana Banana	4 oz	120	0	–
SNACKS				
All About Almonds	1 pkg (1 oz)	170	0	4
Buzzworthy Banana	1 pkg (1.1 oz)	140	0	2

FOOD	PORTION	CALS	CHOL	FIBER
Calypso Cashews	1 pkg (1.1 oz)	170	1	1
Chocolate Twisted Bliss	1 pkg (1.4 oz)	190	6	1
Debbie Loves Fruit	1 pkg (1 oz)	110	0	1
Got Nuts?	1 pkg (1.1 oz)	180	1	2
Hit The Road Jack	1 pkg (1.1 oz)	130	0	2
Honey I Ate The Peanuts	1 pkg (1 oz)	160	0	1
Jamaican Me Crazy Cranberry Mix	1 pkg (1.1 oz)	100	0	2
Judy's Apple Crisps	1 pkg (1 oz)	140	0	2
Nacho Chips They're Mine	1 pkg (1.1 oz)	120	1	0
Nature Lover's Choice	1 pkg (1.1 oz)	140	0	2
Power Pistachios	1 pkg (1.1 oz)	100	0	2
Reggae Rice Crackers	1 pkg (1.1 oz)	120	0	0
Rockin' Raisins	1 pkg (1.4 oz)	170	4	1
Rocky Mountain Munch	1 pkg (1.1 oz)	120	0	1
Sour Wiggle Giggle	1 pkg (1.5 oz)	150	0	0
Soy Glad You're Healthy	1 pkg (1.1 oz)	160	0	4
Survivor Snacks	1 pkg (1.1 oz)	140	0	2
Swinging Sesame Stix	1 pkg (1.1 oz)	180	0	2
Tammy's Flax Snacks	1 pkg (1.1 oz)	170	0	3
Whassup Wasabi!	1 pkg (1.1 oz)	150	0	2
Yogurt Twisted Bliss	1 pkg (1.4 oz)	190	0	1
You've Got Trail	1 pkg (1.1 oz)	150	0	2
Yummy Gummy In My Tummy	1 pkg (1.4 oz)	150	0	0
Zydeco Cajun Mix	1 pkg (1.1 oz)	108	1	1

FRULLATI CAFE

Smoothie	1 (14 oz)	195	0	tr

GODFATHER'S PIZZA

Breadstick	1	80	0	1
Golden All Meat Combo	1 med slice	300	30	1
Golden Apple Dessert	⅙ sm	202	0	1
Golden Bacon Cheeseburger	1 med slice	270	25	1
Golden Cheese	1 med slice	220	15	1
Golden Cherry Dessert	⅙ sm	206	0	1
Golden Cinnamon Streusel	⅙ sm	226	0	1
Golden Combo	1 med slice	290	25	2
Golden Hawaiian	1 med slice	240	15	1

FOOD	PORTION	CALS	CHOL	FIBER
Golden Hot Stuff	1 med slice	290	25	1
Golden Humble Pie	1 med slice	310	30	1
Golden M&M Streusel Dessert	⅙ sm	249	1	1
Golden Pepperoni	1 med slice	260	20	1
Golden Super Combo	1 med slice	320	35	2
Golden Super Hawaiian	1 med slice	250	20	1
Golden Super Taco	1 med slice	330	40	2
Golden Taco	1 med slice	300	35	2
Golden Veggie	1 med slice	230	15	2
Monkey Bread	⅙	120	0	1
Original All Meat Combo	1 med slice	370	35	2
Original Bacon Cheeseburger	1 med slice	330	35	2
Original Cheese	1 med slice	260	15	1
Original Combo	1 med slice	350	30	3
Original Hawaiian	1 med slice	280	20	1
Original Hot Stuff	1 med slice	360	35	2
Original Humble Pie	1 med slice	380	35	2
Original Pepperoni	1 med slice	290	20	1
Original Super Combo	1 med slice	390	40	3
Original Super Hawaiian	1 med slice	280	20	1
Original Super Taco	1 med slice	390	45	2
Original Taco	1 med slice	360	40	2
Original Veggie	1 med slice	270	15	2
Potato Wedges	1 serv (4 oz)	192	0	4
Thin All Meat Combo	1 med slice	280	30	1
Thin Bacon Cheeseburger	1 med slice	250	30	1
Thin Cheese	1 med slice	180	15	1
Thin Combo	1 med slice	250	25	1
Thin Hawaiian	1 med slice	200	15	1
Thin Hot Stuff	1 med slice	270	30	1
Thin Humble Pie	1 med slice	270	30	1
Thin Pepperoni	1 med slice	220	20	1
Thin Super Combo	1 med slice	300	35	2
Thin Super Hawaiian	1 med slice	230	20	1
Thin Super Taco	1 med slice	310	10	2
Thin Taco	1 med slice	260	35	1
Thin Veggie	1 med slice	190	15	1

FOOD	PORTION	CALS	CHOL	FIBER
HAAGEN-DAZS				
FROZEN YOGURT				
Pinapple Coconut	½ cup	230	90	0
Soft Serve Nonfat Chocolate	½ cup	110	0	0
Soft Serve Nonfat Chocolate Mousse	½ cup	80	0	1
Soft Serve Nonfat Coffee	½ cup	110	<5	0
Soft Serve Nonfat Strawberry	½ cup	110	0	0
Soft Serve Nonfat Vanilla	½ cup	110	<5	0
Soft Serve Nonfat Vanilla Mousse	½ cup	70	<5	0
Soft Serve Nonfat White Chocolate	½ cup	110	<5	0
Vanilla Fudge	½ cup	160	<5	0
Vanilla Raspberry Swirl	½ cup	130	<5	tr
ICE CREAM				
Bailey's Irish Cream	½ cup	270	115	0
Bar Chocolate	1 (2.7 oz)	200	85	tr
Bar Chocolate & Dark Chocolate	1 (3.6 oz)	350	85	2
Bar Coffee	1 (2.7 oz)	190	85	0
Bar Coffee & Almond Crunch	1 (3.7 oz)	370	90	tr
Bar Vanilla	1 (2.7 oz)	190	85	0
Bar Vanilla & Almonds	1 (3.7 oz)	380	90	1
Bar Vanilla & Milk Chocolate	1 (3.5 oz)	340	90	tr
Belgian Chocolate Chocolate	½ cup	330	85	2
Brownies A La Mode	½ cup	280	90	tr
Butter Pecan	½ cup	300	105	tr
Cappuccino Commotion	½ cup	310	100	1
Chocolate	½ cup	269	110	1
Chocolate Chocolate Chip	½ cup	300	100	2
Chocolate Chocolate Mint	½ cup	300	95	1
Chocolate Swiss Almond	½ cup	300	100	2
Coffee	½ cup	250	115	0
Coffee Mocha Chip	½ cup	270	105	tr
Cookie Dough Dynamo	½ cup	310	95	0

FOOD	PORTION	CALS	CHOL	FIBER
Cookies & Cream	½ cup	270	105	0
Cookies & Fudge	½ cup	180	15	tr
Deep Chocolate Peanut Butter	½ cup	350	80	4
Dulce De Leche Caramel	½ cup	270	95	0
Lowfat Coffee Fudge	½ cup	170	25	0
Macadamia Brittle	½ cup	280	105	0
Macadamia Nut	½ cup	320	110	0
Mint Chip	½ cup	280	105	tr
Pistachio	½ cup	280	110	tr
Pralines & Cream	½ cup	280	95	0
Rum Raisin	½ cup	260	105	0
Strawberry	½ cup	250	90	tr
Vanilla	½ cup	250	115	0
Vanilla Chocolate Chip	½ cup	290	100	tr
Vanilla Swiss Almond	½ cup	290	100	tr
SORBET				
Bar Raspberry & Vanilla	1 (2.5 oz)	90	0	tr
Mango	½ cup	120	0	tr
Orange	½ cup	120	0	tr
Raspberry	½ cup	120	0	2
Soft Serve Raspberry	½ cup	110	0	2
Strawberry	½ cup	120	0	1
Zesty Lemon	½ cup	120	0	tr

HARDEE'S
BEVERAGES

FOOD	PORTION	CALS	CHOL	FIBER
Barq's Root Beer	1 sm (20 oz)	290	0	0
Cherry Coke	1 sm (20 oz)	260	0	0
Coca-Cola	1 sm (20 oz)	260	0	0
Coffee Black	1 sm (12 oz)	5	0	0
Diet Coke	1 sm (20 oz)	0	0	0
Dr Pepper	1 sm (20 oz)	260	0	0
Hi-C Fruit Punch	1 sm (20 oz)	260	0	0
Hi-C Orange	1 sm (20 oz)	280	0	0
Lemonade Minute Maid	1 sm (20 oz)	250	0	0
Mello Yellow	1 sm (20 oz)	265	0	0
Milk 2%	1 (10 oz)	150	15	0
Orange Juice	1 serv (10 oz)	150	0	0
Shake Chocolate	1 (16 oz)	700	100	1

FOOD	PORTION	CALS	CHOL	FIBER
Shake Strawberry	1 (16 oz)	700	100	0
Shake Vanilla	1 (16 oz)	710	100	0
Sprite	1 sm	260	0	0
BREAKFAST SELECTIONS				
Big Country Breakfast Platter Bacon	1 serv	980	435	3
Big Country Breakfast Platter Breaded Pork Chop	1 serv	1220	465	4
Big Country Breakfast Platter Chicken	1 serv	1140	480	4
Big Country Breakfast Platter Country Ham	1 serv	970	460	3
Big Country Breakfast Platter Country Steak	1 serv	1150	455	4
Big Country Breakfast Platter Grilled Pork Chop	1 serv	1130	465	3
Big Country Breakfast Platter Sausage	1 serv	1060	455	4
Biscuit Bacon	1 serv	430	10	0
Biscuit Bacon Egg Cheese	1	560	225	0
Biscuit Breaded Pork Chop	1 serv	690	40	1
Biscuit Chicken Fillet	1 serv	600	55	1
Biscuit Cinnamon 'N' Raisin	1	280	0	0
Biscuit Country Ham	1	440	35	0
Biscuit Country Steak	1 serv	620	35	0
Biscuit Country Steak & Egg	1 serv	690	235	0
Biscuit Egg	1 serv	450	205	0
Biscuit Ham Egg Cheese	1	560	245	0
Biscuit Loaded Omelet	1 serv	640	245	0
Biscuit Made From Scratch	1	370	0	0
Biscuit 'N' Gravy	1	530	10	0
Biscuit Sausage	1	530	30	0
Biscuit Sausage Egg	1	610	235	0
Breakfast Bowl Loaded Biscuit 'N' Gravy	1 serv	770	245	1
Breakfast Bowl Low Carb	1 serv	620	325	2
Burrito Loaded Breakfast	1	780	495	2
Burrito Steak 'N' Egg Breakfast	1	470	255	1
Folded Egg	1 serv	80	205	0

FOOD	PORTION	CALS	CHOL	FIBER
Frisco Breakfast Sandwich	1	410	245	2
Grits	1 serv	110	0	0
Hash Rounds	1 sm	260	0	2
Loaded Omelet	1	270	245	0
Pancake Platter	1 serv	300	25	2
Scrambled Egg	1 serv	160	405	0
Sunrise Croissant	1	210	5	0
Sunrise Croissant w/ Bacon	1	450	240	0
Sunrise Croissant w/ Ham	1	430	250	0
Sunrise Croissant w/ Sausage	1	550	265	0
CHILDREN'S MENU SELECTIONS				
French Fries	1 serv	250	0	3
Kids Meal Cheeseburger	1 serv	600	45	4
Kids Meal Chicken Strips	1 serv	500	35	3
Kids Meal Hamburger	1 serv	560	35	6
DESSERTS				
Apple Turnover	1	290	5	1
Cone Single Scoop	1	285	47	0
Cookie Chocolate Chip	1	290	20	0
Ice Cream Bowl Single Scoop	1 serv	235	47	0
Peach Cobbler	1 serv	280	0	1
MAIN MENU SELECTIONS				
Burger Six Dollar	1	1060	150	3
Cheeseburger	1	680	90	2
Cheeseburger	1	350	45	1
Cheeseburger Double	1	510	90	1
Chicken Strips	3 pieces	380	55	1
Cole Slaw	1 serv	170	10	2
Crispy Curls	1 sm	340	0	4
French Fries	1 sm	390	0	4
Fried Chicken Breast	1 piece	370	75	0
Fried Chicken Leg	1 piece	170	45	0
Fried Chicken Thigh	1 piece	330	60	0
Fried Chicken Wing	1 piece	200	30	0
Grilled Onions	1 serv	35	0	0
Hamburger	1	310	35	1
Hamburger Double	1	420	70	1
Hot Dog	1	420	55	1

FOOD	PORTION	CALS	CHOL	FIBER
Hot Ham 'N' Cheese	1	420	55	2
Hot Ham 'N' Cheese Big	1	520	85	2
Mashed Potatoes	1 sm	90	0	0
Roast Beef Big	1	470	60	2
Roast Beef Regular	1	330	40	2
Sandwich Big Chicken Fillet	1	850	95	3
Sandwich Charbroiled Chicken Club	1	560	100	3
Sandwich Chargrilled BBQ Chicken	1	415	60	4
Sandwich Fish Supreme	1	500	60	1
Thickburger	1	850	105	3
Thickburger Bacon Cheese	1	910	115	3
Thickburger Double	1	1240	195	3
Thickburger Double Bacon Cheese	1	1300	205	3
Thickburger Low Carb	1	420	115	2
Thickburger Monster	1	1410	229	2
Thickburger Mushroom 'N Swiss	1	720	100	2
SAUCES AND TOPPINGS				
Au Jus Sauce	1 serv (3 oz)	10	0	0
Chicken Gravy	1 serv (1.5 oz)	20	0	0
Dipping Sauce BBQ	1 serv (0.5 oz)	15	0	0
Dipping Sauce Honey Mustard	1 serv (1 oz)	110	10	0
Dipping Sauce Ranch Dressing	1 serv (1 oz)	160	15	0
Dipping Sauce Sweet N Sour	1 serv (1 oz)	45	0	0
Gravy Biscuit	1 serv (5 oz)	160	10	0
Horseradish Sauce	1 pkg	25	5	0
Hot Sauce	1 pkg	0	0	0
Jam Grape	1 serv	10	0	0
Jam Strawberry	1 serv	35	0	0
Ketchup	1 pkg	10	0	0
Mayonnaise	1 pkg	90	5	0
Pancake Syrup	1 serv (1 oz)	90	0	0

FOOD	PORTION	CALS	CHOL	FIBER
HUNGRY HOWIE'S				
MAIN MENU SELECTIONS				
Howie Wings	6 (3 oz)	180	70	0
Three Cheeser Bread	1 serv	370	17	1
PIZZA				
Large Cheese	1 slice	175	11	1
Large Cheese + Bacon	1 slice	208	13	1
Large Cheese + Beef	1 slice	197	16	1
Large Cheese + Black Olives	1 slice	181	12	1
Large Cheese + Green Olives	1 slice	181	12	1
Large Cheese + Green Peppers	1 slice	175	11	1
Large Cheese + Ham	1 slice	179	14	1
Large Cheese + Mushrooms	1 slice	175	11	1
Large Cheese + Onions	1 slice	175	12	1
Large Cheese + Pepperoni	1 slice	191	16	1
Large Cheese + Pineapple	1 slice	388	12	1
Large Cheese + Sausage	1 slice	195	14	1
Medium Cheese	1 slice	153	9	1
Medium Cheese + Bacon	1 slice	179	10	1
Medium Cheese + Beef	1 slice	177	14	1
Medium Cheese + Black Olives	1 slice	159	11	1
Medium Cheese + Green Olives	1 slice	159	11	1
Medium Cheese + Green Peppers	1 slice	155	10	1
Medium Cheese + Ham	1 slice	159	12	1
Medium Cheese + Mushrooms	1 slice	155	9	1
Medium Cheese + Onions	1 slice	155	10	1
Medium Cheese + Pepperoni	1 slice	171	14	1
Medium Cheese + Pineapple	1 slice	158	10	1
Medium Cheese + Sausage	1 slice	175	12	1
Small Cheese	1 slice	121	8	1
Small Cheese + Bacon	1 slice	138	9	1

FOOD	PORTION	CALS	CHOL	FIBER
Small Cheese + Beef	1 slice	137	12	1
Small Cheese + Black Olives	1 slice	125	9	1
Small Cheese + Green Olives	1 slice	125	9	1
Small Cheese + Green Peppers	1 slice	122	8	1
Small Cheese + Ham	1 slice	126	11	1
Small Cheese + Mushrooms	1 slice	123	8	1
Small Cheese + Onions	1 slice	122	8	1
Small Cheese + Pepperoni	1 slice	136	12	1
Small Cheese + Pineapple	1 slice	124	8	1
Small Cheese + Sausage	1 slice	136	11	1
SALADS				
Antipasto Salad w/o Dressing	1 lg	101	24	1
Chef Salad w/o Dressing	1 lg	99	24	2
Garden Salad w/o Dressing	1 lg	17	0	2
Greek Salad w/o Dressing	1 lg	109	25	2
SANDWICHES				
Sub Deluxe Italian	½ sub	506	44	2
Sub Ham & Cheese	½ sub	475	44	2
Sub Pizza	½ sub	689	86	3
Sub Pizza Special	½ sub	606	65	3
Sub Steak Cheese Mushroom	½ sub	491	47	2
Sub Turkey	½ sub	466	38	2
Sub Turkey Club	½ sub	556	44	2
Sub Vegetarian	½ sub	530	39	3

IHOP

FOOD	PORTION	CALS	CHOL	FIBER
Pancake Buckwheat	1 (1.7 oz)	110	50	1
Pancake Buttermilk	1 (1.7 oz)	110	30	tr
Pancake Country Griddle	1 (2 oz)	120	35	tr
Pancake Harvest Grain 'N Nut	1 (2.25 oz)	180	40	2

IN-N-OUT BURGER
BEVERAGES

FOOD	PORTION	CALS	CHOL	FIBER
Coca-Cola	1 (16 oz)	198	0	0

FOOD	PORTION	CALS	CHOL	FIBER
Coffee Black	1 (10 oz)	5	0	0
Diet Coke	1 (16 oz)	0	0	0
Dr Pepper	1 (16 oz)	180	0	0
Iced Tea	1 (16 oz)	0	0	0
Lemonade	1 (16 oz)	180	0	0
Milk	1 (10 oz)	108	30	0
Root Beer	1 (16 oz)	222	0	0
Seven Up	1 (16 oz)	200	0	0
Shake Chocolate	1 (15 oz)	690	95	0
Shake Strawberry	1 (15 oz)	690	85	0
Shake Vanilla	1 (15 oz)	680	90	0
MAIN MENU SELECTIONS				
Cheeseburger w/ Onions	1	480	60	3
Cheeseburger w/ Onions Lettuce Bun	1	330	60	3
Cheeseburger w/ Onions Mustard Ketchup No Spread	1	400	60	3
French Fries	1 serv (4.4 oz)	400	0	2
Hamburger Double Double w/ Onions	1	670	120	3
Hamburger Double Double w/ Onions Lettuce Bun	1	520	120	3
Hamburger Double Double w/ Onions Mustard Ketchup No Spread	1	590	115	3
Hamburger w/ Onions	1	390	40	3
Hamburger w/ Onions Lettuce Bun	1	240	40	3
Hamburger w/ Onions Mustard Ketchup No Spread	1	310	35	3

JACK IN THE BOX
BEVERAGES

FOOD	PORTION	CALS	CHOL	FIBER
Barq's Root Beer	1 serv (20 oz)	180	0	0
Coca-Cola Classic	1 serv (20 oz)	170	0	0
Coffee	1 serv (12 oz)	5	0	0
Diet Coke	1 serv (20 oz)	0	0	0
Dr Pepper	1 serv (20 oz)	190	0	0

FOOD	PORTION	CALS	CHOL	FIBER
Ice Cream Shake Caramel	1 serv (16 oz)	660	115	0
Ice Cream Shake Chocolate	1 (16 oz)	660	110	1
Ice Cream Shake Oreo	1 serv (16 oz)	670	110	1
Ice Cream Shake Strawberry	1 serv (16 oz)	640	110	0
Ice Cream Shake Strawberry Banana	1 serv (16 oz)	700	110	0
Ice Cream Shake Vanilla	1 (16 oz)	570	115	0
Iced Tea	1 serv (20 oz)	0	0	0
Lowfat Milk 2%	1 serv (8 oz)	140	20	0
Orange Juice	1 serv (10 oz)	140	0	2
Sprite	1 serv (20 oz)	160	0	0
BREAKFAST SELECTIONS				
Breakfast Sandwich Sourdough	1	440	215	2
Breakfast Sandwich Ultimate	1	730	440	2
Breakfast Jack	1	310	205	1
Croissant Sausage	1	680	250	2
Croissant Supreme	1	570	240	1
French Toast Sticks	4 pieces	430	10	2
Hash Brown	1 serv	150	0	2
Sandwich Extreme Sausage	1	720	280	2
DESSERTS				
Cheesecake	1 serv	310	55	0
Double Fudge Cake	1 serv	310	25	4
MAIN MENU SELECTIONS				
American Cheese	1 slice	45	10	0
Bacon Cheddar Potato Wedges	1 serv	770	45	4
Cheeseburger Bacon Bacon	1	910	100	3
Cheeseburger Bacon Ultimate	1	1120	160	2
Cheeseburger Junior Bacon	1	540	75	1
Cheeseburger Ultimate	1	990	130	2
Chicken Breast Pieces	4	360	80	1
Chicken Breast Strips	1 serv	500	80	3
Chicken Fajita Pita	1	330	55	3
Chicken Sandwich	1	410	35	2
Dipping Sauce Barbeque	1 serv (1.6 oz)	45	0	0
Egg Rolls	1	130	5	2

FOOD	PORTION	CALS	CHOL	FIBER
Fish & Chips	1 serv	610	40	5
French Fries	1 sm	330	0	3
French Fries	1 med	410	0	4
French Fries	1 lg	580	0	6
Hamburger	1	310	45	1
Hamburger w/ Cheese	1	360	60	1
Jumbo Jack	1	600	45	3
Jumbo Jack w/ Cheese	1	690	70	3
Onion Rings	1 serv	500	0	3
Philly Cheesesteak	1	580	90	3
Salsa	1 serv (1 oz)	10	0	0
Sandwich Roasted Turkey	1	580	110	3
Sandwich Ultimate Club	1	640	105	3
Seasoned Curly Fries	1 serv	400	0	5
Sour Cream	1 serv (1 oz)	60	15	0
Sourdough Grilled Chicken Club	1	520	85	3
Sourdough Jack	1	700	80	3
Spicy Crispy Chicken	1	730	70	4
Stuffed Jalapeno	3 pieces	230	20	2
Swiss Style Cheese	1 slice	40	10	0
Taco	1	170	20	2
Taco Monster	1	260	30	3
Turkey Jack	1	700	115	4
SALAD DRESSINGS AND TOPPINGS				
Almonds Roasted Slivered	1 serv (0.7 oz)	130	0	2
Asian Sesame	1 serv (2.5 oz)	230	0	0
Bacon Ranch	1 serv (2.5 oz)	320	30	0
Balsamic Vinaigrette Low Fat	1 serv (2.5 oz)	40	0	0
Country Crock Spread	1 pkg	25	0	0
Creamy Southwest Dressing	1 serv (2.5 oz)	270	30	0
Croutons	1 serv (0.5 oz)	60	0	0
Dipping Sauce Buttermilk House	1 serv (0.9 oz)	130	10	0
Dipping Sauce Frank's Red Hot Buffalo	1 serv (1 oz)	10	0	0
Dipping Sauce Sweet & Sour	1 serv (1 oz)	45	0	0
Grape Jelly	1 serv (0.5 oz)	35	0	0

FOOD	PORTION	CALS	CHOL	FIBER
Herb Mayo Sauce Low Fat	1 serv (1.5 oz)	45	0	1
Ketchup	1 pkg (0.3 oz)	10	0	0
Marinara Sauce	1 serv (0.9 oz)	15	0	0
Mustard	1 pkg	0	0	0
Ranch	1 serv (2.5 oz)	390	30	0
Ranch Lite	1 serv (2.5 oz)	190	25	0
Soy Sauce	1 serv (0.3 oz)	5	0	0
Syrup	1 serv (1.5 oz)	130	0	0
Taco Sauce	1 serv (0.3 oz)	0	0	0
Tartar Sauce	1 serv (1.5 oz)	210	20	0
Thousand Island	1 serv (2 oz)	160	15	0
Vinegar	1 serv	0	0	0
Wonton Strips	1 serv (0.7 oz)	110	0	2
SALADS				
Asian Salad	1 serv	140	25	6
Chicken Club Salad	1 serv	290	65	5
Side Salad	1 serv	50	10	2
Southwest Chicken	1 serv	320	60	8

JAMBA JUICE

FOOD	PORTION	CALS	CHOL	FIBER
Acai Supercharger Original	1 (24 oz)	420	0	5
Aloha Pineapple Original	1 (26 oz)	500	5	4
Banana Berry Original	1 (25 oz)	480	0	4
Berry Fulfilling Original	1 (24 oz)	290	5	8
Berry Lime Sublime Original	1 (26 oz)	460	5	5
Caribbean Passion Original	1 (26 oz)	440	5	4
Chocolate Moo'd Original	1 (24 oz)	680	30	2
Citrus Squeeze Original	1 (26 oz)	470	5	4
Coldbuster Original	1 (25 oz)	430	5	5
Grape Escape Original	1 (24 oz)	300	0	5
Mango Mantra Original	1 (25 oz)	310	5	6
Mango-A-Go-Go Original	1 (24 oz)	440	5	4
Matcha Green Tea Blast Original	1 (24 oz)	440	0	1
Matcha Green Tea Mist Original	1 (24 oz)	280	0	1
Mega Mango Original	1 (24 oz)	330	0	5
Mighty Cherry Charger Original	1 (24 oz)	490	0	3
Orange Berry Blitz Original	1 (26 oz)	410	5	5

FOOD	PORTION	CALS	CHOL	FIBER
Orange Dream Machine Original	1 (24 oz)	540	10	tr
Orange-A-Peel Original	1 (25 oz)	440	5	5
Passion Berry Breeze Original	1 (24 oz)	270	0	5
Peach Pleasure Original	1 (25 oz)	460	5	4
Peanut Butter Moo'd Original	1 (24 oz)	840	15	7
Peenya Kowlada Original	1 (26 oz)	690	10	3
Protein Berry Pizazz Original	1 (24 oz)	440	0	5
Raspberry Rainbow Original	1 (24 oz)	300	0	6
Razzmatazz Original	1 (26 oz)	480	5	4
Strawberries Wild Original	1 (25 oz)	450	5	4
Strawberry Nirvana Original	1 (25 oz)	280	5	7
Strawberry Surf Rider Original	1 (25 oz)	490	0	4
Strawberry Whirl Original	1 (24 oz)	310	0	6

JERSEY MIKE'S

FOOD	PORTION	CALS	CHOL	FIBER
Ham On Wheat	1	240	35	2
Ham On White	1	240	35	1
Ham/Turkey Wheat	1	230	30	1
Ham/Turkey White	1	240	30	2
Roast Beef Wheat	1	290	60	2
Roast Beef White	1	280	55	0
Turkey On Wheat	1	230	30	2
Turkey On White	1	230	30	1
Veggie On Wheat	1	170	0	2
Veggie On White	1	170	0	2

KENTUCKY FRIED CHICKEN
BEVERAGES

FOOD	PORTION	CALS	CHOL	FIBER
Diet Pepsi	1 sm	0	0	0
Mountain Dew	1 sm	150	0	0
Pepsi	1 sm (11 oz)	140	0	0

DESSERTS

FOOD	PORTION	CALS	CHOL	FIBER
Cake Double Chocolate Chip	1 slice	400	45	2
Cherry Cheesecake Parfait	1 serv	300	4	2

FOOD	PORTION	CALS	CHOL	FIBER
Lil' Bucket Chocolate Creme	1 serv	270	0	2
Lil' Bucket Fudge Brownie	1	270	30	1
Lil' Bucket Lemon Creme	1 serv	400	5	2
Lil' Bucket Strawberry Shortcake	1 serv	200	20	0
Pie Apple	1 slice	270	0	4
Pie Lemon Meringue	1 slice	310	40	3
Pie Pecan	1 slice	370	40	2
Pie Strawberry Creme	1 slice	270	10	0
MAIN MENU SELECTIONS				
BBQ Beans	1 serv	230	0	7
Biscuit	1	190	2	0
Boneless Wings HBBQ Sauced	7 pieces	600	75	2
Chicken Pot Pie	1 serv	770	115	5
Cole Slaw	1 serv	190	5	3
Corn On The Cob	1 ear (3 in)	70	0	3
Crispy Strips	3	400	75	0
Extra Crispy Breast	1 serv	490	135	0
Extra Crispy Drumstick	1	160	70	0
Extra Crispy Thigh	1	370	120	0
Extra Crispy Whole Wing	1	190	55	0
Green Beans	1 serv	50	5	2
Hot & Spicy Breast	1 serv	460	130	0
Hot & Spicy Drumstick	1	150	65	0
Hot & Spicy Thigh	1	400	125	0
Hot & Spicy Whole Wing	1	180	60	0
Hot Wings	6 pieces	450	145	1
Mac & Cheese	1 serv	130	5	1
Mashed Potatoes w/o Gravy	1 serv	110	0	1
Mashed Potatoes With Gravy	1 serv	120	0	1
Original Recipe Breast	1 serv	380	145	0
Original Recipe Breast w/o Skin Or Breading	1 serv	140	95	0
Original Recipe Drumstick	1	140	75	0
Original Recipe Thigh	1	360	165	0
Original Recipe Whole Wing	1	150	60	0

FOOD	PORTION	CALS	CHOL	FIBER
Popcorn Chicken	1 reg serv	450	50	0
Potato Salad	1 serv	180	5	1
Potato Wedges	1 sm	240	0	3
Sandwich HBBQ	1	300	50	4
Sandwich Original Recipe w/ Sauce	1	450	65	0
Sandwich Tender Roast w/ Sauce	1	390	70	1
Sandwich Tender Roast w/o Sauce	1	260	65	1
Sandwich Twister	1	670	60	3
Sandwich Zinger w/ Sauce	1	680	90	1
Sandwich Zinger w/o Sauce	1	540	75	1
Sandwiches Original Recipe w/o Sauce	1	320	60	0
Wings HBBQ Sauced	6 pieces	540	150	1

KOO-KOO-ROO

FOOD	PORTION	CALS	CHOL	FIBER
Original Breast	1 piece	187	117	0
Original Chicken Dark	3 pieces	320	101	0
Rotisserie Chicken Breast & Wing	1 serv	355	140	tr
Rotisserie Chicken Leg & Thigh	1 serv	300	114	tr
Rotisserie Half Chicken	1 serv	655	254	tr
Sandwich BBQ Chicken	1	562	113	3
Sandwich Chicken Caesar	1	781	138	2
Sandwich Original Chicken	1	661	116	3
Traditional Turkey Dinner	1 serv	692	127	8
Turkey Pot Pie	1 serv	883	98	6
Turkey Sandwich Hand Carved	1	599	122	5
Wrap Caesar Chicken	1	757	97	4
Wrap Chipotle Chicken	1	924	123	6

KRISPY KREME

FOOD	PORTION	CALS	CHOL	FIBER
Apple Fritter	1	380	5	2
Caramel Kreme Crunch	1	350	5	tr
Chocolate Iced Glazed w/ Sprinkles	1	260	3	tr
Chocolate Malted Kreme	1	390	5	tr

FOOD	PORTION	CALS	CHOL	FIBER
Chocolate Iced	1	250	5	tr
Chocolate Iced Cake	1	270	20	tr
Chocolate Iced Creme Filled	1	350	5	tr
Chocolate Iced Cruller	1	290	15	tr
Chocolate Iced Custard Filled	1	300	5	tr
Chocolated Iced w/ Sprinkles	1	290	20	tr
Cinnamon Apple Filled	1	290	5	tr
Cinnamon Bun	1	260	5	tr
Cinnamon Sugar Cake	1	280	20	1
Cinnamon Twist	1	230	5	tr
Coffee & Kreme	1	360	5	tr
Dulce De Leche	1	290	5	tr
Glazed Blueberry	1	340	20	tr
Glazed Creme Filled	1	340	5	tr
Glazed Devil's Food	1	340	20	tr
Glazed Lemon Filled	1	290	5	tr
Glazed Raspberry Filled	1	300	5	tr
Glazed Sour Cream	1	340	20	tr
Glazed Strawberry Filled	1	290	5	tr
Glazed Cinnamon	1	210	5	tr
Glazed Cruller	1	240	15	tr
Glazed Custard Filled	1	290	5	tr
Glazed Filled Blueberry	1	290	5	tr
Glazed Twist	1	210	5	tr
Honey & Oat	1	340	20	tr
Key Lime Pie	1	330	5	tr
Maple Iced	1	240	5	tr
Maple Iced Cake	1	270	20	tr
New York Cheesecake	1	330	10	1
Original Glazed	1	200	5	tr
Powdered Blueberry Filled	1	290	5	tr
Powdered Strawberry Filled	1	260	5	tr
Powdered Cake	1	280	20	tr
Powdered Creme Filled	1	340	5	tr
Powered Raspberry	1	300	5	tr
Pumpkin Spice Cake	1	340	20	tr
Sugar Coated	1	200	5	0

FOOD	PORTION	CALS	CHOL	FIBER
Traditional Cake	1	230	20	tr
Vanilla Iced Creme Fill	1	340	5	tr
Vanilla Iced Glazed	1	240	5	tr
Vanilla Iced Cake w/ Sprinkles	1	270	20	tr
Vanilla Iced Custard Filled	1	290	5	tr
Vanilla Iced Raspberry Filled	1	350	5	tr
Vanilla Iced Raspberry Glazed	1	350	5	tr

KRYSTAL
BEVERAGES

FOOD	PORTION	CALS	CHOL	FIBER
Coca-Cola Classic	1 sm (16 oz)	129	0	0
Coca-Cola Classic frzn	1 (16 oz)	130	0	0
Diet Coke	1 sm (16 oz)	tr	0	0
Sprite	1 sm (16 oz)	126	0	0

BREAKFAST SELECTIONS

FOOD	PORTION	CALS	CHOL	FIBER
Biscuit	1	270	0	0
Biscuit And Gravy	1	280	0	0
Biscuit Bacon Egg & Cheese	1	390	40	0
Biscuit Chik	1	360	20	0
Biscuit Sausage	1	480	40	0
Country Breakfast	1 serv	660	590	8
Kryspers	1 serv	190	10	2
Krystal Sunriser	1	240	255	2
Scrambler	1 serv	440	255	3

DESSERTS

FOOD	PORTION	CALS	CHOL	FIBER
Fried Apple Turnover	1	220	<5	2
Lemon Icebox Pie	1 serv	260	25	2

MAIN MENU SELECTIONS

FOOD	PORTION	CALS	CHOL	FIBER
Chik'n Bites	1 sm	310	55	1
Chik'n Bites Salad	1 serv	290	66	4
Fries	1 med	470	20	7
Fries Chili Cheese	1 serv	540	45	5
Krystal	1	160	20	1
Krystal Bacon Cheese	1	190	25	2
Krystal Cheese	1	180	25	2
Krystal Chik	1	240	25	2

FOOD	PORTION	CALS	CHOL	FIBER
Krystal Chili	1 serv	200	25	7
Krystal Double	1	260	40	2
Krystal Double Cheese	1	310	65	tr
Pup	1	170	25	1
Pup Chili Cheese	1	210	40	2
Pup Corn	1	260	50	1

LITTLE CAESARS
MAIN MENU SELECTIONS

FOOD	PORTION	CALS	CHOL	FIBER
Baby Pan! Pan!	1 piece	360	30	2
Crazy Bread	1 piece	90	tr	0
Crazy Bread Cinnamon	2 pieces	100	tr	0
Crazy Sauce	1 serv (4 oz)	45	0	3
Deli Sandwich Ham & Cheese	1	640	50	3
Deli Sandwich Italian	1	800	90	3
Deli Sandwich Veggie	1	600	30	3
Italian Cheese Bread	1 piece	130	10	0

PIZZA

FOOD	PORTION	CALS	CHOL	FIBER
14 Inch Round Meatsa	1/10 pie	280	30	2
14 Inch Round Supreme	1/10 pie	270	25	3
14 Inch Round Veggie	1/10 pie	240	15	3
14 Inch Thin Crust Cheese	1/10 pie	160	15	0
16 Inch Round Cheese	1/12 pie	220	15	1
18 Inch Round Cheese	1/14 pie	230	15	1
Deep Dish Large	1/8 pie	320	20	2
Deep Dish Medium	1/8 pie	230	15	1

SALAD DRESSINGS

FOOD	PORTION	CALS	CHOL	FIBER
Caesar	1 serv (1.5 oz)	230	55	0
Greek	1 serv (1.5 oz)	270	0	0
Italian	1 serv (1.5 oz)	220	0	0
Italian Fat Free	1 serv (1.5 oz)	25	0	0
Ranch	1 serv (1.5 oz)	230	10	0

SALADS

FOOD	PORTION	CALS	CHOL	FIBER
Antipasto	1 serv	140	20	2
Caesar	1 serv	90	0	3
Greek	1 serv	128	25	3
Tossed Salad	1 serv	100	0	3

TOPPINGS PER SLICE

FOOD	PORTION	CALS	CHOL	FIBER
Bacon	1 serv	41	7	tr

FOOD	PORTION	CALS	CHOL	FIBER
Beef	1 serv	20	2	tr
Extra Cheese	1 serv	26	6	–
Ham	1 serv	5	2	tr
Italian Sausage	1 serv	22	5	tr
Pepperoni	1 serv	26	4	–

LONG JOHN SILVER'S
BEVERAGES

FOOD	PORTION	CALS	CHOL	FIBER
Coca-Cola	1 sm	150	0	0
Diet Coke	1 sm	0	0	0
Sprite	1 sm	140	0	0

DESSERTS

FOOD	PORTION	CALS	CHOL	FIBER
Pie Chocolate Cream	1 pie	310	15	1
Pie Pecan	1 pie	370	40	2
Pie Pineapple Cream	1 pie	290	15	1

MAIN MENU SELECTIONS

FOOD	PORTION	CALS	CHOL	FIBER
Baked Cod	1 piece	120	90	1
Battered Chicken	1 piece	140	20	0
Battered Fish	1 piece	230	30	0
Battered Shrimp	1 piece	45	15	0
Breaded Clams	1 serv	240	10	1
Cheesesticks	3 pieces	140	10	1
Clam Chowder	1 bowl	220	25	tr
Corn Cobbette	1 piece	90	0	3
Crumblies	1 serv	170	0	1
Crunchy Shrimp	21 pieces	330	105	2
Fries	1 reg	230	0	3
Hushpuppy	1 piece	60	0	1
Rice	1 serv	180	0	3
Sandwich Chicken	1	360	25	3
Sandwich Fish	1	440	35	3
Sandwich Ultimate Fish	1	500	50	3
Slaw	1 serv	200	20	3

MAGGIE MOO'S

FOOD	PORTION	CALS	CHOL	FIBER
Ice Cream Fat Free	½ cup	80	0	0
Ice Cream Low Carb Sugar Added	½ cup	100	30	0
Ice Cream Udderly Cream	½ cup	180	45	0
Sorbet	½ cup	90	0	0

FOOD	PORTION	CALS	CHOL	FIBER
MANHATTAN BAGEL				
Blueberry	1	260	0	2
Cheddar Cheese	1	270	10	2
Chocolate Chip	1	290	0	2
Cinnamon Raisin	1	280	0	3
Cranberry Orange	1	270	0	2
Egg	1	270	0	2
Everything	1	290	0	3
Garlic	1	270	0	2
Jalapeno Cheddar	1	260	0	2
Marble	1	260	0	3
Oat Bran	1	260	0	3
Oat Bran Raisin Walnut	1	270	0	3
Onion	1	270	0	2
Plain	1	260	0	2
Poppy	1	300	0	5
Pumpernickel	1	250	0	3
Rye	1	260	0	3
Salt	1	260	0	2
Sesame	1	310	0	3
Spinach	1	270	0	3
Sun-Dried Tomato	1	260	0	3
Whole Wheat	1	260	0	3
MARBLE SLAB CREAMERY				
Cone Honey Wheat	1	130	15	tr
Cone Sugar	1	130	15	0
Cone Vanilla Cinnamon	1	130	15	tr
Frozen Yogurt Nonfat	½ cup	100	0	1
Frozen Yogurt Nonfat No Sugar Added	½ cup	90	0	1
Ice Cream Reduced Fat	1 serv (6.75 oz)	390	80	0
Ice Cream Superpremium	1 serv (6.75 oz)	450	115	0
Sorbet	½ cup	90	0	0
MAUI WOWI				
Smoothie Rip Sticks All Flavors	1	88	0	0
MAX & ERMA'S				
Black Bean Roll Up	1 serv	401	13	8

FOOD	PORTION	CALS	CHOL	FIBER
Black Bean Salsa	½ cup	215	0	5
Fruit Smoothie	1 serv	124	0	1
Garden Grill Sandwich w/ Tex Mex Dressing	1	569	19	14
Garlic Breadstick	1	156	0	0
Hula Bowl w/ Fat Free Honey Mustard Dressing w/o Breadsticks	1 serv	583	111	5
Salad Dressing Fat Free French	2 tbsp	126	0	2
Salad Dressing Fat Free Honey Mustard	2 tbsp	60	0	0
Salad Dressing Tex Mex	2 tbsp	33	5	tr
Sugar Snap Peas w/ Lemon Pepper Butter	1 serv (4 oz)	106	15	3

MCDONALD'S
BEVERAGES

FOOD	PORTION	CALS	CHOL	FIBER
Apple Juice	1 box (6.75 oz)	90	0	0
Chocolate Milk 1% Low Fat	8 oz	170	5	1
Coca-Cola Classic	1 sm (16 oz)	150	0	0
Coffee	1 (12 oz)	0	0	0
Diet Coke	1 sm (16 oz)	0	0	0
Half & Half Creamer	1 pkg	15	5	0
Hi-C Orange	1 sm (16 oz)	160	0	0
Iced Tea Unsweetened	1 (16 oz)	0	0	0
Milk Lowfat 1%	1 serv (8 oz)	100	10	0
Orange Juice	1 sm (12 oz)	140	0	0
Powerade Mountain Blast	1 sm (16 oz)	100	0	–
Sprite	1 sm (16 oz)	150	0	0
Triple Shake Chocolate	1 (16 oz)	580	50	1
Triple Shake Strawberry	1 (16 oz)	560	50	0
Triple Shake Vanilla	1 (16 oz)	550	50	0

BREAKFAST SELECTIONS

FOOD	PORTION	CALS	CHOL	FIBER
Big Breakfast	1 serv	730	456	3
Biscuit	1	240	0	1
Biscuit Bacon Egg Cheese	1	440	245	1
Biscuit Sausage	1	410	30	1
Biscuit Sausage w/ Egg	1	500	250	1
Deluxe Breakfast	1 serv	1220	480	4

FOOD	PORTION	CALS	CHOL	FIBER
English Muffin Buttered	1	150	0	2
Hash Browns	1 serv	140	0	2
Hotcakes Margarine & Syrup	1 serv	600	20	2
Hotcakes & Sausage	1 serv	770	50	2
Hotcakes Plain	1 serv	340	20	2
McGriddles Sausage	1	420	30	1
McGriddles Sausage Egg Cheese	1	560	260	1
McMuffin Egg	1	290	235	2
McMuffin Sausage	1	370	45	2
Sausage	1 patty	170	30	0
Sausage Burrito	1	300	175	1
Scrambled Eggs	2	180	435	0
DESSERTS				
Apple Dippers	1 pkg	35	0	0
Apple Pie Baked	1	250	0	2
Carmel Dip Low Fat	1 pkg	70	5	0
Cinnamon Roll Deluxe Warm	1	590	55	4
Cinnamon Roll Warm	1	420	60	2
Cookie Chocolate Chip	1 pkg	270	35	1
Cookie Chocolate Chip	1 (1.1 oz)	160	10	1
Cookie Oatmeal	1 (1.1 oz)	140	10	1
Cookie Sugar	1 (1.1 oz)	150	5	0
Fruit 'n Yogurt Parfait	1 serv	160	5	1
Ice Cream Cone Reduced Fat Vanilla	1	150	15	0
McDonaldland Cookies	1 pkg	250	0	1
McFlurry M&M	1 (12 oz)	620	55	1
McFlurry Oreo	1 (12 oz)	560	50	0
Peanuts For Sundae	1 serv	45	0	1
Sundae Hot Caramel	1	340	30	0
Sundae Hot Fudge	1	340	25	1
Sundae Strawberry	1	280	25	0
MAIN MENU SELECTIONS				
Big Mac	1	560	80	3
Big N' Tasty	1	470	80	3
Big N' Tasty w/ Cheese	1	520	95	3
Cheeseburger	1	310	40	1
Cheeseburger Double	1	460	80	1

FOOD	PORTION	CALS	CHOL	FIBER
Chicken McNuggets	4 pieces	170	25	0
Chicken Selects	3 pieces	380	55	0
Crispy Chicken Classic	1	500	60	3
Crispy Chicken Club	1	680	100	3
Crispy Chicken Ranch BLT	1	580	70	3
Filet-O-Fish	1	400	40	1
French Fries	1 sm (2.6 oz)	230	0	3
Grilled Chicken Classic	1	420	80	3
Grilled Chicken Club	1	590	120	3
Grilled Chicken Ranch BLT	1	490	90	3
Hamburger	1	260	30	1
McChicken	1	370	50	1
McChicken Hot 'n Spicy	1	380	45	1
Quarter Pounder	1	420	70	3
Quarter Pounder Double w/ Cheese	1	730	160	3
Quarter Pounder w/ Cheese	1	510	95	3
SALAD DRESSINGS AND SAUCES				
Honey	1 pkg (0.5 oz)	50	0	0
Newman's Own Cobb	1 pkg (2 oz)	120	10	0
Newman's Own Creamy Caesar	1 pkg (2 oz)	190	20	0
Newman's Own Low Fat Balsamic Vinaigrette	1 pkg (1.5 oz)	40	0	0
Newman's Own Low Fat Family Recipe Italian	1 pkg (1.6 oz)	50	5	0
Newman's Own Ranch	1 pkg (2 oz)	170	20	0
Sauce Barbecue	1 pkg (1 oz)	45	0	0
Sauce Chipotle Barbecue	1 pkg	70	0	0
Sauce Creamy Ranch	1 pkg (1.5 oz)	200	10	0
Sauce Hot Mustard	1 pkg (1 oz)	50	0	1
Sauce Spicy Buffalo	1 pkg (1.5 oz)	60	0	1
Sauce Sweet 'N Sour	1 pkg (1 oz)	50	0	0
Sauce Tangy Honey Mustard	1 pkg (1.5 oz)	70	0	1
SALADS				
Bacon Ranch w/ Crispy Chicken	1 serv	340	70	3
Bacon Ranch w/ Grilled Chicken	1 serv	260	90	3
Bacon Ranch w/o Chicken	1 serv	140	25	3

FOOD	PORTION	CALS	CHOL	FIBER
Caesar w/ Crispy Chicken	1 serv	300	55	3
Caesar w/ Grilled Chicken	1 serv	220	75	3
Caesar w/o Chicken	1 serv	90	10	3
California Cobb w/ Crispy Chicken	1 serv	360	130	4
California Cobb w/ Grilled Chicken	1 serv	280	150	4
California Cobb w/o Chicken	1 serv	160	85	4
Croutons Butter Garlic	1 pkg	60	0	1
Fruit & Walnut	1 serv	310	5	6
Side Salad	1 serv	20	0	1

MIAMI SUBS

FOOD	PORTION	CALS	CHOL	FIBER
Burger Deluxe	1	784	30	1
Cheeseburger Deluxe	1	859	47	1
Cheeseburger Deluxe Bacon	1	919	61	1
Cheesesteak Classic	1 (6 in)	420	77	2
Cheesesteak Original	1 (6 in)	409	77	1
Cheesesteak Works	1 (6 in)	532	87	2
Chicken Philly Classic	1 (6 in)	551	92	2
Mozzarella Sticks	1 serv	757	60	1
Onion Rings	1 serv	869	0	2
Pita Chicken	1	392	75	5
Pita Gyros	1	662	84	5
Platter Chicken Breast	1 serv	743	80	5
Platter Gyros	1 serv	1420	186	5
Salad Caesar w/ Dressing	1 serv	459	14	4
Salad Chicken Caesar w/ Dressing	1 serv	609	74	4
Salad Chicken Club	1 serv	490	210	5
Salad Garden	1 serv	310	136	5
Salad Greek	1 serv	284	123	5
Salad Greek Side w/ Dressing	1 serv	78	8	1
Spicy Fries	1 reg	532	19	4
Subs 6 Inch Ham And Cheese	1	452	59	2
Subs 6 Inch Italian Deli	1	516	69	2

FOOD	PORTION	CALS	CHOL	FIBER
Subs 6 Inch Meatball	1	491	76	4
Subs 6 Inch Tuna	1	468	67	2
Subs 6 Inch Turkey	1	484	68	2
Wings w/ Fries Celery & Blue Cheese	1 serv	1020	179	4
MR. PITA				
Cranberry Turkey	1 reg	424	45	3
Grilled Raspberry Chicken	1 reg	342	34	1
Grilled Chicken & Broccoli	1 reg	373	41	2
Grilled Chicken Caesar	1 reg	353	42	1
Grilled Hawaiian Chicken	1 reg	375	41	1
Ultra Combo	1 reg	354	43	2
Ultra Grilled Chicken	1 reg	367	41	2
Ultra Supreme	1 reg	350	37	1
Ultra Turkey	1 reg	343	45	2
MRS. FIELDS				
Brownie Double Fudge	1 (2.7 oz)	360	80	2
Brownie Frosted Fudge	1 (3.7 oz)	440	80	2
Brownie Pecan Fudge	1 (2.7 oz)	340	70	2
Brownie Pecan Pie	1 (2.7 oz)	340	70	2
Brownie Walnut Fudge	1 (2.7 oz)	380	80	tr
Bundt Cake Banana Walnut	1 piece (2.9 oz)	350	40	3
Bundt Cake Banana Walnut w/ Chocolate Chips	1 piece (2.9 oz)	370	35	3
Bundt Cake Blueberry	1 piece (2.9 oz)	270	50	1
Bundt Cake Raspberry	1 piece (2.9 oz)	270	50	tr
Bundt Cake White w/ Chocolate Chips	1 piece (2.9 oz)	350	50	tr
Cookie Butter Toffee	1 (2.3 oz)	290	55	tr
Cookie Cinnamon Sugar	1 (2.3 oz)	300	50	tr
Cookie Coconut Macadamia	1 (2.3 oz)	280	20	tr
Cookie Debra's Special	1 (2.3 oz)	280	40	2
Cookie Milk Chocolate	1 (2.3 oz)	280	40	tr
Cookie Milk Chocolate & Walnuts	1 (2.3 oz)	320	40	1
Cookie Milk Chocolate Macadamia	1 (2.3 oz)	320	40	tr
Cookie Oatmeal Chocolate Chip	1 (2.3 oz)	280	35	1

FOOD	PORTION	CALS	CHOL	FIBER
Cookie Oatmeal Raisin & Walnuts	1 (2.3 oz)	280	40	2
Cookie Peanut Butter	1 (2.3 oz)	310	45	tr
Cookie Peanut Butter w/ Milk Chocolate Chips	1 (2.3 oz)	300	40	tr
Cookie Semi-Sweet Chocolate	1 (2.3 oz)	280	30	1
Cookie Semi-Sweet Chocolate & Walnuts	1 (2.3 oz)	310	35	2
Cookie White Chunk Macadamia	1 (2.3 oz)	310	35	tr
Jumbo Cookie Snickerdoodle	1 (5 oz)	640	110	2
Nibbler Cookies	2 (0.9 oz)	110	15	0
Nibbler Cookies Chewy Chocolate Fudge	2 (0.9 oz)	110	10	tr
Nibbler Cookies Cinnamon Sugar	2 (0.9 oz)	120	15	0
Nibbler Cookies Debra's Special	2 (0.9 oz)	100	10	0
Nibbler Cookies M&M	2 (0.9 oz)	110	15	0
Nibbler Cookies Milk Chocolate	2 (0.9 oz)	110	15	tr
Nibbler Cookies Milk Chocolate w/ Walnuts	2 (0.9 oz)	120	10	tr
Nibbler Cookies Peanut Butter	2 (0.9 oz)	110	15	0
Nibbler Cookies Semi-Sweet Chocolate	2 (0.9 oz)	110	10	tr
Nibbler Cookies Triple Chocolate	2 (0.9 oz)	110	15	tr
Nibbler Cookies White Chunk Macadamia	2 (0.9 oz)	120	10	tr

MY FAVORITE MUFFIN
BAGELS

FOOD	PORTION	CALS	CHOL	FIBER
Blueberry	1	320	0	2
Cinnamon Raisin	1	310	0	3
Honey Grain	1	310	0	4
Plain	1	310	0	2

FOOD	PORTION	CALS	CHOL	FIBER
Russian Black Bread	1	320	0	4
Sour Dough	1	310	0	2
Whole Wheat	1	310	0	5
MUFFINS				
Banana Nut	⅓ jumbo	195	21	1
Blueberry	⅓ jumbo	168	24	0
Blueberry Cheesecake	⅓ jumbo	199	38	0
Boston Cream Pie	⅓ jumbo	176	22	0
Cherry Cheesecake	⅓ jumbo	170	30	0
Chocolate Cheesecake	⅓ jumbo	202	20	0
Chocolate Chip	⅓ jumbo	211	25	1
Cinnamon Crumb Cake	⅓ jumbo	212	37	0
Cinnamon Swirl Cheesecake	⅓ jumbo	214	25	0
Deep Dish Apple Pie	⅓ jumbo	177	19	0
Double Chocolate	⅓ jumbo	201	0	1
Fat Free Blueberry	⅓ jumbo	108	0	1
Fat Free Cherry Pie	⅓ jumbo	109	0	0
Fat Free Chocolate Eclair	⅓ jumbo	120	0	1
Fat Free Chocolate Marble	⅓ jumbo	125	0	1
Fat Free Cinnamon Bun	⅓ jumbo	168	0	0
Fat Free Raspberry Amaretto	⅓ jumbo	127	0	1
Golden Corn Bread	⅓ jumbo	197	24	1
Lemon Poppyseed	⅓ jumbo	201	28	0
Pumpkin Spice	⅓ jumbo	181	23	0
NATHAN'S				
¼ Pound Burger	1	537	90	2
¼ Pound Burger w/ Cheese	1	850	136	2
Bacon Cheeseburger	1	707	128	2
Cheesesteak Chicken	1 serv	565	81	5
Cheesesteak Original	1	741	124	4
Cheesesteak Supreme	1 serv	786	124	5
Chicken Tender Pita	1	610	65	2
Chicken Tenders	3 pieces	512	30	3
Cole Slaw	1 serv	213	7	3
Corn Muffin	1	163	0	1
Famous Hot Dog	1	309	35	1

FOOD	PORTION	CALS	CHOL	FIBER
Fish N Chips	1 serv	1538	111	9
French Fries	1 reg	547	0	6
Hot Dog Nuggets	6 pieces	351	20	0
Hush Puppy	2 pieces	277	5	2
Onion Rings	1 sm	559	0	2
Platter Chicken Breast	1 serv	943	84	9
Platter Chicken Tender	1 serv	1301	105	9
Sandwich Chicken Tender	1	725	65	2
Sandwich Fish	1	469	34	13
Sandwich Grilled Chicken	1	524	67	2
Seafood Sampler	1 serv	3379	156	15
Shrimp N Chips	1 serv	2051	222	12
Super Burger	1	864	136	3

NEWPORT CREAMERY

FOOD	PORTION	CALS	CHOL	FIBER
Ice Cream Chocolate No Sugar Added	½ cup	110	10	–
Ice Cream Vanilla No Sugar Added	½ cup	100	15	–
Vanilla Yogurt	½ cup	120	10	–
Vanilla Yogurt Nonfat	½ cup	100	0	–

OLD SPAGHETTI FACTORY
CHILDREN'S MENU SELECTIONS

FOOD	PORTION	CALS	CHOL	FIBER
Grilled Cheese Sandwich	1 serv	360	25	1
Macaroni & Cheese	1 serv	350	10	2
Spaghetti w/ Tomato Sauce	1 serv	300	0	4
Spaghetti w/ Tomato Sauce & Meatballs	1 serv	440	40	4

DESSERTS

FOOD	PORTION	CALS	CHOL	FIBER
Caramel Turtle Pie	1 serv	660	45	0
Mud Pie	1 serv	680	45	3
New York Cheese Cake w/ Strawberry Topping	1 serv	690	180	1

MAIN MENU SELECTIONS

FOOD	PORTION	CALS	CHOL	FIBER
Baked Chicken	1 dinner serv	880	165	4
Caesar Salad	1 sm	330	30	2
Caesar Salad Dinner Chicken	1 serv	1280	250	4
Chicken Marsala	1 dinner serv	960	250	4

FOOD	PORTION	CALS	CHOL	FIBER
Fettuccine Alfredo	1 dinner serv	1130	260	4
Fettuccine Chicken	1 dinner serv	960	220	6
Lasagne	1 dinner serv	630	110	4
Parmigiana Chicken	1 dinner serv	840	80	5
Parmigiana Eggplant	1 dinner serv	670	130	8
Pot Pourri	1 dinner serv	710	95	6
Ravioli Spinach & Cheese	1 dinner serv	480	70	4
Salmon Tuscany	1 dinner serv	680	175	1
Sandwich Meatball	1	860	140	4
Sandwich Sausage	1	730	105	4
Sandwich Tuscan Chicken	1	1060	175	4
Seafood Cheddar Melt	1 serv	790	165	4
Spaghetti w/ Clam Sauce	1 dinner serv	690	125	5
Spaghetti w/ Clam Sauce & Mizithra	1 dinner serv	960	180	5
Spaghetti w/ Meat & Clam Sauces	1 dinner serv	980	70	6
Spaghetti w/ Meat Sauce	1 dinner serv	470	15	6
Spaghetti w/ Meat Sauce & Mizithra	1 dinner serv	850	125	5
Spaghetti w/ Meat Sauce & Sausage	1 dinner serv	830	105	6
Spaghetti w/ Meatballs	1 dinner serv	840	130	5
Spaghetti w/ Mizithra	1 dinner serv	1010	180	4
Spaghetti w/ Mushroom & Clam Sauces	1 dinner serv	830	65	5
Spaghetti w/ Mushroom & Meat Sauces	1 dinner serv	460	10	6
Spaghetti w/ Mushroom Sauce	1 dinner serv	460	0	6
Spaghetti w/ Mushroom Sauce & Mizithra	1 dinner serv	850	120	5
Spaghetti w/ Tomato & Mizithra	1 dinner serv	840	120	5
Spaghetti w/ Tomato & Meat Sauces	1 dinner serv	460	10	6
Spaghetti w/ Tomato Sauce	1 dinner serv	440	0	7
Spaghetti w/ Tomato Sauce & Clam Sauce	1 dinner serv	560	65	6
Starter Garlic Cheese Bread	1 serv	1220	0	5

FOOD	PORTION	CALS	CHOL	FIBER
Starter Meatballs	1 serv	910	245	1
Starter Sausage	1 serv	690	140	tr
Starter Tortellini	1 serv	930	205	2
Tortellini Mortadella & Chicken	1 dinner serv	930	205	2
SOUPS				
Chicken Mulligatawny	1 serv	250	60	2
Chicken Orzo	1 serv	90	20	tr
Clam Chowder	1 serv	380	95	–
Cream Of Broccoli	1 serv	220	40	2
Mediterranean White Bean	1 serv	150	0	6
Minestrone	1 serv	120	5	3

PANDA EXPRESS
MAIN MENU SELECTIONS

FOOD	PORTION	CALS	CHOL	FIBER
BBQ Pork	1 serv	350	85	tr
Beef & Broccoli	1 serv	150	15	1
Beef w/ String Beans	1 serv	170	20	2
Black Pepper Chicken	1 serv	180	40	2
Chicken w/ Mushrooms	1 serv	130	50	2
Chicken w/ Potato	1 serv	220	55	1
Chicken w/ String Beans	1 serv	170	30	3
Egg Roll Chicken	1 (3 oz)	190	25	3
Fried Shrimp	6 pieces	260	65	tr
Mandarin Chicken	1 serv	250	125	2
Mixed Vegetables	1 serv	70	0	1
Orange Chicken	1 serv	480	80	2
Spicy Chicken w/ Peanuts	1 serv	200	70	4
Spring Roll Veggie	1 (1.7 oz)	80	0	tr
Steamed Rice	1 serv	330	0	2
String Beans w/ Fried Tofu	1 serv	180	0	3
Sweet & Sour Chicken	1 serv	310	50	2
Sweet & Sour Pork	1 serv	410	55	3
Vegetable Chow Mein	1 serv	330	0	4
Vegetable Fried Rice	1 serv	390	85	2
SAUCES				
Hot	2 tsp	10	0	0
Hot Mustard	1 serv	18	0	0
Mandarin	1 serv	70	0	0
Soy	1 tbsp	16	0	0
Sweet & Sour	1 serv	60	0	0

FOOD	PORTION	CALS	CHOL	FIBER
PANERA BREAD				
BAGELS AND SPREADS				
Bagel Asiago Cheese	1	330	15	2
Bagel Blueberry	1	320	0	3
Bagel Cinnamon Crunch	1	490	0	3
Bagel Dutch Apple & Raisin	1	340	0	3
Bagel Everything	1	290	0	2
Bagel French Toast	1	340	0	2
Bagel Mochachip Swirl	1	340	0	3
Bagel Nine Grain	1	290	0	3
Bagel Peanut Butter Crunch	1	400	0	3
Bagel Plain	1	280	0	2
Bagel Sesame	1	310	0	3
Cream Cheese Hazelnut Reduced Fat	1 serv (2 oz)	150	35	tr
Cream Cheese Honey Walnut Reduced Fat	1 serv (2 oz)	150	30	tr
Cream Cheese Mocha Reduced Fat	1 serv (2 oz)	160	7	1
Cream Cheese Plain	1 serv (2 oz)	190	55	0
Cream Cheese Plain Reduced Fat	1 serv (2 oz)	130	35	tr
Cream Cheese Raspberry Reduced Fat	1 serv (2 oz)	120	30	0
Cream Cheese Smoked Salmon Reduced Fat	1 serv (2 oz)	120	35	0
Cream Cheese Sun Dried Tomato Reduced Fat	1 serv (2 oz)	140	35	tr
Cream Cheese Veggie Reduced Fat	1 serv (2 oz)	130	35	1
Hummus Roasted Garlic	1 serv (2 oz)	100	0	4
BEVERAGES				
Caffe Mocha	1 serv (11.5 oz)	360	10	2
Homestyle Lemonade	1 serv (16 oz)	80	0	0
Hot Chocolate	1 serv (11 oz)	350	50	2
IC Cappuccino Chip	1 serv (16 oz)	590	70	0
IC Caramel	1 serv (16 oz)	550	80	0
IC Honeydew Green Tea	1 serv (16 oz)	270	30	0
IC Mocha	1 serv (16 oz)	520	75	2
IC Spice	1 serv (16 oz)	470	70	0

FOOD	PORTION	CALS	CHOL	FIBER
Iced Green Tea	1 serv (16 oz)	60	0	0
Latte Caffe	1 serv (8.5 oz)	120	20	0
Latte Caramel	1 serv (11 oz)	400	55	0
Latte Chai Tea	1 serv (10 oz)	210	15	0
Latte House	1 serv (10.8 oz)	320	50	0
BREADS				
Artisan Country	1 slice	120	0	1
Artisan French	1 slice (2 oz)	110	0	tr
Artisan Kalamata Olive	1 slice (2 oz)	140	0	1
Artisan Multigrain	1 slice (2 oz)	120	0	1
Artisan Raisin Pecan	1 slice (2 oz)	140	0	1
Artisan Sesame Semolina	1 slice (2 oz)	120	0	4
Artisan Stone Milled Rye	1 slice (2 oz)	110	0	2
Artisan Three Cheese	1 slice (2 oz)	120	5	tr
Artisan Three Seed	1 slice	130	0	1
Ciabatta	1 (6 oz)	430	0	3
Cinnamon Raisin	1 slice (2 oz)	160	0	1
Focaccia Asiago Cheese	1 slice (2 oz)	150	5	1
Focaccia Basil Pesto	1 slice (2 oz)	150	5	1
Focaccia Rosemary & Onion	1 slice (2 oz)	140	5	1
French	1 slice (2 oz)	130	0	1
French Roll	1 (2.25 oz)	140	0	1
Holiday	1 slice (2 oz)	150	5	tr
Honey Wheat	1 slice (2 oz)	140	0	1
Nine Grain	1 slice (2 oz)	150	0	2
Rye	1 slice (2 oz)	140	0	1
Sourdough	1 slice (2 oz)	120	0	1
Sourdough Roll	1 (2.5 oz)	160	0	1
Sourdough Soup Bowl	1 serv (8 oz)	500	0	4
Sunflower	1 slice (2 oz)	160	0	1
Tomato Basil	1 slice (2 oz)	130	0	1
DESSERTS				
Bear Claw	1	380	70	1
Brownie Caramel Pecan	1	470	80	2
Brownie Chocolate Raspberry	1	370	75	2
Brownie Very Chocolate	1	460	80	2
Cinnamon Roll	1	560	90	3
Cobblestone	1	560	0	4
Coffee Cake Cherry Cheese	1	190	30	1

FOOD	PORTION	CALS	CHOL	FIBER
Cookie Chocolate Chipper	1	420	60	2
Cookie Chocolate Duet w/ Walnuts	1	410	60	3
Cookie Nutty Chocolate Chipper	1	440	55	3
Cookie Nutty Oatmeal Raisin	1	350	45	5
Cookie Shortbread	1	340	60	1
Croissant Apple	1	260	30	1
Croissant Cheese	1	300	45	1
Croissant Chocolate	1	440	35	4
Croissant French	1	265	40	1
Croissant Raspberry Cheese	1	280	35	1
Danish Apple	1	510	85	2
Danish Cheese	1	590	110	1
Danish Cherry	1	520	85	1
Danish Georgia Peach	1	580	85	2
Danish German Chocolate	1	770	85	4
Macaroon Chocolate Hazelnut	1	270	0	3
Mini Bundt Cake Carrot Walnut	1	430	75	2
Mini Bundt Cake Lemon Poppyseed	1	460	90	1
Mini Bundt Cake Pineapple Upside Down	1	450	70	2
Muffie Banana Nut	1	260	15	3
Muffie Chocolate Chip	1	240	15	2
Muffie Pumpkin	1	270	30	1
Muffin Banana Nut	1	470	30	5
Muffin Blueberry	1	450	35	4
Muffin Chocolate Chip	1	540	30	5
Muffin Pumpkin	1	510	60	1
Muffin Low Fat Tripleberry	1	300	30	3
Pecan Roll	1	520	40	2
Scone Cinnamon Chip	1	560	150	2
Scone Orange	1	530	140	3
Strudel Apple Raisin	1	390	0	1
Strudel Cherry	1	400	0	1

FOOD	PORTION	CALS	CHOL	FIBER
SALADS				
Asian Sesame Chicken	1 serv	370	60	5
Caesar	1 serv	350	110	3
Caesar Grilled Chicken	1 serv	470	165	3
Classic Cafe	1 serv	380	0	4
Fandango	1 serv	400	25	6
Greek	1 serv	520	20	5
SANDWICHES				
Asiago Roast Beef	1	730	115	2
Bacon Turkey Bravo	1	770	45	5
Chicken Salad On Artisan Sesame Semolina	1	730	90	6
Chicken Salad On Nine Grain	1	640	90	4
Garden Veggie	1	570	15	5
Italian Combo	1	1050	165	5
Panini Coronado Carnitas	1	810	95	3
Panini Frontega Chicken	1	860	110	5
Panini Portobello & Mozzarella	1	650	40	8
Panini Turkey Artichoke	1	810	25	6
Peanut Butter & Jelly On French	1	450	0	3
Sierra Turkey	1	950	40	4
Smoked Ham On Artisan Stone Milled Rye	1	930	110	6
Smoked Ham On Rye	1	650	110	4
Smoked Turkey Breast On Artisan Country	1	590	10	5
Smoked Turkey On Sourdough	1	440	10	3
Tuna Salad On Artisan Multigrain	1	830	65	5
Tuna Salad On Honey Wheat	1	720	65	4
Turkey Fresco	1	580	0	4
Tuscan Chicken	1	950	80	6
SOUPS				
Baked Potato	1 serv	260	35	1
Boston Clam Chowder	1 serv	210	40	tr

FOOD	PORTION	CALS	CHOL	FIBER
Broccoli Cheddar	1 serv	230	45	1
Cream Of Chicken & Wild Rice	1 serv	200	35	tr
Forest Mushroom	1 serv	140	15	2
French Onion	1 serv	220	20	2
Low Fat Chicken Noodle	1 serv	100	15	1
Low Fat Vegetarian Garden Vegetable	1 serv	90	0	2
Low Fat Vegetarian Black Bean	1 serv	100	0	17
Vegetarian Santa Fe Roasted Corn	1 serv	130	0	3

PAPA JOHNS
OTHER MENU SELECTIONS

FOOD	PORTION	CALS	CHOL	FIBER
Bread Sticks	1 serv	140	0	1
Cheese Sticks	1 serv	180	13	1
Chickenstrips	1	83	13	tr
Cinnapie	1 serv	114	0	0

PIZZA 14 INCH

FOOD	PORTION	CALS	CHOL	FIBER
Original All The Meats	⅛ pie	405	41	2
Original BBQ Chicken & Bacon	⅛ pie	369	31	2
Original Cheese	⅛ pie	290	17	2
Original Chicken Alfredo	⅛ pie	310	31	2
Original Garden Fresh	⅛ pie	287	14	3
Original Hawaiian BBQ Chicken	⅛ pie	376	31	2
Original Pepperoni	⅛ pie	343	27	2
Original Sausage	⅛ pie	336	28	2
Original Spinach Alfredo	⅛ pie	303	25	2
Original The Works	⅛ pie	370	34	3
Thin Crust All The Meat	⅛ pie	371	44	2
Thin Crust BBQ Chicken & Bacon	⅛ pie	336	34	1
Thin Crust Cheese	⅛ pie	238	17	1
Thin Crust Chicken Alfredo	⅛ pie	276	35	1
Thin Crust Garden Fresh	⅛ pie	228	14	2
Thin Crust Hawaiian BBQ Chicken	⅛ pie	324	31	1

FOOD	PORTION	CALS	CHOL	FIBER
Thin Crust Pepperoni	⅛ pie	294	28	2
Thin Crust Sausage	⅛ pie	303	31	2
Thin Crust Spinach Alfredo	⅛ pie	251	26	1
Thin Crust The Works	⅛ pie	315	32	2
SALAD DRESSINGS AND SAUCES				
BBQ Sauce	1 serv	48	0	0
Buffalo Sauce	1 serv	25	0	0
Cheese Sauce	1 serv	60	19	0
Garlic Sauce	1 serv	235	0	0
Honey Mustard Dressing	1 serv	170	10	0
Pizza Sauce	1 serv	25	0	2
Ranch Dressing	1 serv	140	15	0

PAPA MURPHY'S
PIZZA

FOOD	PORTION	CALS	CHOL	FIBER
Deeper Dish Traditional	⅛ pie	440	40	2
Delite Large Cheese	¹⁄₁₀ pie	130	15	0
Delite Large Hawaiian	¹⁄₁₀ pie	140	15	1
Delite Large Meat	¹⁄₁₀ pie	190	25	0
Delite Large Pepperoni	¹⁄₁₀ pie	160	20	0
Delite Large Veggie	¹⁄₁₀ pie	150	15	0
Family Size Cheese	¹⁄₁₂ pie	270	20	2
Gourmet Family Size Chicken Garlic	¹⁄₁₂ pie	320	35	1
Gourmet Family Size Classic Italian	¹⁄₁₂ pie	360	35	2
Gourmet Family Size Veggie	¹⁄₁₂ pie	300	25	2
Papa's Family Size All Meat	¹⁄₁₂ pie	370	40	2
Papa's Family Size Cheese	¹⁄₁₂ pie	270	20	2
Papa's Family Size Cowboy	¹⁄₁₂ pie	370	35	2
Papa's Family Size Favorite	¹⁄₁₂ pie	380	35	2
Papa's Family Size Hawaiian	¹⁄₁₂ pie	290	25	2
Papa's Family Size Murphy's Combo	¹⁄₁₂ pie	480	35	2
Papa's Family Size Pepperoni	¹⁄₁₂ pie	310	30	2
Papa's Family Size Perfect	¹⁄₁₂ pie	300	25	2
Papa's Family Size Rancher	¹⁄₁₂ pie	330	30	2
Papa's Family Size Specialty	¹⁄₁₂ pie	340	30	2

FOOD	PORTION	CALS	CHOL	FIBER
Papa's Family Size Veggie Combo	1/12 pie	300	20	2
Stuffed Big Murphy	1/6 pie	380	30	2
Stuffed Chicago Style	1/6 pie	370	30	2
SALADS				
Club	1 serv	190	50	4
Garden	1 serv	160	20	4
Italian	1 serv	220	30	3

PICCADILLY CAFETERIA
DESSERTS

FOOD	PORTION	CALS	CHOL	FIBER
Gelatin Sugar Free	1 serv	0	0	0
Sugar Free Blueberry Pie	1 serv	314	0	3
Sugar Free Cherry Pie	1 serv	334	0	1
Sugar Free Chocolate Almond Pie	1 serv	611	1	2
MAIN MENU SELECTIONS				
Bass Blackened	1 serv	408	28	1
Bass Cajun Baked	1 serv	260	28	1
Bass Stuffed	1 serv	447	64	1
Beef Chopped Steak	1 serv	382	74	0
Beef Chopped Steak Fried	1 serv	225	59	0
Beef Roast Leg	1 sm serv	353	103	1
Broccoli Florets	1 serv	90	0	3
Broccoli w/ Cheese Sauce	1 serv	55	4	3
Brussels Sprouts	1 serv	92	0	4
Cabbage Steamed Bacon Seasoned	1 serv	108	9	2
Cabbage Steamed Buttered	1 serv	68	0	2
Catfish Filet Blackened	1 serv	523	87	1
Catfish Filet Cajun Baked	1 serv	401	87	1
Catfish Filet Stuffed	1 serv	561	123	1
Cauliflower Buttered	1 serv	73	0	1
Chicken Barbecued Quarters	1 serv	472	255	1
Chicken Grilled Breast	1 serv	345	136	1
Chicken Rotisserie Herb Dark Meat	1 serv	823	276	1
Chicken Rotisserie Herb White Meat	1 serv	602	218	1

FOOD	PORTION	CALS	CHOL	FIBER
Chicken Baked Cajun Boneless Breast	1 serv	428	136	1
Chicken Baked Quarters	1 serv	828	255	1
Chicken Breast Italian Boneless Breast	1 serv	371	139	1
Chicken Breast Mesquite Smoke	1 serv	212	86	1
Chicken Breast Mesquite w/ BBQ Sauce	1 serv	240	86	0
Chicken Breast Southwestern	1 serv	315	133	1
Chicken Half Rotisserie Herb	1 serv	833	478	2
Corn	1 serv	125	0	1
Cottage Cheese	1 serv	117	17	0
Filet Mignon	1 (6 oz)	184	105	0
Green Beans	1 serv	136	12	4
Green Collard Mustard Turnip	1 serv	135	12	2
Greens Turnip w/ Diced Turnips	1 serv	150	14	2
Grouper Filet Baked	1 piece (6 oz)	305	84	1
New York Strip	1 (10 oz)	871	190	0
Okra Creole	1 serv	77	5	3
Okra Fried	1 serv	240	0	4
Peas & Sugar Snapped Mixed	1 serv	102	0	3
Pork Loin Marinated Boneless	1 serv	365	102	0
Pork Loin Roast Bone In	1 serv	373	120	1
Ribeye	1 (10 oz)	1038	193	1
Roast Beef	1 serv	481	141	1
Roll Parker House	1	147	0	1
Roll Whole Wheat	1	231	0	5
Shrimp Fried	1 serv	499	277	0
Tilapia Baked	1 serv	210	0	1
Tilapia Cajun Baked	1 serv	263	0	1
Trout Almondine Baked	1 lg serv	457	167	1
Trout Cajun Baked	1 lg serv	517	167	1
Trout Filet Baked	1 lg serv	464	167	1

FOOD	PORTION	CALS	CHOL	FIBER
Turkey Breast Carved	1 serv	302	123	0
Vegetables Mixed	1 serv	95	0	3
SALAD DRESSINGS AND TOPPINGS				
Au Jus	1 serv	6	0	0
Blue Cheese	2 tbsp	160	20	0
Cheese Sauce	2 oz	35	4	0
French	2 tbsp	130	0	0
Italian	2 tbsp	140	0	0
Ranch	2 tbsp	150	15	0
Ranch Fat Free	2 tbsp	36	0	1
SALADS				
Asparagus & Tomato	1 serv	86	4	2
Caesar	1 serv	141	12	1
Cauliflower	1 serv	118	33	2
Chef	1 sm serv	146	150	1
Cole Slaw Kosher Style	1 serv	140	0	2
Coleslaw Italian	1 serv	163	0	2
Combination	1 serv	63	125	2
Cucumber & Celery	1 serv	74	0	1
Cucumber & Tomato	1 serv	41	0	1
Cucumber Mix	1 serv	61	0	2
Cucumbers & Sour Cream	1 serv	90	22	1
Louisianne Bowl	1 serv	42	9	1
Mexican	1 serv	58	0	1
Piccadilly Bowl	1 serv	27	0	2
Piccadilly Fruit	1 serv	76	0	3
Shrimp Ramoulade	1 serv	521	410	5
Spring Bowl	1 reg serv	24	0	2
Tomato Cucumber & Onion	1 serv	44	0	1
Vegetable Combo w/ Cherry Tomatoes	1 serv	66	0	2
SOUPS				
Gumbo Chicken & Sausage No Rice	1 serv	224	39	1
Gumbo Chicken No Rice	1 serv	89	23	1
PIZZA HUT				
APPETIZERS				
Breadstick	1	150	0	tr
Breadstick Cheese	1	200	15	tr

FOOD	PORTION	CALS	CHOL	FIBER
Hot Wings	2 pieces	110	70	0
Mild Wings	2 pieces	110	70	0
BEVERAGES				
Diet Pepsi	1 med (14 oz)	0	0	0
Mt. Dew	1 med (14 oz)	190	0	0
Pepsi	1 med (14 oz)	180	0	0
DESSERTS				
Apple Pizza	1 slice	260	0	1
Cherry Pizza	1 slice	240	0	1
Cinnamon Sticks	2	170	0	tr
PIZZA				
Fit 'N Delicious Diced Chicken Mushroom Jalapeno	1 med slice	170	15	2
Fit 'N Delicious Diced Chicken Red Onion Green Pepper	1 med slice	170	15	2
Fit 'N Delicious Diced Red Tomato Mushroom Jalapeno	1 med slice	150	10	2
Fit 'N Delicious Green Pepper Red Onion Diced Red Tomato	1 med slice	150	10	2
Fit 'N Delicious Ham Pineapple Diced Red Tomato	1 med slice	160	15	2
Fit 'N Delicious Ham Red Onion Mushroom	1 med slice	160	15	2
Hand Tossed Cheese	1 med slice	240	25	2
Hand Tossed Chicken Supreme	1 med slice	230	25	2
Hand Tossed Ham	1 med slice	220	20	2
Hand Tossed Meat Lover's	1 med slice	300	35	2
Hand Tossed Pepperoni	1 med slice	250	25	2
Hand Tossed Pepperoni Lover's	1 med slice	300	40	2
Hand Tossed Super Supreme	1 med slice	300	35	2
Hand Tossed Supreme	1 med slice	270	25	2

FOOD	PORTION	CALS	CHOL	FIBER
Hand Tossed Veggie Lover's	1 med slice	220	15	2
Pan Cheese	1 med slice	280	25	1
Pan Chicken Supreme	1 med slice	280	25	2
Pan Ham	1 med slice	260	20	1
Pan Meat Lover's	1 med slice	340	35	2
Pan Pepperoni	1 med slice	290	25	2
Pan Pepperoni Lover's	1 med slice	340	40	2
Pan Super Supreme	1 med slice	340	35	2
Pan Supreme	1 med slice	320	25	2
Pan Veggie Lover's	1 med slice	260	15	2
Personal Pan Cheese	1 pie	630	60	4
Personal Pan Chicken Supreme	1 pie	620	55	4
Personal Pan Meat Lover's	1 pie	800	90	5
Personal Pan Pepperoni	1 pie	660	60	4
Personal Pan Pepperoni Lover's	1 pie	800	95	4
Personal Pan Super Supreme	1 pie	790	85	6
Personal Pan Supreme	1 pie	750	70	6
Personal Pan Veggie Lover's	1 pie	580	40	5
Stuffed Crust Cheese	1 lg slice	360	40	2
Stuffed Crust Chicken Supreme	1 lg slice	380	40	3
Stuffed Crust Ham	1 lg slice	340	40	2
Stuffed Crust Meat Lover's	1 lg slice	450	55	3
Stuffed Crust Pepperoni	1 lg slice	370	45	2
Stuffed Crust Pepperoni Lover's	1 lg slice	420	55	3
Stuffed Crust Super Supreme	1 lg slice	440	50	3
Stuffed Crust Supreme	1 lg slice	400	45	3
Stuffed Crust Veggie Lover's	1 lg slice	360	35	3
Thin'N Crispy Cheese	1 med slice	200	25	1
Thin'N Crispy Chicken Supreme	1 med slice	200	25	1
Thin'N Crispy Ham	1 med slice	180	20	1
Thin'N Crispy Meat Lover's	1 med slice	270	35	2
Thin'N Crispy Pepperoni	1 med slice	210	25	1

FOOD	PORTION	CALS	CHOL	FIBER
Thin'N Crispy Pepperoni Lover's	1 med slice	260	40	2
Thin'N Crispy Super Supreme	1 med slice	260	35	2
Thin'N Crispy Supreme	1 med slice	240	25	2
Thin'N Crispy Veggie Lover's	1 med slice	180	15	2
XL Full House Cheese	1 slice	280	25	3
XL Full House Chicken Supreme	1 slice	270	25	3
XL Full House Ham	1 slice	260	25	3
XL Full House Meat Lover's	1 slice	380	45	3
XL Full House Pepperoni	1 slice	290	25	3
XL Full House Pepperoni Lover's	1 slice	310	30	3
XL Full House Super Supreme	1 slice	330	35	3
XL Full House Supreme	1 slice	310	30	3
XL Full House Veggie Lover's	1 slice	280	20	3
SALAD DRESSINGS AND SAUCES				
Dipping Cup White Icing	1 serv	170	0	0
Dipping Sauce Breadstick	1 serv	45	0	2
Dipping Sauce Wing Blue Cheese	1 serv	230	25	0
Dipping Sauce Wing Ranch	1 serv	210	10	0
Dressing Caesar	2 tbsp	150	5	0
Dressing French	2 tbsp	140	0	0
Dressing Italian	2 tbsp	140	0	0
Dressing Ranch	2 tbsp	100	5	0
Dressing Thousand Island	2 tbsp	110	10	0
Dressing Lite Italian	2 tbsp	60	0	0
Dressing Lite Ranch	1 tbsp	70	10	0

POLLO TROPICAL

DESSERTS

Flan	1 serv (4 oz)	390	110	1
Key Lime	1 serv (3.9 oz)	210	90	0
Tres Leches	1 serv (5.4 oz)	410	70	0

FOOD	PORTION	CALS	CHOL	FIBER
MAIN MENU SELECTIONS				
Balsamic Tomato	1 combo	88	0	1
Balsamic Tomato	1 sm	176	0	2
Bananas Tropical	1 serv	437	0	9
Beef Skewers	1 (1 oz)	77	26	tr
Black Beans	1 combo	90	0	7
Black Beans	1 sm	203	0	16
Boiled Yuca	1 combo	188	0	4
Boiled Yuca	1 sm	251	0	5
Caesar Salad	1 combo	130	16	1
Caesar Salad	1 sm	207	25	1
Chicken Boneless Breast	2 pieces	240	160	0
Chicken ¼ Dark Meat	1 serv	291	156	0
Chicken ¼ Dark Meat No Skin	1 serv	191	111	0
Chicken ¼ White Meat	1 serv	323	171	0
Chicken ¼ White Meat No Skin	1 serv	204	120	0
Chicken Caesar Salad	1 serv	669	207	3
Corn	1 combo	121	0	5
French Fries	1 sm	311	0	4
Ribs	¼ rack (2 oz)	200	51	0
Ribs	½ rack (4 oz)	400	102	0
Roast Pork	1 serv	392	143	0
Sandwich Chicken Caesar	1	881	203	5
Sandwich Grilled Chicken	1	827	168	6
Sandwich Roast Pork	1	773	119	5
Steak & Chicken Dark Meat	1 serv	437	205	tr
TropiChop Chicken w/ Yellow Rice & Vegetables	1 serv	341	53	2
TropiChop Chicken w/ White Rice & Black Beans	1 serv	564	53	11
TropiChop Grilled Chicken Deluxe	1 serv	409	94	3
TropiChop Pork w/ White Rice & Black Beans	1 serv	714	72	12

FOOD	PORTION	CALS	CHOL	FIBER
TropiChop Pork w/ Yellow Rice & Vegetables	1 serv	480	72	5
TropiChop Rop Vieja	1 serv	618	65	13
TropiChop Shrimp Creole	1 serv	506	185	3
TropiChop Vegetarian	1 serv	580	0	16
TropiChop Max Chicken w/ Yellow Rice & Vegetables	1 serv	864	202	4
TropiChop Max Chicken w/ White Rice & Black Beans	1 serv	1117	202	16
TropiChop Max Grilled Chicken Deluxe	1 serv	753	187	5
TropiChop Max Pork w/ White Rice & Black Beans	1 serv	1273	158	18
TropiChop Max Pork w/ Yellow Rice & Vegetables	1 serv	1020	158	6
TropiChop Max Ropa Vieja	1 serv	1160	145	20
TropiChop Max Shrimp Creole	1 serv	102	384	7
TropiChop Max Vegetarian	1 serv	950	0	26
White Rice	1 combo	203	0	1
White Rice	1 sm	339	0	2
Wrap Chicken Ceasar	1	901	161	4
Wrap Chicken Classic	1	694	115	5
Wrap Curry Chicken	1	930	97	6
Wrap Steak	1	993	74	6
Yellow Rice w/ Vegetables	1 combo	163	0	1
Yellow Rice w/ Vegetables	1 sm	245	0	2
Yucatan Fries	1 serv	497	0	3
SALAD DRESSINGS AND SAUCES				
BBQ Sauce	1 serv (1.8 oz)	83	0	0
BBQ Sauce Guava	1 serv (1.8 oz)	83	0	0
Dressing Caesar	1 serv (1 oz)	161	24	0
Guacamole Sauce	1 serv (1.8 oz)	75	0	3
Mojo Sauce	1 serv (0.9 oz)	97	0	tr

FOOD	PORTION	CALS	CHOL	FIBER
Mustard Curry Sauce	1 serv (1.8 oz)	265	0	0
Salsa	1 serv (1.8 oz)	8	0	0
SOUPS				
Caribbean Chicken	1 sm (8 oz)	121	14	3
Tropical Shrimp	1 sm (8 oz)	134	59	0

POPEYE'S

FOOD	PORTION	CALS	CHOL	FIBER
Buttermilk Biscuit	1	240	0	1
Cajun Rice	1 reg	180	60	2
Coleslaw	1 serv	230	15	9
Collard Greens	1 serv	50	5	3
Corn On The Cob	1	220	0	4
Etouffee Chicken	1 serv	223	20	2
Etouffee Crawfish	1 serv	200	48	2
French Fries	1 serv	261	7	3
Fried Catfish	1 serv	300	55	0
Fried Crawfish	1 serv	370	185	tr
Green Beans	1 serv	40	5	2
Jambalaya Chicken Sausage	1 serv	257	32	1
Mashed Potatoes & Gravy	1 serv	120	5	2
Mashed Potatoes No Gravy	1 serv	100	0	tr
Mild Breast	1	510	195	0
Mild Breast Skinless	1	280	145	0
Mild Leg	1	200	110	0
Mild Leg Skinless	1	110	100	0
Mild Strips	2	280	55	tr
Mild Strips No Breading	2	200	50	0
Mild Thigh	1	390	150	0
Mild Thigh Skinless	1	210	125	0
Mild Wing	1	220	90	0
Mild Wing Skinless	1	130	70	tr
Naked Chicken Strips	3	170	80	0
Popcorn Shrimp	1 serv	280	95	tr
Red Beans & Rice	1 reg	340	20	16
Sandwich Catfish Fully Dressed	1	640	45	5

FOOD	PORTION	CALS	CHOL	FIBER
Sandwich Deluxe Tame w/ Mayo	1	728	71	3
Sandwich Deluxe Tame w/o Mayo	1	530	55	3
Sandwich Shrimp Fully Dressed	1	740	100	8
Smothered Chicken	1 serv	210	23	1
Spicy Breast	1	530	185	1
Spicy Breast Skinless	1	290	135	tr
Spicy Leg	1	190	85	0
Spicy Leg Skinless	1	120	70	0
Spicy Strips	2	310	55	tr
Spicy Strips No Breading	2	190	55	0
Spicy Thigh	1	390	145	0
Spicy Thigh Skinless	1	200	125	0
Spicy Wing	1	220	85	0
Spicy Wing Skinless	1	140	80	tr
Turnover Cinnamon Apple	1	250	5	2

QUIZNOS

FOOD	PORTION	CALS	CHOL	FIBER
Cookie Oatmeal Chocolate Chip	1	360	25	1
Cookie w/ Reese's Pieces	1	360	20	1
Sub Honey Burbon Chicken	1 sm	329	38	3
Sub Sierra Turkey w/ Raspberry Chipotle Sauce	1 sm	350	25	3
Sub Turkey Lite	1 sm	334	19	3
Sub Tuscan Chicken Salad	1 sm	326	35	4

RANCH 1
MAIN MENU SELECTIONS

FOOD	PORTION	CALS	CHOL	FIBER
Baked Potato w/ Broccoli	1 serv	510	0	12
Baked Potato w/ Cheese	1 serv	790	50	11
Baked Potato w/ Chicken	1 serv	610	55	11
Chicken Tenders	1 serv	370	140	0
Fajita Grilled Chicken	1	330	50	4
Fruit Cup	1 serv	90	0	2
Hot Pasta Grilled Chicken	1 serv	590	60	6
Platter Grilled Chicken & Vegetables	1 serv	790	105	16

FOOD	PORTION	CALS	CHOL	FIBER
Ranch Fries	1 reg	350	0	5
Ranch Fries	1 lg	420	0	7
Sandwich American Rancher	1	390	50	3
Sandwich Grilled Chicken Philly	1	450	50	3
Sandwich Ranch Classic	1	370	50	3
Sandwich Spicy Grilled Chicken	1	420	35	3
Sandwich Club	1	470	60	3
SALADS				
Gourmet Greens	1 serv	220	10	5
Gourmet Greens w/ Chicken	1 serv	350	70	5
Zesty Caesar	1 serv	180	5	4
Zesty Chicken Caesar	1 serv	290	50	4

RAX
MAIN MENU SELECTIONS

FOOD	PORTION	CALS	CHOL	FIBER
Baked Potato	1	207	0	–
Baked Potato w/ Butter	1	306	0	–
Baked Potato w/ Cheese	1 serv	270	4	–
Baked Potato w/ Cheese Bacon	1 serv	336	82	–
Baked Potato w/ Cheese Broccoli	1 serv	281	4	–
Baked Potato w/ Sour Cream Topping	1 serv	257	0	–
BBC Sandwich	1	716	102	–
BBQ Beef Sandwich	1	399	40	–
Cheddar Melt	1	346	41	–
Deluxe Sandwich	1	521	68	–
Grilled Chicken Sandwich	1	526	69	–
Jr. Deluxe Sandwich	1	367	42	–
Mushroom Melt	1	599	104	–
Philly Melt	1	537	79	–
Regular Rax	1	388	54	–
Turkey Bacon Club	1	680	76	–
Turkey Sandwich	1	484	50	–
SALAD DRESSINGS				
1000 Island	1 serv	130	10	–

FOOD	PORTION	CALS	CHOL	FIBER
Blue Cheese	1 serv	145	25	–
Buttermilk Ranch	1 serv	175	0	–
Catalina Fat Free	1 serv	32	0	–
Creamy Caesar	1 serv	140	5	–
Honey French	1 serv	140	0	–
Italian Fat Free	1 serv	12	0	–
Ranch Fat Free	1 serv	30	0	–
Vinaigrette	1 serv	30	0	–
SALADS				
Garden	1 serv	220	5	–
Grilled Chicken	1 serv	160	50	–
Side Salad	1 serv (19 oz)	40	0	–
SOUPS				
Chicken Noodle	1 serv	113	45	–
Chili	1 serv	158	31	–
Cream Of Broccoli	1 serv	95	1	–
RITA'S				
Cream Ice	1 reg	312	1	1
Cream Ice Kids	1 serv	193	1	0
Custard	1 reg	385	125	1
Custard Kids	1 serv	285	93	1
Gelati w/ Chocolate Custard	1 reg	351	65	1
Gelati w/ Vanilla Custard	1 reg	120	85	0
Gelati w/ Cream Ice w/ Chocolate Custard	1 reg	368	66	1
Gelati w/ Cream Ice w/ Vanilla Custard	1 reg	392	86	0
Ice	1 reg	263	0	0
Ice Kids	1 serv	165	0	0
Misto w/ Chocolate Custard	1 reg	409	35	1
Misto w/ Vanilla Custard	1 reg	420	45	0
Misto w/ Cream Ice w/ Chocolate Custard	1 reg	463	37	1
Misto w/ Cream Ice w/ Vanilla Custard	1 reg	473	47	0
Sugar Free Gelati w/ Chocolate Custard	1 reg	268	65	1
Sugar Free Gelati w/ Vanilla Custard	1 reg	288	85	0

FOOD	PORTION	CALS	CHOL	FIBER
Sugar Free Ice	1 reg	160	0	0
Sugar Free Ice Kids	1 serv	63	8	0
Sugar Free Misto w/ Chocolate Custard	1 reg	233	36	1
Sugar Free Misto w/ Vanilla Custard	1 reg	245	46	0

ROBEKS
FREEZES AND SHAKES
800 Lb Gorilla	12 oz	375	27	2
Freeze Lemon	12 oz	279	9	0
Freeze Orange	12 oz	242	0	1
Shake Bananasplit	12 oz	302	0	2
Shake P-Nut Power	12 oz	422	0	4

SMOOTHIES
Acai Energizer	12 oz	167	3	2
Awesome Acai	12 oz	183	3	2
Banzai Blueberry	12 oz	175	3	3
Berry Brillance	12 oz	194	3	2
Big Wednesday	12 oz	172	3	1
Cardio Cooler	12 oz	215	3	3
Citrus Stinger	12 oz	194	3	2
Cranberry Quest	12 oz	173	3	1
Dr. Robeks	12 oz	181	3	3
Guava Lava	12 oz	180	3	2
Hummingbird	12 oz	185	3	1
Infinite Orange	12 oz	181	0	3
Mahalo Mango	12 oz	174	3	1
Malibu Peach	12 oz	153	0	1
Outrageous Raspberry	12 oz	174	3	2
Passionfruit Cove	12 oz	168	3	1
Pina Koolada	12 oz	261	3	3
Polar Pineapple	12 oz	164	3	1
Pomegranate Passion	12 oz	196	0	1
Pomegranate Power	12 oz	211	3	1
Pro Arobek	12 oz	265	3	3
Raspberry Romance	12 oz	172	0	2
Robeks MuscleMax	12 oz	202	15	2
Robeks Rejuvenator	12 oz	193	3	2
South Pacific Squeeze	12 oz	188	3	3

FOOD	PORTION	CALS	CHOL	FIBER
Strawnana Berry	12 oz	179	0	2
Venice Burner	12 oz	231	3	4
Zen Berry	12 oz	190	0	5

RUBIO'S
MAIN MENU SELECTIONS

FOOD	PORTION	CALS	CHOL	FIBER
Black Beans	1 serv	220	5	12
Burritos Baja Carne Asada	1	710	100	5
Burritos Baja Carnitas	1	660	85	5
Burritos Baja Chicken	1	640	85	5
Burritos Carne Asada Especial w/ Black Beans	1	970	65	13
Burritos Carne Asada Especial w/ Pinto	1	950	65	14
Burritos Chicken Especial w/ Black Beans	1	920	50	13
Burritos Chicken Especial w/ Pinto	1	900	50	14
Burritos Fish	1	780	50	7
Burritos HealthMex Chicken	1	520	40	9
Burritos HealthMex Veggie	1	470	0	13
Burritos Lobster	1	660	190	9
Burritos Mahi	1	630	65	5
Burritos Shrimp	1	650	170	6
Carne Asada	1 serv	1430	170	19
Chips	1 serv	430	0	7
Grilled Grande Bowl Asada Black Beans	1 serv	770	85	11
Grilled Grande Bowl Asada Pinto	1 serv	760	85	12
Grilled Grande Bowl Chicken Black Beans	1 serv	710	75	11
Grilled Grande Bowl Chicken Pinto	1 serv	700	75	12
Guacamole	1 sm	170	0	5
Nachos Grande	1 serv	1270	120	19
Nachos Grande w/ Chicken	1 serv	1380	160	19
Pinto Beans	1 serv	190	5	16
Quesadillas Carne Asada	1	1010	175	4

FOOD	PORTION	CALS	CHOL	FIBER
Quesadillas Cheese	1	860	125	4
Quesadillas Grilled Chicken	1	860	165	4
Quesadillas Lobster	1	820	280	5
Quesadillas Shrimp	1	810	285	4
Roasted Chipotle	1 serv (1.5 oz)	10	0	1
Salsa Picante	1 serv (1.5 oz)	30	0	2
Salsa Regular	1 serv (1.5 oz)	15	0	1
Salsa Verde	1 serv (1.5 oz)	5	0	1
Tacos Carne Asada	1	220	25	2
Tacos Fish	1	310	20	2
Tacos Fish Especial	1	370	35	3
Tacos Grilled Chicken	1	300	30	2
Tacos Grilled Fish	1	310	30	2
Tacos HealthMex w/ Chicken	1	170	15	2
Taquitos	3	310	45	5
SALADS AND SALAD DRESSINGS				
Grilled Chicken Chopped Salad	1 serv	540	75	5
HealthMex Chicken	1 serv	220	40	2
Low Carb Chicken	1 serv	480	95	5
Serrano Grape Dressing	1 serv (1.3 oz)	10	0	0

SALADWORKS
SALAD DRESSINGS

FOOD	PORTION	CALS	CHOL	FIBER
Balsamic Vinaigrette	1 serv (2 oz)	192	0	0
Blue Cheese	1 serv (2 oz)	192	13	0
Creamy Italian	1 serv (2 oz)	232	11	0
Dijon Honey	1 serv	272	11	0
Fat Free Balsamic w/ Sundried Tomatoes	1 serv (2 oz)	28	0	0
French	1 serv (2 oz)	266	14	0
Herbal Ranch	1 serv (2 oz)	198	25	0
Italian Vinaigrette	1 serv (2 oz)	255	0	0
Lowfat Ranch	1 serv (2 oz)	34	19	0
Oriental Sesame	1 serv (2 oz)	147	0	0
Royal Caesar	1 serv (2 oz)	266	14	0
Russian	1 serv (2 oz)	221	14	0
SALADS				
B.L.T.	1 serv	262	54	4
Bently	1 serv	340	171	3

FOOD	PORTION	CALS	CHOL	FIBER
Caesar	1 serv	283	240	4
Caesar Chicken	1 serv	423	313	4
Caesar Shrimp	1 serv	350	380	4
Fiesta	1 serv	460	102	6
Garden	1 serv	58	0	5
Mandarin Chicken	1 serv	589	109	6
Newport	1 serv	184	189	4
Nicoise	1 serv	407	253	6
Spinach	1 serv	433	265	2
Tivoli	1 serv	563	61	5
Turkey Club	1 serv	720	60	6

SBARRO
DESSERTS

FOOD	PORTION	CALS	CHOL	FIBER
Black Forest Cake	1 serv (4.6 oz)	480	50	1
Deluxe Carrot Cake	1 serv (5 oz)	540	65	1
Deluxe Cheese Cake	1 serv (5.7 oz)	560	170	1
Deluxe Milk Chocolate Cake	1 serv (4.3 oz)	490	30	1

MAIN MENU SELECTIONS

FOOD	PORTION	CALS	CHOL	FIBER
Baked Ziti w/ Sauce	1 serv (14 oz)	700	135	4
Calzone Cheese	1 (12 oz)	770	90	3
Chicken Francese	1 serv (11 oz)	640	175	2
Chicken Parmigiana	1 serv (11 oz)	520	175	2
Chicken Portofino	1 serv (12 oz)	730	225	1
Chicken Vesuvio	1 serv (11 oz)	690	225	1
Eggplant Rollatini w/ Cheese	1 serv (11 oz)	580	50	4
Garlic Roll	1 (2.2 oz)	170	0	tr
Meat Lasagna	1 serv (13 oz)	650	130	3
Meatballs	1 serv (3.7 oz)	140	30	1
Mixed Vegetables	1 serv (7 oz)	190	0	4
Pasta Milano	1 serv (20 oz)	640	175	6
Pasta Rustica	1 serv (14 oz)	600	70	5
Penne Alla Vodka	1 serv (14 oz)	640	120	5
Penne w/ Sausage & Peppers	1 serv (14 oz)	710	130	4
Pizza Cheese	1 slice	460	30	3
Pizza Chicken Vegetable	1 slice	530	45	5
Pizza Fresh Tomato	1 slice	450	25	3
Pizza Mushroom	1 slice	460	20	4
Pizza Pepperoni	1 slice	730	75	3

FOOD	PORTION	CALS	CHOL	FIBER
Pizza Sausage	1 slice	670	80	3
Pizza Sauteed Spinach & Yellow Pepper	1 slice	670	30	5
Pizza Supreme	1 slice	630	60	3
Pizza White	1 slice	570	55	2
Pizza Gourmet Broccoli & Spinach	1 slice	720	30	6
Pizza Gourmet Cheese	1 slice	660	40	4
Pizza Gourmet Ham Pineapple & Bacon	1 slice	680	45	4
Pizza Gourmet Meat Delight	1 slice	780	80	4
Pizza Gourmet Mushroom	1 slice	610	20	5
Pizza Gourmet Mushroom & Spinach	1 slice	710	30	6
Pizza Gourmet Tomato & Basil	1 slice	700	40	5
Pizza Low Carb Cheese	1 slice	310	25	–
Pizza Low Carb Pepperoni	1 slice	420	60	–
Pizza Low Carb Sausage Pepperoni	1 slice	560	95	–
Pizza Stuffed Pepperoni	1 slice	960	115	4
Pizza Stuffed Philly Cheesesteak	1 slice	830	70	5
Pizza Stuffed Spinach & Broccoli	1 slice	790	50	5
Sausage & Peppers	1 serv (10 oz)	410	55	4
Spaghetti w/ Chicken Parmigiana	1 serv (15 oz)	930	175	6
Spaghetti w/ Chicken Francese	1 serv (15 oz)	800	110	5
Spaghetti w/ Chicken Vesuvio	1 serv (15 oz)	850	145	4
Spaghetti w/ Meatballs	1 serv (18 oz)	680	15	9
Spaghetti w/ Sauce	1 serv (20 oz)	820	0	10
Stromboli Pepperoni	1 (10 oz)	890	80	3
Stromboli Spinach Tomato Broccoli	1 (10 oz)	680	35	5
SALADS				
Caesar	1 serv (8 oz)	80	5	1
Cucumber & Tomato	1 serv (8 oz)	130	0	2

FOOD	PORTION	CALS	CHOL	FIBER
Fruit Salad	1 serv (12 oz)	130	0	3
Greek	1 serv (8 oz)	60	10	tr
Mixed Garden	1 serv (8 oz)	35	0	3
Pasta Primavera	1 serv (8 oz)	190	0	2
Stringbean & Tomato	1 serv (8 oz)	100	0	2

SEASON 52
CHILDREN'S MENU SELECTIONS

Children's Chicken	1 serv	344	131	4
Children's Flatbread	1	468	40	1
Children's Pasta	1 serv	177	2	2

DESSERTS

Boston Cream Pie	1 serv	188	14	0
Carrot Cake	1 serv	320	51	2
Chocolate & Peanut Butter Harlequin	1 serv	330	41	0
Fresh Spring Fruit	1 serv	35	0	3
Key Lime Pie	1 serv	283	113	0
Pecan Pie	1 serv	263	26	2
Sorbet w/ Fruit	1 serv	213	0	7
Strawberry Shortcake	1 serv	154	39	0
Strawberry Mango Cheesecake	1 serv	226	93	1
Toasted Almond Amaretto	1 serv	324	161	1

FLATBREADS

Artichoke & Goat Cheese	1	469	22	4
Garlic Chicken	1	474	57	2
Parmesan Crispbread	1	363	37	1
Spicy Shrimp	1	474	106	3
Steak & Mushroom	1	474	50	2
Tomato	1	460	26	3

MAIN MENU SELECTIONS

Appetizer Goat Cheese Ravioli	1 serv	473	112	2
Appetizer Grilled Artichokes	1 serv	185	5	10
Appetizer Grilled Asparagus	1 serv	186	19	5
Appetizer Roasted Potato Wedges	1 serv	333	0	6
Appetizer Shrimp Cocktail	1 serv	221	332	1

FOOD	PORTION	CALS	CHOL	FIBER
Appetizer Shrimp Stuffed Mushrooms	1 serv	302	177	1
Appetizer Steak Skewers w/ Thai Salad	1 serv	438	78	6
Appetizer Steamed Mussels	1 serv	472	92	4
Cedar Salmon	1 serv	472	99	6
Chicken Boccone Pasta	1 serv	434	82	8
Chicken Breast	1 serv	403	131	5
Filet Mignon	1 serv	473	108	5
Grilled Rainbow Trout	1 serv	410	110	5
Grilled Scallops	1 serv	471	71	10
Pork Tenderloin	1 serv	392	130	4
Sandwich Chicken Breast	1	472	115	5
Sandwich Fresh Fish	1	437	63	6
Sandwich Grilled Steak	1	463	95	4
Sandwich Vegetable Stack	1	461	26	8
Shrimp Stuffed w/ Crab	1 serv	470	948	3
Soup Chicken Tortilla	1 serv (8 oz)	181	29	3
Soup Vegetable	1 serv (8 oz)	153	5	3
Spring Vegetable Plate	1 serv	465	1	17
Tuna w/o Soy Sauce	1 serv	175	49	2
Turkey Skewer	1 serv	404	110	5
Yellowfin Tuna	1 serv	466	84	10
SALADS				
Chicken Cobb	1 entree	474	125	4
Greek	1 entree	478	51	6
Mesclun Greens	1 side	315	11	3
Portobello & Romaine	1 entree	270	34	4
Salmon	1 entree	470	101	5
Spinach	1 side	272	5	4
Spring Greens	1 side	240	0	4
Tabbouleh	1 side	417	0	12
Tomato & Blue Cheese Stack	1 side	352	21	5

SEE'S CANDIES

FOOD	PORTION	CALS	CHOL	FIBER
Bridge Mix	14 pieces (1.4 oz)	200	10	1
Dark Chocolate Bordeaux	2 (1.4 oz)	170	25	1
Dark Chocolates	2 (1.2 oz)	160	10	2
Marshmints	3 (1.4 oz)	140	0	tr
Milk Chocolate Bordeaux	2 (1.4 oz)	170	15	tr

FOOD	PORTION	CALS	CHOL	FIBER
Milk Chocolate Butter	2 (1.4 oz)	190	15	tr
Milk Chocolate Buttercreams	2 (1.4 oz)	180	15	0
Milk Chocolate California Brittle	2 (1.3 oz)	220	25	0
Milk Chocolate Nuts & Chews	3 (1.7 oz)	250	15	2
Milk Chocolate Peanuts	3 (1.5 oz)	230	5	2
Milk Chocolate Soft Centers	2 (1.4 oz)	170	15	tr
Milk Chocolates	2 (1.2 oz)	160	10	tr
Nuts & Chews	3 (1.6 oz)	240	10	2
Peanut Brittle	1.5 oz	230	25	0
Pecan Buds	3 (1.7 oz)	270	10	tr
P-Nut Crunch	2 (1.4 oz)	220	10	1
Red Hot Swamp Goo	3 pieces (1.4 oz)	140	0	tr
Soft Centers	2 (1.4 oz)	170	10	tr
Truffles Black or Gold	2 (1.4 oz)	180	10	1
Truffles Mint	3 (1.6 oz)	200	15	tr
Victoria Toffee	1.5 oz	250	20	1

SIZZLER

FOOD	PORTION	CALS	CHOL	FIBER
Grilled Salmon w/ Broccoli	1 serv	393	117	7
Hibachi Chicken w/ Broccoli	1 serv	290	109	6
Petite Steak w/ Broccoli	1 serv	520	159	6

SKIPPERS
CHILDREN'S MENU SELECTIONS

FOOD	PORTION	CALS	CHOL	FIBER
Kids Catch Chicken Tenderloin + Chips & Kids Side	1 serv	560	30	1
Kids Catch Fish Bites + Chips & Kids Side	1 serv	490	0	3
Kids Catch Sandwich Grilled Cheese + Chips & Kids Side	1 serv	620	20	3
Kids Catch Shrimp + Chips & Kids Side	1 serv	520	50	2

MAIN MENU SELECTIONS

FOOD	PORTION	CALS	CHOL	FIBER
Baked Potato Plain	1	210	0	4

FOOD	PORTION	CALS	CHOL	FIBER
Basket Chicken & Fish + Chips & Slaw	1 serv	620	45	1
Basket Chicken & Shrimp + Chips & Slaw	1 serv	760	120	1
Basket Chicken + Chips & Slaw	1 piece	730	70	0
Basket Clam Strips + Chips & Slaw	1 serv	890	75	12
Basket Clams & Fish + Chips & Slaw	1 serv	740	50	8
Basket Original Recipe Shrimp + Chips & Slaw	1 serv	800	165	3
Basket Popcorn Shrimp + Chips & Slaw	1 serv	750	180	2
Basket Prawn & Fish + Chips & Slaw	1 serv	730	235	2
Basket Prawn Seafood + Chips & Slaw	1 serv	720	280	tr
Basket Shrimp & Fish + Chips & Slaw	1 serv	650	90	2
Basket Shrimp Trio + Chips & Slaw	1 serv	1040	305	4
Clam Chowder	1 cup	120	5	tr
Clam Strips	1 serv	270	30	6
Fish Bites + Chips & Slaw	6 pieces	490	0	7
French Fries	1 reg	180	0	0
Grilled Veggies	1 serv	35	0	3
Halibut + Chips & Slaw	1 serv	580	45	0
Homestyle Chicken Tenderloin	1 piece	190	30	0
Hush Puppies	3 pieces	240	0	3
Original Fish Fillet	1 piece	80	0	1
Original Fish + Chips & Slaw	2 pieces	510	15	2
Original Shrimp	9 pieces	220	75	1
Sandwich Fish + Chips & Slaw	1 serv	800	20	4
Sandwich Fried Chicken + Chips & Slaw	1	1260	105	3

FOOD	PORTION	CALS	CHOL	FIBER
Sandwich Grilled Chicken + Chips & Slaw	1	1070	145	3
Skipper's Platter + Chips & Slaw	1 serv	930	12	8
SALADS				
Caesar	1 sm	150	5	2
Caesar w/ Chicken	1 sm	340	100	2
Caesar w/ Salmon	1 sm	350	80	2
Green Salad w/o Dressing	1 sm	25	0	2

SMOOTHIE KING

FOOD	PORTION	CALS	CHOL	FIBER
Activator Chocolate	1 (20 oz)	429	2	4
Activator Strawberry	1 (20 oz)	559	2	5
Activator Vanilla	1 (20 oz)	429	2	4
Banana Boat	1 (20 oz)	520	80	5
Coconut Surprise	1 (20 oz)	457	3	5
Coffee Smoothie Hazelnut	1 (20 oz)	118	1	tr
Coffee Smoothies Amaretto	1 (20 oz)	118	1	tr
Coffee Smoothies French Roast	1 (20 oz)	164	1	tr
Coffee Smoothies French Vanilla	1 (20 oz)	118	1	tr
Coffee Smoothies Irish Creme	1 (20 oz)	118	1	tr
Coffee Smoothies Mocha	1 (20 oz)	206	1	1
HeaterZ Banana Nut	1	400	5	3
HeaterZ Blueberry Muffin	1	370	<5	9
HeaterZ Chocolate Peanut Butter Cup	1	380	5	6
HeaterZ Cinnamon Oatmeal Raisin	1	420	0	9
HeaterZ Coconut	1	440	5	3
HeaterZ Coffee Amaretto	1 (12 oz)	177	1	4
HeaterZ Coffee French Roast	1 (12 oz)	172	1	4
HeaterZ Coffee French Vanilla	1 (12 oz)	177	1	4
HeaterZ Coffee Hazelnut	1 (12 oz)	177	1	4
HeaterZ Coffee Irish Creme	1 (12 oz)	177	1	4
HeaterZ Coffee Mocha	1 (12 oz)	266	1	5
High Protein Almond Mocha	1 (20 oz)	402	17	4

FOOD	PORTION	CALS	CHOL	FIBER
High Protein Banana	1 (20 oz)	412	14	6
High Protein Chocolate	1 (20 oz)	401	17	4
High Protein Lemon	1 (20 oz)	390	12	3
High Protein Pineapple	1 (20 oz)	380	12	7
Hot Coffee Amaretto	1 (12 oz)	168	1	tr
Hot Coffee French Roast	1 (12 oz)	164	1	tr
Hot Coffee French Vanilla	1 (12 oz)	168	1	tr
Hot Coffee Hazelnut	1 (12 oz)	168	1	tr
Hot Coffee Irish Creme	1 (12 oz)	168	1	tr
Hot Coffee Mocha	1 (12 oz)	209	1	1
Iced Coffee Amaretto	1 (20 oz)	168	1	tr
Iced Coffee French Roast	1 (20 oz)	164	1	tr
Iced Coffee French Vanilla	1 (20 oz)	168	1	tr
Iced Coffee Hazelnut	1 (20 oz)	168	1	tr
Iced Coffee Irish Creme	1 (20 oz)	168	1	tr
Iced Coffee Mocha	1 (20 oz)	209	1	1
Kid Cup Berry Interesting	1	150	0	2
Kid Cup Choc-A-Laka	1	210	0	2
Kid Cup Gimmi-Grape	1	170	0	1
Kid Cup Smarti Tarti	1	150	0	0
Low Carb All Flavors	1 (20 oz)	225	6	2
Low Fat Angel Food	1 (20 oz)	330	2	4
Low Fat Blackberry Dream	1 (20 oz)	343	0	3
Low Fat Carribean Way	1 (20 oz)	392	0	5
Low Fat Celestial Cherry High	1 (20 oz)	285	0	4
Low Fat Cherry Picker	1 (20 oz)	360	0	2
Low Fat Cranberry Supreme	1 (20 oz)	577	24	3
Low Fat Cranberry Cooler	1 (20 oz)	538	0	3
Low Fat Grape Expectations	1 (20 oz)	399	0	2
Low Fat Grape Expectations II	1 (20 oz)	529	0	4
Low Fat Healthy Apple	1 (20 oz)	380	25	2
Low Fat Immune Builder	1 (20 oz)	333	24	4
Low Fat Instant Vigor	1 (20 oz)	359	0	2
Low Fat Island Treat	1 (20 oz)	334	0	5
Low Fat Lemon Twist Banana	1 (20 oz)	339	0	2
Low Fat Lemon Twist Strawberry	1 (20 oz)	399	0	2

FOOD	PORTION	CALS	CHOL	FIBER
Low Fat Light & Fluffy	1 (20 oz)	389	0	4
Low Fat Mangofest	1 (20 oz)	320	0	2
Low Fat Muscle Punch	1 (20 oz)	339	2	4
Low Fat Muscle Punch Plus	1 (20 oz)	340	2	5
Low Fat Orange Ka-BAM	1 (20 oz)	320	0	3
Low Fat Peach Slice	1 (20 oz)	341	2	3
Low Fat Peach Slice Plus	1 (20 oz)	471	2	5
Low Fat Pep Upper	1 (20 oz)	334	0	5
Low Fat Pineapple Pleasure	1 (20 oz)	331	0	4
Low Fat Pineapple Surf	1 (20 oz)	440	3	4
Low Fat Raspberry Sunrise	1 (20 oz)	335	0	4
Low Fat Strawberry X-Treme	1 (20 oz)	370	0	4
Low Fat Strawberry Kiwi Breeze	1 (20 oz)	300	0	2
Low Fat Youth Fountain	1 (20 oz)	267	0	5
Malts	1 (20 oz)	887	166	tr
Mo'cuccino	1 (20 oz)	420	75	1
Peanut Power	1 (20 oz)	502	2	4
Peanut Power Plus Grape	1 (20 oz)	703	2	4
Peanut Power Plus Strawberry	1 (20 oz)	632	2	5
Pina Colada Island	1 (20 oz)	550	5	6
Power Punch	1 (20 oz)	430	2	4
Power Punch Plus	1 (20 oz)	499	2	4
Shakes	1 (20 oz)	875	166	0
Slim-N-Trim Chocolate	1 (20 oz)	270	4	3
Slim-N-Trim Orange Vanilla	1 (20 oz)	199	0	1
Slim-N-Trim Strawberry	1 (20 oz)	357	2	3
Slim-N-Trim Vanilla	1 (20 oz)	227	2	2
Super Punch	1 (20 oz)	425	0	6
Super Punch Plus	1 (20 oz)	516	0	6
The Hulk Chocolate	1 (20 oz)	846	102	6
The Hulk Strawberry	1 (20 oz)	953	102	6
The Hulk Vanilla	1 (20 oz)	846	102	5
Yogurt D-Lite	1 (20 oz)	335	43	0

SONIC DRIVE-IN
ADD-ONS

FOOD	PORTION	CALS	CHOL	FIBER
Bacon	1 serv (0.5 oz)	80	15	0
Cheddar Cheese Shredded	1 serv (1 oz)	104	28	0

FOOD	PORTION	CALS	CHOL	FIBER
Cheese	1 serv (0.7 oz)	70	15	0
Chili	1 serv (1 oz)	52	8	0
Cone Coat Chocolate	1 serv (1 oz)	143	0	1
Green Chilies	1 serv (1 oz)	10	0	0
Honey Mustard Dressing	1 serv (1.1 oz)	110	10	0
Jalapenos Nachos Sliced	1 serv (1 oz)	5	0	1
Malt	1 serv (1 oz)	104	0	–
Maraschino Cherry	1 serv (8 g)	10	0	0
Marinara Sauce	1 serv (1 oz)	15	0	1
Ranch Dressing	1 serv (1 oz)	147	5	0
Slaw	1 serv (0.9 oz)	45	0	1
Sweet Pickle Relish	1 serv (1.1 oz)	40	0	0
Syrup Blue Coconut	1 serv (1 oz)	65	0	0
Syrup Cherry	1 serv (1 oz)	64	0	0
Syrup Chocolate	1 serv (1 oz)	74	0	0
Syrup Grape	1 serv (1 oz)	63	0	0
Syrup Vanilla	1 serv (1 oz)	61	0	0
Syrup Watermelon	1 serv (1 oz)	71	0	0
Thousand Island Dressing	1 serv (1 oz)	150	10	0
Topping Pineapple	1 serv (1.5 oz)	108	0	0
Topping Strawberry	1 serv (1.2 oz)	38	0	1
Topping Strawberry	1 serv (1 oz)	101	0	0
BEVERAGES				
Barqs Root Beer	1 sm	160	0	0
Barqs Root Beer	1 lg	333	0	0
Coca-Cola	1 sm	139	0	0
Coca-Cola	1 lg	291	0	0
Diet Coke	1 sm	1	0	0
Diet Coke	1 lg	3	0	0
Diet Sprite	1 sm	4	0	0
Diet Sprite	1 lg	8	0	0
Dr Pepper	1 sm	144	0	0
Dr Pepper	1 lg	300	0	0
Float or Flurry Blue Coconut Slush	1 reg	424	30	0
Limeade	1 sm	143	0	1
Limeade	1 lg	303	0	2
Limeade Cherry	1 sm	169	0	1
Limeade Cherry	1 lg	361	0	2
Limeade Strawberry	1 sm	172	0	1

FOOD	PORTION	CALS	CHOL	FIBER
Limeade Strawberry	1 lg	341	0	2
Slush Blue Coconut	1 lg	521	0	0
Slush Watermelon	1 lg	526	0	0
Sprite	1 sm	138	0	0
Sprite	1 lg	288	0	0
BREAKFAST SELECTIONS				
Breakfast Burrito	1	731	167	3
Fruit Taquitos	1 serv	302	0	3
Sunrise	1 reg	224	0	1
Sunrise	1 lg	368	0	2
Toaster Bacon Egg & Cheese	1	500	156	2
Toaster Ham Egg & Cheese	1	436	174	2
Toaster Sausage Egg & Cheese	1	570	126	2
DESSERTS				
Banana Split	1 serv	467	23	3
Chocolate Covered Shake Banana	1 reg	625	46	2
Chocolate Covered Shake Cherry	1 reg	587	46	1
Chocolate Covered Shake Peanut Butter	1 reg	678	46	1
Chocolate Covered Shake Strawberry	1 reg	608	46	1
Cream Pie Shake Banana	1 reg	775	47	2
Cream Pie Shake Chocolate	1 reg	795	47	1
Cream Pie Shake Coconut	1 reg	721	47	1
Dish Of Vanilla	1 serv	265	26	0
Float or Flurry Cherry Slush	1 reg	421	30	0
Float or Flurry Coca-Cola	1 reg	379	30	0
Float or Flurry Dr Pepper	1 reg	377	30	0
Float or Flurry Grape Slush	1 reg	423	30	0
Float or Flurry Orange Slush	1 reg	422	30	0
Float or Flurry Rootbeer	1 reg	386	30	0
Float or Flurry Watermelon Slush	1 reg	427	30	0
Ice Cream Cone	1	285	26	0
Shake Banana	1 reg	508	45	1
Shake Chocolate	1 reg	564	45	0
Shake Pineapple	1 reg	615	45	1

FOOD	PORTION	CALS	CHOL	FIBER
Shake Strawberry	1 reg	510	45	1
Shake Vanilla	1 reg	454	45	0
Sonic Blast Butterfinger	1 reg	636	46	1
Sonic Blast M&M	1 reg	641	50	1
Sonic Blast Oreo	1 reg	638	45	1
Sonic Blast Reese's	1 reg	658	47	1
Sundae Chocolate	1 serv	362	26	0
Sundae Hot Fudge	1 serv	392	27	0
Sundae Pineapple	1 serv	399	26	0
Sundae Strawberry	1 serv	322	26	1
MAIN MENU SELECTIONS				
Ched'R'Peppers	1 serv	256	28	4
Cheese Fries	1 reg	265	15	4
Cheese Fries	1 lg	322	15	5
Cheese Tater Tots	1 reg	329	15	3
Cheese Tots	1 lg	435	15	4
Chicken Strip Dinner	1 serv	749	47	5
Chicken Strip Snack	1 serv	272	35	0
Chicken Strips	2	184	23	0
Chili Cheese Fries	1 reg	299	22	4
Chili Cheese Fries	1 lg	357	22	5
Chili Cheese Tater Tots	1 reg	363	22	3
Chili Cheese Tots	1 lg	547	37	5
Corn Dog	1	262	15	1
Extra Long Coney Cheese	1	666	87	2
Extra Long Coney Plain	1	483	50	1
French Fries	1 reg	195	0	4
French Fries	1 lg	252	0	5
Fritos Chili Pie	1 serv	611	53	36
Hot Dog Plain	1	262	30	1
Jr. Burger	1	353	45	1
Mozzarella Sticks	1 serv	382	50	0
No.1 Hamburger	1	577	37	2
No.1 Sonic Cheeseburger	1	647	52	2
No.2 Hamburger	1	481	29	2
No.2 Sonic Cheeseburger	1	551	44	2
Onion Rings	1 reg	331	0	7
Onion Rings	1 lg	507	0	10
Regular Coney Cheese	1	366	52	1
Regular Coney Plain	1	262	30	1

FOOD	PORTION	CALS	CHOL	FIBER
Sandwich Breaded Chicken	1	582	53	2
Sandwich Country Fried Steak	1	748	60	2
Sandwich Grilled Chicken	1	343	70	2
Super Sonic No.1	1	929	964	2
Super Sonic No.2	1	839	88	3
SuperSonic Onion Rings	1 serv	706	1	11
SuperSonic Tots	1 serv	485	0	5
SuperSonic Fries	1 serv	358	0	7
Tater Tots	1 reg	259	0	3
Tater Tots	1 lg	365	0	4
Toaster Sandwich Bacon Cheddar Burger	1	675	59	4
Toaster Sandwich BLT	1	581	47	3
Toaster Sandwich Chicken Club	1	675	85	3
Toaster Sandwich Country Fried Steak	1	708	60	3
Toaster Sandwich Grilled Cheese	1	282	15	2
Wrap Chicken Strip	1	574	28	2
Wrap Grilled Chicken	1	539	70	2
Wrap w/o Ranch Chicken Strip	1	428	23	2
Wrap w/o Ranch Grilled Chicken	1	393	65	2

SOUPLANTATION
BREADS AND MUFFINS

FOOD	PORTION	CALS	CHOL	FIBER
Bread Low Fat Sourdough	1 slice	150	0	0
Breads Indian Grain Low Fat	1 slice	200	15	0
Cornbread Buttermilk Low Fat	1 piece	140	10	2
Focaccia Big Hearth Pizza	1	140	10	1
Focaccia Bruschetta	1 piece	130	5	1
Focaccia Pepperoni	1 piece	160	15	1
Focaccia Roasted Potato	1 piece	150	10	2
Focaccia Sauteed Vegetables	1 piece	150	10	1
Focaccia Tomatillo	1 piece	140	10	1

FOOD	PORTION	CALS	CHOL	FIBER
Focaccia Low Fat Garlic Parmesan	1 piece	100	0	1
Muffin Apple Cinnamon Bran 96% Fat Free	1	80	0	1
Muffin Apple Raisin	1	150	10	1
Muffin Banana Nut	1	150	10	1
Muffin Big Blue Blueberry	1	310	20	2
Muffin Black Forest	1	230	10	1
Muffin Cappuccino Chip	1	160	25	1
Muffin Caribbean Key Lime	1	170	10	1
Muffin Cherry Nut	1	150	10	1
Muffin Chocolate Brownie	1	170	10	1
Muffin Chocolate Chip	1	170	10	1
Muffin Country Blackberry	1	170	15	1
Muffin French Quarter Praline	1	290	20	2
Muffin Georgia Peach Poppyseed	1	150	10	1
Muffin Lemon	1	140	10	1
Muffin Macadamia Nut Spice	1	220	20	1
Muffin Maple Walnut	1	230	5	1
Muffin Nutty Peanut Butter	1	170	10	1
Muffin Pumpkin Raisin	1 piece	150	10	1
Muffin Strawberry Buttermilk	1	140	10	1
Muffin Sweet Orange & Cranberry	1	200	5	1
Muffin Taffy Apple	1	160	10	1
Muffin Tropical Papaya Coconut	1	180	10	1
Muffin Zucchini Nut	1	150	10	1
Muffin 96% Fat Free Cranberry Orange Bran	1	80	0	1
Muffin 96% Fat Free Fruit Medley Bran	1	80	0	1
Muffin Low Fat Chile Corn	1	140	10	2
DESSERTS				
Cobbler Apple	½ cup	350	0	1
Cobbler Blissful Blueberry	½ cup	380	0	3
Cobbler Cherry	½ cup	340	0	2

FOOD	PORTION	CALS	CHOL	FIBER
Cobbler Cranberry Apple	½ cup	370	0	3
Cobbler Peach	½ cup	360	0	2
Cookie Chocolate Chip	1 sm	70	5	0
Fat Free Apple Medley	½ cup	70	0	1
Fat Free Banana Royale	½ cup	80	0	1
Fat Free Frozen Yogurt Chocolate	½ cup	95	0	0
Jello Fat Free All Flavors	½ cup	80	0	0
Jello Fat Free Sugar Free All Flavors	½ cup	10	0	0
Pudding Banana	½ cup	160	10	1
Pudding Vanilla	½ cup	140	10	0
Pudding Low Fat Butterscotch	½ cup	140	10	0
Pudding Low Fat Chocolate	½ cup	140	10	0
Pudding Low Fat Rice	½ cup	110	10	1
Soft Serve Reduced Fat Vanilla	½ cup	140	20	0
Tapioca Low Fat	½ cup	140	10	0
MAIN MENU SELECTIONS				
Alfredo Broccoli w/ Basil	1 cup	380	40	1
Alfredo Fettuccine	1 cup	390	50	2
Alfredo Four Cheese	1 cup	390	30	3
Alfredo Roasted Garlic & Asiago	1 cup	330	25	2
Alfredo Roasted Mushroom w/ Rosemary	1 cup	380	35	2
Alfredo Southwestern	1 cup	350	50	1
Beef Stroganoff	1 cup	340	75	2
Carbonara Pasta	1 cup	280	20	2
Chili Arizona	1 cup	220	20	7
Chili Longhorn Beef	1 cup	190	20	4
Chili Rock N' Mole	1 cup	240	25	5
Chili Santa Fe Black Bean Low Fat	1 cup	190	0	8
Chili Texas Red	1 cup	240	20	7
Chili Three Bean Turkey Low Fat	1 cup	140	20	5
Chili Vegetarian	1 cup	150	0	6
Chili Cheatin' Heart	1 cup	300	60	6

FOOD	PORTION	CALS	CHOL	FIBER
Chili Deep Kettle House Low Fat	1 cup	230	15	7
Creamy Herb Chicken	1 cup	310	80	2
Creamy Pepper Jack	1 cup	290	50	2
Garden Vegetable w/ Italian Sausage	1 cup	300	20	3
Garen Vegetable w/ Meatballs	1 cup	270	10	3
Greek Mediterranean	1 cup	290	15	2
Italian Vegetable Beef	1 cup	270	10	4
Italian Sausage w/ Red Pepper Puree	1 cup	250	45	2
Lemon Cream & Asparagus	1 cup	230	0	1
Linguini w/ Clam Sauce	1 cup	380	40	1
Low Fat Oriental Green Bean & Noodle	1 cup	240	0	2
Macaroni & Cheese	1 cup	260	15	2
Nutty Mushroom	1 cup	390	45	2
Pasta Florentine	1 cup	360	15	7
Penne Arrabbiatta	1 cup	340	20	3
Pesto Cilantro Lime	1 cup	370	20	2
Roasted Eggplant Marinara	1 cup	340	20	3
Smoked Salmon & Dill	1 cup	360	45	2
Tuscany Sausage w/ Capers & Olives	1 cup	240	15	2
Vegetable Ragu	1 cup	250	10	3
Vegetarian Marinara w/ Basil	1 cup	260	10	3
Walnut Pesto	1 cup	310	10	2
SALAD DRESSINGS				
Bacon	2 tbsp	120	0	0
Balsamic Vinaigrette	1 tbsp	180	0	0
Basil Vinaigrette	2 tbsp	160	0	0
Blue Cheese	1 tbsp	140	10	0
Creamy Italian	2 tbsp	120	10	0
Fat Free Honey Mustard	2 tbsp	45	10	0
Honey Mustard	2 tbsp	150	10	0
Italian Fat Free	2 tbsp	20	0	0
Kahlena French	2 tbsp	120	0	0
Parmesan Pepper Cream	2 tbsp	160	5	0

FOOD	PORTION	CALS	CHOL	FIBER
Ranch	2 tbsp	130	10	0
Ranch Fat Free	2 tbsp	50	0	0
Reduced Calorie Cucumber	2 tbsp	80	0	0
Roasted Garlic	2 tbsp	140	5	0
Thousand Island	2 tbsp	110	5	0
SALADS				
Ambrosia w/ Cocount	½ cup	170	5	2
Antipasto w/ Peppered Salami	1 cup	140	10	2
Artichoke Rice	½ cup	160	3	2
Aunt Doris' Red Pepper Slaw Fat Free	½ cup	70	0	3
Baja Bean & Cilantro Low Fat	½ cup	180	0	5
Bartlett Pear & Walnut	1 cup	180	5	2
BBQ Julienne Chopped	1 cup	190	20	3
BBQ Smokehouse w/ Bacon & Peanuts	1 cup	190	10	3
Caesar Asiago	1 cup	190	10	1
California Cobb	1 cup	180	25	2
Cape Cod Spinach w/ Walnuts	1 cup	170	5	4
Carrot Ginger w/ Herb Vinaigrette	½ cup	150	0	3
Carrot Raisin Low Fat	½ cup	90	5	2
Chicken Tortilla	1 cup	180	20	2
Chinese Krab	½ cup	160	3	3
Citrus Noodle w/ Snow Peas	½ cup	140	0	2
Country French w/ Bacon	1 cup	210	20	2
Ensalada Azteca	1 cup	130	15	4
Field Corn & Very Wild Rice	½ cup	170	0	3
Greek	1 cup	120	10	2
Greek Couscous w/ Feta	½ cup	170	4	3
Italian Garden Vegetable	½ cup	110	0	2
Italian Sub Salad w/ Turkey & Salami	1 cup	260	20	2
Italian White Bean	½ cup	140	0	4
Joan's Blue BLT	1 cup	250	25	3
Joan's Broccoli Madness	½ cup	180	10	3

FOOD	PORTION	CALS	CHOL	FIBER
Lemon Rice w/ Cashews	½ cup	160	0	1
Mandarin Noodles w/ Broccoli Low Fat	½ cup	120	0	2
Mandarin Shells w/ Almonds	½ cup	120	0	2
Mandarin Spinach w/ Carmelized Walnuts	1 cup	170	0	3
Marinated Summer Vegetables Fat Free	½ cup	80	0	4
Mediterranean	1 cup	150	5	4
Monterey Blue w/ Peanuts	1 cup	200	5	2
Moroccan Marinated Vegetables Low Fat	½ cup	90	0	2
Old Fashioned Macaroni Salad w/ Ham	½ cup	180	10	3
Oriental Ginger Slaw w/ Krab Low Fat	½ cup	70	2	4
Penne w/ Chicken In Citrus Vinaigrette Low Fat	½ cup	130	5	2
Pesto Orzo w/ Pinenuts	1 cup	220	10	2
Pesto Pasta	½ cup	160	2	2
Pineapple Coconut Slaw	½ cup	150	15	2
Poppyseed Coleslaw	½ cup	120	10	3
Potato BBQ	½ cup	160	5	2
Potato Dijon w/ Garlic Dill Vinaigrette	½ cup	150	0	3
Potato German	½ cup	120	0	2
Potato Jalapeno	½ cup	140	0	2
Potato Picnic	½ cup	150	80	2
Potato Southern Dill Low Fat	½ cup	120	5	2
Ragin' Cajun	1 cup	200	15	2
Ranch House BLT Salad w/ Turkey	1 cup	180	15	6
Red Potato & Tomato	½ cup	120	5	3
Roasted Vegetables w/ Feta & Olives	1 cup	140	10	4
Roasted Potato Salad w/ Chipotle Chili Vinaigrette	½ cup	140	0	4

FOOD	PORTION	CALS	CHOL	FIBER
Roma Tomatoes Mozzarella & Basil	1 cup	120	10	1
San Francisco Herb Rice	½ cup	170	5	1
Shrimp & Seafood	½ cup	200	20	2
Smoked Turkey & Spinach w/ Almonds	1 cup	190	15	2
Sonoma Spinach w/ Honey Dijon Vinaigrette	1 cup	210	10	2
Southern Black Eyed Pea	½ cup	130	0	3
Southwestern Rice & Beans	½ cup	90	0	3
Spiced Pecans & Roasted Vegetables	1 cup	180	15	2
Spicy Southwestern Pasta Low Fat	½ cup	130	0	4
Spinach Gorgonzola w/ Spiced Pecans	1 cup	210	10	4
Strawberry Fields w/ Carmelized Walnuts	1 cup	130	0	3
Summer Barley w/ Black Beans Low Fat	½ cup	110	0	4
Summer Lemon w/ Spiced Pecans	1 cup	220	10	2
Thai Noodle w/ Peanut Sauce	½ cup	170	0	3
Three Bean Marinade	½ cup	170	0	3
Tomato Cucumber Marinade	½ cup	80	0	1
Traditional Spinach w/ Bacon	1 cup	160	40	3
Tuna Tarragon	½ cup	240	10	3
Turkey Chutney Pasta	½ cup	230	30	2
Watercress & Orange	1 cup	90	0	2
Wild Rice & Chicken	½ cup	300	20	1
Won Ton Chicken Happiness	1 cup	150	10	2
Zesty Tortellini	½ cup	190	10	2
SOUPS				
Albino Bean Chicken	1 cup	190	40	4
Albondigas Locas	1 cup	210	30	2

FOOD	PORTION	CALS	CHOL	FIBER
Autumn Root Vegetable w/ Wild Rice	1 cup	80	0	2
Baked Potate & Cheese w/ Bacon	1 cup	290	50	2
Be Wild With Mushroom	1 cup	220	50	2
Big Chunk Chicken Noodle Low Fat	1 cup	160	20	2
Black Bean Sausage Fling	1 cup	350	60	5
Black Bean & Chorizo	1 cup	230	15	6
Bombay Lentil Low Fat	1 cup	160	0	9
Broc On	1 cup	220	60	2
Broccoli Cheese	1 cup	280	50	2
Butternut Squash	1 cup	140	17	4
Cheese Stuffed Cappelletti	1 cup	130	10	1
Chesapeake Corn Chowder	1 cup	280	35	2
Chicken Got Smoked	1 cup	350	85	2
Chicken Tortilla w/ Jalapeno Chiles & Tomatoes Low Fat	1 cup	100	20	1
Chunky Potato Cheese w/ Thyme	1 cup	210	30	2
Classical French Onion	1 cup	130	5	2
Classical Minestrone Low Fat	1 cup	120	0	3
Classical Shrimp Bisque	1 cup	240	70	1
Country Corn & Red Potato Chowder	1 cup	160	15	4
Cream Of Broccoli	1 cup	210	25	7
Cream of Mushroom	1 cup	290	30	2
Cream Of Rosemary Potato	1 cup	270	50	2
Cream Of Chicken	1 cup	260	55	1
Creamy Vegetable Chowder	1 cup	200	20	3
Devotion To The Ocean	1 cup	220	100	2
El Paso Lime & Chicken	1 cup	160	15	2
Field Of Creams Cauliflower w/ Cheese	1 cup	260	40	1
Field Of Creams Celery	1 cup	210	30	2
Field Of Creams Spinach	1 cup	280	45	2
Field Of Creams Tomato Basil	1 cup	220	30	2

FOOD	PORTION	CALS	CHOL	FIBER
Fire Roasted Green Chili & Corn Chowder	1 cup	230	25	1
Garden Fresh Vegetable Low Fat	1 cup	110	0	4
Garlic Kickin Roasted Chicken	1 cup	140	30	3
Hungarian Vegetable Low Fat	1 cup	120	0	2
Irish Potato Leek	1 cup	250	35	1
Living On The Veg	1 cup	90	0	3
Manhattan Clam Chowder	1 cup	130	20	2
Mulligatawny	1 cup	210	40	2
Navy Bean w/ Ham	1 cup	340	40	6
Neighbor Joe's Gumbo	1 cup	280	50	3
Posole	1 cup	150	35	2
Ratatouille Provencale Fat Free	1 cup	110	0	2
Roasted Mushroom w/ Sage	1 cup	320	50	1
Spicy Sausage & Pasta	1 cup	310	30	5
Split Pea w/ Ham	1 cup	350	40	6
Tomato Chipotle Bisque	1 cup	240	40	2
Tomato Parmesan & Vegetables Low Fat	1 cup	120	5	3
Toot Your Horn For Crab & Corn	1 cup	290	90	2
Vegetarian Lentils & Brown Rice Low Fat	1 cup	130	0	6
Yankee Clipper Clam Chowder w/ Bacon	1 cup	330	80	2

SOUTHERN TSUNAMI SUSHI BAR
SALADS

FOOD	PORTION	CALS	CHOL	FIBER
Calamari	1 serv (4 oz)	148	307	1
Edamame	1 serv (4 oz)	124	0	1
Harusame	1 serv (5 oz)	148	0	0
Seabreeze	1 serv (4 oz)	113	0	0

SUSHI

FOOD	PORTION	CALS	CHOL	FIBER
California Roll	1 (0.8 oz)	31	0	tr
Cream Cheese Roll w/ Salmon	1 piece (0.8 oz)	43	6	tr

FOOD	PORTION	CALS	CHOL	FIBER
Crunchy Shrimp Roll	1 piece (0.9 oz)	42	9	tr
Dragon Roll	1 piece (0.8 oz)	42	8	1
Freshwater Eel Roll	1 piece (0.8 oz)	41	9	tr
Green Horseradish	1 tsp	7	0	0
Inari	1 piece (1.9 oz)	105	0	0
Nigiri Cuttlefish	1 piece (1 oz)	42	6	0
Nigiri Egg Cake	1 piece (1.4 oz)	73	28	0
Nigiri Fish Roe	1 piece (1.4 oz)	61	31	0
Nigiri Fresh Salmon	1 piece (1.3 oz)	68	8	0
Nigiri Fresh Water Eel	1 piece (1.6 oz)	108	32	0
Nigiri Ostopus	1 piece (1.1 oz)	57	14	0
Nigiri Sea Eel	1 piece (1.6 oz)	90	31	0
Nigiri Shrimp	1 piece (1.1 oz)	44	9	0
Nigiri Smoked Salmon	1 piece (1.3 oz)	68	8	0
Nigiri Tilapia	1 piece (1.2 oz)	49	5	0
Nigiri Tuna	1 piece (1.3 oz)	60	9	0
Nigiri Yellowtail	1 piece (1.2 oz)	54	6	0
Ocean Crab Roll	1 piece (0.8 oz)	33	7	tr
Orange Roll	1 piece (0.8 oz)	32	5	tr
Pickled Ginger	1 tbsp	9	0	0
Rainbow Roll	1 piece (1 oz)	41	5	tr
Sea Eel Roll	1 piece (0.8 oz)	36	9	tr
Soy Sauce	1 pkg	16	0	0
Spicy Roll Salmon	1 piece (0.8 oz)	40	4	tr
Spicy Roll Shrimp	1 piece (0.8 oz)	31	9	tr
Spicy Roll Tuna	1 piece (0.8 oz)	37	4	tr
Tempura Roll	1 piece (0.9 oz)	44	9	tr
Tofu Roll	1 piece (0.8 oz)	27	0	tr
Tusnami Roll Crab & Fish Roe	1 piece (0.8 oz)	39	5	tr

STARBUCKS
BAKED SELECTIONS

FOOD	PORTION	CALS	CHOL	FIBER
Baby Bundt Cake Chocolate	1	330	25	4
Bagel	1	430	0	3
Bagel Cinnamon Raisin	1	440	0	3
Bagel Sesame	1	440	0	6
Bar Caramel Apple	1	310	40	2
Bar Carrot Cake	1	420	85	tr
Bar Lemon	1	310	140	0

FOOD	PORTION	CALS	CHOL	FIBER
Bar Oreo Dream	1	420	65	2
Bar Toffee Crunch	1	430	50	1
Biscotti Chocolate Hazelnut	1	110	25	1
Biscotti Vanilla Almond	1	110	25	1
Brownie Caramel	1	580	100	2
Brownie Enrobed Espresso	1	430	75	3
Brownie Espresso	1	370	85	2
Brownie Milk Chocolate Peanut Butter	1	460	50	2
Bundt Cake Lemon Yogurt	1 serv	350	55	tr
Caramel Pecan Sticky Roll	1	730	40	7
Cinnamon Roll	1	620	45	3
Cinnamon Twist	1	320	25	1
Coffee Cake	1 serv	570	75	2
Coffee Cake Apple Walnut	1 serv	320	55	1
Coffee Cake Blueberry Walnut	1 serv	340	60	1
Coffee Cake Cinnamon Walnut	1 serv	360	65	1
Coffee Cake Crumble Berry	1 serv	520	75	2
Coffee Cake Hazelnut	1 serv	630	125	2
Coffee Cake Sour Cream	1 serv	420	95	1
Cookie Black And White	1	430	50	2
Cookie Double Chocolate Chunk	1 serv	430	15	3
Cookie Oatmean Raisin	1	390	15	3
Cookie White Chocolate Macadamia Nut	1	470	15	2
Crisp Cinnamon Twist	1	60	0	0
Croissant Almond	1	330	30	2
Croissant Butter w/ Apricot Glaze	1	320	25	1
Croissant Chocolate	1	350	30	2
Croissant Raspberry & Cream Cheese	1	260	30	1
Crumb Cake	1 serv	670	115	1
Crumb Cake Key Lime	1 serv	550	190	1
Danish Apple w/ Mocha Swirls	1	370	25	2

FOOD	PORTION	CALS	CHOL	FIBER
Danish Cheese w/ Mocha Swirls	1	460	50	1
Danish Raspberry w/ Mocho Swirls	1	370	25	1
Graham Dark Chocolate	1	140	<5	tr
Graham Milk Chocolate	1	140	<5	tr
Madeline	1	80	25	0
Muffin Blueberry	1	380	70	1
Muffin Chocolate Cream Cheese	1	450	80	1
Muffin Cranberry Orange	1	410	70	2
Muffin Morning Sunrise	1	330	35	2
Pound Cake Banana	1 serv	360	100	1
Pound Cake Cranberry Walnut	1 serv	390	110	1
Pound Cake Iced Carrot	1 serv	540	35	3
Pound Cake Iced Lemon	1 serv	500	145	tr
Pound Cake Marble	1 serv	400	130	tr
Pound Cake Orange Poppy	1 serv	490	140	2
Pound Cake Pumpkin	1 serv	310	65	2
Pound Cake Zucchini	1 serv	370	55	2
Pullman Banana	1 serv	400	65	2
Pullman Chocolate	1	380	55	2
Pullman Cranberry Walnut	1	360	25	2
Pullman Lemon Glazed	1	370	90	tr
Pullman Marble Chocolate Chip	1	440	95	1
Pullman Orange Poppy Cheese	1	450	110	1
Pullman Pumpkin	1	370	60	2
Scone Blueberry	1	460	50	3
Scone Butterscotch Pecan	1	520	50	2
Scone Cinnamon Chip w/ Icing	1	510	50	2
Scone Maple Oat w/ Icing	1	490	45	2
Scone Apricot Currant	1	450	60	3
Scone Raspberry	1	440	50	2
Shortbread	1	100	15	0
BEVERAGES				
Apple Juice	1 grande	230	0	0

FOOD	PORTION	CALS	CHOL	FIBER
Blended Coffee Of The Week	1 grande	10	0	0
Cafe Americano	1 grande	150	0	0
Cafe Au Lait Nonfat Milk	1 grande	90	<5	0
Cafe Au Lait Soy Milk	1 grande	110	0	tr
Cafe Latte Whole Milk	1 grande	260	55	0
Cafe Misto Cafe Au Lait Whole Milk	1 grande	140	30	0
Cafe Mocha Whip Whole Milk	1 grande	400	80	2
Caffe Latte Nonfat Milk	1 grande	160	10	0
Caffe Latte Soy Milk	1 grande	210	0	2
Caffe Mocha No Whip Nonfat Milk	1 grande	230	5	2
Caffe Mocha No Whip Soy Milk	1 grande	260	0	3
Caffe Mocha No Whip Whole Milk	1 grande	300	40	2
Caffe Mocha Whip Nonfat Milk	1 grande	330	45	2
Caffe Mocha Whip Soy Milk	1 grande	360	40	3
Cappuccino Nonfat Milk	1 grande	100	<5	0
Cappucino Soy Milk	1 grande	120	0	tr
Caramel Apple Cider No Whip	1 grande	300	0	0
Caramel Apple Cider Whip	1 grande	410	40	0
Caramel Macchiato Nonfat Milk	1 grande	230	15	0
Caramel Macchiato Soy Milk	1 grande	300	5	1
Caramel Macchiato Whole Milk	1 grande	320	55	0
Caramel Mocha No Whip Nonfat Milk	1 grande	300	5	2
Caramel Mocha No Whip Soy Milk	1 grande	340	0	3
Caramel Mocha No Whip Whole Milk	1 grande	370	35	2
Caramel Mocha Whip Nonfat Milk	1 grande	410	45	2

FOOD	PORTION	CALS	CHOL	FIBER
Caramel Mocha Whip Soy Milk	1 grande	440	40	3
Caramel Mocha Whip Whole Milk	1 grande	470	75	2
Chocolate Nonfat Milk	1 grande	240	10	2
Chocolate Whole Milk	1 grande	340	50	2
Cinnamon Spice Mocha No Whip Nonfat Milk	1 grande	250	5	tr
Cinnamon Spice Mocha No Whip Whole Milk	1 grande	330	45	tr
Cinnamon Spice Mocha Whip Nonfat Milk	1 grande	350	45	tr
Cinnamon Spice Mocha Whip Whole Milk	1 grande	430	85	tr
Cinnamon Spice No Whip Soy Milk	1 grande	290	0	2
Cinnamon Spice Whip Soy Milk	1 grande	390	40	2
Espresso Decaf Coffee Of The Week	1 grande	10	0	0
Frappuccino Blended Coffee	1 grande	230	10	0
Frappuccino Blended Coffee Mocha Coconut No Whip Whole Milk	1 grande	400	15	2
Frappuccino Caramel Blended Coffee No Whip	1 grande	280	15	0
Frappuccino Caramel Blended Coffee Whip	1 grande	430	65	0
Frappuccino Chocolate Blended Creme Whip	1 grande	530	55	1
Frappuccino Chocolate Blended Creme No Whip	1 grande	400	<5	1
Frappuccino Chocolate Brownie Blended Coffee No Whip	1 grande	370	15	2
Frappuccino Chocolate Brownie Blended Coffee Whip	1 grande	510	65	2
Frappuccino Chocolate Malt Blended Creme No Whip	1 grande	470	15	2

FOOD	PORTION	CALS	CHOL	FIBER
Frappuccino Chocolate Malt Blended Creme Whip	1 grande	610	65	2
Frappuccino Mocha Blended Coffee No Whip	1 grande	290	15	0
Frappuccino Mocha Blended Coffee Whip	1 grande	420	65	0
Frappuccino Mocha Coconut Blended Coffee Whip	1 grande	550	65	2
Frappuccino Mocha Malt Blended Coffee No Whip	1 grande	430	20	1
Frappuccino Mocha Malt Blended Coffee Whip	1 grande	570	75	1
Frappuccino Tazo Chai Creme Blended Tea No Whip	1 grande	370	<5	0
Frappuccino Tazo Chai Creme Blended Tea Whip	1 grande	500	55	0
Frappuccino Tazoberry Blended Tea	1 grande	190	0	tr
Frappuccino Tazoberry Creme Blended Tea No Whip	1 grande	330	0	tr
Frappuccino Tazoberry Creme Blended Tea Whip	1 grande	460	50	tr
Frappuccino Vanilla Blended Creme No Whip	1 grande	350	<5	0
Frappuccino Vanilla Blended Creme Whip	1 grande	480	55	0
Frappuccino White Chocolate Mocha Blended Coffee No Whip	1 grande	320	15	0
Frappuccino White Chocolate Mocha Blended Coffee Whip	1 grande	450	65	0
Hot Chocolate No Whip Whole Milk	1 grande	340	50	2
Hot Chocolate No Whip Nonfat Milk	1 grande	240	10	2
Hot Chocolate Whip Nonfat Milk	1 grande	340	45	2

FOOD	PORTION	CALS	CHOL	FIBER
Hot Chocolate Whip Whole Milk	1 grande	440	90	2
Iced Cafe Latte Whole Milk	1 grande	160	30	0
Iced Cafe Mocha Whip Nonfat Milk	1 grande	310	55	2
Iced Cafe Mocha Whip Soy Milk	1 grande	330	50	3
Iced Caffe Americano	1 grande	20	0	0
Iced Caffe Latte Nonfat Milk	1 grande	100	<5	0
Iced Caffe Latte Soy Milk	1 grande	120	0	tr
Iced Caffe Mocha No Whip Whole Milk	1 grande	220	25	2
Iced Caffe Mocha No Whip Nonfat Milk	1 grande	180	<5	2
Iced Caffe Mocha No Whip Soy Milk	1 grande	200	0	3
Iced Caffe Mocha Whip Whole Milk	1 grande	350	75	2
Iced Caramel Macchiato Nonfat Milk	1 grande	100	10	0
Iced Caramel Macchiato Soy Milk	1 grande	230	<5	1
Iced Caramel Macchiato Whole Milk	1 grande	270	40	0
Iced Shaken Coffee	1 grande	80	0	0
Iced Tazo Chai Nonfat Milk	1 grande	230	0	0
Iced Tazo Chai Whole Milk	1 grande	270	25	0
Iced White Chocolate Mocha No Whip Soy Milk	1 grande	340	<5	tr
Iced White Chocolate Mocha No Whip Whole Milk	1 grande	360	25	0
Iced White Chocolate Mocha Whip Nonfat Milk	1 grande	450	55	0
Iced White Chocolate Mocha Whip Soy Milk	1 grande	470	55	tr
Iced White Chocolate Mocha Whip Whole Milk	1 grande	490	75	0
Iced White Chocolate No Whip Nonfat Milk	1 grande	320	5	0
Milk Nonfat	1 grande	160	10	0

FOOD	PORTION	CALS	CHOL	FIBER
Steamed Apple Cider	1 grande	230	0	0
Steamed Nonfat Milk	1 grande	160	0	0
Steamed Whole Milk	1 grande	270	60	0
Tazo Chai Whole Milk	1 grande	290	30	0
Tazo Chai Nonfat Milk	1 grande	230	5	0
Tazo Iced Tea	1 grande	80	0	0
Tazo Tea Lemonade	1 grande	120	0	0
Vanilla Creme Whip Nonfat Milk	1 grande	340	50	0
Vanilla Creme Whip Whole Milk	1 grande	440	95	0
Vanilla Creme No Whip Nonfat Milk	1 grande	240	10	0
Vanille Creme No Whip Whole Milk	1 grande	340	60	0
White Chocolate Mocha No Whip Nonfat Milk	1 grande	340	10	0
White Chocolate Mocha No Whip Whole Milk	1 grande	410	45	0
White Chocolate Mocha Whip Nonfat Milk	1 grande	440	45	0
White Chocolate Mocha Whip Whole Milk	1 grande	510	80	0
White Chocolate No Whip Soy Milk	1 grande	370	0	1
White Chocolate Whip Soy Milk	1 grande	440	20	1
White Hot Chocolate No Whip Nonfat Milk	1 grande	390	10	0
White Hot Chocolate No Whip Whole Milk	1 grande	480	55	0
White Hot Chocolate Whip Nonfat Milk	1 grande	490	50	0
White Hot Chocolate Whip Whole Milk	1 grande	580	95	0
Whole Milk	1 grande	270	60	0
TOPPINGS				
Caramel	1 tbsp	15	0	0
Chocolate	1 tsp	5	0	0
Flavored Sugar Free Syrup	1 pump	0	0	0

FOOD	PORTION	CALS	CHOL	FIBER
Flavored Syrup	1 pump	20	0	0
Mocha Syrup	1 pump	25	0	0
Sprinkles	1 serv	0	0	0

STEAK ESCAPE
BEVERAGES

FOOD	PORTION	CALS	CHOL	FIBER
Coca-Cola	12 oz	110	0	–
Coca-Cola	44 oz	430	0	–
Diet Coke	12 oz	0	0	0
Diet Coke	44 oz	0	0	0
Hi-C Fruit Punch	12 oz	116	0	–
Hi-C Fruit Punch	44 oz	452	0	–
Lemonade	12 oz	126	0	–
Lemonade	44 oz	488	0	–
Sprite	12 oz	110	0	–
Sprite	44 oz	430	0	–

CHILDREN'S MENU SELECTIONS

FOOD	PORTION	CALS	CHOL	FIBER
Kids Fries	1 serv	249	0	–
Kids Tenders	2 pieces	240	35	–
Sandwich Chicken	1	205	32	–
Sandwich Ham	1	183	13	–
Sandwich Steak	1	210	13	–
Sandwich Turkey	1	183	13	–

MAIN MENU SELECTIONS

FOOD	PORTION	CALS	CHOL	FIBER
12 Inch Sandwich Grand Cobbler	1	680	60	–
12 Inch Sandwich Grand Escape	1	776	100	–
12 Inch Sandwich Grandest Chicken	1	770	110	–
12 Inch Sandwich Great Escape	1	776	100	–
12 Inch Sandwich Hambrosia	1	684	60	–
12 Inch Sandwich Ragin' Cajun	1	756	110	–
12 Inch Sandwich Turkey Club	1	675	70	–
12 Inch Sandwich Vegetarian	1	524	0	–

FOOD	PORTION	CALS	CHOL	FIBER
12 Inch Sandwich Wild West BBQ	1	841	100	–
7 Inch Sandwich Grand Cobbler	1	380	30	–
7 Inch Sandwich Grand Escape	1	435	50	–
7 Inch Sandwich Grandest Chicken	1	425	55	–
7 Inch Sandwich Great Escape	1	428	50	–
7 Inch Sandwich Hambrosia	1	382	30	–
7 Inch Sandwich Ragin' Cajun	1	418	55	–
7 Inch Sandwich Turkey Club	1	390	40	–
7 Inch Sandwich Vegetarian	1	302	0	–
7 Inch Sandwich Wild West BBQ	1	469	50	–
Fries	1 serv (32 oz)	996	0	–
Fries	1 serv (12 oz)	498	0	–
Fries Loaded Bacon Bacon & Cheddar	1 serv	905	29	–
Fries Loaded Ranch & Bacon	1 serv	1044	39	–
Smashed Potatoes Loaded Bacon & Cheddar	1 serv	636	24	–
Smashed Potatoes Loaded Ranch & Bacon	1 serv	692	29	–
Smashed Potatoes Plain	1 serv	246	0	–
Smashed Potatoes w/ Chicken	1 serv	318	55	–
Smashed Potatoes w/ Ham	1 serv	336	30	–
Smashed Potatoes w/ Steak	1 serv	391	50	–
Smashed Potatoes w/ Turkey	1 serv	336	30	–
SALAD DRESSINGS AND TOPPINGS				
American Cheese	1 slice	101	26	–
Bacon	1 serv (1 oz)	80	10	0

FOOD	PORTION	CALS	CHOL	FIBER
BBQ Sauce	1 serv (1 oz)	40	0	–
Black Olives	1 serv (1 oz)	32	0	–
Brown Mustard	1 serv (1 oz)	0	0	0
Cheddar Cheese	1 slice	116	30	–
Dressing Italian	1 serv (0.5 oz)	51	0	–
Dressing Ranch	1 serv (0.5 oz)	83	5	0
Lettuce	1 serv (1 oz)	2	0	0
Margarine	1 serv (1 oz)	203	0	0
Mayonnaise	1 serv (1 oz)	101	5	0
Peppers Jalapeno	1 serv (1.5 oz)	11	0	–
Peppers Mild	1 serv (1.5 oz)	11	0	–
Provolone Cheese	1 slice	80	15	–
Sour Cream	1 serv (1 oz)	61	13	–
Swiss Cheese	1 slice	100	26	–
Tomatoes	1 serv (2 oz)	24	0	–
SALADS				
Grilled Salad w/ Chicken	1 serv	175	55	–
Grilled Salad w/ Ham	1 serv	130	30	–
Grilled Salad w/ Steak	1 serv	185	50	–
Grilled Salad w/ Turkey	1 serv	130	30	–
Side	1 serv	40	0	–

SUBWAY
BEVERAGES

FOOD	PORTION	CALS	CHOL	FIBER
Fruizle Smoothie Berry Lishus	1 sm (13 oz)	113	15	1
Fruizle Smoothie Berry Lishus w/ Banana	1 sm (17 oz)	221	15	4
Fruizle Smoothie Peach Pizazz	1 sm (12 oz)	103	0	0
Fruizle Smoothie Pineapple Delight w/ Banana	1 sm (17 oz)	241	0	4
Fruizle Smoothie Pineapple Delite	1 sm (13 oz)	133	0	1
Fruizle Smoothie Sunrise Refresher	1 sm (12 oz)	119	0	1
COOKIES				
Chocolate Chip	1	215	13	1
Chocolate Chunk	1	217	12	1

FOOD	PORTION	CALS	CHOL	FIBER
Double Chocolate	1	209	15	1
M&M	1	215	13	1
Oatmeal Raisin	1	210	14	2
Peanut Butter	1	221	12	1
Sugar	1	227	17	0
White Macadamia Nut	1	221	15	1
SALAD DRESSINGS				
Fat Free French	1 serv (2 oz)	70	0	0
Fat Free Italian	1 serv (2 oz)	20	0	0
Fat Free Ranch	1 serv (2 oz)	60	0	0
SALADS				
BMT	1 serv	275	55	3
Cold Cut Trio	1 serv	234	57	3
Ham	1 serv	112	25	3
Meatball	1 serv	320	56	4
Roast Beef	1 serv	117	25	3
Roasted Chicken Breast	1 serv	130	50	3
Seafood & Crab	1 serv	197	24	4
Steak & Cheese	1 serv	181	37	4
Subway Club	1 serv	146	33	3
Subway Melt	1 serv	203	44	3
Tuna	1 serv	238	42	3
Turkey Breast	1 serv	105	20	3
Turkey Breast & Ham	1 serv	117	26	3
Veggie Delight	1 serv	50	0	3
SANDWICHES				
6 Inch Steak & Cheese	1	362	37	4
6 Inch Subway Melt	1	384	44	3
6 Inch Sub BMT	1	456	55	3
6 Inch Sub Cold Cut Trio	1	415	57	3
6 Inch Sub Ham	1	261	25	3
6 Inch Sub Meatball	1	501	56	4
6 Inch Sub Roast Beef	1	267	20	3
6 Inch Sub Roasted Chicken Breast	1	291	46	3
6 Inch Sub Seafood & Crab	1	378	24	3
6 Inch Sub Subway Club	1	296	33	3
6 Inch Sub Tuna	1	419	42	3
6 Inch Sub Turkey Breast	1	254	20	3

FOOD	PORTION	CALS	CHOL	FIBER
6 Inch Sub Turkey Breast & Ham	1	267	26	3
6 Inch Sub Veggie Delight	1	200	0	3
American Cheese Triangles	2	41	10	0
Asiago Caesar Sauce	1.5 tbsp	110	10	0
Bacon Strips	2	45	8	0
Breakfast Bacon & Egg	1	321	184	3
Breakfast Cheese & Egg	1	317	187	3
Breakfast Ham & Egg	1	338	201	3
Breakfast Western Egg	1	300	182	3
Cheddar Triangles	2	59	15	0
Cucumber Slices	3	2	0	0
Deli Ham	1	210	12	3
Deli Roast Beef	1	223	13	3
Deli Tuna	1	325	26	3
Deli Turkey Breast	1	215	13	3
Deli Style Roll	1	165	0	3
Dijon Horseradish	1.5 tbsp	91	8	0
Dijon Horseradish Melt	6 in	465	52	4
Fat Free Red Wine Vinaigrette	1.5 tbsp	29	1	0
Fat Free Sweet Onion	1.5 tbsp	38	0	0
Green Pepper Strips	3 (0.2 oz)	2	0	0
Hearty Italian Bread	6 in	207	0	3
Honey Mustard	1.5 tbsp	28	0	0
Honey Mustard Ham	6 in	311	25	4
Honey Oat Bread	6 in	249	0	4
Italian Bread	6 in	178	0	2
Lettuce	1 serv (0.7 oz)	3	0	0
Mayonnaise	1 tbsp	111	9	0
Mayonnaise Light	1 tbsp	46	6	0
Moneterey Cheddar Bread	6 in	235	10	3
Mustard	2 tsp	7	0	0
Olive Oil Blend	1 tsp	45	0	0
Olive Rings	3 (3 g)	3	0	0
Onions	1 serv (0.5 oz)	5	0	0
Parmesan Oregano Bread	6 in	211	0	3
Pepperjack Cheese Triangles	2	40	11	0
Pickle Chips	3 pieces (0.3 oz)	1	0	0
Provolone Circles	2 halves	51	11	0

FOOD	PORTION	CALS	CHOL	FIBER
Red Wine Vinaigrette Club	6 in	350	33	4
Roasted Garlic Bread	6 in	225	0	4
Sourdough Bread	6 in	208	0	3
Southwest Sauce	1.5 tbsp	86	7	0
Southwest Turkey Bacon	6 in	407	35	4
Sweet Onion Chicken Teriyaki	6 in	374	50	4
Swiss Triangles	2	53	13	0
Tomato Slices	3 (1.2 oz)	7	0	0
Vinegar	1 tsp	1	0	0
Wheat Sub	6 in	186	0	3
SOUPS				
Black Bean	1 cup	180	5	15
Brown & Wild Rice w/ Chicken	1 cup	190	20	2
Cheese w/ Ham & Bacon	1 cup	230	20	2
Chicken & Dumplings	1 cup	130	30	1
Cream Of Broccoli	1 cup	130	15	1
Cream Of Potato w/ Bacon	1 cup	210	20	4
Golden Broccoli Cheese	1 cup	180	10	9
Hearty Chili Beef	1 cup	250	20	9
Minestrone	1 cup	70	5	0
New England Clam Chowder	1 cup	140	15	1
Potato Cheese Chowder	1 cup	210	25	2
Roasted Chicken Noodle	1 cup	90	20	1
Tomato Bisque	1 cup	90	0	3
Vegetable Beef	1 cup	90	5	2

TACO BELL

FOOD	PORTION	CALS	CHOL	FIBER
Bean Burrito	1	370	10	8
Border Bowl Zesty Chicken	1 serv	730	45	12
Border Bowl Zesty Chicken w/o Dressing	1 serv	500	30	12
Burrito 7 Layer	1	530	25	10
Burrito Chili Cheese	1	390	40	3
Burrito Grilled Chicken	1	680	70	7
Burrito Spicy Chicken	1	430	30	4
Burrito Supreme Beef	1	440	40	5
Burrito 1/2 Lb Bean Especial	1	600	15	12
Burrito 1/2 Lb Beef & Potato	1	530	40	4

FOOD	PORTION	CALS	CHOL	FIBER
Burrito ½ Lb Combo Beef	1	470	45	5
Burrito Fiesta Chicken	1	370	30	3
Burrito Fiesta Steak	1	370	25	4
Burrito Supreme Chicken	1	410	45	5
Burrito Supreme Steak	1	420	35	6
Chalupa Baja Beef	1	430	30	2
Chalupa Baja Chicken	1	400	40	2
Chalupa Baja Steak	1	400	30	2
Chalupa Nacho Cheese Beef	1	380	20	1
Chalupa Nacho Cheese Chicken	1	350	25	1
Chalupa Nacho Cheese Steak	1	350	20	2
Chalupa Supreme Beef	1	390	35	4
Chalupa Supreme Chicken	1	370	45	1
Chalupa Supreme Steak	1	370	35	2
Cheesy Fiesta Potatoes	1 serv	280	20	2
Cinnamon Twists	1 serv	160	0	0
Empanada Caramel Apple	1	290	<5	1
Enchirito Beef	1	380	45	5
Enchirito Chicken	1	350	55	5
Enchirito Steak	1	360	45	5
Express Taco Salad	1 serv	630	65	10
Express Taco Salad w/o Chips	1 serv	410	65	8
Fiesta Taco Salad	1 serv	870	65	12
Fiesta Taco Salad w/o Shell	1 serv	500	65	10
Gordita Baja Beef	1	350	30	2
Gordita Baja Chicken	1	320	40	2
Gordita Baja Steak	1	320	30	2
Gordita Nacho Cheese Beef	1	300	20	2
Gordita Nacho Cheese Chicken	1	270	25	2
Gordita Nacho Cheese Steak	1	270	20	2
Gordita Supreme Beef	1	310	35	2
Gordita Supreme Chicken	1	290	45	2
Gordita Supreme Steak	1	280	35	2
Mexican Pizza	1 serv	550	45	5
Mexican Rice	1 serv	210	15	3

FOOD	PORTION	CALS	CHOL	FIBER
MexiMelt	1 serv	290	40	2
Nacho Supreme	1 serv	450	35	5
Nachos	1 serv	320	<5	2
Nachos Bellgrande	1 serv	780	35	11
Pintos 'n Cheese	1 serv	180	15	6
Quesadilla Cheese	1 serv	490	55	3
Quesadilla Chicken	1	540	80	3
Quesadilla Steak	1	540	70	3
Soft Taco Beef	1	210	25	tr
Soft Taco Grande	1	450	45	2
Soft Taco Grilled Steak	1	280	30	1
Soft Taco Ranchero Chicken	1	270	35	2
Soft Taco Supreme Beef	1	260	35	1
Southwest Steak Bowl	1 serv	700	55	13
Taco	1	170	25	tr
Taco Double Decker	1	340	25	5
Taco Spicy Chicken	1	180	20	2
Taco Supreme	1	220	35	1
Taco Supreme Double Decker	1	380	40	5
Tostada	1	250	15	7

TACO JOHN'S
DESSERTS

Apple Grande	1 serv	240	5	0
Choco Taco	1 serv	300	15	1
Churro	1 serv	230	10	1
Cinnamon Mini Swirl	1 piece	10	0	0

MAIN MENU SELECTIONS

Burrito Bean	1	380	15	10
Burrito Beefy	1	430	55	8
Burrito Chicken & Potato	1	460	35	8
Burrito Combination	1	400	35	9
Burrito Meat & Potato	1	490	30	9
Burrito Super	1	450	40	10
Crispy Taco	1 serv	180	25	3
Mexican Rice	1 serv	250	0	2
Nachos	1 serv	380	10	tr
Potato Oles	1 lg	790	0	8
Potato Oles	1 sm	440	0	5

FOOD	PORTION	CALS	CHOL	FIBER
Potato Oles Bravo	1 serv	580	20	6
Potato Oles Super	1 serv	980	60	10
Potato Oles w/ Nacho Cheese	1 serv	550	10	5
Quesadilla Cheese	1	480	50	6
Quesadilla Chicken	1	540	75	7
Refried Beans	1 serv	400	15	11
Sierra Taco Beef	1	430	45	4
Sierra Taco Chicken	1	390	50	3
Softshell Taco	1	220	25	4
Softshell Taco Chicken	1	190	30	4
Super Nachos	1 serv	830	60	5
Super Nachos Chicken	1 serv	780	90	3
Taco Bravo	1 serv	340	25	8
Taco Burger	1	280	35	3
Texas Chili	1 serv	270	35	4
SALAD DRESSINGS AND TOPPINGS				
Bacon Ranch Dressing	1 serv (3 oz)	250	20	0
Barbecue Sauce	1 serv (2 oz)	70	0	0
Chipotle Cream Sauce	1 serv (3 oz)	450	30	0
Creamy Italian Dressing	1 serv (3 oz)	260	0	0
Guacamole	1 serv (2 oz)	90	0	–
Hot Sauce	1 serv (1 oz)	5	0	0
House Dressing	1 serv (3 oz)	140	0	tr
Jalapenos	1 serv (2 oz)	15	0	1
Mild Sauce	1 serv (1 oz)	5	0	0
Nacho Cheese	1 serv (3 oz)	120	10	0
Pico De Gallo	1 serv (2 oz)	15	0	tr
Ranch Dressing	1 serv (3 oz)	280	45	0
Salsa	1 serv (2 oz)	20	0	0
Sour Cream	1 serv (2 oz)	120	25	0
Super Hot Sauce	1 serv (1 oz)	10	0	tr
SALADS				
Chicken Festiva w/o Dressing	1 serv	400	70	4
Chicken Taco w/o Dressing	1	530	70	3
Side w/o Dressing	1 serv	80	5	1
Taco w/o Dressing	1 serv	580	60	4

FOOD	PORTION	CALS	CHOL	FIBER
TACOTIME				
DESSERTS				
Cinnamon Crustos	1 serv	373	0	–
Fruit Filled Empanada	1 serv	250	0	–
MAIN MENU SELECTIONS				
Burrito Beef Bean & Cheese	1 serv	617	63	18
Burrito Casita	1 serv	647	89	16
Burrito Chicken & Black Bean	1 serv	400	36	5
Burrito Chicken BLT	1 serv	580	50	5
Burrito Crisp Bean	1 serv	427	12	9
Burrito Crisp Chicken	1	422	54	2
Burrito Crisp Meat	1 serv	552	58	7
Burrito Soft Bean	1	380	15	13
Burrito Soft Meat	1 serv	491	56	12
Burrito Veggie	1 serv	491	24	10
Burrito Big Juan Beef	1 serv	640	60	15
Burrito Big Juan Chicken	1 serv	620	65	12
Cheddar Melt	1 serv	205	30	1
Mexi-Rice	1 serv	159	0	1
Nachos	1 serv	680	78	11
Nachos Deluxe	1 serv	1048	109	17
Refritos Cheese Sauce Chips	1 serv	326	22	13
Stuffed Fries	1 sm	490	20	3
Stuffed Fries	1 lg	990	35	6
Taco Cheeseburger	1	633	66	7
Taco Crisp	1	295	48	5
Taco Soft	1 serv	316	48	5
Taco Soft ½ lb	1 serv	512	63	12
Taco Soft ½ lb Chicken	1 serv	387	48	7
Taco Super Soft	1 serv	510	60	11
SALAD DRESSINGS AND TOPPINGS				
1000 Island Dressing	1 serv (1 oz)	120	5	0
Green Sauce	1 serv (1 oz)	5	0	tr
Original Hot Sauce	1 serv (1 oz)	10	0	0
Salsa Fresca	1 serv (1 oz)	65	0	0
SALADS				
Chicken Fiesta	1 serv	390	45	4
Taco	1 reg	479	63	7
Taco Salad Chicken	1 serv	370	48	3
Tostada	1 serv	628	82	13

FOOD	PORTION	CALS	CHOL	FIBER
TASTI D-LITE				
Vanilla	1 sm (4 oz)	40	7	3
TCBY				
FROZEN YOGURT AND SORBET				
Hand Scooped Butter Butter Pecan Perfection	½ cup	110	10	tr
Hand Scooped Chocolate Chocolate Swirl	½ cup	120	15	tr
Hand Scooped Chocolate Chunk Cookie Dough	½ cup	160	15	0
Hand Scooped Cookies & Cream	½ cup	140	10	0
Hand Scooped Cotton Candy	½ cup	120	15	0
Hand Scooped Mint Chocolate Chunk	½ cup	140	10	0
Hand Scooped Mocha Almond	½ cup	150	10	tr
Hand Scooped No Sugar Added Chocolate Chocolate Swirl	½ cup	90	0	6
Hand Scooped No Sugar Added Vanilla	½ cup	80	0	5
Hand Scooped No Sugar Added Vanilla Fudge Brownie	½ cup	100	10	5
Hand Scooped Pralines & Cream	½ cup	140	10	0
Hand Scooped Psychedelic Sorbet	½ cup	290	0	0
Hand Scooped Rainbow Cream	½ cup	120	15	0
Hand Scooped Rocky Road	½ cup	220	5	1
Hand Scooped Strawberries & Cream	½ cup	120	10	0
Hand Scooped Vanilla Chocolate Chunk	½ cup	140	10	0
Hand Scooped Vanilla Bean	½ cup	120	15	0
Soft Serve Frozen Yogurt All Flavors 96% Fat Free	½ cup	140	15	0

FOOD	PORTION	CALS	CHOL	FIBER
Soft Serve Frozen Yogurt All Flavors No Sugar Added Nonfat	½ cup	90	<5	0
Soft Serve Frozen Yogurt All Flavors Nonfat	½ cup	110	<5	0
Soft Serve Frozen Yogurt Low Carb	½ cup	110	25	7
Soft Serve Sorbet All Flavors Nonfat Nondairy	½ cup	100	0	0
SMOOTHIES				
A Lotta Coloda w/ Yogurt	1 (20 oz)	550	0	2
A Lotta Coloda w/o Yogurt	1 (20 oz)	380	0	3
Berry Slim w/ Yogurt	1 (20 oz)	410	10	2
Berry Slim w/o Yogurt	1 (20 oz)	300	0	2
Healthy Balance w/ Yogurt	1 (20 oz)	410	10	2
Healthy Balance w/o Yogurt	1 (20 oz)	300	0	2
Holy-Cal w/ Yogurt	1 (20 oz)	470	10	3
Holy-Cal w/o Yogurt	1 (20 oz)	360	0	3
Peachy Lean w/ Yogurt	1 (20 oz)	470	10	tr
Peachy Lean w/o Yogurt	1 (20 oz)	360	0	tr
Raspberry Delite w/ Yogurt	1 (20 oz)	360	10	4
Raspberry Delite w/o Yogurt	1 (20 oz)	240	0	3
Raspberry Revitalizer w/ Yogurt	1 (20 oz)	370	10	3
Raspberry Revitalizer w/o Yogurt	1 (20 oz)	300	0	6
Tropical Replenisher w/ Yogurt	1 (20 oz)	370	10	1
Tropical Replenisher w/o Yogurt	1 (20 oz)	240	0	2
Workout Whey w/ Yogurt	1 (20 oz)	460	10	1
Workout Whey w/o Yogurt	1 (20 oz)	340	0	1

TIM HORTONS
BAGELS AND CREAM CHEESE

FOOD	PORTION	CALS	CHOL	FIBER
Blueberry	1	200	0	3
Cinnamon Raisin	1	300	0	4
Cream Cheese Light	1.5 oz	90	20	0
Cream Cheese Plain	1.5 oz	140	45	0
Everything	1	300	0	3

FOOD	PORTION	CALS	CHOL	FIBER
Multigrain	1	300	0	6
Onion	1	295	0	3
Plain	1	290	0	3
Poppy Seed	1	300	0	4
Sesame Seed	1	300	0	4
Whole Wheat & Honey	1	300	0	6
BAKED SELECTIONS				
Biscuit Southern Country Cranberry	1	470	0	2
Biscuit Southern Country Raspberry	1	470	0	2
Cake Black Forest	1 serv	500	0	3
Cake Celebration	1 serv	500	5	1
Cake Chocolot Fantasy	1 serv	420	35	3
Cake Shadow	1 serv	430	35	2
Cookie Chocolate Chip	1	150	20	1
Cookie Macaroon	1	140	0	3
Cookie Oatcakes	1	190	0	1
Cookie Oatmeal Raisin	1	150	15	1
Cookie Peanut Butter	1	170	20	1
Cookie Peanut Butter Chocolate Chunk	1	170	15	1
Croissant Butter	1	210	30	1
Croissant Cheese	1	240	20	1
Danish Cherry Cheese	1	380	45	1
Donut Apple Fritter	1	300	0	2
Donut Chocolate Dip	1	230	0	0
Donut Chocolate Glazed	1	360	10	1
Donut Dutchie	1	280	0	1
Donut Honey Dip	1	230	0	0
Donut Maple Dip	1	250	0	0
Donut Old Fashion Glazed	1	270	15	0
Donut Old Fashion Plain	1	220	15	0
Donut Sour Cream Plain	1	280	20	0
Donut Sugar Twist	1	230	0	0
Donut Walnut Crunch	1	320	10	2
Donut Filled Angel Cream	1	280	0	0
Donut Filled Blueberry	1	220	0	0
Donut Filled Boston Cream	1	230	0	0

FOOD	PORTION	CALS	CHOL	FIBER
Donut Filled Canadian Maple	1	230	0	0
Donut Filled Strawberry	1	220	0	0
Donuts Honey Stick	1	280	30	0
Muffin Blueberry Bran	1	300	10	5
Muffin Carrot Whole Wheat	1	410	10	4
Muffin Chocolate Chip	1	390	20	2
Muffin Oatbran Carrot 'n Raisin	1	340	0	4
Muffin Oatbran 'n Apple	1	350	0	4
Muffin Oatmeal Raisin	1	430	20	3
Muffin Raisin Bran	1	380	10	6
Muffin Wild Blueberry	1	330	15	2
Muffin Low Fat Carrot	1	260	0	6
Muffin Low Fat Cranberry	1	260	0	6
Muffin Low Fat Honey	1	290	0	6
Pie Apple	1 serv	540	0	3
Pie Banana Cream	1 serv	440	0	1
Pie Cherry	1 serv	570	0	2
Pie Chocolate Cream	1 serv	490	10	1
Tart Fresh Strawberry	1 serv	220	0	2
Tart Raisin Butter	1 serv	330	15	1
Tea Biscuit Plain	1	220	0	1
Tea Biscuit Raisin	1	250	0	2
Timbits Chocolate Glazed	1	70	5	0
Timbits Dutchie	1	60	0	0
Timbits Honey Dip	1	50	0	0
Timbits Old Fashion Plain	1	45	5	0
Timbits Filled Banana Cream	1	45	0	0
Timbits Filled Lemon	1	50	0	0
Timbits Filled Spiced Apple	1	80	0	0
Timbits Filled Strawberry	1	50	0	0
BEVERAGES				
Apple Juice	1 (9 oz)	140	0	0
Cafe Mocha	1 (10 oz)	250	0	0
Cappuccino English Toffee	1 (10 oz)	130	0	0
Cappuccino French Vanilla	1 (10 oz)	130	0	0
Cappuccino Iced	(16 oz)	430	80	0
Chocolate Milk	1 (14 oz)	280	15	0

FOOD	PORTION	CALS	CHOL	FIBER
Coffee Decaffeinated + Sugar & Cream	1 (10 oz)	80	12	0
Coffee + Sugar & Cream	1 (10 oz)	80	12	0
Coke	1 (14 oz)	170	0	0
Diet Coke	1 (14 oz)	1	0	0
Fruit Punch	1 (10 oz)	150	0	0
Hot Chocolate	1 (10 oz)	200	0	0
Iced Tea	1 (14 oz)	130	0	0
Milk 2%	1 (14 oz)	210	30	0
Orange Juice	1 (10 oz)	140	0	0
Sprite	1 (14 oz)	160	0	0
Tea + Sugar & Milk	1 (10 oz)	45	0	0
SANDWICHES				
Albacore Tuna Salad	1 serv	350	15	3
Black Forest Ham & Swiss	1 serv	640	75	2
Chunky Chicken Salad	1 serv	380	45	3
Fireside Roast Beef	1 serv	470	36	2
Garden Vegetable	1 serv	460	45	3
Harvest Turkey Breast	1 serv	470	30	2
SOUPS				
Barley & Wild Rice	1 serv	120	6	1
Chicken Noodle	1 serv	100	14	1
Chili	1 serv	320	65	8
Cream Of Broccoli	1 serv	190	6	1
Cream of Mushroom	1 serv	195	8	1
Hearty Vegetable	1 serv	130	0	2
Minestrone	1 serv	125	1	2
Potato Bacon	1 serv	195	5	1
Vegetable Beef Barley	1 serv	110	9	2

TJ CINNAMONS

FOOD	PORTION	CALS	CHOL	FIBER
Cinnachips	1 bag (10 oz)	1130	42	3
Cinnamon Twist	1	260	5	10
Coffee Black	1 (12 oz)	0	0	0
Mocha Chill w/ Whipped Cream	1 (12.5 oz)	310	25	10
Mocha Chill w/o Whipped Cream	1 (12.5 oz)	260	15	10
Original Roll w/o Icing	1	500	30	0

FOOD	PORTION	CALS	CHOL	FIBER
Original Roll w/ Cream Cheese Icing	1	651	40	0
Pecan Sticky Roll	1	690	32	0

TOGO'S
SALAD DRESSINGS

FOOD	PORTION	CALS	CHOL	FIBER
1000 Island	1 serv (2.3 oz)	231	30	0
Caesar	1 serv (2.3 oz)	241	20	0
Oriental	1 serv (2.3 oz)	221	5	0
Ranch	1 serv (2.3 oz)	321	15	0
Reduced Calorie Italian	1 serv (2.3 oz)	60	0	0
Reduced Calorie Ranch	1 serv (2.3 oz)	191	25	0

SALADS

FOOD	PORTION	CALS	CHOL	FIBER
Caesar Salad	1 serv	471	72	2
Garden Salad	1 serv	256	214	2
Oriental Salad	1 serv	499	41	3
Potato Salad	1 serv (4 oz)	215	11	0
Taco Salad	1 serv	943	71	11

SANDWICHES

FOOD	PORTION	CALS	CHOL	FIBER
Albacore Tuna	1 sm	701	67	3
Avocado & Turkey	1 sm	675	80	6
Avocado & Alfalfa Sprouts	1 sm	637	85	7
Bar-B-Q Beef	1 sm	724	88	3
California Roasted Chicken	1 sm	510	65	3
Cheese Swiss American Provolone	1 sm	859	107	3
Chunky Chicken Salad	1 sm	636	42	3
Egg Salad w/ Cheese	1 sm	728	456	3
Ham & Cheese	1 sm	661	68	3
Hot Pastrami	1 sm	705	72	3
Hummus	1 sm	668	9	4
Italian Salami & Cheese	1 sm	770	118	3
Italian Salami Capicolla Mortadella Cotto & Provolone	1 sm	736	85	3
Meatballs w/ Pizza Sauce & Parmesan	1 sm	707	97	4
Pastrami Reuben	1 sm	875	111	2
Roast Beef Hot & Cold	1 sm	552	84	3
Turkey & Cranberry	1 sm	623	49	4

FOOD	PORTION	CALS	CHOL	FIBER
Turkey & Bacon Club	1 sm	667	81	3
Turkey & Cheese	1 sm	638	71	3
Turkey & Ham w/ Cheese	1 sm	670	76	3

WENDY'S
BEVERAGES

FOOD	PORTION	CALS	CHOL	FIBER
Chocolate Milk 1%	8 oz	170	15	0
Coca Cola	1 med (12 oz)	140	0	0
Dasani Water	1 bottle	0	0	0
Diet Coke	1 med (11 oz)	0	0	0
Frosty	1 sm (8 oz)	330	35	0
Milk 2%	8 oz	120	20	0
Sprite	1 med (12 oz)	130	0	0

CHILDREN'S MENU SELECTIONS

FOOD	PORTION	CALS	CHOL	FIBER
French Fries	1 serv (3.2 oz)	280	0	3
Kid's Meal Cheeseburger	1	320	40	1
Kid's Meal Ham & Cheese	1 serv	240	30	1
Kid's Meal Hamburger	1	270	30	1
Kid's Meal Turkey & Cheese	1 serv	250	25	1
Kids'Meal Chicken Nuggets	4 pieces	180	25	0

SALAD DRESSINGS AND TOPPINGS

FOOD	PORTION	CALS	CHOL	FIBER
Ancho Chipotle Ranch	1 pkg	110	15	0
Blue Cheese	1 pkg	260	35	0
Buttery Best Spread	1 pkg	50	0	0
Caesar	1 pkg	120	20	0
Cheddar Cheese Shredded	2 tbsp	70	15	0
Creamy Ranch	1 pkg	230	15	0
Creamy Ranch Reduced Fat	1 pkg	100	15	1
Crispy Noodles	1 pkg	60	0	0
Croutons Homestyle Garlic	1 pkg	70	0	0
Dipping Sauce Deli Honey Mustard	1 pkg	170	15	0
Dipping Sauce Heartland Ranch	1 pkg	200	15	0
Dipping Sauce Spicy Southwest Chipotle	1 pkg	150	25	0
Dipping Sauce Sweet & Sour Hawaiian	1 pkg	70	0	0
Dipping Sauce Wild Buffalo Ranch	1 pkg	180	10	0

OD	PORTION	CALS	CHOL	FIBER
French Fat Free	1 pkg	80	0	0
Granola Topping	1 pkg	110	0	1
Honey Mustard	1 pkg	280	25	0
Honey Mustard Low Fat	1 pkg	110	0	0
Hot Chili Seasoning	1 pkg	5	0	0
Italian Vinaigrette	1 pkg	140	0	0
Ketchup	1 tsp	7	0	0
Mayonnaise	1 tsp	30	5	0
Mustard	½ tsp	5	0	0
Nuggets Sauce Barbeque	1 pkg	45	0	0
Nuggets Sauce Honey Mustard	1 pkg	130	10	0
Nuggets Sauce Sweet & Sour	1 pkg	50	0	0
Oriental Sesame	1 pkg	190	0	0
Roasted Almonds	1 pkg	130	0	2
Saltines	2	25	0	0
Sour Cream Reduced Fat	1 pkg	45	10	0
Thousand Island	1 pkg	260	20	0
SALADS				
Caesar Chicken w/o Dressing & Croutons	1 serv	180	70	4
Ceasar Side Salad w/o Dressing & Croutons	1 serv	70	15	2
Chicken BLT w/o Dressing & Croutons	1 serv	340	105	4
Mandarin Chicken w/o Dressing	1 serv	170	60	3
Side Salad w/o Dressing	1	35	0	2
Southwest Taco w/o Dressing Tortilla Strip & Sour Cream	1 serv	440	80	9
SANDWICHES AND SIDES				
Baked Potato Plain	1	270	0	7
Baked Potato w/ Sour Cream & Chives	1 serv	320	10	7
Big Bacon Classic	1	580	95	3
Chicken Nuggets	5 pieces	220	35	0
Chili	1 sm (8 oz)	220	35	5
Classic Single w/ Everything	1	420	65	2
French Fries	1 med (5 oz)	440	0	5

FOOD	PORTION	CALS	CHOL	FIBE
Frescata Black Forest Ham & Swiss	1	480	65	4
Frescata Club	1	440	50	4
Frescata Roasted Turkey & Basil Pesto	1	420	40	4
Frescata Roasted Turkey & Swiss	1	490	60	4
Hamburger	1	280	30	1
Homestyle Chicken Strips	3 pieces	410	60	0
Jr. Bacon Cheeseburger	1	370	50	2
Jr. BBQ Cheeseburger	1	330	40	1
Jr. Cheeseburger	1	320	40	1
Jr. Cheeseburger Deluxe	1	360	45	2
SANDWICHES AND SIDES				
Mandarin Orange Cup	1 serv	80	0	1
Sandwich Crispy Chicken	1	380	35	1
Sandwich Spicy Chicken Fillet	1	510	55	2
Sandwich Ultimate Chicken Grill	1	360	75	2
Yogurt Low Fat Strawberry	1 pkg	140	5	0
WETZEL'S PRETZELS				
Original w/ Butter	1	320	10	2
Original w/o Butter	1	280	0	2
WHATABURGER				
BEVERAGES				
Cherry Coke	1 sm (20 oz)	169	0	0
Cherry Coke	1 lg (44 oz)	343	0	0
Coca-Cola Classic	1 sm (20 oz)	161	0	0
Coca-Cola Classic	1 lg (44 oz)	327	0	0
Coffee	1 sm (8 oz)	30	0	0
Creamer Nondairy	1 pkg	15	0	0
Diet Coke	1 sm (20 oz)	0	0	0
Diet Coke	1 lg (44 oz)	0	0	0
Diet Dr Pepper	1 sm (20 oz)	0	0	0
Dr Pepper	1 sm (20 oz)	147	0	0
Fanta Strawberry	1 sm (20 oz)	177	0	0
Fanta Strawberry	1 lg (44 oz)	360	0	0
Fruit Drink	1 sm (20 oz)	121	0	0

...D	PORTION	CALS	CHOL	FIBER
...ruit Drink	1 lg (44 oz)	244	0	0
Lemonade	1 sm (20 oz)	158	0	0
Lemonade	1 lg (44 oz)	320	0	0
Lipton Iced Tea	1 med	0	0	0
Milk 2%	8 oz	120	20	0
Orange Juice	1 serv	140	0	0
Orange Soda	1 sm (20 oz)	173	0	0
Orange Soda	1 lg (44 oz)	350	0	0
Shake Chocolate	1 sm (20 oz)	616	61	0
Shake Strawberry	1 sm (20 oz)	620	61	0
Shake Vanilla	1 sm (20 oz)	559	65	0
Sprite	1 sm	158	0	0
Sprite	1 lg (44 oz)	320	0	0
CHILDREN'S MENU SELECTIONS				
Kid's Justaburger	1	306	40	1
Kid's Chicken Strips	1 serv	382	33	4
MAIN MENU SELECTIONS				
Biscuit Buttermilk	1	300	0	0
Biscuit w/ Bacon	1	375	12	0
Biscuit w/ Bacon Egg & Cheese	1	476	252	0
Biscuit w/ Egg & Cheese	1	446	250	0
Biscuit w/ Sausage	1	517	35	1
Biscuit w/ Sausage Egg & Cheese	1	663	285	1
Biscuit w/ Sausage Gravy	1	491	19	tr
Breakfast Platter w/ Bacon	1 serv	698	466	3
Breakfast Platter w/ Sausage	1 serv	840	489	4
Breakfast On A Bun Ranchero w/ Bacon	1	404	262	3
Breakfast On A Bun Ranchero w/ Sausage	1	546	285	3
Breakfast On A Bun w/ Bacon	1	398	262	2
Breakfast On A Bun w/ Sausage	1	540	285	2
Chicken Strips	2	382	33	4
Cinnamon Roll	1	860	50	4
Croutons Njoy Seasoned	1 pkg	35	0	0
French Fries	1 sm	257	0	3

FOOD	PORTION	CALS	CHOL	
French Fries	1 lg	514	0	
Grape Jelly	1 pkg	35	0	0
Gravy White Peppered	1 serv	53	0	0
Hashbrown Sticks	1 serv	140	0	3
Honey	1 pkg	25	0	0
Hot Apple Pie	1	240	5	1
Justaburger	1	309	40	1
Ketchup	1 pkg	40	0	0
Margarine	1 pkg	23	0	0
Onion Rings	1 med	201	0	1
Pancake Syrup	1 pkg	120	0	0
Pancakes	1 serv	614	0	3
Pancakes w/ Bacon	1 serv	689	12	3
Pancakes w/ Sausage	1 serv	831	35	5
Picante Sauce	1 serv	5	0	0
Sandwich Egg	1	323	250	1
Sandwich Grilled Chicken	1	473	82	4
Sandwich Grilled Chicken Not Bun	1	190	73	1
Sandwich Whatacatch	1	473	59	2
Sandwich Whatachick'n	1	523	49	5
Strawberry Jam	1 pkg	40	0	0
Taquito Bacon & Egg	1	387	352	1
Taquito Potato & Egg	1	382	340	4
Taquito Sausage & Egg	1	389	354	1
Taquito w/ Bacon Egg & Cheese	1	432	362	1
Taquito w/ Potato Egg & Cheese	1	427	350	4
Taquito w/ Sausage Egg & Cheese	1	434	364	1
Texas Toast	1 serv	328	0	2
Whataburger	1	607	75	3
Whataburger Double Meat	1	857	150	3
Whataburger Double Meat No Bun	1	520	150	1
Whataburger Jr.	1	315	40	2
Whataburger No Bun	1	270	75	1
Whataburger Triple Meat	1	1107	225	4

	PORTION	CALS	CHOL	FIBER
...aburger w/ Bacon & Cheese	1	810	113	3
Whatacatch	2 pieces	814	147	2
SALAD DRESSINGS				
Low Fat Ranch	1 pkg	66	19	2
Low Fat Vinaigrette	1 pkg	35	0	0
Ranch	1 pkg	310	20	0
Thousand Island	1 pkg	150	20	0
SALADS				
Chicken Strips	1 serv	419	33	7
Chicken Strips w/ Cheddar Cheese	1 serv	600	76	8
Chicken Strips w/ Cheddar Cheese & Bacon	1 serv	675	88	8
Garden Salad	1	49	0	4
Garden w/ Cheddar Cheese	1 serv	218	43	4
Garden w/ Cheddar Cheese & Bacon	1 serv	293	55	4
Grilled Chicken	1 serv	229	73	5
Grilled Chicken w/ Cheddar Cheese	1 serv	398	115	4
Grilled Chicken w/ Cheddar Cheese & Bacon	1 serv	473	127	5

WHITE CASTLE

BEVERAGES				
Coca-Cola	16 oz	200	0	–
Coffee Black	1 sm	6	0	–
Diet Coke	16 oz	0	0	0
Iced Tea	16 oz	90	0	–
Shake Chocolate	16 oz	250	30	–
Shake Vanilla	16 oz	260	30	–
MAIN MENU SELECTIONS				
Bacon Cheeseburger	1	200	25	3
Cheese Sticks	3	250	25	2
Cheeseburger	1	160	15	2
Chicken Rings	6	210	50	0
Double Cheeseburger	1	290	30	5

FOOD	PORTION	CALS	CHc	
Double Hamburger	1	240	20	
Hamburger	1	140	10	
Onion Rings	6	260	0	3
Sandwich Breakfast	1	340	130	0
Sandwich Chicken	1	190	20	–
Sandwich Chicken Ring	1	180	25	0
Sandwich Fish	1	180	10	1

INDEX

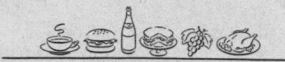